MEDICAL-
SURGICAL
NURSING

Assessment and Management
of Clinical Problems

CLINICAL COMPANION

MEDICAL-SURGICAL NURSING

Assessment and Management
of Clinical Problems

EIGHTH EDITION

Prepared by

SHANNON RUFF DIRKSEN, RN, PhD
Associate Professor
College of Nursing and Health Innovation
Arizona State University
Phoenix, Arizona

SHARON L. LEWIS, RN, PhD, FAAN
MARGARET MCLEAN HEITKEMPER, RN,
    PhD, FAAN
LINDA BUCHER, RN, PhD, CEN

ELSEVIER
MOSBY

by Mosby, Inc., an affiliate of Elsevier Inc.

Notices

Knowledge and best practice in this field are constantly changing. As new research and experience broaden our understanding, changes in research methods, professional practices, or medical treatment may become necessary.

Practitioners and researchers must always rely on their own experience and knowledge in evaluating and using any information, methods, compounds, or experiments described herein. In using such information or methods they should be mindful of their own safety and the safety of others, including parties for whom they have a professional responsibility.

With respect to any drug or pharmaceutical products identified, readers are advised to check the most current information provided (i) on procedures featured or (ii) by the manufacturer of each product to be administered, to verify the recommended dose or formula, the method and duration of administration, and contraindications. It is the responsibility of practitioners, relying on their own experience and knowledge of their patients, to make diagnoses, to determine dosages and the best treatment for each individual patient, and to take all appropriate safety precautions.

To the fullest extent of the law, neither the Publisher nor the authors, contributors, or editors, assume any liability for any injury and/or damage to persons or property as a matter of products liability, negligence or otherwise, or from any use or operation of any methods, products, instructions, or ideas contained in the material herein.

Nursing Diagnoses—Definitions and Classification 2009-2011 © 2009, 2007, 2005, 2003, 2001, 1998, 1996, 1994 NANDA International. Used by arrangement with Wiley-Blackwell Publishing, a company of John Wiley & Sons, Inc. In order to make safe and effective judgments using NANDA-I diagnoses it is essential that nurses refer to the definitions and defining characteristics of the diagnoses listed in this work.

Previous editions copyrighted 2007, 2004, 2000, 1996

Library of Congress Cataloging-in-Publication Data

Clinical companion to Medical-surgical nursing : assessment and management of clinical problems / prepared by Shannon Ruff Dirksen ... [et al.]. — 8th ed.
    p. ; cm.
    Rev. ed. of: Clinical companion, Medical-surgical nursing / prepared by Patricia Graber O'Brien ... [et al.]. 7th ed. 2007.
    Companion vol. to: Medical-surgical nursing / Sharon L. Lewis ... [et al.]. 8th ed. c2011.
    Includes index.
    ISBN 978-0-323-06662-4 (pbk. : alk. paper)
    1. Nursing — Handbooks, manuals, etc. 2. Surgical nursing — Handbooks, manuals, etc. I. Dirksen, Shannon Ruff. II. Medical-surgical nursing.
III. Clinical companion, Medical-surgical nursing.
    [DNLM: 1. Perioperative Nursing — Handbooks. 2. Nursing Process — Handbooks. WY 49]
    RT41.M488 2011 Suppl.
    610.73 — dc22
                                                        2010036054

Senior Acquisitions Editor: Kristin Geen
Senior Developmental Editor: Jamie Horn
Publishing Services Manager: Jeff Patterson
Project Manager: Bill Drone
Design Direction: Teresa McBryan

Printed in the United States of America

Last digit is the print number: 9   8   7   6   5   4   3   2   1

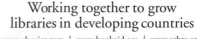

Working together to grow
libraries in developing countries

www.elsevier.com | www.bookaid.org | www.sabre.org

ELSEVIER   BOOK AID International   Sabre Foundation

The *Clinical Companion* to Lewis, Dirksen, Heitkemper, Bucher, and Camera's *Medical-Surgical Nursing: Assessment and Management of Clinical Problems,* eighth edition, has been expanded and updated as a condensed reference of essential information on nearly 200 medical-surgical patient problems and clinically related topics. The eighth edition of this pocket-sized book provides nurses and nursing students with quick access to current, concise, and important information when caring for patients.

The *Clinical Companion* can be used separately as a standalone reference or in conjunction with *Medical-Surgical Nursing: Assessment and Management of Clinical Problems,* eighth edition.

The book is divided into three sections. Part One contains commonly encountered medical-surgical patient problems that are arranged alphabetically and organized in an easy-to-use format. The disorders are extensively cross-referenced to *Medical-Surgical Nursing,* eighth edition, for the reader who desires additional information. Part Two contains brief explanations of common medical-surgical treatments and procedures (e.g., pacemakers, oxygen therapy) in which the role of the nurse is emphasized. Part Three contains reference material that is frequently used in clinical nursing practice (e.g., heart and breath sounds, medication administration, and blood and urine laboratory values). This section also contains a list of commonly used abbreviations and key phrases translated into Spanish. An extensive index is provided for easy location of information, and content updates and weblinks may be found at http://evolve.elsevier.com/Lewis/medsurg.

We hope the *Clinical Companion* will become an invaluable source of information and serve as a resource in helping nurses meet the challenges of caring for patients and their caregivers during states of altered health and well-being.

Shannon Ruff Dirksen
Sharon L. Lewis
Margaret McLean Heitkemper
Linda Bucher

"Enjoy the little things in life, for one day you may look back and realize they were the big things."

— **Antonio Smith**

CONTENTS

Contents

Part Two
Treatments and Procedures

Part Three
Reference Appendix

PART ONE

Disorders

ABDOMINAL PAIN, ACUTE

Description

Acute abdominal pain is a symptom associated with tissue injury. It can arise from damage to abdominal or pelvic organs and blood vessels. The most common causes of acute abdominal pain are listed in Table 1. Certain causes (e.g., hemorrhage, obstruction, perforation) can be life threatening because large fluid losses can lead to shock and abdominal compartment syndrome.

Clinical Manifestations

Pain is the most common symptom of an acute abdominal problem. Patients may also complain of nausea, vomiting, diarrhea, constipation, flatulence, fatigue, fever, and an increase in abdominal girth.

Diagnostic Studies

- Diagnosis begins with a complete history and physical examination. Physical examination should include both a rectal and pelvic examination in addition to an abdominal examination.
- Complete blood count (CBC), urinalysis, abdominal x-ray, and an electrocardiogram (ECG) are done initially, along with an ultrasound or computed tomography (CT) scan.
- Pregnancy tests should be performed on women of childbearing age with acute abdominal pain to rule out ectopic pregnancy.

Collaborative Care

The goal of management is to identify and treat the cause and monitor and treat complications, especially shock.

Table 1	Common Causes of Acute Abdominal Pain
■ Abdominal compartment syndrome
■ Appendicitis
■ Bowel obstruction
■ Cholecystitis
■ Diverticulitis
■ Gastroenteritis
■ Pelvic inflammatory disease
■ Perforated gastric or duodenal ulcer
■ Peritonitis
■ Ruptured abdominal aneurysm
■ Ruptured ectopic pregnancy

- A minimally invasive diagnostic laparoscopy may be performed to inspect the surface of abdominal organs, obtain biopsy specimens, perform laparoscopic ultrasounds, and provide treatment.
- Open surgery is used when laparoscopic management techniques are inadequate. If the cause of the acute abdomen can be surgically removed (e.g., inflamed appendix) or surgically repaired (e.g., ruptured abdominal aneurysm), surgery is considered definitive therapy.

Nursing Management

Goals

The patient will have resolution of inflammation, relief of abdominal pain, freedom from complications (especially hypovolemic shock), and normal nutritional status.

Nursing Diagnoses

- Acute pain
- Risk for deficient fluid volume
- Imbalanced nutrition: less than body requirements
- Anxiety

Nursing Interventions

General care for the patient involves monitoring and managing fluid and electrolyte balance, pain, and anxiety. Assess the quality and intensity of pain at regular intervals, and provide medication and other comfort measurements. Maintain a calm environment and provide information to help allay anxiety. Conduct ongoing assessments of vital signs, intake and output, and level of consciousness, which are key indicators of hypovolemic shock.

If the patient has an exploratory laparotomy or other surgery, provide preoperative and postoperative care.

- Preoperative emergency preparation of the patient with acute abdominal pain may include a CBC count, typing and crossmatching of blood, and clotting studies. Catheterization, preparation of abdominal skin, and insertion of a nasogastric (NG) tube may be done in the emergency department (ED) or operating room (OR).

Postoperative care depends on the type of surgical procedure performed. Laparoscopic procedures result in lower rates of postoperative complications (e.g., poor wound healing, paralytic ileus), earlier diet advancement, and shorter hospital stays as compared to open procedures. A general nursing care plan for the postoperative patient is presented online at http://evolve.elsevier.com/Lewis/medsurg.

An NG tube with low suction may be used to empty the stomach and prevent gastric dilation. If the upper GI tract has been entered, drainage from the NG tube may be dark brown to dark red for the first 12 hours. Later it should be light yellowish brown or greenish. If a dark red color continues or if bright red blood is observed, the health care provider should be notified at once of the possibility of hemorrhage. "Coffee ground" granules in the drainage indicate blood that has been modified by acidic gastric secretions.

- Nausea and vomiting are not uncommon after abdominal surgery and may be caused by the surgery and pain medication. Antiemetics such as prochlorperazine (Compazine), ondansetron (Zofran), or trimethobenzamide (Tigan) may be ordered (see Nausea and Vomiting, p. 441).
- Swallowed air and decreased peristalsis from decreased mobility, manipulation of abdominal organs during surgery, and anesthesia can lead to abdominal distention and gas pains. Early ambulation helps restore peristalsis and eliminate flatus and gas pain. For severe gas pain, a medication (e.g., metoclopramide [Reglan]) may be given to stimulate peristalsis. Inform the health care provider of abdominal distention and rigidity. Gradually, as intestinal activity increases, distention and gas pain disappear.

▼ **Patient and Caregiver Teaching**

Preparation for discharge begins soon after surgery. Teach the patient and caregiver about any modifications in activity, care of the incision, diet, and drug therapy.

- Clear liquids are given initially after surgery, and if tolerated, the patient progresses to a regular diet.
- Normal activities should be resumed gradually with planned rest periods.
- The patient and caregiver should be aware of possible complications after surgery and instructed to notify the physician immediately if vomiting, pain, weight loss, incisional drainage, or changes in bowel function occur.

ACUTE CORONARY SYNDROME

Description

When ischemia is prolonged and not immediately reversible, acute coronary syndrome (ACS) develops and encompasses the spectrum of unstable angina (UA), non–ST-segment-elevation myocardial infarction (NSTEMI), and ST-segment-elevation myocardial infarction (STEMI) (see Fig 1). Although each remains a distinct diagnosis, this nomenclature (ACS) reflects the relationships among the pathophysiology, presentation, diagnosis, prognosis, and interventions for these disorders.

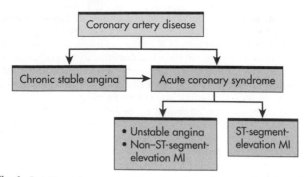

Fig. 1. Relationships among coronary artery disease, chronic stable angina, and acute coronary syndrome. *MI*, Myocardial infarction.

Pathophysiology

ACS is associated with deterioration of a once stable atherosclerotic plaque. The plaque then ruptures, exposing the intima to blood and stimulating platelet aggregation and vasoconstriction with thrombus formation. This unstable lesion may be partially occluded by a thrombus (manifesting as UA or NSTEMI) or totally occluded by a thrombus (manifesting as STEMI).

What causes a coronary plaque to suddenly become unstable is not well understood, but systemic inflammation is thought to play a role.

Unstable angina. The patient with chronic stable angina may develop UA, or UA may be the first clinical manifestation of CAD. Unlike chronic stable angina, UA is unpredictable and represents an emergency.

- The patient with previously diagnosed chronic stable angina will describe a significant change in the pattern of angina. It will occur with increasing frequency and is easily provoked by minimal or no exertion, during sleep, or even at rest.
- The patient without previously diagnosed angina will describe anginal pain that has progressed rapidly in the last few hours, days, or weeks, often culminating in pain at rest.

Myocardial infarction. A myocardial infarction (MI) occurs as a result of sustained ischemia, causing irreversible myocardial cell death (necrosis). Thrombus formation is responsible for 80% to 90% of all acute MIs. When a thrombus develops, perfusion to the myocardium distal to the occlusion is blocked, resulting in an infarction. Contractile function of the heart stops in the necrotic

areas. The degree of altered function depends on the area of the
heart involved and the size of the infarction. Most MIs involve
some portion of the left ventricle.

Cardiac cells can withstand ischemic conditions for approximately 20 minutes before cellular death (necrosis) begins. If ischemia persists, it takes approximately 4 to 6 hours for the entire
thickness of the heart muscle to become necrosed.

- Infarctions are usually described by the area of occurrence as
  anterior, inferior, lateral, or posterior wall infarctions. Damage
  can occur in more than one location (e.g., anterolateral MI,
  anteroseptal MI). The location correlates with the involved
  coronary circulation. For example, inferior wall infarctions
  result from occlusions in the right coronary artery.
- The degree of preestablished collateral circulation also determines the infarction's severity. In an individual with a history
  of CAD, adequate collateral channels may have been established that provide the area surrounding the infarction site with
  a blood supply.

The body's response to cell death is the inflammatory process.
Within 24 hours, leukocytes infiltrate the area. Enzymes are
released from the dead cardiac cells and are important diagnostic
indicators of MI. Proteolytic enzymes from neutrophils and macrophages remove all necrotic tissue by the fourth day.

- The necrotic zone is identifiable by electrocardiogram (ECG)
  changes and by nuclear scanning after the onset of symptoms.
- At 10 to 14 days after an MI, the new scar tissue is still weak.
  The myocardium is vulnerable to increased stress because of
  the unstable state of the healing heart wall.
- Changes in the infarcted muscle also alter the unaffected myocardium as well. In an attempt to compensate for the infarcted
  muscle, the normal myocardium will hypertrophy and dilate.
  Remodeling of normal myocardium can lead to the development of late heart failure (HF).

Clinical Manifestations

Unstable angina. The chest pain associated with UA is new in
onset, occurs at rest, or has a worsening pattern. Women have
prodromal symptoms such as fatigue, shortness of breath, indigestion, and anxiety that are early manifestations of CAD. Because
these symptoms are not recognized as manifestations of CAD,
many women present with UA before CAD has been diagnosed.

Myocardial infarction. Severe, immobilizing, and persistent chest
pain not relieved by rest or nitrate administration is the hallmark
of an MI.

- Persistent pain unlike any other pain; it is usually described as a heaviness, pressure, burning, crushing, tightness, or constriction.
- Common locations are epigastric, substernal, or retrosternal. The pain may radiate to the neck, jaw, and arms or to the back. It may occur while the patient is active or at rest, asleep or awake, and commonly occurs in the early morning hours.
- The pain usually lasts for 20 minutes or more and is more severe than usual anginal pain. When epigastric pain is present, the patient may take antacids without relief.
- Some patients may not have pain but may have "discomfort," weakness, fatigue, or shortness of breath. Women may experience atypical discomfort, shortness of breath, or fatigue.

Additional manifestations may include nausea and vomiting, diaphoresis, and constriction of peripheral blood vessels. On physical examination, the patient's skin is ashen, clammy, and cool (cold sweat). Fever occurs within the first 24 hours (up to 100.4° F [38° C]) and may continue for 1 week. Blood pressure (BP) and pulse rate are also elevated initially. BP then drops, with decreased urine output, lung crackles, hepatic engorgement, and peripheral edema. Jugular veins may be distended with obvious pulsations.

Complications

Dysrhythmias are the most common complication after an MI and are the most common cause of death in patients in the prehospital period. Dysrhythmias are caused by any condition that affects the myocardial cell's sensitivity to nerve impulses, such as ischemia, electrolyte imbalances, and sympathetic nervous system stimulation. The intrinsic rhythm of the heartbeat is disrupted, causing either a very fast heart rate (HR) (tachycardia), a very slow HR (bradycardia), or an irregular HR. Life-threatening dysrhythmias occur most often with anterior wall infarction, heart failure, and shock. Complete heart block is seen in massive infarction (see Dysrhythmias, p. 200).

- Ventricular fibrillation, a common cause of sudden death, is a lethal dysrhythmia that most often occurs within the first 4 hours after the onset of pain. Premature ventricular contractions may precede ventricular tachycardia and fibrillation. Ventricular dysrhythmias need immediate treatment.

Heart failure (HF) occurs when the pumping power of the heart has diminished. Depending on the severity and extent of the injury, HF occurs initially with subtle signs such as slight dyspnea, restlessness, agitation, or slight tachycardia. Pulmonary congestion, crackles in the lungs, S_3 or S_4 heart sounds, and jugular vein distention are additional signs.

Cardiogenic shock occurs when inadequate oxygen and nutrients are supplied to the tissues because of severe left ventricular failure. Cardiogenic shock requires aggressive management, including control of dysrhythmias, intraaortic balloon pump therapy, and support of contractility with vasoactive drugs.

Diagnostic Studies

In addition to the patient's history of pain, risk factors, and health history, the primary diagnostic studies used to determine whether a person has UA or an MI, and the type of MI, include an ECG and serum cardiac markers.

- Changes in the QRS complex, ST segment, and T wave caused by ischemia and infarction can help differentiate among UA, STEMI, and NSTEMI.
- Patients with STEMI tend to have a more extensive MI that is associated with prolonged and complete coronary occlusion and the development of a pathologic Q wave on the ECG.
- Patients with UA or NSTEMI usually have transient thrombosis or incomplete coronary occlusion and usually do not develop pathologic Q waves.
- Because an MI evolves over time, the ECG can reveal the time sequence of ischemia, injury, infarction, and resolution of the infarction.
- When the ECG is normal or nondiagnostic at the time the patient presents with chest pain, the ECG may change to reflect an infarction within a few hours.

Certain proteins, called *serum cardiac markers,* are released into the blood in large quantities from necrotic heart muscle after an MI.

- The MB band of creatine kinase (CK-MB) and troponin are two important specific markers that can indicate the presence and extent of cardiac damage.

Other diagnostic measures can include coronary angiography, exercise stress testing, and echocardiograms.

Collaborative Care

It is extremely important that a patient with ACS is rapidly diagnosed and treated to preserve cardiac muscle. Initial management of the patient with chest pain most often occurs in the emergency department (ED).

- You establish an intravenous (IV) route and initiate O_2 by nasal cannula at a rate of 2 to 4 L/min and ECG and pulse oximetry monitoring.
- Sublingual nitroglycerin and chewable aspirin are given if not done by emergency medical personnel prior to arrival at the ED. Morphine sulfate is given IV for pain unrelieved by nitroglycerin.
- The patient will receive ongoing care in a critical care or telemetry unit where continuous ECG monitoring is available and dysrhythmias can be treated.
- Monitor vital signs, including pulse oximetry, frequently during the first few hours after admission and closely thereafter. Maintain bed rest and limitation of activity for 12 to 24 hours with a gradual increase in activity unless contraindicated.
- For patients with UA or NSTEMI with negative cardiac markers and ongoing angina, a combination of aspirin, heparin, and a glycoprotein IIb/IIIa inhibitor (e.g., eptifibatide [Integrilin]) is recommended. *Percutaneous coronary intervention* (PCI) is considered once the patient is stabilized and angina is controlled, or if angina returns and increases in severity.
- For patients with STEMI or NSTEMI with positive cardiac markers, reperfusion therapy is indicated.

Reperfusion therapy can include emergent PCI or fibrinolytic (thrombolytic) therapy. The goal in treatment of acute MI is to salvage as much myocardial muscle as possible.

- Emergent PCI is recommended as the first line of treatment for patients with confirmed MI. The patient undergoes cardiac catheterization to evaluate the blockage, and stents may be placed (see Angina, Chronic Stable, p. 45).

Fibrinolytic therapy can be performed in facilities that do not have an interventional cardiac catheterization lab and when another facility with these services is not nearby. Treatment of MI with fibrinolytic therapy (e.g., reteplase [Retavase]) is aimed at stopping the infarction process by dissolving the thrombus in the coronary artery and reperfusing the myocardium. To be of the most benefit, thrombolytics must be given as soon as possible, ideally within the first hour after onset of symptoms and preferably within the first 6 hours after the onset of symptoms. Contraindications and complications with thrombolytic therapy are described in Lewis et al, *Medical-Surgical Nursing,* ed 8, pp. 782 to 783.

Drug therapy includes IV nitroglycerin (Tridil), aspirin, β-adrenergic blockers, and systemic anticoagulation with either low-molecular-weight heparin given subcutaneously or IV

A

unfractionated heparin as initial drug treatments of choice. ACE inhibitors are added for select patients following MI, and calcium channel blockers may be used if the patient is already taking adequate doses of β-adrenergic blockers or does not tolerate β-adrenergic blockers. Morphine sulfate is used for chest pain unrelieved by nitroglycerin. It also decreases cardiac workload and reduces anxiety and fear. Antidysrhythmic drugs are used to treat life-threatening dysrhythmias.

Coronary artery bypass graft (CABG) surgery consists of the placement of new vessels to transport blood between the aorta, or other major arteries, and the myocardium distal to the obstructed coronary artery (or arteries). It requires a sternotomy (opening of the chest cavity) and the use of cardiopulmonary bypass (CPB). It is a palliative treatment for CAD and not a cure. Newer techniques include minimally invasive direct coronary artery bypass and trans-myocardial laser revascularization. These surgical procedures and related nursing care are further discussed in Lewis et al, *Medical-Surgical Nursing,* ed 8, pp. 783 to 785.

Nursing Management
Goals
The patient with an MI will experience relief of pain, preservation of myocardium, immediate and appropriate treatment, effective coping with illness-associated anxiety, participation in a rehabilitation plan, and reduction of risk factors.

See NCP 34-1 for the patient with acute coronary syndrome, Lewis et al, *Medical-Surgical Nursing,* ed 8, pp. 786 to 787.

Nursing Diagnoses
- Acute pain
- Decreased cardiac output
- Anxiety
- Activity intolerance
- Ineffective self-health management

Nursing Interventions
Priorities for nursing interventions in the initial phase include pain assessment and relief, physiologic monitoring, promotion of rest and comfort, alleviation of stress and anxiety, and understanding of the patient's emotional and behavioral reactions. Proper management of these priorities decreases the O_2 needs of a compromised myocardium. In addition, you should institute measures to avoid the hazards of immobility while encouraging rest.

- Provide nitroglycerin, morphine, and O_2 as needed to eliminate or reduce chest pain. Once pain is relieved, you may have to deal with denial in a patient who interprets the absence of pain as an absence of cardiac disease.

- You must be competent in ECG interpretation so that dysrhythmias and/or ischemia causing further deterioration of the cardiovascular status can be identified and treated.
- In addition to frequent vital signs, intake and output should be evaluated at least once per shift, and physical assessment should be carried out to detect deviations from the patient's baseline parameters; included are the assessment of lung and heart sounds and inspection for evidence of early heart failure (e.g., dyspnea, tachycardia, pulmonary congestions, distended neck veins).
- Assessment of the patient's oxygenation status is helpful, especially if the patient is receiving O_2. The nares also should be checked for irritation or dryness (see Oxygen Therapy, p. 743).
- It is important to plan nursing and therapeutic actions to ensure adequate rest periods free from interruption.
- Anxiety is present in all patients with ACS in various degrees. Your role is to identify the source of anxiety and assist the patient in reducing it. If the patient is afraid of being alone, a caregiver should be allowed to sit quietly by the bedside or to check in frequently with the patient. If a source of anxiety is fear of the unknown, you should explore these concerns with the patient.

▼ **Patient and Caregiver Teaching**

Patient teaching begins with you and continues at every stage of the patient's hospitalization and recovery (e.g., ED, telemetry unit, home care). The purpose of teaching is to give the patient and caregiver the tools they need for successful rehabilitation (Table 2).

- Anticipatory guidance involves preparing the patient and caregiver for what to expect in the course of recovery and rehabilitation. By learning what to expect during treatment and recovery, the patient gains a sense of control over his or her life.
- Teach the patient the parameters within which to exercise and how to check pulse rate. Tell the patient the maximum HR that should be present at any point. If the HR exceeds this level or does not return to the rate of the resting pulse within a few minutes, instruct the patient to stop. Also instruct the patient to stop exercising if pain or shortness of breath occurs. Basic physical activity guidelines following ACS are presented in Table 34-21, Lewis et al, *Medical-Surgical Nursing*, ed 8, p. 792.
- You should discuss participation in an outpatient cardiac rehabilitation program with all patients. These programs are

| Table 2 | Patient and Caregiver Teaching Guide: Acute Coronary Syndrome | A |

You should include the following information in the teaching plan for the patient (with acute coronary syndrome) and caregiver:

- Signs and symptoms of angina and MI and what to do should they occur (e.g., take NTG)*
- When and how to seek help (e.g., contact EMS)
- Anatomy and physiology of the heart and coronary arteries
- Cause and effect of coronary artery disease
- Definition of terms (e.g., CAD, angina, MI, sudden cardiac death, HF)
- Identification of and plan to decrease risk factors* (see Table 34-3, Lewis et al., *Medical-Surgical Nursing,* ed. 8, p. 767)
- Rationale for tests and treatments (e.g., ECG monitoring, blood tests, angiography), activity limitations/rest, diet, and medications*
- Appropriate expectations about recovery and rehabilitation (anticipatory guidance)
- Resumption of work, physical activity, sexual activity
- Measures to take to promote recovery and health
- Importance of the gradual, progressive resumption of activity*

CAD, Coronary artery disease; *ECG,* electrocardiogram; *EMS,* emergency medical services; *HF,* heart failure; *MI,* myocardial infarction; *NTG,* nitroglycerin.
* Identified by patients as most important to learn before discharge.

beneficial, but not all patients choose or are able to participate in them (e.g., location). Home-based cardiac rehabilitation programs can be an alternative.

- It is important to include sexual counselling for cardiac patients and their partners. Reading material on resumption of sexual activity may be presented to the patient to facilitate discussion. Calmly and matter-of-factly introducing the subject of resumption of sexual activity during teaching about physical activity has positive effects of eliciting questions and concerns that might not have otherwise surfaced.

ACUTE RESPIRATORY DISTRESS SYNDROME

Description

Acute respiratory distress syndrome (ARDS) is a sudden and progressive form of acute respiratory failure in which the alveolar-capillary membrane becomes damaged and more permeable to intravascular fluid. The alveoli fill with fluid, resulting in severe dyspnea, hypoxemia refractory to supplemental oxygen (O_2), reduced lung compliance, and diffuse pulmonary infiltrates.

The incidence of ARDS in the United States is estimated at more than 150,000 cases annually. Despite supportive therapy, mortality from ARDS is approximately 50%. Patients who have both gram-negative septic shock and ARDS have a mortality rate of 70% to 90%.

- Table 3 lists conditions that predispose patients to the development of ARDS. The most common cause is sepsis. Patients with multiple risk factors are 3 or 4 times more likely to develop ARDS.

Table 3	Conditions Predisposing to Acute Respiratory Distress Syndrome

Direct Lung Injury
Common Causes
- Aspiration of gastric contents or other substances
- Viral/bacterial pneumonia
- Sepsis

Less Common Causes
- Chest trauma
- Embolism: fat, air, amniotic fluid, thrombus
- Inhalation of toxic substances
- Near-drowning
- O_2 toxicity
- Radiation pneumonitis

Indirect Lung Injury
Common Causes
- Sepsis (especially gram-negative infection)
- Severe massive trauma

Less Common Causes
- Acute pancreatitis
- Anaphylaxis
- Cardiopulmonary bypass
- Disseminated intravascular coagulation
- Nonpulmonary systemic diseases
- Opioid drug overdose (e.g., heroin)
- Severe head injury
- Shock states
- Transfusion-related acute lung injury (e.g., multiple blood transfusions)

- Direct lung injury may cause ARDS, or ARDS may develop as a consequence of the systemic inflammatory response syndrome (SIRS). ARDS may also develop as a result of multiple organ dysfunction syndrome (MODS) (see Systemic Inflammatory Response Syndrome and Multiple Organ Dysfunction Syndrome, p. 624).

Pathophysiology

An exact cause for damage to the alveolar-capillary membrane is not known. However, many changes are thought to be caused by stimulation of the inflammatory and immune systems, which causes an attraction of neutrophils to the pulmonary interstitium. The neutrophils cause a release of biochemical, humoral, and cellular mediators that produce changes in the lung, including increased pulmonary capillary membrane permeability, destruction of elastin and collagen, formation of pulmonary microemboli, and pulmonary artery vasoconstriction. Pathophysiologic changes in ARDS are divided into three phases: injury or exudative, reparative or proliferative, and fibrotic.

The *injury* or *exudative phase* occurs approximately 1 to 7 days (usually 24 to 48 hours) after the initial direct lung injury or host insult. The primary changes of this phase are interstitial and alveolar edema (noncardiogenic pulmonary edema) and atelectasis

- Initially, there is engorgement of the peribronchial and perivascular interstitial space, which produces interstitial edema. Intrapulmonary shunt develops because the alveoli fill with fluid, and blood passing through them cannot be oxygenated.
- Alveolar cells that produce surfactant are damaged by the changes caused by ARDS. This damage, in addition to further fluid and protein accumulation, results in surfactant dysfunction. Widespread atelectasis further decreases lung compliance, compromises gas exchange, and contributes to hypoxemia
- Hyaline begins to line the alveolar membrane. Hyaline membranes contribute to fibrosis and atelectasis, leading to a decrease in gas exchange capability and lung compliance.
- Severe ventilation-perfusion (V/Q) mismatch and shunting of pulmonary capillary blood result in hypoxemia unresponsive to increasing concentrations of O_2 *(refractory hypoxemia).*

The *reparative* or *proliferative phase* begins 1 to 2 weeks after the initial lung injury. During this phase there is an influx of granulocytes, monocytes, and lymphocytes and fibroblast proliferation.

- Increased pulmonary vascular resistance and pulmonary hypertension may occur in this stage because fibroblasts and inflammatory cells destroy the pulmonary vasculature.
- Lung compliance continues to decrease, and hypoxemia worsens because of the thickened alveolar membrane.
- If this phase persists, widespread fibrosis results. If this phase is arrested, the lesions resolve.

The *fibrotic phase* occurs approximately 2 to 3 weeks after the initial lung injury. This phase is also called the chronic or late phase of ARDS. By this time the lung is completely remodeled by collagenous and fibrous tissues. Diffuse scarring and fibrosis result in decreased lung compliance and decreased surface area for gas exchange. Pulmonary hypertension results from fibrosis.

Progression of ARDS varies among patients. Some persons survive the acute phase of lung injury; pulmonary edema resolves, and complete recovery occurs in a few days. Others go on to the fibrotic (late or chronic) phase requiring long-term mechanical ventilation, with a poor chance of survival.

Clinical Manifestations

At the time of initial injury and for several hours to 1 to 2 days afterward, the patient may not exhibit respiratory symptoms.

- The patient may exhibit dyspnea, cough, and restlessness. Chest auscultation may be normal or reveal fine, scattered crackles. Arterial blood gases (ABGs) usually demonstrate mild hypoxemia and respiratory alkalosis. Chest x-ray may be normal or exhibit evidence of minimal scattered interstitial infiltrates. Edema may not manifest until there is a 30% increase in lung fluid content.
- As ARDS progresses, symptoms worsen because of increased fluid accumulation in the lungs and decreased lung compliance. Tachycardia, tachypnea, diaphoresis, changes in sensorium with decreased mentation, cyanosis, and pallor may be present. Chest auscultation usually reveals scattered to diffuse crackles and rhonchi.
- Hypoxemia, despite increased fraction of inspired oxygen concentration (FIO_2) by mask, cannula, or endotracheal tube, is a hallmark of ARDS. Hypercapnia signifies that hypoventilation is occurring.
- As ARDS progresses, profound respiratory distress occurs, requiring endotracheal intubation and positive pressure ventilation (PPV). The chest x-ray reveals *whiteout* or *white lung* because consolidation and coalescing infiltrates pervade the lungs, leaving few recognizable air spaces.

- Pleural effusions may be present. Severe hypoxemia, hypercapnia, and metabolic acidosis, with symptoms of target organ or tissue hypoxemia, may ensue if prompt therapy is not instituted.

Complications may develop as a result of ARDS itself or its treatment. The major cause of death in ARDS is MODS, often accompanied by sepsis. The vital organs most commonly involved are the kidneys, liver, and heart. The organ systems most often involved are the central nervous system (CNS) and hematologic and gastrointestinal systems.

Diagnostic Studies

There are no precise criteria that define ARDS. ARDS is considered to be present if the patient presents with refractory hypoxemia, a chest x-ray with new bilateral interstitial or alveolar infiltrates, and a pulmonary artery wedge pressure <18 mm Hg and no evidence of heart failure.

Nursing and Collaborative Management

Goals

With appropriate therapy, the overall goals for the patient with ARDS include a partial pressure of oxygen in arterial blood (PaO_2) of at least 60 mm Hg and adequate lung volume to maintain normal pH. A patient recovering from ARDS will experience a PaO_2 within limits of normal for age or baseline values on room air (FIO_2 of 21%), oxygen saturation in arterial blood (SaO_2) >90%, a patent airway, and clear lungs on auscultation.

The collaborative care for acute respiratory failure is applicable to ARDS (see nursing care plan for acute respiratory failure [http://evolve.elsevier.com/Lewis/medsurg]). Patients with ARDS are commonly cared for in critical care units.

Nursing Diagnoses

Nursing diagnoses for the patient with ARDS may include, but are not limited to, those described under Respiratory Failure, Acute (p. 542).

Respiratory Therapy

O_2 *administration.* The goal of O_2 therapy is to correct hypoxemia (see Oxygen Therapy, p. 743). Masks with high-flow systems that deliver higher O_2 concentrations are initially utilized to maximize O_2 delivery. The general standard for O_2 administration is to give the lowest concentration that results in a PaO_2 of 60 mm Hg or greater. When FIO_2 exceeds 60% for more than 48 hours, the risk for O_2 toxicity increases. Patients with ARDS need intubation with mechanical ventilation (see Artificial Airways: Endotracheal

Tubes, p. 699) because the PaO_2 cannot otherwise be maintained at acceptable levels.

Mechanical ventilation. Endotracheal intubation and mechanical ventilation provide additional respiratory support. In patients with ARDS, positive expiratory-end pressure (PEEP) is often used. When PEEP is applied, the lung is kept partially expanded, which prevents alveoli from totally collapsing. If hypoxemic failure persists in spite of high levels of PEEP, alternative modes and therapies may be used. These include airway pressure release ventilation, pressure-control inverse ratio ventilation, high-frequency ventilation, and permissive hypercapnia (low tidal volumes that allow $PaCO_2$ to increase slowly).

Extracorporeal membrane oxygenation (ECMO) and extracorporeal carbon dioxide (CO_2) removal pass blood across a gas-exchanging membrane outside the body and then return oxygenated blood back to the body.

Positioning. Some patients with ARDS demonstrate a marked improvement in PaO_2 when turned from the supine to the prone position (e.g., PaO_2 70 mm Hg supine, PaO_2 90 mm Hg prone) with no change in inspired O_2 concentration. The response may be sufficient to allow a reduction in inspired O_2 concentration or PEEP. When this positioning is used, there must be a plan in place for immediate positioning for cardiopulmonary resuscitation (CPR) in the event of a cardiac arrest.

Another positioning strategy that can be considered for patients with ARDS is continuous lateral rotation therapy. The purpose of this therapy is to provide continuous, slow, side-to-side turning of the patient by rotating the actual bed frame. You should maintain the lateral movement of the bed for 18 of every 24 hours to stimulate postural drainage and help to mobilize pulmonary secretions. In addition, the bed may also contain a vibrator pack that can provide chest physiotherapy to further assist with secretion mobilization and removal.

Medical Supportive Therapy

Maintenance of cardiac output and tissue perfusion. Patients on PPV and PEEP frequently experience decreased cardiac output. Continuous hemodynamic monitoring is essential to detect these changes and titrate therapy. An arterial catheter is inserted for continuous monitoring of blood pressure (BP) and to withdraw blood for ABGs. Use of inotropic drugs, such as dobutamine (Dobutrex) or dopamine (Intropin), may be necessary.

Maintenance of nutrition and fluid balance. Maintenance of nutrition and fluid balance is challenging in the patient with ARDS. Parenteral or enteral feedings are started to meet the high energy requirements of these patients. Leaky pulmonary capillaries cause increased fluid in the lungs, resulting in pulmonary edema. At the same time, the patient may be volume depleted and therefore prone to hypotension and decreased cardiac output from mechanical ventilation and PEEP. Controversy exists as to the benefits of fluid replacement with crystalloids versus colloids. To limit pulmonary edema, the pulmonary artery wedge pressure is kept as low as possible without impairing cardiac output. The patient is usually placed on mild fluid restriction, and diuretics are used as necessary.

▼ **Patient and Caregiver Teaching**

Fear of suffocation or death is not uncommon in patients with ARDS.

- Providing reassurance, spending time with the patient, and ensuring that help can be received immediately (e.g., call light is readily available) may help to decrease patient anxiety level. Anxiety also may be reduced through instruction and use of progressive relaxation, guided imagery, and music therapy.

- It is helpful to explain to the patient any possible sensations that may be encountered with each new experience (e.g., suctioning, drawing ABGs) so that coping strategies can be purposefully selected.

ADDISON'S DISEASE

Description

Addison's disease is a primary adrenocortical insufficiency in which all three classes of adrenal steroids (glucocorticoids, mineralocorticoids, and androgens) are reduced because of hypofunction of the adrenal cortex. In secondary adrenocortical insufficiency, which is caused by a lack of pituitary adrenocorticotropic hormone (ACTH) secretion, corticosteroids and androgens are deficient but mineralocorticoids rarely are. The most common cause of Addison's disease is an autoimmune disorder; adrenal tissue is destroyed by antibodies against the patient's own adrenal cortex. Often, other endocrine conditions are present and Addison's disease is considered a component of *polyendocrine deficiency syndrome.* Other causes include infarction, fungal infections (e.g., histoplasmosis), acquired immunodeficiency syndrome (AIDS), and metastatic cancer. Iatrogenic Addison's disease may be caused by adrenal hemorrhage (often related to anticoagulant therapy), antineoplastic chemotherapy, ketoconazole (Nizoral) therapy for AIDS, or bilateral adrenalectomy.

Clinical Manifestations

Manifestations have a very slow (insidious) onset and include progressive weakness, fatigue, weight loss, and anorexia. Skin hyperpigmentation, a striking feature, is seen primarily in sun-exposed areas of the body, at pressure points, over joints, and in creases, especially palmar creases.

- Other frequent manifestations are orthostatic hypotension, hyponatremia, hyperkalemia, nausea and vomiting, and diarrhea.

Patients with adrenocortical insufficiency are at risk for acute adrenal insufficiency *(addisonian crisis),* a life-threatening emergency caused by insufficient adrenocortical hormones or a sudden, sharp decrease in these hormones.

- The most dangerous feature is hypotension, which may cause shock, especially during stress. Circulatory collapse from this cause is often unresponsive to the usual treatment (vasopressors and fluid replacement) and requires corticosteroid administration.
- Addisonian crisis may be triggered by stress (e.g., from infection, surgery, trauma, or psychologic distress), sudden cessation of corticosteroid hormone replacement therapy (often done by a patient who lacks knowledge regarding replacement therapy), adrenal surgery, or sudden pituitary gland destruction.

Diagnostic Studies

- In Addison's disease, plasma cortisol levels are subnormal or fail to rise over basal levels with an ACTH stimulation test.
- A positive response to ACTH stimulation indicates a functioning adrenal gland and points to pituitary disease rather than adrenal disease.
- Free cortisol levels in the urine are decreased.
- Serum electrolytes show hyperkalemia, hypochloremia, and hyponatremia.
- Computed tomography (CT) and magnetic resonance imaging (MRI) are used to localize tumors or identify adrenal changes.

Collaborative Care

Treatment is focused on management of the underlying cause when possible. The mainstay of treatment is replacement therapy with corticosteroids (e.g., hydrocortisone) with glucocorticoid and mineralocorticoid activity. Mineralocorticoid replacement with fludrocortisone acetate (Florinef) is administered daily with increased salt in the diet.

A

- When any illness or stress occurs, whether mild or acute, the corticosteroid dosage must be increased to prevent adrenal crisis. The patient usually is instructed to take 2 to 3 times the usual dose.

If vomiting or diarrhea occurs, as may happen with influenza, the health care provider must be notified immediately because electrolyte replacement may be necessary. In addition, these symptoms may be early indicators of crisis.

Management of addisonian crisis requires immediate aggressive management. Treatment must be directed toward shock management and high-dose hydrocortisone replacement. Large volumes of 0.9% saline solution and 5% dextrose are administered to reverse hypotension and electrolyte imbalances until blood pressure returns to normal.

Nursing Management

When the patient with Addison's disease is hospitalized, whether for diagnosis, an acute crisis, or some other health problem, frequent nursing assessment is necessary.

- Vital signs and signs of fluid volume deficit and electrolyte imbalance should be assessed every 30 minutes to 4 hours for the first 24 hours, depending on the patient's instability.
- Nursing interventions include daily weights, corticosteroid administration, protection against exposure to infection (reverse isolation), and assistance with daily hygiene.
- The patient should be protected from noise, light, and environmental temperature extremes. The patient cannot cope with these stresses because corticosteroids cannot be produced.
- If hospitalization was due to an adrenal crisis, patients usually respond by the second day and can start oral corticosteroid replacement.
- Because discharge frequently occurs before the usual maintenance dose of corticosteroids is reached, the patient should be instructed on the importance of keeping scheduled follow-up appointments.

▼ **Patient and Caregiver Teaching**

Because of the serious nature of the disease and the need for lifelong replacement therapy, a well-organized and carefully presented teaching plan is important (Table 4).

- Patients must be taught the signs and symptoms of corticosteroid deficiency and excess and to report these to their health care provider so that the dose can be adjusted to each patient's need.

Table 4	Patient and Caregiver Teaching Guide: Addison's Disease

You should include the following information in the teaching plan for Addison's disease:

1. Names, dosages, and actions of drugs
2. Symptoms of overdosage and underdosage
3. Conditions requiring increased medication (e.g., trauma, infection, surgery, emotional crisis)
4. Course of action to take relative to changes in medication
   - Increase in dose of corticosteroid
   - Administration of large dose of corticosteroid intramuscularly, including demonstration and return demonstration
   - Consultation with health care provider
5. Prevention of infection and need for prompt and vigorous treatment of existing infections
6. Need for lifelong replacement therapy
7. Need for lifelong medical supervision
8. Need for medical identification device

- It is critical that the patient wear an identification bracelet (Medic-Alert) and carry a wallet card stating the patient has Addison's disease so that appropriate therapy can be initiated in case of an unexpected trauma, accident, or crisis.
- Patients should carry an emergency kit with them at all times. The kit should consist of 100 mg of intramuscular (IM) hydrocortisone (Solu-Medrol), syringes, and instructions for use.
- The patient and significant others should be instructed in how to give an IM injection if replacement therapy cannot be taken orally. The patient should verbalize instructions, practice IM injections with saline, and have written instructions as to when to alter the dose.

ALZHEIMER'S DISEASE

Description

Alzheimer's disease (AD) is a chronic, progressive, degenerative disease of the brain. It is the most common form of dementia, accounting for more than 60% of all cases of dementia. Dementia is a syndrome characterized by dysfunction or loss of memory, orientation, attention, language, judgment, and reasoning. Approximately 5.3 million people in the United States have AD.

Most patients live 4 to 6 years after being diagnosed, although some patients live for 20 years.

Pathophysiology

The exact etiology of AD is unknown. AD is not a normal part of aging. When AD develops in someone younger than 60 years, it is referred to as *early-onset AD*. AD that becomes evident in individuals after the age of 60 years is called *late-onset AD*.

Characteristic findings of AD include the abnormal presence of amyloid plaques and neurofibrillary tangles in the brain, loss of connections among cells, and cell death.

- Amyloid plaques consist of clusters of insoluble deposits of a protein called β-amyloid, other proteins, remnants of neurons, nonnerve cells such as microglia, and other cells. In AD the plaques develop first in brain areas used for memory and cognitive function, and eventually the cerebral cortex areas responsible for language and reasoning are affected.
- Neurofibrillary tangles are abnormal collections of twisted protein threads inside nerve cells. The main component of these structures is a protein called *tau*. Normally tau proteins maintain cellular structure by holding intracellular microtubules together. In AD the tau protein is altered, and as a result, the microtubules twist together in a helical fashion, ultimately forming neurofibrillary tangles.
- The third feature of AD, the gradual loss of connections among neurons, causes damage and death of neurons. This causes the brain shrinkage (atrophy) seen in AD.

Genetic factors may play a critical role in how the brain processes the β-amyloid protein. Other etiologic factors being studied included the role of inflammation in the development of AD, links between cardiovascular disease and AD, and lifestyle factors such as dietary patterns, leisure activities, and educational attainment.

Clinical Manifestations

Pathologic changes often precede clinical manifestations of dementia by 5 to 20 years. (Early warning signs of AD are listed in Table 5.)

- An initial sign is subtle deterioration in memory. Inevitably this progresses to more profound memory loss that interferes with the patient's ability to function. Recent events and new information cannot be recalled. Personal hygiene deteriorates as does the ability to maintain attention.
- Behavioral manifestations (e.g., agitation) and psychotic manifestations (e.g., delusion, illusions) may occur as a

Table 5	Patient and Caregiver Teaching Guide: Early Warning Signs of Alzheimer's Disease (AD)

You should include the following information in the teaching plan for the patient with Alzheimer's disease.

1. Memory loss that affects job skills
   - Frequent forgetfulness or unexplainable confusion at home or in the workplace may signal that something is wrong.
   - This type of memory loss goes beyond forgetting an assignment, colleague's name, deadline, or phone number.
2. Difficulty performing familiar tasks
   - It is not abnormal for most people to become distracted and to forget something (e.g., leave something on the stove too long).
   - People with AD may cook a meal but then forget not only to serve it but also that they made it.
3. Problems with language
   - Most people have trouble with finding the "right" word from time to time.
   - Persons with AD may forget simple words or substitute inappropriate words, making their speech difficult to understand.
4. Disorientation to time and place
   - While most individuals occasionally forget the day of the week or what they need from the store, people with AD can become lost on their own street, not knowing where they are, how they got there, or how to get back home.
5. Poor or decreased judgment
   - Many individuals from time to time may choose not to dress appropriately for the weather (e.g., not bringing a coat or sweater on a cold evening).
   - Person with AD may dress inappropriately in more noticeable ways, such as wearing a bathrobe to the store or a sweater on a hot day.
6. Problems with abstract thinking
   - For the person with AD, this goes beyond challenges such as balancing a checkbook.
   - Person with AD may have difficulty recognizing numbers or doing even basic calculations.
7. Misplacing things
   - For many individuals, temporarily misplacing keys, purses, or wallets is a normal albeit frustrating event.
   - Person with AD may put items in inappropriate places (e.g., eating utensils in clothing drawers) but have no memory of how they got there.

Table 5	Patient and Caregiver Teaching Guide: Early Warning Signs of Alzheimer's Disease (AD)—cont'd

8. Changes in mood or behavior
   - Most individuals experience mood changes.
   - Person with AD tends to exhibit more rapid mood swings for no apparent reason.
9. Changes in personality
   - As most individuals age, they may demonstrate some change in personality (e.g., become less tolerant).
   - Person with AD can change dramatically, either suddenly or over time.
   - For example, someone who is generally easygoing may become angry, suspicious, or fearful.
10. Loss of initiative
   - Person with AD may become and remain uninterested and uninvolved in many or all of his or her usual pursuits.

Adapted from Alzheimer's Association: *Early warning signs*, Chicago, Alzheimer's Association.

result of changes in the brain and are neither intentional nor controllable by the patient with AD.
- Later in the disease, long-term memories cannot be recalled, and patients lose the ability to recognize family members. Eventually the ability to communicate and perform activities of daily living (ADLs) is lost.
- In the late or final stages, the patient is unresponsive and incontinent and requires total care.

Diagnostic Studies

The diagnosis of AD is a diagnosis of exclusion. When all other possible conditions that can cause mental impairment have been ruled out and manifestations of dementia persist, the diagnosis of AD can be made.
- A computed tomography (CT) scan or magnetic resonance imaging (MRI) may show brain atrophy and enlarged ventricles in the later stages of the disease, although this finding occurs in other diseases and in persons without cognitive impairment.
- Newer techniques, including single photon emission computed tomography (SPECT), magnetic resonance spectroscopy (MRS), and positron emission tomography (PET), allow for detection of changes early in the disease, as well as monitoring treatment response.

- Laboratory tests may be used to examine genetic markers and to rule out other causes of cognitive impairment (e.g., thyroid disease, anemia, renal disease).
- Definitive diagnosis of AD can be made only at autopsy when the presence of neurofibrillary tangles and neuritic plaques is observed.

Collaborative Care

Management of AD is aimed at improving or controlling the decline in cognition and undesirable symptoms that the patient may exhibit and providing support for the caregiver. Table 60-8, Lewis et al, *Medical-Surgical Nursing,* ed 8, p. 1526 details drug therapy for AD. These drugs do not cure or reverse the progression of the disease.

- Cholinesterase inhibitors block cholinesterase, the enzyme responsible for the breakdown of acetylcholine in the synaptic cleft. Cholinesterase inhibitors include donepezil (Aricept), rivastigmine (Exelon), and galantamine (Razadyne). Rivastigmine is available as a patch.
- Memantine (Namenda) protects brain nerve cells by blocking the damaging effects of glutamate, which is released in large amounts by cells damaged by AD.
- Although antipsychotic drugs are approved for treating psychotic conditions (e.g., schizophrenia), they have been used for the management of behavioral problems (e.g., agitation, aggressive behavior) that occur in patients with AD. However, these drugs have been shown to increase the risk of death in elderly dementia patients.
- Treating the depression associated with AD may improve cognitive ability. These drugs include selective serotonin reuptake inhibitors (SSRIs) such as fluoxetine (Prozac), sertraline (Zoloft), fluvoxamine (Luvox), and citalopram (Celexa).

Nursing Management
Goals

The patient with AD will maintain functional ability for as long as possible, be maintained in a safe environment with a minimum of injuries, have personal care needs met, and have dignity maintained.

See NCP 60-1 for the patient with AD, Lewis and others, *Medical-Surgical Nursing,* ed 8, pp. 1528 to 1529.

Nursing Diagnoses

- Impaired memory
- Self-care deficit
- Risk for injury
- Wandering

Nursing Interventions

Although there is no current treatment for reversing AD, there is a need for ongoing monitoring of both the patient and the patient's caregiver. An important nursing responsibility is to work collaboratively with the patient's health care provider to manage symptoms effectively as they change over time. You are often responsible for teaching the caregiver to perform the many tasks that are required to manage the patient's care. You must consider both the patient with AD and the caregiver as patients with overlapping but unique problems.

- Adult day care is one of the options available to the person with AD. Common goals of all day-care programs are to provide respite for the family and a protective environment for the patient.
- As the disease progresses, the demands on the caregivers eventually exceed the resources. The person with AD may need to be placed in a long-term care facility, where special units to care for persons with AD are becoming increasingly common.
- Patients with AD are subject to acute and other chronic illnesses. Their inability to communicate health symptoms and problems places responsibility for assessment and diagnosis on caregivers and health professionals. Hospitalization of the patient can be a traumatic event for both patient and caregiver and can precipitate a worsening of the disease.
- Support groups for caregivers and family members have been formed throughout the United States and other countries to provide an atmosphere of understanding and to give current information about the disease itself and related topics such as safety, legal, ethical, and financial issues.

A family and caregiver teaching guide based on the disease stages is provided in Table 6.

Table 6	**Family and Caregiver Teaching Guide: Alzheimer's Disease**

You should include the following instructions when teaching families and caregivers the management of the patient with Alzheimer's disease:

Mild Stage
1. Confirm the diagnosis. Many treatable (and potentially reversible) conditions can mimic Alzheimer's disease (see Table 60-2, Lewis et al., *Medical-Surgical Nursing,* ed. 8, p. 1520).
2. Get the person to stop driving. Confusion and poor judgment can impair driving skills and potentially put others at risk.

Continued

Table 6	Family and Caregiver Teaching Guide: Alzheimer's Disease—cont'd

3. Encourage activities such as visiting with friends and family, listening to music, participating in hobbies, and exercising.
4. Provide cues in the home, establish a routine, and determine specific location where essential items (e.g., glasses) need to be kept.
5. Do not correct misstatements or faulty memory.
6. Register with MedicAlert + Safe Return, a program established by the Alzheimer's Association to locate individuals who may wander from their homes.
7. Make plans for the future in terms of advance directives, care options, financial concerns, and personal preference for care.

Moderate Stage
1. Install door locks for patient safety.
2. Provide protective wear for urinary and fecal incontinence.
3. Ensure that the home has good lighting, install handrails in stairways and bathroom, and remove area rugs or ensure that they are tacked down.
4. Label drawers and faucets (hot and cold) to ensure safety.
5. Develop strategies such as distraction and diversion to cope with behavioral problems. Identify and reduce potential triggers (e.g., reduce stress, extremes in temperature) for disruptive behavior.
6. Provide memory triggers, such as pictures of family and friends.

Late Stage
1. Provide a regular schedule for toileting to reduce incontinence.
2. Provide care to meet needs, including oral care and skin care.
3. Monitor diet and fluid intake to ensure their adequacy.
4. Continue communication through talking and touching.
5. Consider placement in a long-term care facility when providing total care becomes too difficult.

AMYOTROPHIC LATERAL SCLEROSIS

Amyotrophic lateral sclerosis (ALS) is a rare, progressive neurologic disease characterized by loss of motor neurons. This disease became known as Lou Gehrig's disease when the famous baseball player was stricken with it in the early 1940s. The onset is between the ages of 40 and 70 years, and twice as many men as women are affected. ALS usually leads to death within 2 to 6 years of diagnosis.

- For unknown reasons, motor neurons in the brainstem and spinal cord gradually degenerate in ALS. Consequently, messages originating in the brain never reach the muscles to activate them.
- Typical symptoms are weakness of the upper extremities, dysarthria, and dysphagia. Muscle wasting and fasciculations result from denervation of the muscles and lack of stimulation and use.
- Death usually results from respiratory infection secondary to compromised respiratory function.
- There is no cure for ALS. This illness is devastating because the patient remains cognitively intact while wasting away.
- Riluzole (Rilutek) slows the progression of ALS. This drug works to decrease the amount of glutamate (an excitatory neurotransmitter) in the brain.

The challenge of nursing care is to support the patient's cognitive and emotional functions by facilitating communication, reducing risk of aspiration, decreasing pain secondary to muscle weakness, decreasing risk of injury related to falls, providing diversional activities such as reading and human companionship, and helping the patient and family with anticipatory grieving related to loss of motor function and ultimately death.

ANEMIA

Description

Anemia is a deficiency in the number of red blood cells (RBCs) or erythrocytes, the quantity of hemoglobin (Hb), and/or the volume of packed red cells (hematocrit). Anemia can be caused by blood loss, impaired production of erythrocytes, or increased destruction of erythrocytes.

- Because RBCs transport oxygen (O_2), erythrocyte disorders can lead to tissue hypoxia. This hypoxia accounts for many of the signs and symptoms of anemia.
- Anemia is not a specific disease; it is a manifestation of a pathologic process.
- Anemia is identified and classified by laboratory evaluation.
- Anemia can result from primary hematologic problems or can develop as a secondary consequence of defects in other body systems.

The different types of anemia can be classified according to either morphology (cell characteristics) or etiology.

Table 7	Etiologic Classification of Anemia

Decreased RBC Production
Decreased Hemoglobin Synthesis
- Iron deficiency
- Thalassemias (decreased globin synthesis)
- Sideroblastic anemia (decreased porphyrin)

Defective DNA Synthesis
- Cobalamin (vitamin B_{12}) deficiency
- Folic acid deficiency

Decreased Number of RBC Precursors
- Aplastic anemia
- Anemia of myeloproliferative diseases (e.g., leukemia) and myelodysplasia
- Chronic diseases or disorders
- Medications (e.g., chemotherapy)

Blood Loss
Acute
- Trauma
- Blood vessel rupture

Chronic
- Gastritis
- Menstrual flow
- Hemorrhoids

Increased RBC Destruction (Hemolytic Anemias)
Intrinsic
- Abnormal hemoglobin (Hb S-sickle cell anemia)
- Enzyme deficiency (G6PD)
- Membrane abnormalities (paroxysmal nocturnal hemoglobinuria, hereditary spherocytosis)

Extrinsic*
- Physical trauma (prosthetic heart valves, extracorporeal circulation)
- Antibodies (isoimmune and autoimmune)
- Infectious agents and toxins

DNA, Deoxyribonucleic acid; *G6PD*, glucose-6-phosphate dehydrogenase; *Hb S*, hemoglobin S.
* Result in acquired hemolytic anemia.

- *Morphologic classification* is based on erythrocyte size and color.
- *Etiologic classification* is related to clinical conditions causing the anemia (Table 7).
- Although the morphologic system is the most accurate means of classifying anemia, it is easier to discuss patient

Table 8	Relationship of Morphologic Classification and Etiologies of Anemia	A

Morphology	Etiology
Normocytic, normochromic (normal size and color) MCV 80-100 fl, MCH 27-34 pg	Acute blood loss, hemolysis, chronic kidney disease, chronic disease, cancers, sideroblastic anemia, refractory anemia, diseases of endocrine dysfunction, aplastic anemia, sickle cell anemia, pregnancy
Microcytic, hypochromic (small size, pale color) MCV <80 fl, MCH <27 pg	Iron-deficiency anemia, thalassemia, lead poisoning
Macrocytic (megaloblastic), normochromic (large size, normal color) MCV >100 fl, MCH >34 pg	Cobalamin (vitamin B_{12}) deficiency, folic acid deficiency, liver disease (including effects of alcohol abuse), postsplenectomy

MCH, Mean corpuscular hemoglobin; *MCHC*, mean corpuscular hemoglobin concentration; *MCV*, mean corpuscular volume.

care by focusing on the etiologic problem. Table 8 relates morphologic classifications to various etiologies.

- Although the Hb level is decreased in all anemias, other laboratory findings are characteristic of specific anemias (Table 9).

Clinical Manifestations

- Manifestations of anemia are caused by the body's response to tissue hypoxia. The specific manifestations vary depending on the rate at which it has evolved, severity of anemia, and the presence of coexisting disease. Hb levels may determine the severity of anemia.
- *Mild anemia* (Hb 10 to 14 g/dL [100 to 140 g/L]) may exist without causing symptoms. If symptoms develop, they are usually caused by an underlying disease or a compensatory response to heavy exercise. These symptoms include palpitations, dyspnea, and mild fatigue.
- In *moderate anemia* (Hb 6 to 10 g/dL [60 to 100 g/L]), cardiopulmonary symptoms (e.g., increased heart rate) may be present with rest as well as activity.
- In *severe anemia* (Hb <6 g/dL [<60 g/L]) patients display many clinical manifestations involving multiple body systems (Table 10).

Table 9   Laboratory Study Findings in Anemias

Etiology of Anemia	Hb/Hct	MCV	Reticulocytes	Serum Iron	TIBC	Transferrin	Ferritin	Bilirubin
Iron deficiency	↓	↓	N or slight ↓ or ↑	↓	↑	N or ↓	↓	N or ↓
Thalassemia major	↓ ↓	N or ↓ ↑	↑	↑	N	→	N or ↑	↑
Cobalamin deficiency	↓	↑	N or ↓	N or ↑	N	Slight ↑	↑	N or slight ↑
Folic acid deficiency	↓ ↓	↑	N or ↓	N or ↑	N	Slight ↑	↑	N or slight ↑
Aplastic anemia	↓	N or slight ↑	↓	N or ↑	N or ↑	N	N	N
Chronic disease	↓	N or ↓	N or ↓	N or ↓	↓	N or ↓	N or ↑	N
Acute blood loss	↓	N or ↓	N or ↑	N	N	N	N	N
Chronic blood loss	↓	↓	N or ↑	↓	↑	N	N	N or ↓
Sickle cell anemia	↓ ↓	N	↑	N or ↑	N or →	N	N	↑
Hemolytic anemia	↓	N or ↑	↑	N or ↑	N or →	N	N or ↑	↑

Hb, Hemoglobin; *Hct,* hematocrit; *MCV,* mean corpuscular volume; *N,* normal; *TIBC,* total iron-binding capacity.

A

Table 10   Clinical Manifestations of Anemia

Body System	Severity of Anemia		
	Mild (Hb 10-12 g/dL [100-120 g/L])	Moderate (Hb 6-10 g/dL [60-100 g/L])	Severe (Hb <6 g/dL [<60 g/L])
Integument	None	None	Pallor, jaundice,* pruritus*
Eyes	None	None	Icteric conjunctiva and sclera,* retinal hemorrhage, blurred vision
Mouth	None	None	Glossitis, smooth tongue
Cardiovascular	Palpitations	Increased palpitations, "bounding pulse"	Tachycardia, increased pulse pressure, systolic murmurs, intermittent claudication, angina, HF, MI
Pulmonary	Exertional dyspnea	Dyspnea	Tachypnea, orthopnea, dyspnea at rest
Neurologic	None	"Roaring in the ears"	Headache, vertigo, irritability, depression, impaired thought processes
Gastrointestinal	None	None	Anorexia, hepatomegaly, splenomegaly, difficulty swallowing, sore mouth
Musculoskeletal	None	None	Bone pain
General	None or mild fatigue	Fatigue	Sensitivity to cold, weight loss, lethargy

HF, Heart failure; *Hb,* hemoglobin; *MI,* myocardial infarction.
* Caused by hemolysis.

Nursing Management

Goals
The patient with anemia will assume normal activities of daily living (ADLs), maintain adequate nutrition, and develop no complications related to anemia. See NCP 31-1 for the patient with anemia, Lewis et al, *Medical-Surgical Nursing,* ed 8, pp. 664 to 665.

Nursing Diagnoses
- Fatigue
- Altered nutrition: less than body requirements
- Ineffective self-health management

Nursing Interventions
The numerous causes of anemia necessitate different nursing interventions specific to patient needs. General components of care for all patients with anemia may include:
- Dietary and lifestyle changes that may reverse some anemias.
- Acute interventions such as blood or blood product transfusions, drug therapy (e.g., erythropoietin, vitamin supplements), and O_2 therapy.
- Assessing the patient's knowledge regarding adequate nutritional intake.

Specific types of anemia are listed under separate headings.

ANEMIA, APLASTIC

Description
Aplastic anemia is a disease in which the patient has peripheral blood pancytopenia (decrease of all blood types: red blood cells [RBCs], white blood cells [WBCs], and platelets) and hypocellular bone marrow. Signs and symptoms can range from a chronic condition managed with erythropoietin or blood transfusions to a critical condition with hemorrhage and sepsis.

Pathophysiology
- There are various etiologic classifications for aplastic anemia, but they can be divided into two major groups: congenital (idiopathic) or acquired.
- Congenital aplastic anemia is caused by chromosomal alterations.
- Acquired aplastic anemia is a result of exposure to radiation, chemical agents (e.g., benzene, insecticides, arsenic, alcohol), viral and bacterial infections (e.g., hepatitis, parvovirus), and drugs (e.g., alkylating agents, antiseizure medications, antimetabolites, antimicrobials, gold).

- Approximately 70% of the acquired aplastic anemias are idiopathic and thought to be autoimmune.

Clinical Manifestations

Aplastic anemia may develop abruptly over days or insidiously over weeks and months. It can vary from mild to severe. Clinically the patient may have symptoms caused by suppression of any or all bone marrow elements.

- General manifestations of anemia such as fatigue and dyspnea, as well as cardiovascular and cerebral signs, may be seen (Table 9).
- The patient with neutropenia (low neutrophil count) is susceptible to infection and is at risk for septic shock and death. Even a low grade temperature (>100.4° F) should be considered a medical emergency.
- Thrombocytopenia may be manifested by petechiae, ecchymoses, and epistaxis.

Diagnostic Studies

Diagnosis is confirmed by laboratory studies.

- All marrow elements are affected: hemoglobin (Hb), WBC, and platelet values are often decreased (see Table 9).
- Reticulocyte count is low, and bleeding time is prolonged
- Serum iron and total iron-binding capacity (TIBC) are elevated as initial signs of erythroid suppression.
- Bone marrow examination may be done for any anemic state, but findings are especially important in aplastic anemia because the marrow is hypocellular with increased yellow marrow (fat content).

Nursing and Collaborative Management

Management of aplastic anemia is based on identifying and removing the causative agent (when possible) and providing supportive care until pancytopenia reverses.

Nursing interventions appropriate for the patient with pancytopenia from aplastic anemia are presented in the nursing care plans for patients with anemia, thrombocytopenia, and neutropenia (see NCPs 31-1, pp. 664 to 665, 31-2, p. 683, and 31-3, p. 693, Lewis et al, *Medical-Surgical Nursing,* ed 8). Nursing actions are directed at preventing complications from infection and hemorrhage.

- Prognosis of untreated aplastic anemia is poor (approximately 70% fatal). However, advances in medical management, including hematopoietic stem cell transplant (HSCT) and immunosuppressive therapy with antithymocyte globulin (ATG) and cyclosporine or high-dose cyclophosphamide

(Cytoxan), have improved outcomes significantly. ATG is a horse serum containing polyclonal antibodies against human T cells. Rationale for this therapy is that aplastic anemia is an immune-mediated disease.

- Treatment of choice for adults <45 years old who do not respond to immunosuppressive therapy and who have a human leukocyte antigen (HLA)-matched donor is HSCT. Best results occur in younger patients who have not had previous blood transfusions. Prior transfusions increase the risk of graft rejection.
- For the older adult or the patient without an HLA-matched donor, the treatment of choice is immunosuppression with ATG or cyclosporine or high-dose cyclophosphamide. This therapy may be only partially beneficial.

ANEMIA, COBALAMIN (VITAMIN B_{12}) DEFICIENCY

Description

Anemia resulting from a cobalamin (vitamin B_{12}) deficiency is a type of megaloblastic anemia caused by impaired DNA synthesis. When DNA synthesis is impaired, defective red blood cell (RBC) maturation results in large, abnormal RBCs. Normally a protein known as *intrinsic factor* (IF) is secreted by parietal cells of the gastric mucosa. IF is required for cobalamin (extrinsic factor) absorption in the distal ileum. Therefore if IF is not secreted, cobalamin cannot be absorbed.

- In *pernicious anemia,* the most common cause of cobalamin deficiency, the gastric mucosa does not secrete IF.
- Other causes of cobalamin deficiency include gastrointestinal (GI) surgery and diseases that impair secretion of IF, nutritional deficiency, chronic alcoholism, and hereditary enzymatic defects of cobalamin utilization.

Pathophysiology

Cobalamin deficiency can occur in patients who have had GI surgery, such as gastrectomy; patients who have had a small bowel resection involving the ileum; and patients with Crohn's disease, ileitis, diverticuli of the small intestine, and/or chronic atrophic gastritis. In these cases, cobalamin deficiency results from the loss of IF-secreting gastric mucosal surface or impaired absorption of cobalamin in the distal ileum. Cobalamin deficiency is also found in long-term users of H_2-histamine receptor blockers and proton pump inhibitors and those who are strict vegetarians.

Pernicious anemia is caused by an absence of IF, either from gastric mucosal atrophy or autoimmune destruction of parietal cells. This results in a decrease of hydrochloric acid secretion by the stomach.

Clinical Manifestations

Manifestations of anemia related to cobalamin deficiency develop because of tissue hypoxia (see Table 9). It may take several months for manifestations to develop.

- GI manifestations include a sore tongue, anorexia, nausea, vomiting, and abdominal pain.
- Neuromuscular manifestations include weakness, paresthesias of feet and hands, reduced vibratory and position senses, ataxia, muscle weakness, and impaired thought processes ranging from confusion to dementia.

Diagnostic Studies

Laboratory data reflective of cobalamin deficiency anemia are presented in Table 9.

- Erythrocytes appear large (macrocytic) and have abnormal shapes. This structure contributes to erythrocyte destruction because the cell membrane is fragile.
- Serum cobalamin levels are reduced.
- A Schilling test can be used to assess parietal cell function and is diagnostic of pernicious anemia if orally administered radioactive cobalamin is absorbed following the parenteral administration of IF.

Collaborative Care

Regardless of how much cobalamin is ingested, the patient is not able to absorb it if IF is lacking or if there is impaired ileum absorption, so diet management is not used for cobalamin replacement.

- Lifelong administration of cobalamin is needed. It can be given IM (cyanocobalamin or hydroxocobalamin) or intranasally (Nascobal, CaloMist). A typical treatment schedule consists of 1000 mg cobalamin IM daily for 2 weeks, then weekly until hematocrit is normal, and then monthly for life. Regular supplemental cobalamin can reverse the anemia, but long-standing neuromuscular complications may not be reversible.
- High-dose oral cobalamin and sublingual cobalamin are also available for those in which GI absorption is intact.

Nursing Management

- Nursing interventions for the patient with anemia are appropriate for the patient with cobalamin deficiency (see Anemia, p. 29). In addition to these measures, ensure that the patient is protected from burns and trauma because of a diminished sensation to heat and pain as a result of neurologic impairment.
- Ongoing care is primarily related to ensuring good patient compliance with treatment. There must be careful follow-up evaluation to assess for neurologic difficulties that were not fully corrected by cobalamin replacement therapy. Because the potential for gastric cancer is increased in patients with atrophic gastritis-related pernicious anemia, the patient should have frequent and appropriate screenings.

ANEMIA, FOLIC ACID DEFICIENCY

Folic acid is required for DNA synthesis leading to red blood cell (RBC) (erythrocyte) formation and maturation. Common causes of folic acid deficiency are (1) dietary deficiency, especially a lack of leafy green vegetables and citrus fruits; (2) malabsorption syndromes; (3) drugs that interfere with absorption/use of folic acid (e.g., methotrexate), antiseizure medications (e.g., phenobarbital, phenytoin [Dilantin]); (4) alcohol abuse and anorexia; and (5) hemodialysis treatments, because folic acid is lost during dialysis.

Clinical Manifestations

Clinical manifestations of folic acid deficiency are similar to those of cobalamin deficiency. The disease develops insidiously, and the patient's symptoms may be attributed to other coexisting problems, such as cirrhosis or esophageal varices.

- Gastrointestinal (GI) disturbances include dyspepsia and a smooth, beefy red tongue.
- Absence of neurologic problems is an important diagnostic finding; this lack of neurologic involvement differentiates folic acid deficiency from cobalamin deficiency.
- Diagnostic findings for folic acid deficiency are presented in Table 9. The serum folate level is low (normal is 3 to 25 mg/mL [7 to 57 mol/L]), and the serum cobalamin is normal.

Folic acid deficiency is treated by replacement therapy with the usual dose of 1 mg/day by mouth. In malabsorption states, up to 5 mg/day may be required. Duration of treatment depends on the reason for the deficiency. Encourage the patient to eat foods containing large amounts of folic acid.

Nursing interventions for the patient with anemia are appropriate for the patient with folic acid deficiency (see Anemia, p. 29).

ANEMIA, IRON DEFICIENCY

Description

Iron deficiency anemia, one of the most common chronic hematologic disorders, is found in up to 30% of the world's population. In the United States, those most susceptible to iron deficiency anemia are the very young, those on poor diets, and women in their reproductive years.

Pathophysiology

Iron deficiency may develop from inadequate dietary intake, malabsorption, blood loss, or hemolysis. Dietary iron is adequate to meet the needs of men and older women, but it may be inadequate for those individuals who have higher iron needs (e.g., menstruating or pregnant women).

Iron absorption occurs in the duodenum, and absorption can be altered after surgical procedures that involve removal of or bypass of the duodenum. Malabsorption syndromes may also involve disease of the duodenum, affecting iron absorption.

Blood loss is a major cause of iron deficiency in adults. Major sources of chronic blood loss are from the gastrointestinal (GI) and genitourinary (GU) systems.

- GI bleeding is often not apparent and therefore may exist for a considerable time before the problem is identified. Loss of 50 to 75 mL of blood from the upper GI tract is required to cause stools to appear black (melena). This color results from iron in the red blood cells (RBCs).
- Common causes of GI blood loss are peptic ulcer, esophagitis, diverticula, hemorrhoids, and neoplasia. GU blood loss occurs primarily from menstrual bleeding. The average monthly menstrual blood loss is about 45 mL, which causes a loss of about 22 mg of iron.
- In addition to the anemia of chronic kidney disease, dialysis treatment may induce iron deficiency anemia because of the blood lost in the dialysis equipment and frequent blood sampling.

Clinical Manifestations

In the early course of iron deficiency anemia, the patient may be free of symptoms. As the disease becomes chronic, general manifestations of anemia may develop (see Table 10). In addition, specific clinical symptoms related to iron deficiency anemia may occur.

- Pallor is the most common finding, and glossitis (inflammation of tongue) is the second most common; another finding is cheilitis (inflammation of lips).
- In addition, the patient may report headache, paresthesias, and a burning sensation of the tongue, all of which are caused by lack of iron in the tissues.

Diagnostic Studies

Laboratory abnormalities characteristic of iron deficiency anemia are presented in Table 9. Other diagnostic studies are done to determine the cause of iron deficiency. For example, endoscopy and colonoscopy may be used to detect GI bleeding.

Collaborative Care

The main goal is to treat the underlying cause of reduced iron intake (e.g., malnutrition, alcoholism) or absorption of iron. Efforts are directed toward replacing iron.

- Teach the patient which foods are good sources of iron. If nutrition is adequate, increasing iron intake by dietary means may not be practical. Consequently, oral or occasionally parenteral iron supplements are used.
- Drug therapy with iron supplements requires special considerations related to administration and side effects (see Drug Therapy, Iron Deficiency Anemia, Lewis et al, *Medical-Surgical Nursing,* ed 8, pp. 666 to 667).
- If iron deficiency is from acute blood loss, transfusion of packed RBCs may be required.

Nursing Management

It is important to recognize groups of individuals who are at increased risk for development of iron deficiency anemia, including premenopausal and pregnant women, persons from low socioeconomic backgrounds, older adults, and individuals experiencing blood loss. Diet teaching, with an emphasis on foods high in iron and how to maximize absorption, is important for these groups.

Appropriate nursing measures are presented in NCP 31-1, Lewis et al, *Medical-Surgical Nursing,* ed 8, pp. 664 to 665.

▼ **Patient and Caregiver Teaching**

- Discuss with the patient the need for diagnostic studies to identify the cause of anemia. Reassess the hemoglobin (Hb) level and RBC count to evaluate response to therapy.
- Emphasize compliance with dietary and drug therapy. To replenish the body's iron stores, the patient should take iron therapy for 2 to 3 months after the Hb level returns to normal.
- Monitor patients who require lifelong iron supplementation for potential liver problems related to the iron storage.

ANEURYSM

Description

An aneurysm is an outpouching or dilation of the arterial wall and is a common problem involving the aorta. Aneurysms of peripheral arteries also develop but are less common. Aortic aneurysms may involve the aortic arch, thoracic aorta, and/or abdominal aorta. Most aneurysms are found in the abdominal aorta below the level of the renal arteries. Over time, the dilated aortic wall becomes lined with thrombi that can embolize, leading to acute ischemia in distal arteries. Growth rates are unpredictable, but the larger the aneurysm, the greater the risk of rupture.

Pathophysiology

The most common etiology of descending and abdominal aneurysms is atherosclerosis. Atherosclerotic plaque formation is thought to cause degenerative changes in the media leading to loss of elasticity, weakening, and dilation.

- Male gender, age 65 years or older, and tobacco use are the major risk factors for abdominal aortic aneurysms (AAAs) of atherosclerotic origin. Other risk factors include the presence of coronary or peripheral artery disease, high blood pressure (BP), and high cholesterol. A strong genetic component may exist in the development of AAAs. Less common causes of aneurysms include blunt or penetrating trauma and inflammatory or infectious aortitis.

Aneurysms are classified as true and false aneurysms.

- A *true aneurysm* is one in which the wall of the artery forms the aneurysm, with at least one vessel layer still intact. True aneurysms are further subdivided into fusiform and saccular dilations. A fusiform aneurysm is circumferential and relatively uniform in shape; a saccular aneurysm is pouchlike, with a narrow neck connecting the bulge to one side of the arterial wall.

- A *false aneurysm,* or *pseudoaneurysm,* is not an aneurysm but a disruption of all layers of all wall layers with bleeding that is contained by surrounding anatomic structures. False aneurysms may result from trauma or infection, or after peripheral artery bypass graft surgery at the site of the graft-to-artery anastomosis. They may also result from arterial leakage after removal of cannulae (e.g., upper or lower extremity arterial catheters, intraaortic balloon pump devices).

Clinical Manifestations

Thoracic aorta aneurysms are usually asymptomatic. When present, the most common symptom is deep, diffuse chest pain that may extend to the interscapular area.

Aneurysms in the ascending aorta and aortic arch can produce angina from disruption of blood flow to the coronary arteries and hoarseness as a result of pressure on the recurrent laryngeal nerve. Pressure on the esophagus can cause dysphagia. If the aneurysm presses on the superior vena cava, it can cause distended neck veins and head and arm edema.

AAAs are often asymptomatic and frequently found on routine physical examination or when the patient is being examined for an unrelated problem (e.g., abdominal x-ray). A pulsatile mass in the periumbilical area slightly to the left of midline may be present. Bruits may be auscultated over the aneurysm. Physical findings may be more difficult to detect in obese individuals.

- AAA symptoms may mimic pain associated with any abdominal or back disorders. Compression of nearby anatomic structures may cause symptoms such as back pain from lumbar nerve compression or epigastric discomfort and/or altered bowel elimination from bowel compression.
- Occasionally aneurysms spontaneously embolize plaque causing "blue toe syndrome," in which patchy mottling of the feet and toes occurs in the presence of peripheral pulses.

Complications

The most serious complication is rupture.

- If rupture occurs into the retroperitoneal space, bleeding may be tamponaded by surrounding structures, preventing exsanguination and death. In this case the patient has severe back pain and may have back and/or flank ecchymosis *(Grey Turner's sign).*

- If rupture occurs into the thoracic or abdominal cavity, most patients die from massive hemorrhage. The patient who reaches the hospital will be in hypovolemic shock with tachycardia; hypotension; pale, clammy skin; decreased urine output; altered sensorium; and abdominal tenderness.

Diagnostic Studies

- Chest x-ray reveals abnormal widening of the thoracic aorta.
- Echocardiography assesses function of the aortic valve.
- Ultrasonography is useful to screen for aneurysms and to serially monitor aneurysm size.
- An electrocardiogram (ECG) is done to rule out a myocardial infarction (MI) since thoracic aneurysm symptoms can mimic angina.
- Computed tomography (CT) determines anterior-posterior, cross-sectional diameter, and the presence of thrombus in the aneurysm.
- Magnetic resonance imaging (MRI) may also be used to diagnose and assess severity of the aneurysm.

Collaborative Care

The goal of management is to prevent aneurysm rupture and extension of the dissection. Therefore early detection and prompt treatment are imperative.

Surgical repair is done for aneurysms ≥5.5 cm for men and ≥5 cm for women. Surgical intervention may occur sooner in younger, low-risk patients or if the aneurysm expands rapidly (i.e., >1 cm diameter increase per year), becomes symptomatic, or if the risk of rupture is high. If the aneurysm has ruptured, immediate surgical intervention is required.

- All AAA resections require aortic cross-clamping proximal and distal to the aneurysm. Most resections are done in 30 to 45 minutes, after which time the clamps are removed and blood flow is restored. Surgical repair of an AAA is presented in Fig. 38-4 in Lewis et al, *Medical-Surgical Nursing,* ed 8, p. 869.
- An alternative to conventional surgical repair is the minimally invasive endovascular grafting technique. This technique involves placement of a sutureless aortic graft into the abdominal aorta inside the aneurysm via a femoral artery cutdown.

Nursing Management

Goals

The patient undergoing aortic surgery will have normal tissue perfusion, intact motor and sensory function, and no complications related to surgical repair, such as infection or thrombosis.

Nursing Diagnoses

- Ineffective peripheral tissue perfusion
- Risk for infection

Nursing Interventions

Encourage the patient to reduce cardiovascular risk factors, including BP control, smoking cessation, increasing physical activity, and maintaining normal body weight and serum lipid levels. These measures also help to ensure continued graft patency after surgical repair.

- During the preoperative period, you need to provide emotional support and education to the patient and caregiver and thoroughly assess all body systems. Preoperative teaching includes a brief explanation of the disease process, the planned surgical procedure(s), preoperative routines, what to expect immediately after surgery (e.g., recovery room, tubes/drains), and usual postoperative timelines.
- In the postoperative period, in addition to the usual goals of care for a postoperative patient (e.g., maintaining adequate respiratory function, fluid and electrolyte balance, and pain control), monitor graft patency and renal perfusion. Also monitor for and intervene to limit or treat dysrhythmias, infections, and neurologic complications.
- A nursing care plan for the patient with an aneurysm repair is available at http://evolve.elsevier.com/Lewis/medsurg.

▼ Patient and Caregiver Teaching

Instruct the patient and caregiver to gradually increase activities after they get home. Fatigue, poor appetite, and irregular bowel habits are common.

- Teach the patient to avoid heavy lifting for 6 weeks after surgery. Any redness, swelling, increased pain, drainage from incisions, or fever greater than 100° F (37.8° C) should be reported to a health care provider.
- Teach the patient and caregiver to observe for changes in color or warmth of the extremities. Patients and caregivers can learn to palpate peripheral pulses to assess changes in their quality.
- Sexual dysfunction in male patients is common after aortic surgery. Preoperatively, document baseline sexual function and recommend counseling as appropriate. A referral to a urologist may be useful if erectile dysfunction occurs.

ANGINA, CHRONIC STABLE   A

Description
Angina, or chest pain, is the clinical manifestation of reversible myocardial ischemia that occurs when the demand for myocardial oxygen exceeds the ability of the coronary arteries to supply the heart muscle with oxygen. The primary cause of myocardial ischemia is insufficient blood flow to the myocardium through coronary arteries narrowed by atherosclerosis (see Coronary Artery Disease, p. 155). Chronic stable angina is a clinical manifestation of coronary artery disease (CAD).

Chronic Stable Angina
Chronic stable angina refers to chest pain that occurs intermittently over a long period with the same pattern of onset, duration, and intensity of symptoms. The pain usually lasts for only a few minutes (5 to 15 minutes) and commonly subsides when the precipitating factor is relieved. Pain at rest is unusual.
- An electrocardiogram (ECG) usually reveals ST-segment depression and/or T wave inversion, indicating ischemia.
- Chronic stable angina is controlled with medications on an outpatient basis. Because stable angina is often predictable, medications can be timed to provide peak effects during the time of day when angina is likely to occur.

Variants of chronic stable angina include:
- *Silent ischemia,* in which ischemia occurs in the absence of any subjective symptoms
- *Nocturnal ischemia,* which occurs only at night but not necessarily when the person is lying down or sleeping
- *Angina decubitus,* which is chest pain that occurs only when the person is lying down and is usually relieved by standing or sitting
- *Prinzmetal's angina* (variant angina) often occurs at rest, usually in response to spasm of a major coronary artery. It is a rare form of angina frequently seen in patients with a history of migraine headaches and Raynaud's phenomenon. Calcium channel blockers and/or nitrates are used to control the angina.
- *Microvascular angina* also occurs in the absence of significant coronary atherosclerosis or coronary spasm, especially in women. In these patients chest pain is related to myocardial ischemia associated with abnormalities of the coronary microcirculation. This is known as coronary microvascular

disease (MVD). Prevention and treatment of MVD follow the same recommendations as for CAD.

Pathophysiology

On the cellular level the myocardium becomes cyanotic within the first 10 seconds of coronary occlusion. With total occlusion of the coronary arteries, contractility ceases after several minutes, depriving myocardial cells of oxygen and glucose for aerobic metabolism. Myocardial nerve fibers are irritated by the lactic acid formed by anaerobic metabolism and transmit a pain message to cardiac nerves and upper thoracic posterior roots (the reason for referred cardiac pain to the left shoulder and arm).

- Under ischemic conditions, cardiac cells are viable for about 20 minutes. With restoration of blood flow, aerobic metabolism resumes and contractility is restored. Cellular repair begins.

Clinical Manifestations

When questioned, some patients may deny feeling pain but will refer to a vague sensation, pressure, or ache in the chest. It is an unpleasant feeling, often described as a constrictive, squeezing, heavy, choking, or suffocating sensation. Table 11 provides a memory device to assess the characteristics of angina.

| Table 11 | PQRST Assessment of Angina |

Use the following memory aid to obtain information from the patient who has chest pain.

	Factor	Questions to Ask Patient
P	Precipitating events	What events or activities precipitated the pain (e.g., argument, exercise, resting)?
Q	Quality of pain	What does the pain feel like (e.g., pressure, dull, aching, tight, squeezing, heaviness)?
R	Radiation of pain	Where is the pain located? Does the pain radiate to other areas (e.g., back, neck, arms, jaw, shoulder, elbow)?
S	Severity of pain	On a scale of 0 to 10, with 10 being the most severe pain you could imagine, how would you rate the pain?
T	Timing	When did the pain begin? Has the pain changed since this time? Have you had pain like this before?

- Many persons complain of severe indigestion or burning. Although discomfort is usually felt substernally, the sensation may occur in the neck or radiate to various locations, including the jaw, shoulders, and down the arms.
- Often people will complain of pain between the shoulder blades and dismiss it as not being related to the heart.
- Relief of chronic stable angina pectoris is usually obtained with rest or relief of the precipitating factor.

Diagnostic Studies

Diagnostic studies used to evaluate angina are the same as those used to diagnose CAD (see Coronary Artery Disease, p. 155). For patients with known CAD and chronic stable angina, two studies are commonly used to evaluate coronary artery perfusion.

- Exercise treadmill testing is important because ST-segment and T-wave changes that occur during exercise are an indirect assessment of coronary perfusion. Severely abnormal ECGs during exercise testing indicate a significant disease process and may indicate the need for coronary angiography.
- Cardiac catheterization and coronary angiography can identify a coronary lesion that may be amenable to an intervention that can be done at the time of the catheterization.

Collaborative Care

The treatment of chronic stable angina is aimed at decreasing oxygen demand and/or increasing oxygen supply. Continued emphasis on reduction of CAD risk factors is a priority. In addition to antiplatelet and cholesterol-lowering drug therapy, the most common therapeutic interventions for chronic stable angina are the use of nitrate therapy, beta blockers, and calcium channel blockers to optimize myocardial perfusion. Emergency care of the patient with chest pain is presented in Table 34-13, Lewis et al, *Medical-Surgical Nursing*, ed 8, p. 782. Treatment of chronic stable angina may also include percutaneous coronary intervention with balloon angioplasty and stent placement.

Drug Therapy

- Aspirin is given in the absence of contraindications.
- Short-acting nitrates are first-line therapy for the treatment of angina. Nitrates produce their principal effects by dilating peripheral blood vessels, coronary arteries, and collateral vessels. Sublingual nitroglycerin will usually relieve pain in approximately 3 minutes and has a duration of approximately 30 to 60 minutes. If symptoms are unchanged or worse after 5 minutes, the patient should activate the emergency medication

services system. Nitroglycerin sublingually can be used prophylactically before undertaking an activity that the patient knows may precipitate an anginal attack.

- Long-acting nitrates such as isosorbide dinitrate (Isordil) and isosorbide mononitrate (Imdur) can be used to reduce the incidence of anginal attacks. Longer-acting nitrates are available in oral preparations, ointments, and transdermal controlled-release patches.

- β-Adrenergic blocking agents, such as propranolol (Inderal) and metoprolol (Lopressor), are preferred drugs for management of chronic stable angina. These drugs decrease myocardial contractility, heart rate, systemic vascular resistance (SVR), and blood pressure (BP), all of which reduce myocardial O_2 demand.

- Calcium blocking agents, such as nifedipine (Procardia), verapamil (Calan), diltiazem (Cardizem), and nicardipine (Cardene) are used if β-adrenergic blocking agents are contraindicated, poorly tolerated, or do not control symptoms. The primary effects of calcium channel blockers are systemic vasodilation with decreased SVR, decreased myocardial contractility, and coronary vasodilation.

Percutaneous Coronary Intervention
If a coronary lesion is amenable to an intervention during cardiac catheterization, coronary revascularization with an elective percutaneous coronary intervention (PCI) is done.

- During this procedure, which is called balloon angioplasty, a catheter equipped with a balloon tip is inserted into the appropriate coronary artery. When the blockage is located, the catheter is passed through, the balloon is inflated, and the atherosclerotic plaque is compressed, resulting in vessel dilation.

- Intracoronary stents are often inserted in conjunction with balloon angioplasty. Stents are used to treat abrupt or threatened abrupt closure and restenosis after balloon angioplasty. Stents are expandable, meshlike structures designed to maintain vessel patency by compressing arterial walls and resisting vasoconstriction. Because stents are thrombogenic, the patient is treated with oral antiplatelet agents (e.g., clopidogrel [Plavix], prasugrel [Effient], aspirin) until the intimal lining grows over the stent and provides a smooth vascular surface.

The most serious complications of PCI are abrupt closure and vascular injury. Other less common complications include acute MI, stent embolization, coronary spasm, and emergent coronary artery bypass graft (CABG) surgery. The possibility of dysrhythmias during and after the procedure is always present.

Nursing Management

Goals
The patient with chronic stable angina will experience pain relief, have reduced anxiety, have adequate knowledge of the problem and prescribed treatment, and modify or alter risk factors.

Nursing Diagnoses
- Acute pain
- Anxiety

Nursing Interventions
- If you are present during an anginal attack, institute the following measures: (1) administer O_2 and place the patient in an upright position unless contraindicated, (2) assess vital signs, (3) obtain a 12-lead ECG, (4) provide prompt pain relief with a nitrate first followed by an opioid analgesic if needed, and (5) auscultate heart sounds.

▼ **Patient and Caregiver Teaching**
Reassure the patient with a history of chronic stable angina that a long, productive life is possible.

- Teaching tools, such as pamphlets, films at the bedside, a heart model, and especially written information, are important components of patient and caregiver education.
- Assist the patient to identify factors that precipitate angina and give instructions on how to avoid or control these factors.
- Assist the patient to identify personal risk factors in CAD. Once known, discuss the various methods of decreasing any modifiable risk factors with the patient.
- Teach the patient and caregiver about diets that are low in sodium and reduced in saturated fats. Maintaining ideal body weight is important in controlling angina, because excess weight increases myocardial workload.
- Adhering to a regular, individualized exercise program that conditions the myocardium rather than overstressing it is important. For example, advise patients to walk briskly on a flat surface at least 30 minutes a day, most days of the week, if not contraindicated.
- It is important to teach the patient and caregiver the proper use of nitroglycerin.
- If needed, arrange for counseling to assess psychologic adjustment of the patient and caregiver to the diagnosis of CAD and resulting angina. Many patients feel a threat to their identity and self-esteem.

ANGINA, UNSTABLE

See Acute Coronary Syndrome.

ANKYLOSING SPONDYLITIS

Description

Ankylosing spondylitis (AS) is a chronic inflammatory disease that primarily affects the axial skeleton, including the sacroiliac joints, intervertebral disk spaces, and costovertebral articulations. The HLA-B27 antigen is found in approximately 80% to 90% of persons with AS. The highest incidence of AS is in persons 25 to 34 years of age. Men are more likely to develop AS than women.

Pathophysiology

The cause of AS is unknown. Genetic predisposition appears to play an important role in disease pathogenesis, but the precise mechanisms are unknown. Aseptic synovial inflammation in joints and adjacent tissue causes the formation of granulation tissue (pannus) and the development of dense fibrous scars that lead to fusion of articular tissues. Extraarticular inflammation can affect the eyes, lungs, heart, kidneys, and peripheral nervous system.

Clinical Manifestations

Symptoms of inflammatory spine pain are usually the first indications of AS. These include lower back pain, stiffness, and limitation of motion that are worse during the night and in the morning but improve with mild activity. General symptoms such as fever, fatigue, anorexia, and weight loss are rarely present.

Uveitis (intraocular inflammation) is the most common nonskeletal symptom. It can appear as an initial presentation of the disease years before arthritic symptoms develop.

Severe postural abnormalities and deformity can lead to significant disability. Aortic insufficiency and pulmonary fibrosis are frequent complications. Cauda equina syndrome can also result, contributing to lower extremity weakness and bladder dysfunction.

Diagnostic Studies

- Pelvic x-rays demonstrate sacroiliac changes ranging from subtle erosion to completely fused joints in which joint spaces have been obliterated.

- Laboratory testing is not specific, but an elevated erythrocyte sedimentation rate (ESR) and mild anemia may be seen.
- When the suspicion of AS is high, the presence of the HLA-B27 antigen improves the likelihood of this diagnosis.

Collaborative Care

Prevention of AS is not possible; however, families with other diagnosed HLA-B27-positive rheumatic diseases (e.g., acute anterior uveitis, juvenile spondyloarthritis) should be alert to signs of lower back pain and arthritis symptoms so that early therapy can be initiated.

Care of the patient is aimed at maintaining maximal skeletal mobility while decreasing pain and inflammation. Heat applications, nonsteroidal antiinflammatory drugs (NSAIDs) and salicylates, and disease-modifying antirheumatic drugs (DMARDs), such as sulfasalazine (Azulfidine) or methotrexate, can help in relieving symptoms. Etanercept (Enbrel), a biologic therapy, inhibits the action of tumor necrosis factor (TNF) and has been shown to reduce active inflammation and improve spinal mobility.

Postural control with stretching exercises of the back, neck, and chest is important to minimize spinal deformity. Surgery may be indicated for severe deformity and mobility impairment. Spinal osteotomy and total joint replacement are the most commonly performed procedures.

Nursing Management

A key responsibility is to educate the patient about the nature of the disease and principles of therapy. The home management program consists of local moist heat, regular exercise, and knowledgeable use of medications.

- Discourage excessive physical exertion during periods of active inflammation.
- Proper positioning at rest is essential. The mattress should be firm, and the patient should sleep on the back with a flat pillow, avoiding positions that encourage flexion deformity.
- Postural training emphasizes avoiding spinal flexion (e.g., leaning over a desk), heavy lifting, and prolonged walking, standing, or sitting. Encourage sports that facilitate natural stretching, such as swimming and racquet games.
- Family counseling and vocational rehabilitation are important.

ANORECTAL ABSCESS

Anorectal abscesses are collections of perianal pus resulting from obstruction of the anal glands, leading to infection and abscess formation.

- Common causative organisms are *Escherichia coli,* staphylococci, and streptococci. Manifestations include local pain and swelling, foul-smelling drainage, tenderness, and elevated temperature. Sepsis can occur as a complication. Diagnosis is by rectal examination.
- Surgical therapy consists of abscess drainage. If packing is used, it should be impregnated with petroleum jelly and the area should be allowed to heal by granulation. The packing is changed every day, and moist, hot compresses are applied to the area. Care must be taken to avoid soiling the dressing during urination or defecation. A low-fiber diet is given. The patient may leave the hospital with the area still open.
- Teach the patient about wound care, importance of sitz baths, thorough cleaning after bowel movements, and follow-up visits to a health care provider.

AORTIC DISSECTION

Description

Aortic dissection, often misnamed "dissecting aneurysm," is not a type of aneurysm. Rather, dissection results from the creation of a false lumen (between the intima and media) through which blood flows. Classification is based on anatomical location (ascending versus descending aorta) and duration of onset (acute versus chronic).

- Approximately 60% to 70% of dissections involve the ascending aorta and are acute in onset. Acute aortic dissections (i.e., diagnosed within 14 days of symptom onset) carry a mortality rate as high as 1% per hour.
- Aortic dissection affects men 2 to 5 times more often than women and occurs most frequently in the sixth and seventh decades of life. Predisposing factors include age, aortitis (e.g., syphilis), blunt trauma, congenital heart disease (e.g., bicuspid aortic valve, coarctation of the aorta), connective tissue disorders (e.g., Marfan syndrome), cocaine use, history of cardiac surgery, atherosclerosis, pregnancy, hypertension, and Turner syndrome.

Pathophysiology

Most nontraumatic aortic dissections are attributed to the degeneration of the elastic fibers in the medial layer. Chronic hypertension accelerates the degradation process. Aortic dissection is believed to arise from an intimal tear.

As the heart contracts, each systolic pulsation causes increased pressure, which further increases dissection. Extension of the dissection may cut off blood supply to critical areas such as the brain, kidneys, spinal cord, and extremities.

Clinical Manifestations and Complications

The majority of patients with an acute ascending aortic dissection report sudden, severe onset of excruciating chest and/or back pain radiating to the neck or shoulders. Patients with acute descending aortic dissection are more likely to report pain in their back, abdomen, or legs. The pain is frequently described as "sharp" and "worst ever" followed less frequently by "tearing" or "ripping." Dissection pain can be differentiated from MI pain that is more gradual in onset and has increasing intensity.

- If the aortic arch is involved, the patient may exhibit neurologic deficiencies, including altered level of consciousness, dizziness, and weakened or absent carotid and temporal pulses.
- An ascending aortic dissection usually produces some disruption of coronary blood flow and aortic valvular insufficiency.
- When either subclavian artery is involved, pulse quality and blood pressure (BP) readings may differ between the left and right arms.
- As dissection progresses down the aorta, the abdominal organs and lower extremities demonstrate evidence of altered tissue perfusion.

A severe complication of dissection of the ascending aortic arch is cardiac tamponade, which occurs when blood from the dissection leaks into the pericardial sac. Clinical manifestations include hypotension, narrowed pulse pressure, distended neck veins, muffled heart sounds, and pulsus paradoxus.

- Because the aorta is weakened by medial dissection, it may rupture. Hemorrhage may occur into the mediastinal, pleural, or abdominal cavities.
- Dissection can lead to occlusion of the arterial supply to many vital organs, including the spinal cord, kidneys, and abdominal structures. Ischemia of the spinal cord produces symptoms varying from weakness to paralysis in lower extremities and decreased pain sensation. Renal ischemia

can lead to renal failure. Signs of abdominal ischemia include abdominal pain, decreased bowel sounds, and altered bowel elimination.

Diagnostic Studies

- Chest x-ray indicates widening of the mediastinal silhouette and pleural effusion.
- 3-D CT scanning and transesophageal echocardiography (TEE) have become the standard tests for a diagnosis of acute aortic dissection.
- CT scan can provide information on the presence and severity of the dissection.
- Although MRI has the highest accuracy for detecting aortic dissection, it is contraindicated in some patients (e.g., metallic implants, hemodynamically unstable) and may not be available on an emergency basis.

Collaborative Care

The goals of therapy for aortic dissection without complications are BP control and pain management.

- An intravenous (IV) β-adrenergic blocker (e.g., esmolol) is typically used to decrease the BP and the force of left ventricular contraction. Esmolol is particularly useful since it has a rapid onset and a short half-life.
- Other antihypertensive agents, such as calcium channel blockers and angiotensin-converting enzyme (ACE) inhibitors, may also be used.

An acute ascending aortic dissection is considered a surgical emergency. Otherwise, surgery is indicated when drug therapy is ineffective or when complications (e.g., heart failure) occur. Since the aorta is fragile following dissection, surgery is delayed for as long as possible to allow time for edema to decrease and to permit clotting of the blood in the false lumen.

- Surgery involves resection of the aortic segment containing the intimal tear and replacement with synthetic graft.
- Endovascular repair is the standard modality to treat acute descending aortic dissections with complications (e.g., hemodynamic instability, peripheral ischemia).

Nursing Management

Preoperatively, nursing management includes keeping the patient in bed in a semi-Fowler's position and maintaining a quiet environment. These measures help to keep the systolic BP at the lowest possible level that maintains vital organ perfusion (typically between 110-120 mm Hg). Opioids and sedatives are administered as ordered. Manage pain and anxiety for patient comfort and because these symptoms can cause elevations in the systolic BP.

- IV administration of antihypertensive agents requires close supervision. This requires continuous ECG and intraarterial BP monitoring. Monitor vital signs frequently, sometimes as often as every 2 to 3 minutes until target BP is reached. You should observe for changes in peripheral pulses and signs of increasing pain, restlessness, and anxiety.

Postoperative care after surgery to correct the dissection is similar to that after aortic aneurysm repair (see Nursing Management of Aortic Aneurysms in Lewis et al, *Medical-Surgical Nursing,* ed 8, p. 872).

▼ Patient and Caregiver Teaching

- The therapeutic regimen at discharge includes antihypertensive drugs. The patient needs to understand that these drugs must be taken to control BP. β-Adrenergic blockers (e.g., metoprolol [Toprol-XL]) can be taken orally to continue to decrease myocardial contractility.
- Follow-up with regularly scheduled MRIs or CTs is essential.
- You must instruct patients that if the pain or other symptoms return, they should activate Emergency Medical Services (EMS) for immediate care.

APPENDICITIS

Description
Appendicitis is an inflammation of the appendix, a narrow blind tube that extends from the inferior part of the cecum. Appendicitis occurs in 7% to 12% of the world's population, most commonly in young adults.

Pathophysiology
The most common causes of appendicitis are obstruction of the lumen by a fecalith (accumulated feces), foreign bodies, a tumor of the cecum or appendix, or intramural thickening resulting from hypergrowth of lymphoid tissue. Obstruction results in distention, venous engorgement, and the accumulation of mucus and bacteria, which can lead to gangrene and perforation.

Clinical Manifestations and Complications
Appendicitis typically begins with periumbilical pain, followed by anorexia, nausea, and vomiting. The pain is persistent and continuous, eventually shifting to the right lower quadrant and localizing

at McBurney's point (located halfway between the umbilicus and right iliac crest).

- Further assessment reveals localized and rebound tenderness with muscle guarding. The patient usually prefers to lie still, often with right leg flexed. Low-grade fever may be present, and coughing aggravates the pain. Rovsing's sign may be elicited by palpation of the left lower quadrant, causing pain to be felt in the right lower quadrant.

Complications of acute appendicitis are perforation, peritonitis, and abscesses.

Diagnostic Studies
- White blood cell (WBC) count is usually elevated.
- Urinalysis may be done to rule out genitourinary conditions that mimic manifestations of appendicitis.
- CT scan and ultrasound may be used.

Collaborative Care
If diagnosis and treatment are delayed, the appendix can rupture, and the resulting peritonitis can be fatal. Treatment is immediate surgical removal (appendectomy) if the inflammation is localized. If the appendix has ruptured and there is evidence of peritonitis or an abscess, conservative treatment, consisting of antibiotic therapy and parenteral fluids, may be used to prevent sepsis and dehydration for 6 to 8 hours before an appendectomy is performed.

Nursing Management
Encourage the patient with abdominal pain to see a health care provider and to avoid self-treatment, particularly the use of laxatives and enemas. Increased peristalsis from these procedures may cause perforation.

- Nothing should be taken by mouth (NPO) to ensure the stomach will be empty if surgery is needed.
- An ice bag may be applied to the right lower quadrant to decrease the flow of blood to the area and impede the inflammatory process. Heat can cause the appendix to rupture.

Surgery is performed, generally laparoscopically, as soon as a diagnosis is made. Postoperative nursing management is similar to postoperative care of a patient after laparotomy (see Abdominal Pain, Acute, p. 3). In addition, observe the patient for evidence of peritonitis. Ambulation begins the day of surgery or the first postoperative day. Diet is advanced as tolerated.

- The patient is usually discharged on the first or second postoperative day, and normal activities are resumed 2 to 3 weeks after surgery.

ASTHMA

Description

Asthma is a chronic inflammatory disease of the airways. The chronic inflammation leads to recurrent episodes of wheezing, breathlessness, chest tightness, and cough, particularly at night and in the early morning. These episodes are associated with widespread but variable airflow obstruction that is usually reversible, either spontaneously or with treatment. The clinical course of asthma is unpredictable, ranging from periods of adequate control, to exacerbations with very poor control.

- Asthma affects an estimated 16 million adult Americans. Mortality and morbidity rates from asthma appear to have plateaued and/or decreased, yet there are about 4000 deaths per year from asthma.

Pathophysiology

The primary pathophysiologic process in asthma is persistent but variable airway inflammation that leads to airway hyperresponsiveness (hyperreactivity) and acute airflow limitation. Exposure to allergens or irritants initiates the inflammatory cascade (Table 12).

- As the inflammatory process begins, mast cells in the bronchial wall degranulate and release multiple inflammatory mediators. Common inflammatory mediators are leukotrienes, histamine, cytokines, prostaglandins, and nitric oxide.
- The resulting inflammatory process results in vascular congestion; edema formation; production of thick, tenacious

Table 12	Triggers of Acute Asthma Attacks

- Allergen inhalation
- Air pollutants
- Viral upper respiratory infection
- Sinusitis
- Exercise and cold, dry air
- Stress
- Drugs
- Occupational exposure
- Food additives
- Hormones/menses
- Gastroesophageal reflux disease (GERD)

mucus; bronchial muscle spasm; thickening of airway walls; and increased bronchial hyperresponsiveness.

- This process can occur within 30 to 60 minutes after exposure to a trigger or irritant and is sometimes referred to as the *early-phase response* in asthma.

Symptoms can recur 4 to 10 hours after the initial attack because of eosinophil and lymphocyte activation and further release of more inflammatory mediators.

- This delayed response is called the *late-phase response* in asthma. It can be more severe than the early-phase response and can persist for 24 hours or more. Only about 30% to 50% of patients experience this delayed response.
- A self-sustaining cycle of inflammation occurs, limiting airflow as a result of airway swelling with or without bronchoconstriction. Corticosteroids are effective in treating this inflammation.

Chronic, untreated inflammation may result in structural changes in the bronchial wall known as remodeling.

- A progressive loss of lung function occurs that is not prevented or fully reversed by therapy.

During an asthma attack, decreased perfusion and ventilation of the alveoli and increased alveolar gas pressure lead to ventilation-perfusion abnormalities in the lungs.

- The patient will be hypoxemic early on with decreased $PaCO_2$ and increased pH (respiratory alkalosis) as a result of hyperventilation.
- As the airflow limitation worsens with air trapping, the $PaCO_2$ normalizes and then rises to produce respiratory acidosis, which is an ominous sign signifying respiratory failure.

Clinical Manifestations

Asthma attacks may have an abrupt onset but usually symptoms present more gradually, and may last a few minutes to several hours; a person may be asymptomatic with normal pulmonary function between attacks.

- Characteristic manifestations are wheezing, cough, dyspnea, and chest tightness. Expiration may be prolonged with an inspiratory/expiratory (I/E) ratio of 1:3 or 1:4.
- Wheezing is an unreliable sign to gauge the severity of an attack because many patients with minor attacks wheeze loudly, whereas others with severe attacks do not wheeze.
- In some patients with asthma, cough is the only symptom. The cough may be nonproductive because secretions may

A

be so thick, tenacious, and gelatinous that their removal is difficult.

- During an acute attack, the patient usually sits upright or slightly bent forward using accessory muscles of respiration. The more difficult the breathing becomes, the more anxious the patient feels.
- Signs of hypoxemia include restlessness, increased anxiety, inappropriate behavior, increased pulse and blood pressure (BP), and *pulsus paradoxus* (a drop in systolic pressure during the inspiratory cycle greater than 10 mm Hg).
- Percussion reveals hyperresonance of the lungs. Auscultation usually reveals inspiratory or expiratory wheezing.
- Diminished breath sounds, or a "silent chest," are an ominous sign, indicating severe obstruction and impending respiratory failure. Diminished or absent breath sounds may also indicate atelectasis or pneumothorax.

Classification of Asthma

Asthma can be classified as intermittent, mild persistent, moderate persistent, or severe persistent (Table 13). Patients may progress up or down in asthma level severity over the course of their disease.

Complications

Severe asthma exacerbations occur when the patient is dyspneic at rest and they talk in words, not sentences, because of the difficulty breathing. They are usually sitting forward to maximize the diaphragmatic movement with prominent wheezes and a respiratory rate >30/minute and pulse >120/minute.

- Accessory muscles in the neck are straining to try to lift the chest wall and the patient is often agitated. The peak flow (PEFR [peak expiratory flow rate]) is 40% of the personal best or <150 mL.
- Neck vein distention and a pulsus paradoxus of ≥40 mm Hg may result. Usually it is difficult to auscultate pulsus paradoxus secondary to a noisy chest or increased work of breathing. These patients usually are seen in emergency departments or hospitalized.

A few patients perceive asthma symptoms poorly and may have a significant decrease in lung function without any change in symptoms. Patients with life-threatening asthma are typically too dyspneic to speak and will be perspiring profusely. The breath sounds may be very difficult to hear, and no wheezing is apparent as the airflow is exceptionally limited.

- If the patient has been wheezing and then there is an absence of a wheeze (i.e., silent chest) and the patient is obviously

Table 13   Classification of Asthma Severity

Components 92% of Severity		Intermittent	Classification of Asthma Severity		
			Persistent		
			Mild	**Moderate**	**Severe**
Impairment	Symptoms	≤2 days/week	>2 days/week, not daily	Daily	Continuous
	Nighttime Awakenings	≤2×/month	3-4×/month	>1×/wk, not nightly	Often, 7×/week
	SABA Use for Symptoms	≤2 days/week	>2 days/week, not daily	Daily	Several times per day
	Interference with Normal Activity	None	Minor limitation	Some limitation	Extremely limited
	Lung Function*	■ Normal FEV_1 between exacerbations ■ FEV_1 >80% ■ FEV_1/FVC normal	■ FEV_1, >80% predicted ■ FEV_1/FVC normal	■ FEV_1 60%-80% predicted ■ FEV_1/FVC reduced by 5%	■ FEV_1 <60% predicted ■ FEV_1/FVC reduced by 5%

Risk	Exacerbations Requiring Oral Corticosteroids	0-1/year	≥2/year even in the absence of impairment
		Consider severity and interval since last exacerbation.	
		Frequency and severity may fluctuate over time.	
		Relative annual risk of exacerbation may be related to FEV₁	
Recommended Step for Initiating Treatment		Step 1	Step 2	Step 3**	Step 4 or 5**
		Reevaluate asthma control in 2-6 weeks and adjust therapy accordingly

Source: Adapted from *Expert Panel Report 3: Guidelines for the Diagnosis and Management of Asthma*. National Asthma Education and Prevention Program, National Heart, Lung, and Blood Institute, 2007.

* Percent predicted values for forced expiratory volume in 1 second (FEV₁) or ratio of FEV₁/forced vital capacity (FVC).

Normal FEV₁/FVC:
8-19 yr, 85%
20-39 yr, 80%
40-59 yr, 75%
60-80 yr, 70%

** Consider short corticosteroid therapy.

FEV_1, Forced expiratory volume; FVC, forced vital capacity; $SABA$, short-acting bronchodilator.

Guidelines for Using Table

Patients should be assigned to the most severe step in which any feature occurs. Clinical features for individual patients may overlap across steps. Determine level of severity by assessment of both impairment and risk. Assess impairment by patient's recall of previous 2-4 weeks and spirometry results.

An individual's classification should change over time as treatment is initiated. After treatment, the focus switches to level of control, not the classification of severity. Patients at any level of severity of chronic asthma can have mild, moderate, or severe exacerbations of asthma. Some patients with intermittent asthma experience severe and life-threatening exacerbations separated by long periods of normal lung function and no symptoms.

struggling, this is a life-threatening situation that may require mechanical ventilation.

Diagnostic Studies

Underdiagnosis of asthma is common. In general, the health care provider should consider the diagnosis of asthma if various indicators (i.e., clinical manifestations, health history, and peak flow variability or spirometry) are positive.

- Detailed history may help identify asthma triggers.
- Pulmonary function tests can be used to determine the reversibility of bronchoconstriction and thus establish the diagnosis of asthma.
- Sputum specimen, if indicated, can rule out bacterial infection.
- Elevated serum IgE levels and eosinophil count are highly suggestive of allergic tendency.
- Chest x-ray during an attack shows hyperinflation.
- Arterial blood gases (ABGs) with mild attack show respiratory alkalosis with an arterial O_2 pressure (PaO_2) near normal. Hypercapnia and respiratory acidosis indicate severe disease.
- Nitric oxide levels are increased in the breath of people with asthma.
- Serial peak expiratory flow rates (PEFR), oximetry, and ABGs provide information about severity of attack and response to treatment.
- Allergy skin testing may be of some value to determine sensitivity to specific allergens.

Collaborative Care

The goal of asthma treatment is to achieve and maintain control of the disease. Guidelines for the diagnosis and management of asthma are presented in Table 13 on pp. 60 to 61 and in Fig. 29-4 and Table 29-5, Lewis et al, *Medical-Surgical Nursing,* ed 8, pp. 594 and 595. The current guidelines focus on (1) assessing the severity of the disease at diagnosis and initial treatment and then (2) monitoring periodically to achieve control of the disease.

At initial diagnosis a patient may have severe asthma and require asthma medication. After treatment the patient is assessed for level of control (i.e., well controlled, not well controlled, or very poorly controlled). As the patient achieves symptom control, the health care provider steps down the medication or steps it up as the symptoms worsen.

- Achieving rapid control of the symptoms is the goal in order to return the patient to daily functioning at the best possible level.
- The level of control is based on the patient's responses to symptoms, nighttime awakenings, interferences with normal activity, and use of rescue or reliever medication.

Intermittent and persistent asthma. The classification of severity of asthma at initial diagnosis helps determine which types of medications are best suited to control the asthma symptoms (see Table 13).

- Patients in all classifications of asthma will require a short-term (rescue or reliever) medication. The short-acting β_2-adrenergic agonists (SABA) (e.g., albuterol) are the gold standard and most effective. Patients with persistent asthma must be on a long-term or controller medication.
- Inhaled corticosteroids (ICS) (e.g., fluticasone [Flovent]) are the most effective class of drugs to combat the inflammation.

Acute asthma exacerbations. Asthma exacerbations may be mild to life threatening. With mild exacerbations, patients have difficulty breathing only with activity and may feel they "can't get enough air." Peak flow is >70% of their personal best and symptoms often are relieved at home promptly with a short-acting β agonist (SABA) such as albuterol delivered via a nebulizer or MDI with a spacer.

- With a moderate exacerbation, dyspnea interferes with usual activities and peak flow is 40% to 60% of personal best. In this situation, the patient usually comes to the ED or a health care provider's office to get help. Relief is provided with the SABA delivered as in the mild exacerbation and oral corticosteroids are needed. Symptoms may persist for several days even after corticosteroids are started. Oxygen can be used with both mild and moderate exacerbations.

Severe and life-threatening asthma exacerbations Management of the patient with severe and life-threatening asthma focuses on correcting hypoxemia and improving ventilation. The goal is to keep the O_2 saturation $\geq 90\%$. Continuous monitoring of the patient is critical.

- Many therapeutic measures are the same as those for acute asthma. Repetitive or continuous SABA administration is provided in the ED. Initially three treatments of SABA (spaced 20 to 30 minutes apart) are given. Then more SABA is given depending on the patient's airflow, improvement, and side effects from the SABA.

- In life-threatening asthma, corticosteroids are administered IV and are usually tapered rapidly. IV corticosteroids (methylprednisolone) are administered every 4 to 6 hours. Adjunctive medications such as IV magnesium sulfate may be administered in certain adults with very low FEV_1 or peak flow (<40% of predicted or personal best at presentation) or those who fail to respond to initial treatment.
- Supplemental O_2 is given by mask or nasal prongs to achieve a PaO_2 of at least 60 mm Hg or an O_2 saturation >90%. An arterial catheter may be inserted to facilitate frequent ABG monitoring.

Occasionally asthma exacerbations are life threatening and respiratory arrest is pending or actually occurring. Therefore the patient will require intubation and mechanical ventilation if there is no response to treatment. The patient will be provided with 100% oxygen, hourly or continuously nebulized SABA, IV corticosteroids, and possible other adjunctive therapies as noted above.

Drug Therapy

- A stepwise approach to drug therapy is based initially on the asthma severity and then on level of control. Persistent asthma requires daily long-term therapy in addition to appropriate medications to manage acute symptoms. Medications are divided into two general classifications: (1) quick-relief or rescue medications to treat symptoms and exacerbations, such as SABA and (2) long-term control medications to achieve and maintain control of persistent asthma such as ICS. Some of the controllers are used in combination to gain better asthma control (e.g., fluticasone/salmeterol [Advair]) (see Table 29-7, Lewis et al, *Medical-Surgical Nursing,* ed 8, pp. 598 to 599). One of the major factors determining success in asthma management is the correct administration of drugs.
- Information about medications should include the name, purpose, dosage, method of administration, and schedule, taking into consideration activities of daily living (ADLs) which require energy expenditure and thus oxygen, such as bathing.
- Medication teaching should also include side effects, appropriate action if side effects occur, how to properly use and clean devices, and consequences for breathing if not taking medications as prescribed.

Nursing Management

A

Goals
The patient with asthma will maintain >80% of personal best PEFR or FEV_1 and will have minimal symptoms during the day and night, acceptable activity levels (including exercise and other physical activity), no recurrent exacerbations of asthma, and adequate knowledge to participate in and carry out management.

See NCP 29-1 for the patient with asthma, Lewis et al, *Medical-Surgical Nursing,* ed 8, p. 605.

Nursing Diagnoses
- Ineffective airway clearance
- Anxiety
- Deficient knowledge

Nursing Interventions
A goal in asthma care is to maximize the ability of the patient to safely manage acute asthma exacerbations via an asthma action plan developed in conjunction with the health care provider (see Table 29-13, Lewis et al, *Medical-Surgical Nursing,* ed 8, p. 606).

During an acute attack of asthma, it is important for you to monitor the patient's respiratory and cardiovascular systems. This includes auscultating lung sounds; taking pulse rate, respiratory rate, and BP; and monitoring ABGs, pulse oximetry, and peak flow.

- The patient can take two to four puffs of a SABA every 20 minutes three times as a rescue plan. Depending on the response with alleviation of symptoms or improved peak flow, continued SABA use and/or oral corticosteroids may be a part of the home management plan at this point. If symptoms persist or if the patient's peak flow is <50% of the personal best, the health care provider or EMS needs to be immediately contacted.
- An important nursing goal during an acute attack is to decrease the patient's sense of panic. A calm, quiet, reassuring attitude may help the patient relax. The patient should be positioned comfortably (usually sitting) to maximize chest expansion. You need to stay with the patient and be available to provide additional comfort.
- In a firm, calm voice coach the patient to use pursed-lip breathing, which keeps the airways open by maintaining positive pressure and abdominal breathing, which slows the respiratory rate and encourages deeper breaths.

▼ **Patient and Caregiver Teaching**
- Teach the patient to avoid known personal triggers for asthma (e.g., cigarette smoke, pet dander) and irritants (e.g., cold air, aspirin, foods, cats). If cold air cannot be avoided, dressing properly with a scarf or mask helps reduce the risk of an asthma attack. Aspirin and NSAIDs should be avoided if they are known to precipitate an attack. Many over-the-counter (OTC) drugs contain aspirin, and the patient should be instructed to read labels carefully.
- Nonselective β blockers (e.g., propranolol [Inderal]) are contraindicated because they inhibit bronchodilation.
- Prompt diagnosis and treatment of upper respiratory tract infections and sinusitis may prevent an exacerbation of asthma.
- If exercise is planned or if the patient only has asthma with exercise, the health care provider can suggest a medication regimen for pretreatment or long-term control of symptoms to prevent bronchospasm. Physical exercise (e.g., swimming, walking, stationary cycling) within the patient's limit of tolerance can be performed with the use of preexercise bronchodilators.
- The drug regimen can be confusing and complex. Teach patients the need and importance of monitoring their responsiveness to medication.

It is very important to involve the patient's caregiver or family. These persons should know where the patient's inhalers, oral medications, and emergency phone numbers are located. Instruct them on how to decrease the patient's anxiety if an asthma attack occurs. When the patient is stabilized or controlled, the caregiver can gently remind the patient about doing daily PEFR by asking

Table 14	Patient and Caregiver Teaching Guide: Asthma

Teaching Topic
- What Is Asthma?
- What Is Good Asthma Control?
- Hindrances to Asthma Treatment and Control
- Environmental/Trigger Control
- Medications
- Correct Use of Metered-Dose Inhaler, Dry Powder Inhaler, Spacer, and Nebulizer
- Breathing Techniques
- Correct Use of Peak Flowmeter
- Asthma Action Plan

questions such as, "What zone are you in? How's your peak flow today?"

A patient and caregiver teaching guide for the patient with asthma is presented in Table 14.

B

BELL'S PALSY

Description

Bell's palsy (peripheral facial paralysis, acute benign cranial polyneuritis) is a disorder characterized by a disruption of motor branches of the facial nerve (CN VII) on one side of the face in the absence of any other disease, such as a stroke. It can affect any age group, but it is more commonly seen in the 20- to 60-year-old age range. Despite its good prognosis, Bell's palsy leaves more than 8000 people a year in the United States with permanent, potentially disfiguring facial weakness.

- The exact etiology is not known; activation of herpes simplex virus (HSV) may be involved. Reactivation of HSV causes inflammation, edema, ischemia, and eventual demyelination of the nerve, creating pain and alterations in motor and sensory function.
- Bell's palsy is considered benign, with full recovery after 6 months in most patients, especially if treatment is instituted immediately.

Clinical Manifestations

Paralysis of the motor branches of the facial nerve typically results in a flaccidity of the affected side of the face, with drooping of the mouth accompanied by drooling. Inability to close the eyelid, with an upward movement of the eyeball when closure is attempted, is also evident.

- A widened palpebral fissure (opening between the eyelids); flattening of the nasolabial fold; unilateral loss of taste; and inability to smile, frown, or whistle are also common.
- Decreased muscle movement may alter chewing ability, and some patients may experience a loss of tearing or excessive tearing.
- Pain may be present behind the ear on the affected side, especially before the onset of paralysis.

Complications can include psychologic withdrawal because of changes in appearance, malnutrition and dehydration, mucous membrane trauma, corneal abrasions, and facial spasms and contractures.

Diagnosis of Bell's palsy is one of exclusion. Diagnosis and prognosis are indicated by observation of the typical pattern of onset and the testing of percutaneous nerve excitability by electromyogram (EMG).

Collaborative Care

Methods of treatment include moist heat, gentle massage, and electrical stimulation of the nerve. Stimulation may maintain muscle tone and prevent atrophy. Care is primarily focused on relief of symptoms, protection of the eye on the affected side, and prevention of complications.

- Corticosteroids, especially prednisone, are started immediately, and best results are obtained if corticosteroids are initiated before paralysis is complete. When the patient improves to the point that corticosteroids are no longer necessary, they should be tapered off over 2 weeks. Usually corticosteroid treatment decreases edema and pain, but mild analgesics can be used if necessary.
- Because HSV is implicated in many cases of Bell's palsy, treatment with acyclovir (Zovirax) alone or in conjunction with prednisone may be used. Valacyclovir (Valtrex) and famciclovir (Famvir) have also been used.

Nursing Management

Early recognition of the possibility of Bell's palsy is important. Because HSV is a possible etiologic factor, tell any person who is prone to herpes simplex to seek health care if pain occurs in or around the ear. Assess facial muscles for any signs of weakness.

- Mild analgesics can relieve pain. Hot wet packs can reduce discomfort of herpetic lesions, aid circulation, and relieve pain.
- Tell the patient to protect the face from cold and drafts because trigeminal hyperesthesia (extreme sensitivity to pain or touch) may accompany the syndrome.
- Maintenance of good nutrition is important. Teach the patient to chew on the unaffected side of the mouth to avoid trapping food and to improve taste. Thorough oral hygiene must be carried out after each meal to prevent development of parotitis, caries, and periodontal disease from accumulated residual food.
- Dark glasses may be worn for protective and cosmetic reasons. Artificial tears (methylcellulose) should be instilled frequently during the day to prevent corneal drying. Ointment and an impermeable eye shield can be used at night to

retain moisture. In some patients taping the lids closed at night may be necessary to provide protection.

- A facial sling may be helpful to support affected muscles, improve lip alignment, and facilitate eating. Vigorous massage can break down tissues, but gentle upward massage has psychologic benefits. When function begins to return, active facial exercises are performed several times per day.

- The change in physical appearance as a result of Bell's palsy can be devastating. Reassure the patient that a stroke did not occur and that chances for a full recovery are good. It is important to share with the patient that most patients recover within about 6 weeks of the onset of symptoms.

BENIGN PAROXYSMAL POSITIONAL VERTIGO

Description

Approximately 50% of the cases of vertigo may be caused by benign paroxysmal positional vertigo (BPPV). In this condition, free floating debris in the semicircular canal causes vertigo with specific head movements, such as getting out of bed, rolling over in bed, and sitting up from lying down. The debris ("ear rocks") is composed of small crystals of calcium carbonate that may occur in the inner ear due to head trauma, infection, or the aging process. In many cases, a cause cannot be found.

Symptoms are intermittent and include dizziness, vertigo, light-headedness, loss of balance, and nausea. There is no hearing loss. The symptoms of BPPV may be confused with those of Ménière's disease. Diagnosis is based on auditory and vestibular testing results.

Although BPPV is a bothersome problem, it is rarely serious unless a person falls. Repositioning maneuvers and procedures may help in providing symptom relief for many patients. (See Lewis et al, *Medical-Surgical Nursing*, ed 8, p. 428 for a description of these procedures.)

BENIGN PROSTATIC HYPERPLASIA

Description

Benign prostatic hyperplasia (BPH) is an enlargement of the prostate gland. It is the most common urologic problem in male adults.

- BPH occurs in about 50% of men older than 50 years and 90% of men older than 80 years. Approximately 25% of men require treatment by age 80 years.

- Prostatic hyperplasia does not predispose a patient to the development of prostate cancer.

Pathophysiology

Although the cause is not completely understood, it is thought that BPH results from endocrine changes associated with aging.

- Possible causes include the excessive accumulation of dihydroxytestosterone (the principal intraprostatic androgen), which can lead to an overgrowth of prostate tissue; or a decrease in testosterone, which occurs with aging, resulting in a greater proportion of estrogen. This imbalance may lead to prostatic cell growth.
- The enlargement of the gland gradually compresses the urethra, causing partial or complete obstruction. The location of the enlargement rather than the size of the prostate is most significant in the development of obstructive symptoms.
- Risk factors for BPH other than aging have not been clearly identified.

Clinical Manifestations

Early symptoms are often minimal because the bladder can compensate for a small amount of resistance to urine flow. Symptoms gradually worsen as the degree of urethral obstruction increases. Symptoms fall into one of two groups: obstructive symptoms and irritative symptoms.

- Obstructive symptoms of BPH develop as a result of urinary retention and include a decrease in the caliber and force of the urinary stream, difficulty in initiating voiding, and dribbling at the end of urination.
- Irritative symptoms, including urinary frequency, urgency, dysuria, bladder pain, nocturia, and incontinence, are related to inflammation and infection.

Complications are uncommon and are a result of urinary obstruction and urinary retention.

- Acute urinary retention is a complication manifested as a sudden and painful inability to urinate. Treatment involves the insertion of a catheter to drain the bladder. Surgery may also be indicated.
- Urinary tract infection can result from incomplete bladder emptying, which provides a favorable environment for bacterial growth.
- Calculi may develop in the bladder because of alkalinization of the residual urine.

- Hydronephrosis and pyelonephritis caused by back pressure of urine in an obstructed system may lead to renal failure.

Diagnostic Studies

- Physical examination including digital rectal examination (DRE) for prostate size, symmetry, and consistency
- Urinalysis with culture to identify infection or inflammation
- Postvoid residual urine volume to assess degree of urine flow obstruction
- Prostate-specific antigen (PSA) measured to rule out prostate cancer
- Uroflowmetry flow studies and transrectal ultrasound scan of prostate
- Cystoscopy to visualize the urethra and bladder

Collaborative Care

The initial conservative treatment for BPH is referred to as "watchful waiting." If the patient begins to have signs or symptoms that are bothersome or indicate a complication, further treatment is indicated. There are numerous treatment options for BPH.

Drug therapy. Drugs are often used to treat BPH with variable results.

- 5-α-Reductase inhibitors reduce the size of the prostate gland. Finasteride (Proscar) blocks the enzyme needed to convert testosterone to dihydroxytestosterone, the principal intraprostatic androgen. This results in a regression of hyperplastic tissue. Dutasteride (Avodart) has the same effect as finasteride and may also be used.
- α₁-Adrenergic receptor blockers cause smooth muscle relaxation in prostate tissue, which ultimately facilitates urinary flow through the urethra. α₁-Adrenergic receptor blockers, such as silodosin (Rapaflo), terazosin (Hytrin), and tamsulosin (Flomax), are currently being used.

Minimally invasive therapy. Minimally invasive therapies generally do not require hospitalization or catheterization and have few adverse events. When compared to invasive techniques many of these therapies are less effective in improving urine flow and symptoms, which may necessitate retreatment. Advantages and disadvantages of the various minimally invasive and invasive treatment options are compared in Table 55-3, Lewis et al, *Medical-Surgical Nursing,* ed 8, p. 1381.

Transurethral microwave thermotherapy (TUMT) is an outpatient procedure that involves the delivery of microwaves directly to the prostate through a transurethral probe. The temperature of the prostate tissue is raised to about 113° F (45° C) causing necrosis, thus relieving the obstruction.

Transurethral needle ablation (TUNA) is another outpatient procedure that increases the temperature of prostate tissue, thus causing localized necrosis. TUNA differs from TUMT in that only prostate tissue in direct contact with the needle is affected, allowing greater precision in removal of the target tissue.

Laser procedures to treat BPH are used in a variety of approaches. The laser beam is delivered transurethrally through a fiber instrument and is used for cutting, coagulation, and vaporization of prostatic tissue. Examples of this technique include photovaporization and interstitial laser coagulation.

Invasive therapy. Invasive therapy is indicated when there is a decrease in urine flow sufficient to cause discomfort, persistent residual urine, acute urinary retention because of obstruction with no reversible precipitating cause, or hydronephrosis.

- Invasive treatment of symptomatic BPH primarily involves resection or ablation of the prostate. The selection of a surgical approach depends on size and position of the prostatic enlargement as well as surgical risk.

Transurethral resection of the prostate (TURP) is a surgical procedure involving removal of prostate tissue using a resectoscope inserted through the urethra. TURP has been considered the "gold standard" surgical treatment of obstructing BPH. Although this procedure remains commonly performed, there has recently been a decrease in the number of TURP procedures done due to the development of less invasive technologies. After the procedure, a large three-way indwelling catheter with a 30-mL balloon containing sterile water is usually inserted into the bladder to provide hemostasis and facilitate urinary drainage. The bladder is irrigated, either continuously or intermittently, for at least 24 hours to prevent obstruction from mucous threads and blood clots.

Transurethral incision of the prostate (TUIP) is performed with the patient under local anesthesia and is indicated for men with moderate to severe symptoms and small prostates who are poor surgical candidates. TUIP is as effective as TURP in relieving symptoms.

Nursing Management

Because you will be most directly involved with the care of patients having prostatic surgery, the focus of nursing management is on preoperative and postoperative care.

Goals

Overall preoperative goals for the patient having prostatic surgery are to have restoration of urinary drainage, treatment of any urinary tract infection, and understanding of the upcoming surgery. Overall postoperative goals are that the patient will have no complications, restoration of urinary control, and satisfying sexual expression.

See NCP 55-1 for the patient undergoing prostate surgery, Lewis et al, *Medical-Surgical Nursing,* ed 8, pp. 1384 to 1385.

Nursing Diagnoses

Preoperative

- Acute pain
- Risk for infection

Postoperative

- Acute pain
- Impaired urinary elimination
- Deficient knowledge

Nursing Interventions

The cause of BPH is largely attributed to the aging process. The focus of health promotion is on early detection and treatment. When symptoms of prostatic hyperplasia become evident, further diagnostic screening may be necessary.

- Some men find that ingestion of alcohol and caffeine tends to increase prostatic symptoms because of the diuretic effect that increases bladder distention.
- Advise patients with obstructive symptoms to urinate every 2 to 3 hours or when they first feel the urge to minimize urinary stasis and acute urinary retention.

Preoperative care. Urinary drainage must be restored before surgery; a urethral catheter such as a coudé (curved-tip) catheter may be needed.

- Any infection of the urinary tract must be treated before surgery. Restoring drainage and encouraging a high fluid intake (2 to 3 L/day) are helpful.
- The patient is usually concerned about the impact of impending surgery on sexual function. Provide an opportunity for the patient and his partner to express their concerns.

Postoperative care. The plan of care should be adjusted to the type of surgery, reasons for surgery, and patient response to surgery.

- Postoperatively, some form of irrigation (continuous or intermittent) may be used for 24 hours or until no clots are noted draining from the bladder. Monitor the inflow and outflow of the irrigant. The infusion of the continuous bladder irrigation fluid should be at a rate to keep the urine drainage light pink without clots.
- Blood clots are normal for the first 24 to 36 hours. However, large amounts of bright red blood in the urine can indicate hemorrhage.

- The catheter should be connected to a closed drainage system and not disconnected unless it is being removed, changed, or irrigated. Secretions that accumulate around the meatus can be cleansed daily with soap and water.
- Painful bladder spasms occur as a result of irritation of the bladder mucosa from insertion of a resectoscope, presence of a catheter, or clots leading to obstruction of the catheter. Instruct the patient not to attempt to urinate around the catheter because this increases the likelihood of spasm. If bladder spasms develop, check the catheter for clots. If present, remove the clots by irrigation so urine can flow freely. Belladonna and opium suppositories, along with relaxation techniques, are used to relieve pain and decrease spasm.
- Sphincter tone may be poor immediately after catheter removal, resulting in urinary incontinence or dribbling. Sphincter tone can be strengthened by having the patient practice Kegel exercises (pelvic floor muscle technique). Continence can improve for up to 12 months.
- Observe the patient for signs of postoperative infection. If an external wound is present, the area should be observed for redness, heat, swelling, and purulent drainage. Rectal procedures, such as rectal temperatures and enemas (except insertion of well-lubricated belladonna and opium suppositories), should be avoided.
- Dietary intervention and stool softeners are important to prevent straining while having bowel movements. A diet high in fiber facilitates the passage of stool.
- Activities that increase abdominal pressure, such as sitting or walking for prolonged periods and straining to have a bowel movement (Valsalva maneuver), should be avoided.

▼ **Patient and Caregiver Teaching**

Discharge planning and home care issues are important aspects of care after prostate surgery.

- Instructions include (1) caring for an indwelling catheter, if one is in place; (2) managing urinary incontinence; (3) maintaining oral fluids between 2 and 3 L/day; (4) observing for signs and symptoms of urinary tract and wound infection; (5) preventing constipation; (6) avoiding heavy lifting (>10 lb [>4.5 kg]); and (7) refraining from driving or sexual intercourse as directed by the physician.
- Many men experience retrograde ejaculation because of trauma to the internal sphincter. Semen is discharged into the bladder at orgasm and may produce cloudy urine when the patient urinates after orgasm. Discuss these changes with

the patient and his partner and allow them to ask questions and express their concerns.

- Sexual counseling and treatment options may be necessary if erectile dysfunction becomes a chronic or permanent problem.
- The bladder may take up to 2 months to return to its normal capacity. The patient should be instructed to drink at least 2 L of fluid per day and to urinate every 2 to 3 hours to flush the urinary tract. Bladder irritants such as caffeine products, citrus juices, and alcohol should be avoided or limited to small amounts.
- Advise the patient to have yearly digital rectal examinations (DREs) if he has had any procedure other than complete removal of the prostate. Hyperplasia or cancer can occur in the remaining prostatic tissue.

BLADDER CANCER

Description

The most frequent malignant tumor of the urinary tract is transitional cell carcinoma of the bladder, which accounts for nearly 1 in every 20 cancers diagnosed in the United States. Cancer of the bladder is most common between the ages of 60 and 70 years and is at least 3 times as common in men as in women.

Risk factors for bladder cancer include cigarette smoking, exposure to dyes used in the rubber and cable industries, and chronic use of phenacetin-containing analgesics. Individuals with chronic, recurrent renal calculi and chronic lower urinary tract infections also have an increased risk of squamous cell bladder cancer. Women treated with radiation for cervical cancer and patients receiving cyclophosphamide (Cytoxan) also have an increased risk; the reason is unknown.

Clinical Manifestations

Microscopic or gross, painless hematuria (chronic or intermittent) is the most common clinical finding. Bladder irritability with dysuria, frequency, and urgency may also occur.

Diagnostic Studies

- When cancer is suspected, urine specimens for cytology determine the presence of neoplastic or atypical cells.
- Bladder cancer detected by ultrasound, computed tomography (CT), or magnetic resonance imaging (MRI). Bladder cancer is confirmed by cystoscopy and biopsy.

Clinical staging is determined by depth of invasion of the bladder wall and surrounding tissue. Bladder tumors are staged using the Jewett-Strong-Marshall system. This system broadly classifies bladder cancer as superficial, invasive, or metastatic disease.

- Pathologic grading systems are used to classify the malignant potential of tumor cells, indicating a scale ranging from well differentiated to anaplastic.
- Low-stage, low-grade, superficial bladder cancers are most common and most responsive to treatment. Periodic surveillance is important as 30% of patients have tumor recurrence within 5 years and nearly 95% have recurrence by 15 years.

Nursing and Collaborative Management

Surgical therapy may involve a variety of procedures including the following:

- Transurethral resection with fulguration (electrocautery) is used for diagnosis and treatment of superficial lesions with a low recurrence rate. This procedure is also used to control bleeding in patients who are poor operative risks or who have advanced tumors.
- Laser photocoagulation can be repeated a number of times for superficial bladder cancer and recurrence. Advantages of this procedure include bloodless destruction of lesions, minimal risk of perforation, and the lack of a need for a urinary catheter.
- Open loop resection (snaring of polyp-type lesions) with fulguration is used to control bleeding for large superficial tumors and multiple lesions. Treatment of large lesions entails a segmental resection of the bladder.

Postoperative management of the patient who has had one of these surgical procedures includes instructions to drink large amounts of fluid each day for the first week after the procedure, avoid alcoholic beverages, use opioid analgesics and stool softeners if necessary, and take sitz baths to promote muscle relaxation and reduce urinary retention.

- You should also help the patient and family cope with fears about cancer, surgery, and sexuality and should emphasize the importance of regular follow-up care. Frequent routine cystoscopies are required.

When the tumor is invasive or involves the trigone (area where ureters insert into the bladder) and the patient is free from metastases beyond the pelvic area, a partial or radical cystectomy with urinary diversion is the treatment of choice.

- A partial cystectomy includes resection of that portion of the bladder wall containing the tumor, along with a margin of normal tissue.
- A radical cystectomy involves removal of the bladder, prostate, and seminal vesicles in men and the bladder, uterus, cervix, urethra, and ovaries in women.

Radiation therapy is used with cystectomy or as the primary therapy when the cancer is inoperable or when surgery is refused. Increasingly, radiation therapy is being combined with systemic chemotherapy.

- Cisplatin (Platinol), vinblastine (Velban), doxorubicin (Adriamycin), and methotrexate are chemotherapeutic agents that may be used systemically before surgery, before radiation, or for distant metastases.

Chemotherapy with local instillation of chemotherapeutic or immune-stimulating agents can be delivered into the bladder through a urethral catheter, usually at weekly intervals for 6 to 12 weeks.

- These intravesical agents are instilled directly into the patient's bladder and retained for about 2 hours; position of the patient may be changed every 15 minutes for maximum contact in all areas of the bladder.
- Bacille Calmette-Guérin (BCG), a weakened strain of *Mycobacterium bovis,* is the treatment of choice for carcinoma in situ. When BCG fails, α-interferon, thiotepa (Thioplex) and/or valrubicin (Valstar) may be used.
- Most patients have irritative voiding symptoms and hemorrhagic cystitis following intravesical therapy.

Encourage the patient to increase daily fluid intake and to quit smoking. Assess the patient for secondary urinary infection, and stress to the patient the need for routine urology follow-up care. The patient may have fears or concerns about sexual activity or bladder function that will also need to be addressed.

BONE CANCER

Description

Primary bone cancer is rare in adults. Metastatic bone cancer in which the cancer has spread from another site is a more common problem. Primary bone cancer is called *sarcoma.* The more common types of primary bone cancer are osteosarcoma, chondrosarcoma, Ewing's sarcoma, and chordoma.

Osteosarcoma

Osteogenic sarcoma is a primary bone tumor that is extremely aggressive and rapidly metastasizes to distant sites. It usually occurs in the metaphyseal region of long bones of the extremities, particularly in regions of the distal femur, proximal tibia, and proximal humerus, as well as the pelvis. It is the most common malignant bone tumor affecting children and young adults.

Clinical manifestations are usually associated with a gradual onset of pain and swelling, especially around the knee. A minor injury does not cause the tumor but rather serves to bring the pre-existing condition to medical attention.

Diagnosis is confirmed from tissue biopsy, elevation of serum alkaline phosphatase and calcium levels, x-ray, computed tomography (CT) or positron emission tomography (PET) scans, and magnetic resonance imaging (MRI). Metastasis is present in 10% to 20% of individuals on diagnosis.

Major advances continue to be made in treatment. Preoperative chemotherapy is used to decrease tumor size. As a result, limb-salvage surgical procedures are being used more frequently. Amputation (see p. 697) may be necessary. Adjunct chemotherapy after surgery has increased the survival rate.

Metastatic Bone Cancer

The most common type of malignant bone tumor occurs as a result of metastasis from a primary tumor. Common sites for the primary tumor include the breast, prostate, lungs, kidney, and thyroid. Metastatic bone lesions are commonly found in the vertebrae, pelvis, femur, humerus, or ribs.

- Pathologic fractures at the site of metastasis are common because of a weakening of the involved bone. High serum calcium levels result as calcium is released from damaged bones.
- Once a primary lesion has been identified, radionuclide bone scans are often done to detect metastatic lesions before they are visible on x-ray. Metastatic bone lesions may occur at any time (even years later) following diagnosis and treatment of the primary tumor.
- Metastasis to the bone should be suspected in any patient who has local bone pain and a past history of cancer.
- Treatment may be palliative and consists of radiation and pain management. Surgical stabilization of the fracture may be indicated if there is a fracture or pending fracture. Prognosis depends on the extent of metastasis and location.

Nursing Management

Goals

The patient with bone cancer will have satisfactory pain relief; maintain preferred activities as long as possible; demonstrate acceptance of body image changes resulting from chemotherapy, radiation, and surgery; be free from injury; and verbalize a realistic idea of disease progression and prognosis.

Nursing Diagnoses

- Acute pain
- Impaired physical mobility
- Disturbed body image
- Grieving
- Risk for injury
- Impaired home maintenance

Nursing Interventions

Nursing care of the patient with a malignant bone tumor does not differ significantly from care given to the patient with a malignant disease of any other body system. However, special attention is required to reduce complications associated with prolonged bed rest and to prevent pathologic fractures. To prevent pathologic fractures, careful handling and support of the affected extremity and logrolling for those on bed rest is important.

- The patient is often reluctant to participate in therapeutic activities because of weakness and fear of pain. Provide regular rest periods between activities.
- Assist the patient and family in accepting the guarded prognosis associated with bone cancer. Inability to accomplish age-specific developmental tasks can increase the frustrations with this condition. Special attention is necessary for problems of pain and dysfunction, chemotherapy, and specific surgery, such as spinal cord decompression or amputation.

BRAIN TUMORS

Description

Tumors of the brain may be primary, arising from tissues within the brain, or secondary, resulting from a metastasis from a malignant neoplasm elsewhere in the body. Secondary brain tumors are the most common type. Brain tumors are generally classified according to the tissue from which they arise.

- The most common primary brain tumors originate in astrocytes. These tumors are called *gliomas,* including astrocytoma and glioblastoma multiforme. Glioblastoma multiforme

is the most common primary brain tumor, followed by
meningioma and astrocytoma.

- More than half of brain tumors are malignant; they infiltrate
the brain parenchyma and are not amenable to complete
surgical removal. Other tumors may be histologically
benign but are located such that complete removal is not
possible.
- Brain tumors rarely metastasize outside the central nervous
system (CNS) because they are contained by structural
(meninges) and physiologic (blood-brain) barriers. (For a
comparison of the major brain tumors, see Table 57-12,
Lewis et al, *Medical-Surgical Nursing,* ed 8, p. 1446.)
- Unless treated, all brain tumors eventually cause death from
increasing tumor volume leading to increased ICP.

Clinical Manifestations

The appearance of manifestations depends on the location, size,
and rate of tumor growth. A wide range of clinical manifestations
are associated with brain tumors.

- Headache is a common problem. Tumor-related headaches
tend to be worse at night and may awaken the patient. The
headaches are usually dull and constant but occasionally
throbbing.
- Seizures are common in gliomas and brain metastases. Brain
tumors can cause nausea and vomiting from increased ICP.
- Cognitive dysfunction, including memory problems and
mood or personality changes, is common in patients with
brain metastases. As the tumor expands, it may produce
signs of increased ICP, cerebral edema, or obstruction of the
cerebrospinal fluid (CSF) pathways.

Diagnostic Studies

- Extensive history and a comprehensive neurologic examination
are essential in the diagnostic work-up.
- Magnetic resonance imaging (MRI) and positron emission
tomography (PET) scans allow for detection of very small
tumors.
- Computed tomography (CT) and brain scanning assist in tumor
location.
- Other tests include angiography, magnetic resonance spectroscopy, functional MRI, PET scans, and single-photon emission
computed tomography (SPECT).

Correct diagnosis of a brain tumor is made by obtaining tissue
for histologic study. In most patients, tissue is obtained at time of
surgery.

Collaborative Care

Treatment goals are aimed at identifying the tumor type and location, removing or decreasing tumor mass, and preventing or managing increased ICP.

Surgical removal is the preferred treatment for brain tumors (see section on cranial surgery in Chapter 57, Lewis et al, *Medical-Surgical Nursing*, ed 8, pp. 1449 to 1451). Surgical outcome depends on the type, size, and location of the tumor. Meningiomas and oligodendrogliomas can usually be completely removed, whereas more invasive gliomas and medulloblastomas can be only partially removed. Even if complete surgical removal of the tumor is not possible, surgery can reduce tumor mass, which decreases ICP and provides relief of symptoms with an extension of survival time.

Radiation therapy is used as a follow-up measure after surgery. Radiation seeds can also be implanted into the brain. Cerebral edema and rapidly increasing ICP may be a complication of radiation therapy, but this can be managed with high doses of corticosteroids (dexamethasone [Decadron], prednisone).

Normally the blood-brain barrier prohibits the entry of most drugs into brain parenchyma. However, the most malignant brain tumors cause a breakdown of the blood-brain barrier in the tumor area, allowing chemotherapeutic agents to be used. Nitrosoureas such as carmustine (BCNU) and lomustine (CCNU) are used; methotrexate and procarbazine (Matulane) are also used. Temozolomide (Temodar) is the first oral chemotherapy being used that crosses the blood-brain barrier. Chemotherapy-laden biodegradable wafers implanted during surgery can deliver chemotherapy directly to the tumor site. Intrathecal administration also allows direct delivery of chemotherapeutic drugs to the central nervous system.

Bevacizumab (Avastin) is used to treat patients with glioblastoma multiforme when this type of brain cancer continues to progress following standard therapy. Bevacizumab is a targeted therapy that inhibits the action of vascular endothelial growth factor that helps form new blood vessels.

Although progress in treatment has increased the length and quality of survival of patients with gliomas, outcomes remain poor. The 5-year survival rate for these brain tumors is approximately 33%.

Nursing Management

Goals

The patient with a brain tumor will maintain normal ICP, maximize neurologic functioning, achieve control of pain and discomfort, and be aware of the long-term implications with respect to prognosis and cognitive and physical functioning.

Nursing Diagnoses/Collaborative Problems
- Risk for ineffective cerebral tissue perfusion
- Acute pain (headache)
- Self-care deficits
- Anxiety
- Potential complication: seizures
- Potential complication: increased ICP

Nursing Interventions
Behavioral changes associated with a frontal lobe lesion, such as loss of emotional control, confusion, memory loss, and depression, are often not perceived by the patient but can be very disturbing and frightening to the family. You need to assist the family in understanding what is happening.

- The confused patient with behavioral instability can be a challenge. Close supervision of activity, use of side rails, judicious use of restraints, padding of rails, and a calm, reassuring approach are all essential care techniques.
- Minimize environmental stimuli, create a routine, and use reality orientation for the confused patient.
- Seizures often occur with brain tumors, and seizure precautions should be instituted for the protection of the patient (see Seizure Disorders, p. 562).
- Motor and sensory dysfunctions are problems that interfere with the activities of daily living. Alterations in mobility must be managed, and encourage the patient to provide as much self-care as physically possible. Self-image often depends on the patient's ability to participate in care within the limitations of the physical deficits.
- Motor (expressive) or sensory (receptive) dysphasia may occur. Disturbances in communication can be frustrating for the patient and may interfere with your ability to meet patient needs. Make attempts to establish a communication system that can be used by both the patient and staff.
- Nutritional intake may be decreased because of the patient's inability to eat, loss of appetite, or loss of desire to eat. Assessing the nutritional status of the patient and ensuring adequate nutritional intake are important aspects of care. The patient may need encouragement to eat or, in some cases, may have to be fed orally by gastrostomy or nasogastric tube or by parenteral nutrition (PN) (see Enteral Nutrition, p. 731, and Parenteral Nutrition, p. 752).

Social work and home health nurses may be needed to assist the caregiver with discharge planning and to help the family adjust to role changes and psychosocial and socioeconomic factors. Issues related to palliative and end-of-life care need to be discussed with both the patient and the family.

BREAST CANCER

Description
Breast cancer is the most common malignancy in women in the United States except for skin cancer and is second only to lung cancer as the leading cause of death from cancer in women. More than 182,000 new cases of breast cancer are diagnosed in women in the United States each year. About 2000 new cases of breast cancer are diagnosed in men annually.

Patients diagnosed with localized breast cancer with no axillary node involvement have a 5-year survival rate of 98%. Conversely, only 17% of patients diagnosed with advanced-stage breast cancer with metastases to distant sites will survive 5 years or more.

Pathophysiology
Although the etiology is not completely understood, a number of factors are thought to be related to the development of breast cancer. Risk factors appear to be cumulative and interactive. The overall risk for breast cancer may be greatly increased in women with a positive family history and the presence of additional risk factors. Table 15 identifies some of the major risk factors for breast cancer.

- The use of combined hormone replacement therapy (estrogen plus progesterone) increases the risk of breast cancer while also increasing the risk of having a larger, more advanced breast cancer at diagnosis. The use of estrogen replacement therapy alone (for women who have had a prior hysterectomy) does not currently appear to increase breast cancer risk.

The various types of breast cancer identified in Table 16 are based on histologic characteristics and tumor growth pattern. Cancer growth can range from slow to rapid.

- Factors that affect cancer prognosis are tumor size, axillary node involvement (the more nodes involved, the worse the prognosis), tumor differentiation (morphology of malignant cells), estrogen and progesterone receptor status, and human epidermal growth factor receptor 2 (HER-2) status, which is a genetic marker.

Table 15	Risk Factors for Breast Cancer

Increased Risk	Comments
Female	Women account for 99% of breast cancer cases.
Age 50 or over	Majority of breast cancers are found in postmenopausal women. After age 60 greatly elevated increase in incidence.
Family history	Breast cancer in a first-degree relative, particularly when premenopausal or bilateral, increases risk. Gene mutations (BRCA-1 or BRCA-2) play a role in 5%-10% of breast cancer cases.
Personal history of breast cancer, colon cancer, endometrial cancer, ovarian cancer	Personal history significantly increases risk of breast cancer, risk of cancer in other breast, and recurrence.
Early menarche (before age 12); late menopause (after age 55)	A long menstrual history increases the risk of breast cancer.
First full-term pregnancy after age 30; nulliparity	Prolonged exposure to unopposed estrogen increases risk for breast cancer.
Benign breast disease with atypical epithelial hyperplasia, lobular carcinoma in situ	Atypical changes in breast biopsy increase the risk of breast cancer.
Weight gain and obesity after menopause	Fat cells store estrogen.
Exposure to ionizing radiation	Radiation damages DNA (e.g., prior treatment for Hodgkin's lymphoma).
Alcohol consumption	Women who drink ≥ 1 alcoholic beverage per day have an increased risk of breast cancer
Physical inactivity	Breast cancer risk is decreased in physically active women by 33% when compared with sedentary women

Table 16	Types of Breast Cancer	
Type		**Frequency of Occurrence**
Noninvasive		22%
▪ Ductal carcinoma in situ		
Infiltrating Ductal Carcinoma		63%-68%
▪ Colloid (mucinous)		
▪ Inflammatory		
▪ Paget's disease		
▪ Medullary		
▪ Papillary		
▪ Tubular		
Infiltrating Lobular Carcinoma		10%-15%

Clinical Manifestations

Breast cancer is detected as a lump or as a mammographic breast abnormality. It occurs most often in the upper outer quadrant of the breast because that is the location of most of the glandular tissue.

- If palpable, breast cancer is characteristically hard, irregularly shaped, poorly delineated, nonmobile, and nontender.
- A small percentage of breast cancers cause nipple discharge. The discharge is usually unilateral and may be clear or bloody. Nipple retraction may occur.
- Plugging of the dermal lymphatics can cause skin thickening and exaggeration of the usual skin markings, giving skin the appearance of an orange peel (peau d'orange).
- In large cancers, infiltration, induration, and dimpling (pulling in) of the overlying skin may occur.

Recurrence may be local or regional (skin or soft tissue near mastectomy site, axillary lymph nodes) or distant (most commonly bone, lung, brain, and liver).

Diagnostic Studies

Screening

- Physical examination of breast and lymphatics
- Mammography and ultrasound
- Breast magnetic resonance imaging (MRI)
- Biopsy
  - Stereotactic core biopsy
  - Fine needle aspiration

After Diagnosis
- *Axillary node dissection* is often performed. Axillary lymph node involvement is one of the most important prognostic factors in breast cancer. The more nodes involved, the greater the risk of recurrence.
- *Lymphatic mapping and sentinel lymph node dissection (SLND)* helps the surgeon identify the lymph node(s) that drain from the tumor site (sentinel node). Assessment of this node can be used to determine the extent of tumor spread to axillary lymph nodes.
- Tumor size is a valuable prognostic variable: the larger the tumor, the poorer the prognosis. In general, poorly differentiated tumors appear morphologically disorganized and are more aggressive.
- Estrogen and progesterone receptor status is useful to determine treatment decisions and prognosis. Receptor-positive tumors commonly (1) show histologic evidence of being well differentiated, (2) have a lower chance for recurrence, and (3) are frequently responsive to hormonal therapy. Receptor-negative tumors (1) are often poorly differentiated histologically, (2) frequently recur, and (3) are usually unresponsive to hormonal therapy.
- DNA content (ploidy status) correlates with tumor aggressiveness. Diploid tumors have been shown to have a significantly lower risk of recurrence than aneuploid tumors.
- Overexpression of the HER-2 receptor has been associated with a greater risk for recurrence and a poorer prognosis in breast cancer. Between 25% and 30% of metastatic breast cancers produce excessive HER-2.

A patient whose breast cancer tests negative for all three receptors (estrogen, progesterone, and HER-2) has *triple-negative breast cancer*. The incidence of triple-negative breast cancer is higher in Hispanics, African Americans, women who are younger, and women with a BRCA-1 mutation. These patients tend to have a more aggressive tumor with a poorer prognosis.

Collaborative Care

Prognostic factors are considered in treatment decisions, and tumor size (T), nodal involvement (N), and presence of metastasis (M) are used to stage breast cancer with the TNM system (see TNM Classification System, p. 799).

Surgical therapy. Breast conservation surgery (lumpectomy) with radiation therapy and modified radical mastectomy with or without reconstruction are currently the most common options for resectable breast cancer. The overall survival with lumpectomy and radiation is about the same as that with modified radical mastectomy.

Breast-conserving surgery (lumpectomy) involves removal of the entire tumor along with a margin of normal tissue. An axillary lymph node dissection (ALND) is usually done along with a lumpectomy. If there is evidence of systemic disease, chemotherapy may be given before radiation therapy.

- An ALND involves the removal of 12 to 20 nodes and is usually performed if the sentinel lymph node or nodes contain malignant cells. A sentinel lymph node dissection (SLND) has replaced ALND for patients who do not have malignant cells identified in the sentinel nodes.
- One of the main advantages of breast-conserving surgery and radiation is that it preserves the breast, including the nipple. The goal of combined surgery and radiation is to maximize the benefits of both cancer treatment and cosmetic outcome while minimizing risks.

Modified radical mastectomy includes removal of the breast and axillary lymph nodes but preserves the pectoralis major muscle. This surgery is selected over breast-conserving therapy if the tumor is too large to excise with good margins and attain a reasonable cosmetic result. Some patients may select this procedure over lumpectomy when presented with the choice of either procedure. See Table 52-7, Lewis et al, *Medical-Surgical Nursing,* ed 8, p. 1317 for treatment options, side effects, complications, and patient issues related to common surgical procedures to treat breast cancer.

After surgery, the woman must be monitored for the rest of her life at regular intervals. Most women have professional examinations every 6 months for the first 2 years, and then annually thereafter.

- In addition, it is recommended the woman continue to practice monthly breast self-examinations (BSEs) on both breasts or on the remaining breast and mastectomy site. The woman should also have appropriate breast imaging at regular intervals.
- The most common site of cancer recurrence is at the surgical site.

Adjuvant therapy. The decision to recommend adjuvant (additional) therapy after surgery depends on the number of involved nodes, menstrual status, age, cell type, size and extent of the cancer, presence or absence of estrogen and HER-2 receptors, and the underlying health of the patient.

   Adjuvant therapies include local radiation therapy and systemic therapies such as chemotherapy, hormonal therapy, and targeted therapy.

Radiation   therapy. Radiation   therapy   may   be   used   as: (1) primary treatment to prevent local breast recurrences after breast-conserving surgery, (2) adjuvant treatment following mastectomy to prevent local and nodal recurrences, and (3) palliative treatment for pain caused by local recurrence and metastases. Lumpectomy is almost always followed by radiation.

- The MammoSite system is a minimally invasive method of delivering internal radiation therapy. The technique uses a balloon catheter to insert radioactive seeds into the breast after the tumor is removed.

Chemotherapy. Cytotoxic drugs are used to destroy cancer cells. Most breast cancers are responsive to chemotherapy. In some patients, chemotherapy is given preoperatively to decrease the size of the primary tumor. The use of a combination of drugs is superior to the use of a single drug. The incidence and severity of the side effects that accompany chemotherapy are influenced by the specific drug combinations, drug schedule, and dose of the drugs (see Chemotherapy, p. 717).

Hormonal therapy. Estrogen can promote growth of breast cancer cells if cells are estrogen-receptor positive. Hormonal therapy removes or blocks the source of estrogen, thus promoting tumor regression. It may be used as an adjuvant to primary treatment or in patients with recurrent or metastatic cancer. Hormone receptor assays can identify women who are likely to respond to hormone therapy. Women who are postmenopausal are more likely to have hormone-dependent tumors, with significantly greater chances of tumor regression. Tamoxifen (Nolvadex) has been the agent of choice in postmenopausal, estrogen-receptor positive women with all stages of breast cancer (Table 17).

- Aromatase inhibitor drugs interfere with the enzyme that synthesizes endogenous estrogen, and are used in the treatment of breast cancer in postmenopausal women. Aromatase inhibitors do not block the production of estrogen by the ovaries. Thus they are of little benefit in premenopausal women.

Targeted therapy. Trastuzumab (Herceptin) is an antibody that targets HER-2/neu, an antigen that often appears on the surface of breast cancer cells. After the antibody attaches to the antigen, it is taken into the cells and eventually kills them. It can be used alone or in combination with other chemotherapy to treat patients with breast cancer whose tumors overexpress the HER-2 gene. Lapatinib (Tykerb) may be used in combination with capecitabine

Table 17	Drug Therapy: Hormonal Therapy for Breast Cancer	
Mechanism of Action	**Examples**	**Indications for Use**
Blocks estrogen receptors	tamoxifen (Nolvadex)	Prevention, adjuvant, and metastatic disease
	toremifene (Fareston)	Metastatic disease
Destroys estrogen receptors	fulvestrant (Faslodex)	Metastatic disease
Prevents production of estrogen by inhibiting aromatase	anastrozole (Arimidex) letrozole (Femara) exemestane (Aromasin)	Neoadjuvant, adjuvant, and metastatic disease
	aminoglutethimide (Cytadren)	Metastatic disease

(Xeloda) for patients with advanced, metastatic disease who are HER-2 positive. Bevacizumab (Avastin), an angiogenesis inhibitor, given in combination with chemotherapy may extend survival in advanced breast cancer.

Nursing Management
Goals
The patient with breast cancer will actively participate in the decision-making process related to treatment options, comply with the therapeutic plan, manage side effects of adjuvant therapy, and be satisfied with support from significant others and health care providers.

See NCP 52-1 for the patient after a mastectomy or lumpectomy, Lewis et al, *Medical-Surgical Nursing*, ed 8, pp. 1321 to 1322.

Nursing Diagnoses
After a diagnosis of breast cancer and before a treatment plan has been selected, the following diagnoses apply:

- Decisional conflict
- Fear and/or anxiety
- Disturbed body image

If the patient undergoes a lumpectomy or modified radical mastectomy, nursing diagnoses may include:

- Acute pain
- Anxiety

- Disturbed body image
- Ineffective self-health management
- Impaired physical mobility

Nursing Interventions

The time between the diagnosis of breast cancer and the selection of a treatment plan is a difficult period for the woman and her family. Although the primary care provider discusses treatment options, the woman often relies on the nurse to clarify and expand on these options.

- Appropriate nursing interventions during this period include exploring the woman's usual decision-making patterns, helping the woman accurately evaluate the advantages and disadvantages of the options, providing information relevant to the decision, and supporting the patient and family once the decision is made.
- Regardless of the surgery planned, provide the patient with sufficient information to ensure informed consent. Teaching in the preoperative phase includes turning and deep breathing, a review of postoperative exercises, and an explanation of the recovery period from the time of surgery until discharge.

The woman who has breast-conserving surgery usually has an uneventful postoperative course with variable pain intensity. The woman who has had a modified radical mastectomy needs nursing interventions specific to this surgery.

- Restoring arm function on the affected side after mastectomy and axillary lymph node dissection is an important goal.
- Place the woman in a semi-Fowler's position with the arm on the affected side elevated on a pillow. Flexing and extending the fingers should begin in the recovery room, with progressive increases in activity.
- Postoperative arm and shoulder exercises are instituted gradually at the surgeon's direction.
- Postoperative discomfort can be minimized by administering analgesics about 30 minutes before initiating exercises. When able to shower, the warm water on the affected shoulder often has a muscle relaxing effect and reduces joint stiffness.

Whenever possible, the same nurse should work with the woman so that progress can be monitored.

Lymphedema (accumulation of lymph in soft tissue) can occur as a result of excision or radiation of the lymph nodes. The patient may experience heaviness, pain, impaired motor function in the arm, and numbness and paresthesia of the fingers. Help the patient to understand that she is at risk of developing lymphedema for the rest of her life. Teach measures to prevent or reduce lymphedema including:

- The affected arm should never be dependent, even while the person is sleeping.
- Blood pressure (BP) readings, venipunctures, and injections should not be done on the affected arm.
- Instruct the woman to protect the arm on the operative side from even minor trauma such as a pinprick or sunburn.
- If trauma to the arm occurs, the area should be washed thoroughly with soap and water, and a topical antibiotic ointment and bandage should be applied.
- Frequent and sustained elevation of the arm, regular use of a custom-fitted pressure sleeve, and treatment with an inflatable sleeve (pneumomassage) may also be helpful.

Throughout interactions keep in mind the extensive psychologic impact of the disease. All aspects of care must include sensitivity to the woman's efforts to cope with a life-threatening disease. You can help meet the woman's psychologic needs by doing the following:

- Help identify sources of support and strength to her, such as her partner, family, and spiritual practices.
- Encourage her to identify and learn individual coping strengths.
- Provide communication between the patient and her family and/or friends.
- Provide accurate and complete answers to questions about the disease, treatment options, and reproductive or lactation issues (if appropriate).
- Offer information about community resources, such as Reach to Recovery, Y-ME, CanSurmount, Encore, and local support organizations and groups.

▼ **Patient and Caregiver Teaching**
- Emphasize the importance of mammography and breast self-awareness. Future symptoms to report to the clinician include new back pain, weakness, constipation, shortness of breath, and confusion.
- Stress the importance of wearing a well-fitting prosthesis designed for women who have had a mastectomy.
- A preoperative sexual assessment provides baseline data that can be used to plan postoperative interventions. Often the husband, sexual partner, or family members may need assistance in dealing with their emotional reactions to the diagnosis and surgery so that they can act as effective means of support for the patient.

- Depression may occur with the continued stress of a cancer diagnosis. Special nursing interventions are necessary for both psychologic support and self-care if a recurrence is found.

Breast reconstruction is discussed in Chapter 52, Lewis et al, *Medical-Surgical Nursing,* ed 8.

BRONCHIECTASIS

Description
Bronchiectasis is characterized by permanent, abnormal dilation of medium sized bronchi in either a localized or diffuse pattern. The pathophysiologic change is a result of inflammatory changes that destroy elastic and muscular structures supporting the bronchial wall resulting in dilated bronchi.

Stasis of thickened mucus occurs along with impaired clearance by the cilia resulting in a reduced ability to clear mucus from the lungs.

The main cause of diffuse bronchiectasis is bacterial infections of the lungs which are either not treated or treatment is delayed. Other causes include localized endobronchial obstruction or extrinsic compression of the bronchi (tumor), generalized impairment of pulmonary defenses (cystic fibrosis, immunoglobulin deficiencies), systemic effects of inflammatory diseases (ulcerative colitis), or noninfectious causes (heavy metal poisoning).

Clinical Manifestations
The hallmark of bronchiectasis is persistent or recurrent cough with production of purulent sputum. However, some patients with severe disease and upper lobe involvement may have no sputum production and little cough. Hemoptysis occurs in 50% to 70% of the patients and may be massive, necessitating emergency care.
- Other manifestations include dyspnea, fatigue, weight loss, myalgias, and fever.
- Lung auscultation reveals a variety of adventitious sounds (e.g., crackles, wheezes, rhonchi).

Diagnostic Studies
An individual with a chronic productive cough with copious purulent sputum (which may be blood streaked) should be suspected of having bronchiectasis.
- Chest x-rays may show nonspecific abnormalities.
- High-resolution CT (HRCT) scan of the chest is the gold standard for diagnosing bronchiectasis.

- Bronchoscopy but may be used with localized bronchiectasis to diagnose obstruction.
- Sputum may provide additional information regarding severity of impairment and presence of active infection. Patients are frequently colonized with *H. influenzae* or *P. aeruginosa.*
- Pulmonary function studies usually show obstructive pattern including a decrease in FEV_1 and FEV_1/FVC.

Collaborative Care

Bronchiectasis is difficult to treat. Therapy is aimed at treating acute flare-ups and preventing a decline in lung function. Antibiotics are the mainstay of treatment. Concurrent bronchodilator therapy or anticholinergics are given to prevent bronchospasm and stimulate mucociliary clearance.

- Maintaining good hydration is important to liquefy secretions. Chest physiotherapy and other airway clearance techniques facilitate expectoration of sputum. Teach the patient to reduce exposure to excessive air pollutants and irritants, avoid cigarette smoking, and obtain pneumococcal and influenza vaccinations.
- For selected patients who are disabled in spite of maximal therapy, lung transplantation is an option.

Nursing Management

Early detection and treatment of lower respiratory tract infections helps prevent complications such as bronchiectasis. Any obstructing lesion or foreign body should be removed promptly.

An important nursing goal is to promote drainage and removal of bronchial mucus. Various airway clearance techniques can be effectively used to facilitate secretion removal.

- The patient needs to understand the importance of taking the prescribed regimen of drugs to obtain maximum effectiveness.
- Bed rest may be indicated during the acute phase of the illness, especially with hemoptysis. If hemoptysis occurs, patients should know when they should contact the health care provider.
- In the acute care setting if the patient has hemoptysis, you should contact the provider immediately, elevate the head of the bed, and place the patient in a side lying position with the suspected bleeding side down.
- Good nutrition is important and may be difficult to maintain because the patient is often anorexic. Oral hygiene to cleanse

the mouth and remove dried sputum crusts may improve the patient's appetite.

- Unless there are contraindications, instruct the patient to drink at least 3 L of fluid daily.
- Direct hydration of the respiratory system may be beneficial in expectorating secretions. Usually an aerosol with normal saline solution delivered by a jet-type nebulizer is used. Alternatively, hypertonic saline may be ordered for a more aggressive effect.
- Teach the patient and caregiver to recognize significant clinical manifestations to be reported to the health care provider. These manifestations include increased sputum production, bloody sputum, increasing dyspnea, fever, chills, and chest.

BURNS

Description

Burns are tissue injuries caused by heat, chemicals, electric current, or radiation. An estimated 5,000,000 Americans seek medical care each year for burns. The highest fatality rates occur in children 4 years of age and younger, and adults >65 years old.

Pathophysiology

The extent of burn injury is influenced by energy intensity, duration of exposure, and type of tissue injured. Immediately after the injury occurs, there is an increase in blood flow to the area surrounding the wound. This is followed by the release of various vasoactive substances from burned tissue, which results in increased capillary permeability. Fluid then shifts from the intravascular compartment to the interstitial space, producing edema, hypovolemia, and (potentially) shock. After several days, diuresis from fluid mobilization occurs and healing begins.

Types of Burn Injury

Various types of burns may be seen alone or in combination with other burns.

- Thermal injury is the most common type of burn and can be caused by flame, flash, scald, or contact with hot objects.
- Chemical burns are the result of tissue injury and destruction from acids, alkalis (e.g., fertilizer, oven cleaners), and organic compounds such as petroleum products.
- Smoke and inhalation injury results from the inhalation of hot air or noxious chemicals that can cause damage to the

respiratory tract. These injuries include carbon monoxide poisoning, thermal burn above the glottis, or inhalation burn below the glottis.
- Electrical burns result from the intense heat of an electric current.

B

Classification of Burn Injury

The treatment of burns is related to injury severity. A variety of methods exist for determining burn severity.

1. The *depth of burn* is described according to the depth of skin destruction (epidermis, dermis, or subcutaneous tissue) (Table 18).
2. The extent of the burn wound is calculated as the percent of total body surface area (TBSA) affected. Two common methods for determining the extent of a burn include:
   - Lund-Browder chart, which takes into account the patient's age and relative body area.
   - Rule of Nines chart, which is easy to remember and adequate for initial assessment (Fig. 2).
3. Burn location has a direct relationship to the severity of the injury. For example, face and neck burns may inhibit respiratory function; hands, feet, joint, and eye burns may limit self-care and functioning.
4. Patient risk factors include (1) older age, which contributes to slower healing and more difficulty with rehabilitation and (2) preexisting disorders such as cardiovascular, pulmonary, or renal disease that reduce the patient's ability to recover from the tremendous demands of burn injury.

The American Burn Association (ABA) has established referral criteria that recommend which burn injuries should be treated in a burn unit (Table 19).

Clinical Manifestations

Burns can be classified into three phases: emergent (resuscitative), acute, and rehabilitative.
- *Emergent phase:* Characterized by possible shock from pain and hypovolemia, intense thirst, minimal urine output, shivering as a result of heat loss or anxiety, and adynamic ileus. Unconsciousness or altered mental status is not usually the result of a burn, but rather smoke inhalation or head trauma. Complications may include dysrhythmias, airway obstruction, and acute tubular necrosis and renal failure.
- *Acute phase:* Partial-thickness wounds form eschar. When eschar is removed, reepithelialization begins at wound margins and appears as red or pink scar tissue. Wound

Table 18 Classification of Burn Injury Depth

Classification	Clinical Appearance	Possible Cause	Structures Involved
Partial-Thickness Skin Destruction			
▪ Superficial (first-degree)	Erythema, blanching on pressure, pain and mild swelling, no vesicles or blisters (although after 24 hr skin may blister and peel)	Superficial sunburn Quick heat flash	Superficial epidermal damage with hyperemia. Tactile and pain sensation intact.
▪ Deep (second-degree)	Fluid-filled vesicles that are red, shiny, wet (if vesicles have ruptured); severe pain caused by nerve injury; mild to moderate edema	Flame Flash Scald Contact burns Chemical Tar Electrical current	Epidermis and dermis involved to varying depths. Skin elements, from which epithelial regeneration occurs, remain viable.
Full-Thickness Skin Destruction			
▪ (Third- and fourth-degree)	Dry, waxy white, leathery, or hard skin; visible thrombosed vessels; insensitivity to pain because of nerve destruction; possible involvement of muscles, tendons, and bones	Flame Scald Chemical Tar Electric current	All skin elements and local nerve endings destroyed. Coagulation necrosis present. Surgical intervention required for healing.

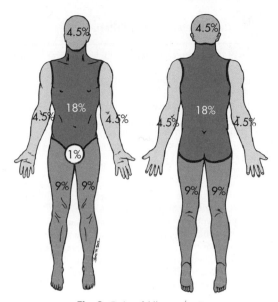

Fig. 2. Rule of Nines chart.

closure and healing usually occur within 10 to 21 days. Separation of eschar from full-thickness wounds takes longer, and these wounds require surgical debridement and skin grafting for healing. Wound infection is a serious complication. Other complications include acute transient neurologic reactions (including extreme disorientation and delirium), contractures, Curling's ulcer, and stress diabetes.

- *Rehabilitative phase:* Mature healing occurs in about 12 months. New scar tissue will shorten, causing a contracture if adequate range of motion (ROM) is not performed. The healing site, which is extremely sensitive to trauma, may itch. Complications are skin and joint contractures and hypertrophic scarring.

Diagnostic Studies

- Serum electrolytes, especially sodium (Na^{++}) and potassium (K^{++}), to monitor fluid and electrolyte shifts
- Chest x-ray, arterial blood gases (ABGs), and sputum for inhalation injury

Table 19	Burn Center Referral Criteria*

Burn injuries that should be referred to a burn center include the following:

1. Partial-thickness burns greater than 10% total body surface area (TBSA)
2. Burns that involve the face, hands, feet, genitalia, perineum, or major joints
3. Third-degree burns in any age group
4. Electrical burns, including lightning injury
5. Chemical burns
6. Inhalation injury
7. Burn injury in patients with preexisting medical disorders that could complicate management, prolong recovery, or affect mortality (e.g., heart or kidney disease)
8. Any patients with burns and concomitant trauma (e.g., fractures) in which the burn injury poses the greatest risk of morbidity or mortality. In such cases, if the trauma poses the greater immediate risk, the patient may be initially stabilized in a trauma center before being transferred to a burn center. The judgment of the health care provider will be necessary in such situations and should be made in consultation with the regional medical control plan and triage protocols.
9. Burn injury in patients who will require special social, emotional, or long-term rehabilitative intervention

Source: Guidelines for the operations of burn centers. In American College of Surgeons, *Committee on Trauma: Resources for optimal care of the injured patient*, 2006. Available at www.ameriburn.org.
*Guidelines from the American Burn Association.

- Urine output and specific gravity to evaluate fluid replacement and detect acute tubular necrosis and/or renal ischemia
- Complete blood count (CBC) to detect anemia and immunologic response to injury
- White blood cell (WBC) count and wound cultures if infection is suspected

Collaborative Care

Burn management can be classified into three phases: emergent (resuscitative), acute, and rehabilitative (Table 20).

Emergent (resuscitative) phase is the period of time required to resolve immediate problems resulting from burn injury. This phase usually lasts up to 72 hours from the time of the burn. The primary concerns are the onset of hypovolemic shock and edema formation. Aggressive fluid resuscitation is required and is based on the

Table 20 Collaborative Care: Patient with Burn Injury

Emergent Phase	Acute Phase	Rehabilitation Phase
Fluid Therapy ■ Assess fluid needs.* ■ Begin IV fluid replacement. ■ Insert urinary catheter. ■ Monitor urine output. **Wound Care** ■ Start daily shower and wound care. ■ Debride as necessary. ■ Assess extent and depth of burns. ■ Administer tetanus toxoid or tetanus antitoxin. **Pain and Anxiety** ■ Assess and manage pain and anxiety. **Physical/Occupational Therapy** ■ Place patient in position that prevents contracture formation and reduces edema. ■ Assess need for splints.	**Fluid Therapy** ■ Continue to replace fluids, depending on patient's clinical response. **Wound Care** ■ Continue daily shower and wound care. ■ Continue debridement (if necessary). ■ Assess wound daily and adjust dressing protocols as necessary. ■ Observe for complications (e.g, infection). **Early Excision and Grafting** ■ Provide temporary homografts. ■ Provide permanent autografts. ■ Care for donor sites. **Pain and Anxiety** ■ Continue to assess for and treat pain and anxiety. **Physical/Occupational Therapy** ■ Begin daily therapy program for maintenance of range of motion. ■ Assess need for splints and anti-contracture positioning. ■ Encourage and assist patient with self-care as possible.	■ Continue to counsel and teach patient and caregiver. ■ Continue to encourage and assist patient in resuming self-care. ■ Continue to prevent or minimize contractures and assess likelihood for scarring (surgery, physical/occupational therapy, splinting, or pressure garments). ■ Discuss possible reconstructive surgery. ■ Prepare for discharge home or transfer to rehabilitation hospital.

Continued

Table 20 **Collaborative Care: Patient with Burn Injury—cont'd**

Emergent Phase	Acute Phase	Rehabilitation Phase
Nutritional Therapy ■ Assess nutritional needs and begin feeding patient by most appropriate route as soon as possible.	**Nutritional Therapy** ■ Continue to assess diet to support wound healing.	
Respiratory Therapy ■ Assess oxygenation needs. ■ Provide supplemental oxygen as needed. ■ Intubate if necessary. ■ Monitor respiratory status.	**Respiratory Therapy** ■ Continue to assess oxygenation needs. ■ Continue to monitor respiratory status. ■ Monitor for signs of complications (e.g., pneumonia).	
Psychosocial Care ■ Provide support to patient and caregiver during initial crisis phase.	**Psychosocial Care** ■ Continue to provide ongoing support/counseling/education to patient and caregiver about physical and emotional aspects of care and recovery. ■ Begin to anticipate discharge needs.	
	Drug Therapy ■ Assess need for medications (e.g., antibiotics). ■ Continue to monitor effectiveness and adjust dosage as needed.	

IV, Intravenous.

*See Tables 25-11 and 25-12, Lewis et al., *Medical-Surgical Nursing*, ed. 8, p. 483.

patient's weight and extent of burn injury. This phase ends when fluid mobilization and diuresis begin.

Acute phase begins with mobilization of extracellular fluid and subsequent diuresis. The acute phase is concluded when the burned area is completely covered by skin grafts or when the wounds are healed. This may take weeks or many months.

Rehabilitation phase begins when the burn wound has healed and the patient is able to assume some self-care activity. This can occur as early as 2 weeks to as long as 7 or 8 months after the injury.

Nursing and Collaborative Management

Emergent phase: patient survival depends on rapid and through assessment and intervention.

- Assess adequacy of airway management and fluid therapy, provide pain medication and wound care, and offer support to patient and family. Begin feeding patient by most appropriate route as soon as possible.

Acute phase: predominant interventions are wound care, excision and grafting, pain management, physical and occupational therapy, nutritional therapy, and psychosocial care.

- Wound care consists of daily observation, assessment, cleansing, debridement, and dressing reapplication.
- A critical function is pain assessment and management.

Rehabilitative phase: goals for this period are to assist the patient in resuming a functional role in society and rehabilitate from functional and cosmetic reconstructive surgery. Both the patient and caregiver are actively encouraged to participate in care.

- Care should be taken to address individual spiritual and cultural needs.
- Responsibility is shared among the health care team to return the patient to optimal functioning.

▼ Patient and Caregiver Teaching

- Describe to the patient and caregiver the burn injury process and the expected signs and symptoms related to phases of burn management.
- Explain therapeutic interventions, precautionary measures, gowning and hand washing, and institution visiting policy to elicit cooperation and decrease anxiety.
- Teach the patient to watch for injuries to new skin.
- Instruct the patient and caregiver about the signs and symptoms of infection so early treatment can be initiated.
- Teach caregivers how to perform dressing changes to ensure proper technique and increase their sense of control.

- Emphasize the importance of exercise and appropriate physical therapy to the patient and caregiver. Plan a daily program with the patient, and offer appropriate resources to provide a continuing activity program as needed.
- Help the patient and caregiver in setting realistic future expectations because anticipatory guidance decreases anxiety and inaccurate perceptions. In addition, they will need anticipatory guidance to know what to expect physiologically as well as psychologically during recovery.
- Assist the patient and caregivers to establish contact with family and patient support groups, such as the Phoenix Society (www. phoenix-society.org).

CARDIOMYOPATHY

Description

Cardiomyopathy (CMP) constitutes a group of diseases that directly affect the structural or functional ability of the myocardium. A diagnosis of CMP is based on the patient's clinical manifestations and diagnostic cardiac procedures.

CMP can be classified as primary or secondary:

- *Primary CMP* refers to those conditions in which the etiology of the heart disease is unknown. The heart muscle in this case is the only portion of the heart involved, and other cardiac structures are unaffected.
- In *secondary CMP* the cause of the myocardial disease is known and is secondary to another disease process. Common causes of secondary CMP are coronary artery disease (CAD), myocarditis, hypertension, cardiotoxic agents (alcohol, cocaine), valve disease, and metabolic and autoimmune disorders.

Three major types of CMP are *dilated, hypertrophic,* and *restrictive.* Each type has its own pathogenesis, clinical presentation, and treatment protocols (Table 21). CMP can lead to cardiomegaly and heart failure (HF), which are the leading causes for heart transplantation.

Dilated Cardiomyopathy

Pathophysiology. Dilated cardiomyopathy is the most common type of CMP. It is characterized by diffuse inflammation and rapid degeneration of myocardial fibers that results in ventricular dilation, impairment of systolic function, atrial enlargement, and stasis of blood in the left ventricle. The ventricular walls do not hypertrophy.

Table 21	Comparison of Major Types of Cardiomyopathy

Dilated	Hypertrophic	Restrictive
Major Manifestations		
Fatigue, weakness, palpitations, dyspnea	Exertional dyspnea, fatigue, angina, syncope, palpitations	Dyspnea, fatigue
Cardiomegaly		
Moderate to marked	Mild to moderate	Mild
Contractility		
↓	↑ or ↓	Normal or ↓
Valvular Incompetence		
Atrioventricular valves, particularly mitral	Mitral valve	Atrioventricular valves
Dysrhythmias		
Sinoatrial tachycardia, atrial and ventricular dysrhythmias	Atrial and ventricular dysrhythmias	Atrial and ventricular dysrhythmias
Cardiac Output		
↓	Normal or ↓	Normal or ↓
Outflow Tract Obstruction		
None	↑	None

- Dilated CMP often follows an infectious myocarditis. Other common causes include alcohol and cocaine, hypertension, and CAD.

Clinical manifestations. The patient may have signs and symptoms of HF including fatigue, dyspnea at rest, paroxysmal nocturnal dyspnea, and orthopnea. Dry cough, abdominal bloating, and anorexia may occur as the disease progresses. Signs can include an irregular heart rate with an abnormal S_3 and/or S_4, pulmonary crackles, edema, pallor, hepatomegaly, and jugular venous distention. Heart murmurs and dysrhythmias are common.

Diagnostic studies. A diagnosis is made on the basis of patient history and ruling out other conditions that cause HF.

- Doppler echocardiography provides the basis for the diagnosis of dilated CMP and distinguishes dilated CMP from other structural abnormalities.

- Chest x-ray may show cardiomegaly with pulmonary venous hypertension and pleural effusion.
- Electrocardiogram (ECG) may reveal dysrhythmias with conduction disturbances.
- Serum levels of b-type natriuretic peptide (BNP) are elevated in the presence of HF.
- Cardiac catheterization confirms or rules out CAD, and multiple gated acquisition (MUGA) nuclear scan determines ejection fraction (EF).

Nursing and collaborative management. Interventions focus on controlling HF by enhancing myocardial contractility and decreasing afterload (similar to treatment for chronic HF).

- Nitrates and loop diuretics decrease preload, and angiotensin-converting enzyme (ACE) inhibitors reduce afterload.
- β-Adrenergic blockers and aldosterone antagonists control the neurohormonal stimulation that occurs in HF.
- Antidysrhythmics and anticoagulants are used as indicated.
- Drug and nutritional therapy and cardiac rehabilitation may help alleviate symptoms of HF and improve cardiac output (CO) and quality of life.
- A patient with secondary dilated CMP must be treated for the underlying disease process. For example, the patient with alcohol-induced dilated CMP must abstain from all alcohol.
- The patient with terminal end-stage CMP may consider heart transplantation.
- Patients with dilated CMP are very ill people with a grave prognosis who need your expert nursing care. The patient's caregivers must learn cardiopulmonary resuscitation (CPR) and when and how to access emergency care.
- Observing for signs and symptoms of worsening HF, dysrhythmias, and embolic formation is paramount in this patient, as is monitoring drug responsiveness.

Hypertrophic Cardiomyopathy

Pathophysiology. Hypertrophic cardiomyopathy (HCM) is asymmetric left ventricular myocardial hypertrophy without ventricular dilation. HCM occurs less commonly than dilated CMP and is more common in men than in women. It is usually diagnosed in young adulthood and is often seen in active, athletic individuals.

- The main characteristics of HCM are massive ventricular hypertrophy, rapid, forceful contraction of the left ventricle, impaired relaxation (diastole) and obstruction to aortic outflow (not present in all patients). The primary defect is diastolic dysfunction caused by left ventricular stiffness.

Decreased ventricular filling and obstruction to outflow result in decreased CO.

Clinical manifestations. Patients may be asymptomatic. The most common symptom is dyspnea, which is caused by an elevated left ventricular diastolic pressure. Other manifestations include fatigue, angina, syncope, and dysrhythmias.

- Common dysrhythmias include atrial fibrillation, ventricular tachycardia, and ventricular fibrillation. Any of these dysrhythmias may lead to syncope or sudden cardiac death (SCD).

Diagnostic studies. Clinical findings on examination may be unremarkable.

- Echocardiogram is the primary diagnostic tool revealing the classic feature of HCM, which is LV hypertrophy; the echocardiogram may also demonstrate wall motion abnormalities and diastolic dysfunction.
- ECG findings usually indicate ventricular hypertrophy, ST-T wave abnormalities, prominent Q waves, and ventricular and atrial dysrhythmias.

Nursing and collaborative management. The goal of therapy is to improve ventricular filling by reducing ventricular contractility and relieving LV outflow obstruction. This can be accomplished with the use of β-adrenergic blockers or calcium channel blockers.

- Antidysrhythmics are used to control dysrhythmias.
- Atrioventricular pacing can reduce the degree of outflow obstruction by causing the septum to move away from the left ventricular wall.
- Patients with severe symptoms unresponsive to therapy with marked obstruction to aortic outflow may be candidates for surgical treatment (ventriculomyotomy and myectomy) of their hypertrophied septum. Most patients have an improvement in symptoms and exercise tolerance after surgery.
- An alternative nonsurgical procedure to reduce symptoms is alcohol-induced, percutaneous transluminal septal myocardial ablation (PTSMA), in which alcohol is used to cause ischemia and septal wall myocardial infarction. Ablation of the septal wall decreases the obstruction to flow, and the patient's symptoms decrease.

Nursing interventions focus on relieving symptoms, observing for and preventing complications, and providing emotional and psychologic support.

- Teaching should focus on helping the patients to adjust their lifestyle to avoid strenuous activity and dehydration. Any activity that causes an increase in systemic vascular resistance (thus increasing obstruction to forward blood flow) is dangerous and should be avoided.

Restrictive Cardiomyopathy

Pathophysiology. Restrictive cardiomyopathy is the least common type of cardiomyopathic conditions. It is a disease of the heart muscle that impairs diastolic filling and stretch.

- A number of pathologic processes may be involved, including myocardial fibrosis, hypertrophy, and infiltration, which produce stiffness of the ventricular wall.
- The ventricles are resistant to filling and therefore demand high diastolic filling pressures to maintain CO.

Clinical manifestations. Classic symptoms of restrictive CMP are fatigue, exercise intolerance, and dyspnea.

- Other manifestations may include angina, orthopnea, syncope, palpations, and signs of HF.

Diagnostic studies. Chest x-ray may be normal or show cardiomegaly with pleural effusions and pulmonary congestion.

- ECG may reveal mild tachycardia at rest. The most common dysrhythmias are atrial fibrillation or atrioventricular block.
- Echocardiography may reveal a left ventricle that is normal size with a thickened wall, a slightly dilated right ventricle, and dilated atria.
- Endomyocardial biopsy, CT scan, and nuclear imaging may help in diagnosis.

Nursing and collaborative management. Currently, no specific treatment for restrictive CMP exists. Interventions are aimed at improving diastolic filling and the underlying disease process. Treatment includes conventional therapy for HF and dysrhythmias. Heart transplant may also be a consideration.

Nursing care is similar to the care of a patient with HF. As in the treatment of patients with HCM, teach patients to avoid situations that impair ventricular filling, such as strenuous activity, dehydration, and increase in systemic vascular resistance such as strenuous activity and dehydration.

CARPAL TUNNEL SYNDROME

Description

Carpal tunnel syndrome (CTS) is a condition caused by compression of the median nerve, which enters the hand through the narrow confines of the carpal tunnel. The carpal tunnel is formed by ligaments and bones. This condition often is caused by pressure from trauma or edema caused by inflammation of a tendon (tenosynovitis), neoplasm, rheumatoid arthritis, or soft tissue masses such as ganglia. CTS is the most common compression neuropathy in the upper extremities.

- This syndrome is associated with hobbies or occupations that require continuous wrist movement (e.g., butchers, computer operators, musicians, painters, carpenters, bowlers, knitters).
- Women are affected more than men, possibly due to a smaller carpal tunnel.

C

Clinical Manifestations
Manifestations include weakness (especially of the thumb), burning pain and numbness, impaired sensation in the distribution of the median nerve, and clumsiness in performing fine hand movements. Numbness and tingling may awaken the patient at night. Shaking the hands will often relieve these symptoms. Physical signs of CTS include Tinel's sign and Phalen's sign.

- *Tinel's sign* can be elicited by tapping over the median nerve as it passes through the carpal tunnel in the wrist. A positive response is a sensation of tingling in the distribution of the median nerve over the hand.
- *Phalen's sign* can be elicited by allowing the wrists to fall freely into maximum flexion and maintain the position for ≥60 seconds. A positive response is a sensation of tingling in the distribution of the median nerve over the hand.

In late stages there is atrophy of the thenar muscles around the base of the thumb resulting in recurrent pain and eventual dysfunction of the hand.

Nursing and Collaborative Management
Prevention of carpal tunnel syndrome involves teaching employees and employers to identify risk factors. Adaptive devices such as wrist splints may be worn to relieve pressure on the median nerve. Special keyboard pads and mouses are available for computer users. Other ergonomic changes include workstation modifications, change in body positions, and frequent breaks from work-related activities.

Early symptoms of CTS can usually be relieved by stopping the aggravating movement and by resting the hand and wrist by immobilizing them in a hand splint. Splints worn at night help keep the wrist in a neutral position and may reduce night pain and numbness. Injection of a corticosteroid drug directly into the carpal tunnel may provide short term relief.

- Because of impaired sensation, teach the patient to avoid hazards such as extremes in heat and cold to prevent thermal injury.

If the problem continues, surgery is generally recommended, which involves severing the band of tissue around the wrist to reduce pressure on the median nerve. Surgery is done under local anesthesia and does not require an overnight hospital stay. Endoscopic carpal tunnel release is performed through a small puncture incision(s) in the wrist and palm.

- After surgery, assess the neurovascular status of the hand regularly.
- Instruct the patient about wound care and the appropriate assessments to perform at home.

CATARACT

Description

A cataract is an opacity within the lens of one or both eyes, causing a gradual decline in vision. Cataracts are the leading cause of blindness worldwide and the major cause of vision loss in the United States. About 50% of the population over 65 years old has some degree of cataract formation, and nearly everyone over age 70 has one. Cataract removal is the most common surgical procedure in the United States.

Pathophysiology

Although most cataracts are age related (senile cataracts), they can be associated with other factors including trauma, congenital factors such as maternal rubella, radiation or ultraviolet (UV) light exposure, certain drugs such as systemic corticosteroids or long-term topical corticosteroids, and ocular inflammation. The patient with diabetes mellitus tends to develop cataracts at a younger age.

- In senile cataract formation, altered metabolic processes within the lens cause water accumulation and alterations in the fiber structure of the lens. These changes affect lens transparency, causing vision changes.

Clinical Manifestations

- The patient may complain of decreased vision, abnormal color perception, and glare.
- Visual decline is gradual, but the rate of cataract development varies from patient to patient.
- Secondary glaucoma may also occur if the enlarging lens causes increased intraocular pressure.

Diagnostic Studies

- Opacity directly observable by ophthalmoscopic or slit lamp microscopic examination
- Visual acuity measurement
- Glare testing
- Keratometry and A-scan ultrasound if surgery is planned

Collaborative Care

The presence of a cataract does not necessarily indicate a need for surgery. For many patients the diagnosis is made long before they actually decide to have surgery. Currently there is no available treatment to "cure" cataracts other than surgical removal.

- Helpful palliative measures include a change in eyeglass prescription, strong reading glasses or magnifiers, an increased amount of light for reading, and avoidance of nighttime driving if glare is worse at night.
- Surgery may be performed when the patient's decreasing vision interferes with normal activities such as driving, reading, and watching television. Removal of the lens may also be medically necessary in patients with increased intraocular pressure and diabetic retinopathy. In these cases the goals of surgery include management of intraocular pressure and visualization of the retina. Surgical treatment can involve lens removal (e.g., phacoemulsification, extracapsular extraction) and correction (e.g., intraocular lens implantation and contact lenses). Almost all patients have an intraocular lens implanted at the time of cataract extraction.

Nursing Management

Goals

Preoperatively, the patient will make informed decisions and experience minimal anxiety. Postoperatively, the patient will understand and comply with therapy, maintain an acceptable level of physical and emotional comfort, and remain free of infection and other complications.

Nursing Diagnoses

- Self-care deficits
- Anxiety

Nursing Interventions

For the patient who chooses not to have surgery, suggest vision enhancement techniques and a modification of activities and lifestyle to accommodate the visual deficit.

For the patient who elects surgery, provide information, support, and reassurance about the surgical and postoperative experience to reduce or alleviate patient anxiety. Inform all patients that they will not have depth perception until their patch is removed (usually within 24 hours).

- Postoperatively, offer mild analgesics for slight scratchiness or mild eye pain. The physician needs to be notified if severe pain, increased or purulent drainage, increased redness, or decreased visual acuity is present.

▼ **Patient and Caregiver Teaching**

- Written and verbal discharge teaching should include postoperative eye care, activity restrictions, medications, follow-up visit schedule, and signs of possible complications (Table 22).
- The patient's family should be included in the instruction, since some patients may have difficulty with self-care activities, especially if vision in the unoperated eye is poor. Provide an opportunity for the patient and family to present return demonstrations of any necessary self-care activities.

Table 22	Patient and Caregiver Teaching Guide: After Eye Surgery

Include the following information in the teaching plan for the patient after eye surgery:

1. Proper hygiene and eye care techniques to ensure that medications, dressings, and/or surgical wound are not contaminated during necessary eye care
2. Signs and symptoms of infection and when and how to report these to allow for early recognition and treatment of possible infection
3. Importance of complying with postoperative restrictions on head positioning, bending, coughing, and Valsalva maneuver to optimize visual outcomes and prevent increased intraocular pressure
4. How to instill eye medications using aseptic techniques and adherence with prescribed eye medication routine to prevent infection
5. How to monitor pain and take medication prescribed for pain and to report pain not relieved by medication
6. Importance of continued follow-up as recommended to maximize potential visual outcomes

Source: American Society of Ophthalmic Registered Nurses: *Core curriculum for ophthalmic nursing*, ed 3, Dubuque, IA, 2004, Kendall-Hunt Publishing.

■ Suggest ways for the patient and caregiver to modify activities and environment to maintain an adequate level of safe functioning for patients with delayed visual correction. Suggestions may include getting assistance with steps, removing area rugs and other potential obstacles, preparing meals for freezing before surgery, and obtaining audio books for diversion until visual acuity improves.

CELIAC DISEASE

Description

Celiac disease is an autoimmune disease characterized by damage to the small intestinal mucosa from the ingestion of wheat, barley, and rye in genetically susceptible individuals. Until recently, celiac disease was considered a relatively rare intestinal disease that began in childhood and was accompanied by symptoms of diarrhea, malabsorption, and malnutrition. It is now known that it is a common disease that occurs at all ages and has a wide variety of symptoms. *Celiac sprue* and *gluten-sensitive enteropathy* are other names for celiac disease.

Celiac disease is not the same as the disease *tropical sprue,* a chronic disorder acquired in tropical areas that is characterized by progressive disruption of jejunal and ileal tissue resulting in nutritional difficulties. Tropical sprue is treated with folic acid and tetracycline.

Incidence is thought to be about 1% of the United States population. High-risk groups include first- or second-degree relatives of someone with celiac disease and people with disorders associated with the disease such as migraine and endocarditis.

■ There is an increased risk of non-Hodgkin's lymphoma and GI cancers in patients with celiac disease.

Pathophysiology

Three factors necessary for the development of celiac disease are a genetic predisposition, gluten ingestion, and an immune-mediated response.

■ About 90% of patients with celiac disease have human leukocyte antigen (HLA) allele HLA-DQ2, and the other 10% have HLA-DQ8. However, not everyone with these genetic markers develops the disease and some people with celiac disease do not have these HLA alleles.

■ Tissue destruction that occurs with celiac disease is the result of chronic inflammation activated by the ingestion of gluten found in wheat, rye, and barley.

- Damage is most severe in the duodenum, probably because it is the site of the highest concentration of gluten. The inflammation lasts as long as gluten ingestion continues.

Clinical Manifestations

Classic signs of celiac disease include foul-smelling diarrhea, steatorrhea, flatulence, abdominal distention, and symptoms of malnutrition. Some people may instead have atypical symptoms such as decreased bone density and osteoporosis, dental enamel hypoplasia, iron and folate deficiencies, peripheral neuropathy, and reproductive problems.

- A pruritic, vesicular skin lesion, called dermatitis herpetiformis, is sometimes present and occurs as a rash on the buttocks, scalp, face, elbows, and knees.
- Poor growth, weight loss, muscle wasting, and other signs of malnutrition may be present. Patients may exhibit lactose intolerance.
- Iron-deficiency anemia is common.
- Celiac disease is also associated with other autoimmune diseases, particularly rheumatoid arthritis, type 1 diabetes mellitus, and thyroid disease.

Diagnostic Studies

Celiac disease is confirmed by (1) histologic evidence when a biopsy is taken from the small intestine and (2) the symptoms and histologic evidence disappear when the person eats a gluten-free diet.

Celiac disease should be ruled out during a diagnostic workup of inflammatory bowel disease, because the symptoms are similar. Many people seek treatment for nonspecific complaints for years before celiac disease is diagnosed.

Nursing and Collaborative Management

Treatment with a gluten-free diet halts the pathologic process. Most patients recover completely within 3 to 6 months of treatment, but they need to maintain a gluten-free diet for life. If the disease is untreated, chronic inflammation and hyperplasia continue.

- Dietary gluten comes from wheat, barley, rye, and oats (oats does not contain gluten but can become contaminated with gluten during milling). Gluten in food additives, preservatives, and stabilizers must also be avoided.
- In patients with refractory celiac disease who do not respond to the gluten-free diet alone, corticosteroids may be used.

▼ **Patient and Caregiver Teaching**

- Maintenance of a gluten-free diet is difficult. Dietary consultation is imperative. The patient needs to know where to purchase gluten-free products and may need financial assistance because of the increased cost of gluten-free products.
- Refer the patient and caregiver to the Celiac Sprue Association (www.csaceliacs.org) for helpful recipes and suggestions for maintaining a gluten-free diet.
- Continuously encourage and motivate patients to continue a gluten-free diet.

C

CERVICAL CANCER

Description
The number of deaths from cervical cancer has fallen steadily over the last 40 years. This is because of earlier and better diagnosis with widespread use of the Pap test. In addition to cancer, the Pap test detects precancerous changes. By treating precancerous lesions, progression to cervical cancer can be prevented.

- An increased risk of cervical cancer is associated with low socioeconomic status, early sexual activity (before 17 years old), multiple sexual partners, infection with human papillomavirus (HPV), immunosuppression, and smoking.

Noninvasive cervical cancer is four times more common than invasive cervical cancer and peaks in women in their early 30s. The average age for women with invasive cervical cancer is 50 years.

Vaccines are now available that reduce the incidence of both cervical-related neoplasia and cervical cancer caused by infection from HPV (types 16 and 18).

Pathophysiology
The progression from normal cervical cells to dysplasia and on to cervical cancer appears to be related to repeated injuries to the cervix. The progression occurs slowly over years rather than months. There is a strong relationship between certain subtypes of HPV and cervical cancer.

Clinical Manifestations
Early cervical cancer is generally asymptomatic, but leukorrhea and intermenstrual bleeding eventually occur.

- A vaginal discharge that is usually thin and watery becomes dark and foul smelling as the disease advances.

- Vaginal bleeding is initially only spotting, but as the tumor enlarges, it becomes heavier and more frequent.
- Pain is a late symptom and is followed by weight loss, anemia, and cachexia.

Diagnostic Studies
- Pap test, colposcopy, and biopsy

Collaborative Care
Treatment is guided by the patient's age, general health, and stage of cervical cancer (see Table 54-11, Lewis et al, *Medical-Surgical Nursing,* ed 8, p. 1364). Four procedures can preserve fertility, an important consideration for younger women. Conization may be the only therapy needed for noninvasive cervical cancer if analysis of removed tissue indicates that a wide area of normal tissue surrounds the excised tissue. Laser treatments can be used to destroy abnormal tissue. Cautery and cryosurgery may also be used.

Invasive cancer of the cervix is treated with surgery, chemotherapy, and/or radiation.

- Surgical procedures include hysterectomy, radical hysterectomy, and, rarely, pelvic exenteration (Table 23). Radiation may be external (e.g., cobalt) or internal (e.g., cesium or radium). Standard radiation treatment is 4 to 6 weeks of external radiation followed by one or two treatments with internal implants (brachytherapy). Cisplatin-based chemotherapy regimens have shown benefit for patients with cancer spread beyond the cervix.

Nursing Management: Cervical Cancer and Other Cancers of the Female Reproductive System
In addition to cervical cancer, malignant tumors of the female reproductive system can be found in the endometrium, ovaries, vagina, and vulva. Management of the patient with any cancer of the female reproductive system includes many similar interventions.

Goals
The patient with a malignant tumor of the female reproductive system will actively participate in treatment decisions, achieve satisfactory pain and symptom management, recognize and report problems promptly, maintain preferred lifestyle as long as possible, and continue to practice cancer detection strategies.

Nursing Diagnoses
- Anxiety
- Acute pain

Table 23	Surgical Procedures Involving the Female Reproductive System

Type of Surgery	Description
Hysterectomy	
Subtotal hysterectomy	Removal of uterus without cervix (rarely done today)
Total hysterectomy	Removal of uterus and cervix
Total abdominal hysterectomy and bilateral salpingo-oophorectomy (TAH-BSO)	Removal of uterus, cervix, fallopian tubes, and ovaries
Radical hysterectomy	Panhysterectomy, partial vaginectomy, and dissection of lymph nodes in pelvis
Laparoscopic-assisted vaginal hysterectomy (LAVH)	Vaginal removal of the uterus with laparoscopic assistance
Vulvectomy	
Simple vulvectomy	Excision of vulva and wide margin of skin
Radical vulvectomy	Excision of tissue from anus to few centimeters above symphysis pubis (skin, labia majora and minora, and clitoris) with superficial and deep lymph node dissection
Vaginectomy	Removal of vagina
Pelvic Exenteration	Radical hysterectomy, total vaginectomy, removal of bladder with diversion of urinary system and resection of bowel with colostomy
Anterior pelvic exenteration	Above operation without bowel resection
Posterior pelvic exenteration	Above operation without bladder removal

C

- Disturbed body image
- Ineffective sexuality patterns
- Grieving

Nursing Interventions

Through your contact with women in a variety of settings, teach women the importance of routine screening for cancers of the reproductive system. Cancer can be prevented when screening reveals precancerous conditions of the vulva, cervix, or endometrium. Assist women to view routine cancer screening as an important self-care activity and recommend vaccination against cervical cancer for those women at high risk.

- Educating women about risk factors for cancers of the reproductive system is also important. Limiting sexual activity during adolescence, using condoms, having fewer sexual partners, and not smoking reduce the risk of cervical cancer.

Hysterectomy. Preoperatively, the patient is prepared for surgery with the standard perineal or abdominal preparation. A vaginal douche and enema may be given according to surgeon preference. The bladder should be emptied before the patient is sent to the operating room. An indwelling catheter is often inserted.

After surgery the patient who has had a hysterectomy will have an abdominal dressing (abdominal hysterectomy) or a sterile perineal pad (vaginal hysterectomy) (see NCP 54-1 for care of a patient after a total abdominal hysterectomy, Lewis et al, *Medical-Surgical Nursing,* ed 8, p. 1369).

- The dressing should be observed frequently for any sign of bleeding during the first 8 hours after surgery. A moderate amount of serosanguineous drainage on the perineal pad is expected after a vaginal hysterectomy.
- Urinary retention may occur postoperatively because of temporary bladder atony resulting from edema or nerve trauma. An indwelling catheter may be used for 1 or 2 days to maintain bladder drainage and prevent strain on the suture line.
- Food and fluids may be restricted if the patient is nauseated. A rectal tube may be prescribed to relieve abdominal flatus. Ambulation is encouraged.
- Special care must be taken to prevent the development of deep vein thrombosis (DVT). Frequent position changes and avoidance of high Fowler's position minimize blood flow stasis and pooling. Encourage leg exercises to promote circulation.

The loss of the uterus may bring about grief responses similar to any great personal loss. The ability to bear children may be essential to a woman's image of being a female. Eliciting the woman's feelings and concerns about her surgery provides needed information to give understanding care.

Prepare the patient for what to expect after surgery (e.g., she will not menstruate). Teaching should include specific activity restrictions. Intercourse should be avoided until the wound is healed (about 4 to 6 weeks). If a vaginal hysterectomy is performed, the woman needs to know that there may be a temporary loss of vaginal sensation.

- Physical restrictions are limited for a short time. Heavy lifting should be avoided for 2 months. Activities that may increase pelvic congestion, such as dancing and brisk walking, should be avoided for several months, whereas activities such as swimming may be both physically and mentally helpful.

Salpingectomy and oophorectomy. Postoperative care of the woman who has undergone removal of a fallopian tube (salpingectomy) or an ovary (oophorectomy) is similar to that for any patient having abdominal surgery. When both ovaries are removed (bilateral oophorectomy), surgical menopause results. Symptoms are similar to those of regular menopause but may be more severe because of the sudden withdrawal of hormones.

Pelvic exenteration. When other forms of therapy are ineffective in controlling cancer spread and no metastases have been found outside the pelvis, pelvic exenteration may be performed. This radical surgery usually involves removal of the uterus, ovaries, fallopian tubes, vagina, bladder, urethra, and pelvic lymph nodes. In some situations the descending colon, rectum, and anal canal may also be removed. Postoperative care involves that of a patient who has had a radical hysterectomy, an abdominal perineal resection, and an ileostomy or colostomy. Physical, emotional, and social adjustments to life on the part of the woman and her family are great. There are urinary or fecal diversions in the abdominal wall, a reconstructed vagina, and the onset of menopausal symptoms.

CHLAMYDIAL INFECTIONS

Description

Chlamydia trachomatis is a gram-negative bacterium recognized as a genital pathogen responsible for a variety of illnesses. Chlamydia can be transmitted during vaginal, anal, or oral sex.

- Different strains of *C. trachomatis* are responsible for urogenital infections (e.g., nongonococcal urethritis [NGU] in men and cervicitis in women), ocular trachoma, and lymphogranuloma venereum.

- In the United States and Canada, chlamydial infections are the most commonly reported sexually transmitted disease (STD).
- Recently chlamydial infections reached their highest level ever with 1.1 million cases reported. Underreporting is significant because many people are asymptomatic and do not seek testing.

Risk factors include women and adolescents, new or multiple sex partners, sexual partners who have had multiple partners, history of STDs and cervical ectopy, coexisting STDs, and inconsistent or incorrect use of a condom.

- Chlamydial infections can cause pelvic inflammatory disease, ectopic pregnancy, and infertility among women.
- Chlamydial infections are closely associated with gonococcal infections, making clinical differentiation difficult. Therefore both infections are usually treated concurrently even without diagnostic evidence.
- Because of the high prevalence of asymptomatic infections in both men and women, screening of high-risk populations is needed to identify those infected.

Clinical Manifestations

As with gonorrhea, chlamydial infections result in a superficial mucosal infection that can become more invasive.

- Symptoms may be absent or minor in most infected women and many men.
- Signs and symptoms in men may include urethritis (dysuria, urethral discharge), epididymitis (unilateral scrotal pain, swelling, tenderness, fever), and proctitis (rectal discharge and pain during defecation).
- Signs and symptoms in women include cervicitis (mucopurulent discharge and hypertrophic ectopy [area that is edematous and bleeds easily]), urethritis (dysuria, pyuria, and frequent urination), dyspareunia (painful intercourse), bartholinitis (purulent exudate), and pelvic inflammatory disease (abdominal pain, nausea, vomiting, fever, abnormal vaginal bleeding, and menstrual abnormalities).

Complications

Complications often develop from poorly managed, inaccurately diagnosed, or undiagnosed chlamydial infections.

- Rare complications in men may result in epididymitis with possible infertility and reactive arthritis.

- Women may develop pelvic inflammatory disease leading to chronic pelvic pain and infertility.

Diagnostic Studies

Chlamydial infections in men can be diagnosed by excluding gonorrhea. The most common diagnostic tests include the nucleic acid amplification test (NAAT), the direct fluorescent antibody (DFA) test, and enzyme immunoassay (EIA). These tests do not require special handling of specimens and are easier to perform than cell cultures. DNA amplification test is the most sensitive diagnostic method available.

Collaborative Care

Chlamydial infections respond to treatment with doxycycline (Vibramycin) or azithromycin (Zithromax). Important teaching for patients includes:

- Advise them to return to their health care provider if symptoms persist or recur.
- Emphasize the importance of treating sex partners.
- Encourage the use of condoms during all sexual contacts.

Nursing Management

See Nursing Management: Sexually Transmitted Diseases, p. 570.

CHOLELITHIASIS/CHOLECYSTITIS

Description

The most common disorder of the biliary system is *cholelithiasis* (stones in the gallbladder). *Cholecystitis* (inflammation of the gallbladder) is usually associated with cholelithiasis. The stones may be lodged in the neck of the gallbladder or in the cystic duct. Cholecystitis may be acute or chronic, with these conditions also occurring together.

Gallbladder disease is a common health problem in the United States. It is estimated that 8% to 10% of adults in the United States have cholelithiasis.

- The incidence of cholelithiasis is higher in women, multiparous women, and persons over 40 years old. Other factors that seem to increase the incidence of gallbladder disease are sedentary lifestyle, familial tendency, and obesity.
- There is an especially high incidence of gallbladder disease in the Native American population, especially in the Navajo and Pima tribes.

Pathophysiology

The actual cause of gallstones is unknown. Cholelithiasis develops when the balance that keeps cholesterol, bile salts, and calcium in solution is altered so that precipitation of these substances occurs. Conditions that upset this balance include infection and disturbances in the metabolism of cholesterol. Mixed cholesterol stones, which are predominantly cholesterol, are the most common gallstones.

The stones may remain in the gallbladder or migrate to the cystic duct or common bile duct. They cause pain as they pass through the ducts and may lodge in the ducts and cause obstruction. Stasis of bile in the gallbladder can lead to cholecystitis.

Cholecystitis is most commonly associated with obstruction resulting from gallstones or biliary sludge. Cholecystitis without obstruction from stones can occur as a result of trauma, extensive burns, prolonged immobility and fasting, and prolonged parenteral nutrition. Bacteria reaching the gallbladder by the vascular or lymphatic route or chemical irritants in the bile can also produce cholecystitis. *Escherichia coli,* streptococci, and salmonellae are the most common causative bacteria. Other etiologic factors include adhesions, neoplasms, anesthesia, and opioid drugs.

- During an acute attack of cholecystitis the gallbladder is edematous and hyperemic. It may be distended with bile or pus. The cystic duct is also involved and may become occluded.
- The wall of the gallbladder becomes scarred after an acute attack. Decreased functioning occurs if large amounts of tissue are fibrosed.

Clinical Manifestations

Cholelithiasis may produce severe symptoms or none at all. Many patients have "silent cholelithiasis." Severity of symptoms depends on whether the stones are stationary or mobile and whether obstruction is present.

- When a stone is lodged in the ducts or when stones are moving through the ducts, spasms may result. This sometimes produces severe pain, which is termed *biliary colic.* The pain can be accompanied by tachycardia, diaphoresis, and prostration. The severe pain may last up to 1 hour, and when it subsides there is residual tenderness in the right upper quadrant.
- The attacks of pain frequently occur 3 to 6 hours after a heavy meal or when the patient lies down.
- When total obstruction occurs, symptoms related to bile blockage are manifested; these include steatorrhea,

pruritus, dark amber urine, bleeding tendencies, and jaundice.

Cholecystitis manifestations may vary from indigestion to moderate to severe pain, leukocytosis, fever, and jaundice. Initial symptoms include indigestion and pain and tenderness in the right upper quadrant, which may be referred to the right shoulder and scapula. Pain may be acute and is accompanied by restlessness, diaphoresis, and nausea and vomiting.

- Symptoms of chronic cholecystitis include a history of fat intolerance, dyspepsia, heartburn, and flatulence.

Complications

Complications of cholecystitis include gangrenous cholecystitis, subphrenic abscess, pancreatitis, *cholangitis* (inflammation of biliary ducts), biliary cirrhosis, fistulas, and rupture of the gallbladder, which can produce bile peritonitis. Many of the same complications can occur from cholelithiasis, including cholangitis, carcinoma, and peritonitis.

Diagnostic Studies

- Ultrasonography is used to diagnose gallstones.
- Endoscopic retrograde cholangiopancreatography (ERCP) allows for visualization of the gallbladder, cystic duct, common hepatic duct, and common bile duct. Bile taken during ERCP is sent for culture to identify any possible infecting organism.
- Percutaneous transhepatic cholangiography may be used to locate stones within the bile ducts.
- Laboratory studies may demonstrate elevated serum enzymes and pancreatic enzymes, increased white blood cell (WBC) count, elevated direct and indirect bilirubin levels, and urinary bilirubin.

Collaborative Care

The treatment of gallstones in cholelithiasis depends upon the stage of disease. Bile acids (cholesterol solvents) such as ursodeoxycholic (ursodiol [Actigall]) and chenodeoxycholic (chenodiol) are used to dissolve stones. Endoscopic retrograde cholangiopancreatography (ERCP) with sphincterotomy (papillotomy) may be used for stone removal. ERCP allows for visualization of the biliary system, as well as the placement of stents and sphincterotomy (papillotomy) if warranted.

Extracorporeal shock-wave lithotripsy (ESWL) may be used to treat cholelithiasis. In this procedure a lithotriptor uses high-energy shock waves to disintegrate gallstones.

Surgical intervention for cholelithiasis is frequently indicated and may consist of one of several procedures.

- Cholecystectomy is the preferred surgical procedure. Most cholecystectomies are now performed laparoscopically. In this procedure the gallbladder is removed through one of four small punctures in the abdomen. Most patients experience minimal postoperative pain and are discharged the day of surgery or the day after. In most cases they are able to resume normal activities and return to work within one week.

During an acute episode of cholecystitis the focus is on control of pain, control of possible infection with antibiotics, and maintenance of fluid and electrolyte balance. Treatment is mainly supportive and symptomatic. A cholecystostomy may be used to drain purulent material from the obstructed gallbladder.

- If nausea and vomiting are severe, gastric decompression may be used to prevent further gallbladder stimulation. Anticholinergics to decrease secretions (which prevents biliary contraction) and counteract smooth muscle spasms may be administered. Analgesics are given to decrease pain.

Drug therapy for gallbladder disease includes analgesics, anticholinergics (antispasmodics), fat-soluble vitamins, and bile salts. Morphine may be used initially for pain management.

Many patients have fewer problems if they eat smaller, more frequent meals with some fat at each meal to promote gallbladder emptying. If obesity is a problem, a reduced-calorie diet is indicated. The diet should be low in saturated fats and high in fiber and calcium.

Nursing Management

Goals
The patient with gallbladder disease will have relief of pain and discomfort, no postoperative complications, and no recurrent attacks of cholecystitis or cholelithiasis.

Nursing Diagnoses
- Acute pain
- Ineffective self-health management

Nursing Interventions
Nursing objectives for the patient undergoing conservative therapy include relieving pain, relieving nausea and vomiting, providing comfort and emotional support, maintaining fluid and electrolyte balance and nutrition, making accurate assessments for effectiveness of treatment, and observing for complications.

The patient with acute cholecystitis or cholelithiasis is frequently experiencing severe pain; medications ordered to relieve pain should be given as required before the pain becomes more severe.

Observe for signs of obstruction of the ducts by stones, including jaundice; clay-colored stools; dark, foamy urine; steatorrhea; fever; and increased WBC count.

Postoperative nursing care after a laparoscopic cholecystectomy includes monitoring for complications such as bleeding, making the patient comfortable, and preparing the patient for discharge.

- A common postoperative problem is referred pain to the shoulder because of the CO_2 that was not released or absorbed by the body. CO_2 can irritate the phrenic nerve and the diaphragm, causing some difficulty breathing. The pain can usually be relieved by nonsteroidal antiinflammatory drugs (NSAIDs) or codeine.
- Placing the patient in Sims' position (left side with right knee flexed) helps move the gas pocket away from the diaphragm. Deep breathing should be encouraged, along with movement and ambulation.

▼ **Patient and Caregiver Teaching**

- When the patient has conservative therapy, dietary teaching is usually necessary. The diet is often low in fat, and sometimes a weight-reduction diet is also recommended. The patient may need to take fat-soluble vitamin supplements.
- Provide instructions about manifestations that may indicate obstruction (stool and urine changes, jaundice, and pruritus).
- The patient who undergoes a laparoscopic cholecystectomy is discharged soon after the surgery, so postoperative teaching is important (Table 24).

Table 24	Patient and Caregiver Teaching Guide: Postoperative Laparoscopic Cholecystectomy

You should include the following instructions in the patient's postoperative teaching plan:

1. Remove the bandages on the puncture site the day after surgery and you can shower.
2. Notify your surgeon if any of the following signs and symptoms occur:
   Redness, swelling, bile-colored drainage or pus from any incision
   Severe abdominal pain, nausea, vomiting, fever, chills
3. You can gradually resume normal activities.
4. Return to work within 1 week of surgery.
5. You can resume your usual diet, but a low-fat diet is usually better tolerated for several weeks following surgery.

CHRONIC FATIGUE SYNDROME

Description

Chronic fatigue syndrome (CFS) is a disorder characterized by debilitating fatigue and a variety of associated complaints. Immune abnormalities are frequently present.

- CFS affects women more often than men and occurs in all ethnic and socioeconomic groups. Prevalence of this syndrome is difficult to determine because of the lack of validated diagnostic tests.

Pathophysiology

Despite numerous attempts to determine the etiology and pathology of CFS, the precise mechanisms remain unknown. There are many theories about the etiology of CFS.

- Neuroendocrine abnormalities have been implicated involving a hypofunction of the HPA (hypothalamic-pituitary-adrenal) axis and HPG (hypothalamic-pituitary-gonadal) axis, which together regulate the stress response and reproductive hormone levels.
- Several microorganisms have been investigated as etiologic agents, including herpes viruses (e.g., Epstein Barr [EBV], cytomegalovirus [CMV]), retroviruses, enteroviruses, *Candida albicans,* and mycoplasma).
- Because cognitive deficits such as decreased memory, attention, and concentration occur in many of the patients, it has been proposed that CFS is caused by changes in the central nervous system.

Clinical Manifestations

It is often difficult to distinguish between CFS and fibromyalgia syndrome (FMS) because many clinical features are similar (Table 25).

In about half of the cases, CFS develops insidiously, or the patient may have intermittent episodes that gradually become chronic.

- Incapacitating fatigue is the most common symptom that causes the patient to seek health care. Associated symptoms (Table 26) may fluctuate in intensity over time.
- The patient may become angry and frustrated with the inability of health care providers to diagnose a problem. The disorder may have a major impact on work and family responsibilities. Some individuals may even need help with activities of daily living.

Table 25	Commonalities Between Fibromyalgia Syndrome and Chronic Fatigue Syndrome
Commonality	**Description**
Occurrence	Previously healthy, young and middle-aged women
Etiology (theories)	Infectious trigger, dysfunction in HPA axis, alteration in CNS
Clinical manifestations	Malaise and fatigue, cognitive dysfunction, headaches, sleep disturbances, depression, anxiety, fever, generalized musculoskeletal pain
Course of disease	Variable intensity of symptoms, fluctuates over time
Diagnosis	No definitive laboratory tests or joint and muscle examinations, mainly a diagnosis of exclusion
Collaborative care	Treatment is symptomatic and may include antidepressant drugs such as amitriptyline (Elavil) and fluoxetine (Prozac). Other measures are heat, massage, regular stretching, biofeedback, stress management, and relaxation training. Patient and caregiver teaching is essential.

CNS, Central nervous system; *HPA,* hypothalamic-pituitary-adrenal.

Diagnostic Studies

Physical examination and diagnostic studies can be used to rule out other possible causes of the patient's symptoms. No laboratory test can diagnose CFS or measure its severity. The Centers for Disease Control and Prevention (CDC) have helped develop diagnostic criteria based on the patient's symptoms (see Table 26). In general, CFS remains a diagnosis of exclusion.

Nursing and Collaborative Management

Because there is no definitive therapy for CFS, supportive management is essential. The patient should be informed about what is known about the disease and all complaints should be taken seriously.

- Nonsteroidal antiinflammatory drugs (NSAIDs) can be used to treat headaches, muscle and joint aches, and fever.

Table 26	Diagnostic Criteria for Chronic Fatigue Syndrome*

Major Criterion
- Unexplained, persistent, or relapsing chronic fatigue of new and definite onset (not lifelong); not caused by ongoing exertion; not substantially alleviated by rest; results in substantial reduction in occupational, educational, social, or personal activities.

Minor Criteria
- Impaired memory or concentration
- Frequent or recurring sore throat
- Tender cervical or axillary lymph nodes
- Muscle pain
- Multijoint pain without joint swelling or redness
- Headaches of a new type, pattern, or severity
- Unrefreshing sleep
- Postexertional malaise
- Adapted from Centers for Disease Control and Prevention: Chronic fatigue syndrome: revised case definition. Available at www.cdc.gov/cfs/cfsdefinitionHCP.htm

*For a diagnosis to be made, the patient must demonstrate the major criterion, plus four or more of the minor criteria for 6 months or more. These criteria were prepared by the Centers for Disease Control and Prevention, National Institutes of Health, and International Chronic Fatigue Syndrome Study Group.

Antihistamines and decongestants can be used to treat allergic symptoms. Tricyclic antidepressants (e.g., doxepin [Sinequan], amitriptyline [Elavil]) and selective serotonin reuptake inhibitors (e.g., fluoxetine [Prozac], paroxetine [Paxil]) can improve mood and sleep disorders. Clonazepam (Klonopin) can also be used to treat sleep disturbances and panic disorders.

- Total rest is not advised, because it can potentiate the self-image of being an invalid. On the other hand, strenuous exertion can exacerbate the exhaustion. Therefore it is important to plan a carefully graduated exercise program.
- Behavioral therapy may be used to promote a positive outlook, as well as improve overall disability, fatigue, and other symptoms.

CFS does not appear to progress. One of the major problems facing many CFS patients is financial instability. When the illness strikes, they cannot work or must decrease the amount of time working.

Although most patients recover or at least improve over time, they experience substantial occupational and psychosocial impairments and loss, including the social pressure and isolation from being characterized as lazy or "crazy."

CHRONIC OBSTRUCTIVE PULMONARY DISEASE: EMPHYSEMA AND CHRONIC BRONCHITIS

C

Description

Chronic obstructive pulmonary disease (COPD) is a disease state characterized by the presence of airway obstruction that is not fully reversible. The limited airflow is usually progressive and is associated with an abnormal inflammatory response of the lungs to noxious particles or gases, primarily cigarette smoke. Previous definitions of COPD encompassed two types of obstructive airway disease *emphysema* and *chronic bronchitis.*

- *Emphysema* is an abnormal permanent enlargement of the air spaces distal to the terminal bronchioles, accompanied by destruction of their walls and without obvious fibrosis.
- *Chronic bronchitis* is the presence of chronic productive cough for 3 months in each of 2 consecutive years in a patient in whom other causes of chronic cough have been excluded.
- Patients with COPD may have a predominance of one of these conditions, but the conditions usually coexist, and COPD is considered one disease state in terms of pathophysiology and management.

More than 12 million persons in the United States have COPD and it is the fourth leading cause of death in the United States.

Etiology

Cigarette smoking is the major risk factor for developing COPD.

- The irritating effect of cigarette smoke causes hyperplasia of cells, which subsequently results in increased mucous production. Hyperplasia reduces airway diameter and increases the difficulty in clearing secretions. Smoking reduces ciliary activity and produces abnormal dilation of the distal air space with destruction of alveolar walls.
- COPD can develop independently of cigarette smoking if a person has intense or prolonged exposure to various dusts, vapors, irritants, or fumes in the workplace.
- High levels of urban air pollution are harmful to persons with existing lung disease, but the effect of outdoor air

pollution as a risk factor for COPD appears to be small compared with the effect of cigarette smoking.

- Severe recurring respiratory tract infections impair normal defense mechanisms, making the bronchioles and alveoli more susceptible to injury and intensifying the pathologic destruction of lung tissue.

α_1-Antitrypsin (AAT) deficiency is a genetic risk factor that leads to COPD. AAT is an autosomal recessive disorder that may affect the lungs or liver. Normally AAT inhibits the breakdown of lung tissues by proteolytic enzymes from neutrophils and macrophages. Emphysema occurs because of the AAT deficiency.

Some degree of emphysema is common in the lungs of older persons, even nonsmokers. Aging results in changes in the lung structure, thoracic cage, and respiratory muscles. However, clinically significant emphysema is usually not caused by aging alone.

Pathophysiology

COPD is characterized by chronic inflammation found in the airways, lung parenchyma (respiratory bronchioles and alveoli), and blood vessels. The pathogenesis of COPD is complex and involves many mechanisms. The defining features of COPD are irreversible airflow limitation during forced exhalation caused by loss of elastic recoil and airflow obstruction caused by mucus hypersecretion, mucosal edema, and bronchospasm.

The inflammatory process starts with inhalation of noxious particles (e.g., cigarette smoke) that causes the release of inflammatory mediators that damage lung tissue. This process causes tissue destruction and disrupts the normal defense mechanisms and repair process of the lung.

- The cascading inflammatory process results in proinflammatory cytokines such as tumor necrosis factor being activated. In addition, growth factors are recruited into the area and activated resulting in structural changes in the lungs.
- After the inhalation of oxidants in tobacco or air pollution, protease activity (which breaks down the connective tissue of the lungs) increases and antiproteases (which protect against the breakdown) are inhibited.
- Inability to expire air is a main characteristic of COPD. As the peripheral airways become obstructed, air is progressively trapped during expiration. The chest hyperexpands and becomes barrel shaped as the respiratory muscles are not able to function effectively.
- Gas exchange abnormalities result in hypoxemia and hypercarbia (increased CO_2). As air trapping worsens and alveoli

are destroyed, bullae (large air spaces in the parenchyma) and blebs (air spaces adjacent to pleurae) can form. There is a significant ventilation/perfusion (V/Q) mismatch and hypoxemia results.

- Excess mucus production is a result of increased number of mucus-secreting goblet cells and enlarged submucosal glands, which respond to the chronic irritation of smoke or other inhalants.

- Pulmonary vascular changes resulting in mild to moderate pulmonary hypertension may occur late in the course of COPD. Pulmonary hypertension may progress and lead to hypertrophy of the right ventricle of the heart or cor pulmonale with or without right-sided heart failure.

COPD has systemic effects, especially in severe disease. These extrapulmonary changes contribute greatly to the clinical findings of the patient and impact survival and management. The mechanisms that cause the changes are unclear and are likely multifaceted. Cachexia is common with a loss of skeletal muscle mass, and weakness is likely caused by increased apoptosis (programmed cell death) and/or muscle disuse. Patients may have muscle weakness in the upper and lower extremities. They also have exercise intolerance, deconditioning, and osteoporosis. Patients with severe COPD may develop chronic anemia, anxiety, and depression.

It is common to find a combination of emphysema and chronic bronchitis in the same person, often with one condition predominating. Patients with COPD may also have asthma, and if they experience poorly reversible airflow limitation, the symptoms may be indistinguishable from COPD, but clinically are treated as asthma.

Clinical Manifestations

Clinical manifestations of COPD typically develop slowly around 50 years of age after 20 pack-years of cigarette smoking.

- A diagnosis of COPD should be considered in any patient who has symptoms of cough, sputum production, or dyspnea, and/or a history of exposure to risk factors for the disease. A chronic intermittent cough usually occurs in the morning and may or may not be productive of small amounts of sticky mucus.

- Dyspnea is often progressive and usually occurs with exertion. In late stages of COPD, dyspnea may be present at rest. Wheezing and chest tightness may be present, but may vary by time of the day or from day to day, especially in patients with more severe disease.

- Even when the patient with advanced COPD has adequate caloric intake, weight loss is still experienced. Fatigue is a prevalent and affects the patient's activities of daily living.
- During physical examination a prolonged expiratory phase of respiration, wheezes, or decreased breath sounds are noted in all lung fields. The anterior-posterior diameter of the chest is increased ("barrel chest") from the chronic air trapping. The patient may assume a tripod position, use pursed-lip breathing, and use accessory muscles of respiration.
- Hypoxemia and hypercapnia may develop later in the disease. The bluish red color of the skin results from polycythemia and cyanosis. Polycythemia develops as a result of increased production of red blood cells as the body attempts to compensate for chronic hypoxemia.

Complications

Cor pulmonale results from pulmonary hypertension. In COPD, pulmonary hypertension is caused primarily by constriction of pulmonary vessels in response to alveolar hypoxia, with acidosis further potentiating vasoconstriction. Increased pulmonary vascular resistance is also caused by inflammatory-induced vascular remodeling, increased viscosity of the blood from polycythemia, and reduction in the pulmonary capillary bed. When pulmonary hypertension develops, the pressure on the right side of the heart must increase to push blood into the lungs. Eventually right-sided heart failure develops (see Cor Pulmonale, p. 154).

A **COPD exacerbation** is an event in the natural course of the disease characterized by a change in the patient's baseline dyspnea, cough, and/or sputum that is beyond the normal day-to-day variations, is acute in onset, and may warrant a change in regular medication in a patient with underlying COPD. Other complaints include malaise, insomnia, increased wheezing, fatigue, depression, confusion, or decreased exercise tolerance. The primary causes of exacerbations are bacterial or viral infection and air pollution/other environmental sources. Exacerbations are managed with bronchodilators, oral systemic corticosteroids, antibiotics, and supplemental oxygen therapy.

- Teach the patient and caregiver early recognition of signs and symptoms of exacerbations to promote early treatment and thus prevent hospitalization and possible respiratory failure.

Acute respiratory failure may occur in patients with severe COPD who have exacerbations (see Acute Respiratory Distress Syndrome, p. 13). Respiratory failure may also be precipitated by cor pulmonale, failure to take respiratory medications, or the use of respiratory depressants such as sedatives and opioids. Surgery or severe, painful illness involving the chest or abdominal organs may lead to splinting and ineffective ventilation and respiratory failure.

Depression and **anxiety** are other complications of COPD. A consult to a mental health specialist may be needed for proper screening and diagnosis of depression or other mental health problems. Treatment consisting of cognitive and behavioral psychotherapy along with COPD education can improve quality of life. Medications may be used to treat both the depression and anxiety.

Diagnostic Studies

Goals of the diagnostic workup are to confirm the diagnosis of COPD via spirometry, evaluate the severity of the disease, and determine the impact of the disease on the patient's quality of life.

- A forced expiratory volume/forced vital capacity (FEV_1/ FVC) <70% establishes the diagnosis of COPD, and the severity of obstruction (FEV_1) determines the stage of COPD.
- Chest x-ray is seldom diagnostic unless bullous emphysema is present.
- Electrocardiogram (ECG) may be normal or indicate right ventricular failure.
- Sputum culture and sensitivity are done if acute exacerbation is present.
- Arterial blood gases (ABGs) in later stages usually indicate low PaO_2, elevated $PaCO_2$, decreased or low normal pH, and increased bicarbonate (HCO_3^-) levels.

Collaborative Care

The primary goals of care for the patient with COPD are to prevent disease progression, relieve symptoms and improve exercise tolerance, prevent and treat complications, promote patient participation in care, prevent and treat exacerbations, and improve quality of life and reduce mortality.

The patient with COPD should have a pneumococcal and influenza virus vaccine yearly and avoid environmental or occupational irritants. Exacerbations of COPD should be treated as soon as possible. Some patients are given a prescription of antibiotics and are instructed to begin taking them at the first signs of an exacerbation.

- Cessation of cigarette smoking in any stage of COPD is the single most effective intervention to reduce the risk of developing COPD and stop the progression of the disease.

Smoking cessation techniques are discussed in Lewis et al, *Medical-Surgical Nursing,* ed 8, pp. 170 to 173, and in Tables 12-4 through 12-7, pp. 171 to 173.

Medications for COPD can reduce or abolish symptoms, increase the capacity to exercise, improve overall health, and reduce the number and severity of exacerbations.

- Bronchodilator medications commonly used are β_2-adrenergic agonists, anticholinergic agents, and methylxanthines (see Table 29-7, Lewis et al, *Medical-Surgical Nursing,* ed 8, pp. 598 to 599). When the patient has mild COPD or intermittent symptoms, a short-acting bronchodilator is used as needed. As symptoms persist or moderate stages of COPD develop, a long-acting bronchodilator is used in addition to a short-acting bronchodilator. Inhaled corticosteroids are beneficial for patients with stage 3 (severe) or stage 4 (very severe) COPD because they reduce the frequency of COPD exacerbations.

Long-term O_2 therapy improves survival, exercise tolerance, cognitive performance, and sleep in hypoxemic patients (see Oxygen Therapy, p. 743).

Breathing exercises may assist the patient during rest and activity (e.g., lifting, walking, stair climbing) by decreasing dyspnea, improving oxygenation, and slowing the respiratory rate. The main types of breathing exercises commonly taught are pursed-lip breathing and diaphragmatic breathing. Airway clearance techniques loosen mucus and secretions so they can be cleared by coughing. A variety of treatments can be used to achieve airway clearance. Respiratory therapy, physical therapy, and nurses are involved in performing these techniques. See Lewis et al, *Medical-Surgical Nursing,* ed 8, pp. 622 to 625 for further information on respiratory care.

- Nutritional therapy is directed toward helping the patient with COPD maintain a body mass index between 21 and 25 kg/m^2. Weight loss and muscle wasting are common in the patient with severe COPD. To decrease dyspnea and conserve energy, the patient should rest at least 30 minutes before eating, use the bronchodilator before meals, and select foods that can be prepared in advance. The patient should eat five or six small, frequent meals to avoid feelings of bloating and early satiety when eating.

Surgical Therapy

Three different surgical procedures have been used in severe COPD. One type of surgery is *lung volume reduction surgery* (LVRS). The goal of this therapy is to reduce the size of the lungs by removing the most diseased lung tissue so the remaining healthy lung tissue can perform better.

Another surgical procedure is a bullectomy. This procedure is used for patients with emphysematous COPD who have large bullae (>1 cm). The bullae are usually resected via thoracoscope. This procedure has resulted in improved lung function and reduction in dyspnea.

A third surgical procedure is lung transplantation that will benefit patients with advanced COPD. Although single-lung transplant is more commonly used because of a shortage of donors, bilateral transplantation can be performed. However, organ rejection, effects of immunosuppressive therapy, and high cost of the surgery remain obstacles to its widespread use in COPD.

Nursing Management

Goals
The patient with COPD will have prevention of disease progression, ability to perform activities of daily living (ADLs), improved exercise tolerance, relief from symptoms, no complications related to COPD, knowledge and ability to implement a long-term treatment regimen, and overall improved quality of life.

See NCP 29-2 for the patient with chronic obstructive pulmonary disease, Lewis et al, *Medical-Surgical Nursing,* ed 8, pp. 626 to 628.

Nursing Diagnoses
- Ineffective airway clearance
- Ineffective breathing pattern
- Impaired gas exchange
- Imbalanced nutrition: less than body requirements
- Risk prone behavior

Nursing Interventions
- You are in an important position to dramatically reduce the incidence of COPD by advocating smoking cessation in all smokers and working to prevent smoking in adolescents.
- Other preventive measures to maintain healthy lungs include avoiding or controlling exposure to pollutants and irritants, early detection of small airway disease, and early diagnosis and treatment of respiratory tract infections. Patients with COPD should maintain influenza and pneumococcal vaccines and avoid exposure to large crowds in peak periods for influenza.
- The patient with COPD will require acute intervention for complications such as exacerbations of COPD, pneumonia, cor pulmonale, and acute respiratory failure. Once the crisis in these situations has been resolved, assess the degree and severity of

the underlying respiratory problem. The information obtained
will help to plan nursing care.

▼ **Patient and Caregiver Teaching**

The most important aspect in long-term care of the patient with
COPD is teaching (Table 27).

Table 27	**Patient and Caregiver Teaching Guide: Chronic Obstructive Pulmonary Disease**

You should include the following information in the teaching plan:

Goal

To assist a patient and caregiver in improving quality of life
through education and promotion of lifestyle practices that
support successful living with chronic obstructive pulmonary
disease (COPD).

Teaching Topic	Resources
Overall Guide	Global Initiative for Lung Disease (GOLD) Patient Guide: What You Can Do about a Lung Disease Called COPD. Available at www.goldcopd.org. Also available in foreign languages
What Is COPD? ■ Basic anatomy and physiology of lung ■ Basic pathophysiology of COPD ■ Signs and symptoms of COPD, exacerbation, cold, flu, pneumonia ■ Tests to assess breathing	*COPD statement: Patient Education Section* (American Thoracic Society [ATS]). Available at www.thoracic.org. (Also in Spanish) *Human Respiratory System* and *Learn about Your Respiratory System* (American Lung Association [ALA]). Available under Your Lungs at www.lungsusa.org
Breathing and Airway Clearance Exercises	
■ Pursed-lip breathing	See Table 29-14, Lewis et al., *Medical-Surgical Nursing*, ed. 8, p. 607
■ Airway clearance technique – Huff cough	See Table 29-23, Lewis et al., *Medical-Surgical Nursing*, ed. 8, p. 623

Table 27	Patient and Caregiver Teaching Guide: Chronic Obstructive Pulmonary Disease—cont'd

Teaching Topic	Resources

Energy Conservation Techniques
- Daily activities (e.g., waking up, bathing, grooming, shopping, traveling)

Consult with physical therapist and occupational therapist
Around the Clock with COPD: Helpful Hints for Respiratory Patients (ALA). Available in COPD Center at www.lungusa.org

Medications
- Types (include mechanism of action, and types of devices)
  - Methylxanthines
  - β_2-adrenergic agonists
  - Corticosteroids
  - Anticholinergics
  - Antibiotics
  - Other medications
- Establishing medication schedule

COPD statement: Patient Education Section: Medications and Other Treatments (ATS). Available at www.thoracic.org
OR
COPD Medicines Chart (ALA). Available in COPD Center at www.lungusa.org
OR
COPD Medications (National Jewish Medicine and Research Center) Available at http://www.nationaljewish.org/
Write out medication list and schedule. Form available at National Jewish link above: "Manage your Medications."

Correct Use of Inhalers, Spacer, and Nebulizer

See Figs. 29-6, 29-7, and 29-8, Lewis et al., *Medical-Surgical Nursing*, ed. 8, pp. 601-602. See Tables 29-8, 29-9, and 29-10, Lewis et al., *Medical-Surgical Nursing*, ed. 8, pp. 602-603.

Home Oxygen
- Explanation of rationale for use
- Guide for home O_2 use and equipment

Around the Clock with COPD: Helpful Hints for Respiratory Patients and Traveling with Oxygen (ALA). Available in COPD Center at www.lungusa.org

Continued

Table 27	Patient and Caregiver Teaching Guide: Chronic Obstructive Pulmonary Disease—cont'd

Teaching Topic	Resources
Psychosocial/Emotional Issues Concerns about interpersonal relationships ■ Dependency ■ Intimacy Problems with emotions ■ Depression, anxiety, panic Treatment decisions ■ Support and rehabilitation groups End-of-life issues	Open discussion (sharing with patient, significant other, and family) COPD Lung NexProfiler (interactive decision support tool via ALA). Available at www.lungusa.org. *Questions about Pulmonary Rehabilitation* (English and Spanish) (ATS). Available at www.thoracic.org *Better Breathers Clubs* and *Living with Lung Disease* (online support group) (ALA). Available at www.lungusa.org
COPD Management Plan ■ Focusing on self-management ■ Need to report changes ■ Cause of flare-ups or exacerbation ■ Recognition of signs and symptoms of respiration infection, heart failure ■ Reduce risk factors, especially smoking cessation ■ Exercise program of walking and arm strengthening ■ Yearly follow-up	Nurse and patient develop and write up COPD management plan that meets individual needs.
Healthy Nutrition ■ Strategies to lose weight (if overweight) ■ Strategies to gain weight (if underweight)	Consultation with dietitian.

Pulmonary rehabilitation should be considered in patients who continue to be disabled by pulmonary symptoms even though getting appropriate and standard medical care. The benefits of rehabilitation include reductions in perceived intensity of breathlessness, number of hospitalizations and days in the hospital, anxiety, and depression.

- A mandatory component of any pulmonary rehabilitation program is exercise that focuses on the muscles used in ambulation. Ideally pulmonary rehabilitation includes exercise training, nutrition counseling, and education. Other important topics include health promotion, psychologic counseling, and vocational rehabilitation. Smoking cessation is critical.

- Energy conservation is an important component in COPD rehabilitation. Exercise training of the upper extremities may improve function and reduce dyspnea. Alternative energy-saving practices for ADLs and scheduled rest periods should be planned.

- Walking or other endurance exercises (e.g., cycling) combined with strength training is likely the best intervention to strengthen muscles and improve the patient's endurance. Coordinated walking with slow, pursed-lip breathing without breath holding is a difficult task that requires conscious effort and frequent reinforcement. Walk with the patient, giving verbal reminders when necessary regarding breathing (inhalation and exhalation) and steps. Encourage the patient to walk 15 to 20 minutes per day with gradual increases.

- Modifying but not abstaining from sexual activity can also contribute to a healthy psychologic well-being. Using an inhaled bronchodilator before sexual activity can help ventilation.

- Adequate sleep is extremely important. The patient who is a restless sleeper, snores, stops breathing while asleep, and has a tendency to fall asleep during the day may need to be tested for sleep apnea.

- Healthy coping is often the most difficult task for a patient with COPD. People with COPD frequently have to deal with many lifestyle changes that may involve decreased ability to care for themselves, decreased energy for social activities, and loss of a job. Support groups at local chapters of the American Lung Association, hospitals, and clinics may be helpful.

CIRRHOSIS

Description

Cirrhosis is a chronic progressive disease of the liver characterized by extensive degeneration and destruction of liver parenchy-
mal cells. It is the third leading cause of death in persons
between 35 and 65 years of age, and is twice as common in men
as women.

- Excessive alcohol ingestion is the single most common
  cause of cirrhosis because alcohol has a direct hepatotoxic
  effect. Environmental factors as well as a genetic predisposition may also lead to the development of cirrhosis, regardless of dietary or alcohol intake.

Pathophysiology

Any chronic (long-term) liver disease can cause cirrhosis. The
specific cause is not determined in all patients. Approximately 20%
of patients with chronic hepatitis C and 10% to 20% of those with
chronic hepatitis B will develop cirrhosis. Chronic inflammation
and cell necrosis result in fibrosis and, ultimately, cirrhosis. The
combination of chronic hepatitis and alcohol ingestion is synergis-
tic in terms of accelerating liver damage.

Biliary causes of cirrhosis include primary biliary cirrhosis
and primary sclerosing cholangitis. *Primary sclerosing cholangitis*
is a chronic inflammatory condition affecting the liver and
bile ducts. The etiology of primary sclerosing cholangitis is
unknown. However, it is strongly associated with ulcerative colitis.
The chronic inflammation can ultimately progress to cirrhosis and
end-stage liver disease.

Clinical Manifestations

The onset of cirrhosis is usually insidious. Occasionally there is an
abrupt onset of symptoms.

- Early symptoms can include anorexia, dyspepsia, flatulence,
  nausea and vomiting, and change in bowel habits (diarrhea
  or constipation). In addition, fever, lassitude, abdominal
  pain, slight weight loss, and enlargement of the liver and
  spleen may occur.
- Later manifestations may be severe and result from liver
  failure and portal hypertension. Jaundice, peripheral edema,
  and ascites develop gradually. Other late symptoms include
  skin lesions, hematologic disorders, endocrine disturbances,
  and peripheral neuropathies. In advanced stages the liver
  becomes small and nodular. (See Fig. 44-6, Lewis et al,

Medical-Surgical Nursing, ed 8, p. 1074, for systemic manifestations of cirrhosis.)

- *Jaundice* occurs as a result of the decreased ability of the liver to conjugate and excrete bilirubin (hepatocellular jaundice).
- *Skin lesions* such as *spider angiomas* that occur on the nose, cheeks, upper trunk, and neck and a redness of the palms of the hands, known as *palmar erythema,* result from an increase in circulating estrogen because the liver cannot metabolize steroid hormones.
- *Hematologic disorders* such as anemia, leukopenia, and thrombocytopenia can result from splenomegaly. Splenomegaly results from backup of blood from the portal vein into the spleen (portal hypertension). Coagulation problems result from the liver's inability to produce prothrombin and other coagulation factors.
- Endocrine problems result because adrenocortical hormones, estrogen, and testosterone cannot be metabolized and inactivated by a damaged liver. Men lose masculine sex characteristics as a result of increased estrogen levels and amenorrhea may occur in women. Sodium and water retention and potassium loss occur as a result of hyperaldosteronism.
- *Peripheral neuropathy* is probably caused by a deficiency of thiamine, folic acid, and cobalamin.

Complications

Major complications are portal hypertension with resultant esophageal and/or gastric varices, peripheral edema and ascites, hepatic encephalopathy (coma), and hepatorenal syndrome.

Portal hypertension and *esophageal* and *gastric varices* result because of structural liver changes from cirrhosis; there is compression and destruction of the portal and hepatic veins and sinusoids. Pathophysiologic changes resulting from portal hypertension include the development of collateral circulation in an attempt to reduce high portal pressure and also to reduce increased plasma volume and lymphatic flow.

- Common areas where collateral channels form are the lower esophagus, anterior abdominal wall, parietal peritoneum, and rectum.
- Varicosities may develop in areas where collateral and systemic circulations communicate, resulting in esophageal and gastric varices, *caput medusae* (ring of varices around the umbilicus), and hemorrhoids.

Esophageal varices are a complex of tortuous veins at the end of the esophagus, which are enlarged and swollen as a result of portal hypertension. *Gastric varices* are located in the upper portion (cardia, fundus) of the stomach. These collateral vessels contain little elastic tissue and are quite fragile. They tolerate high pressure poorly, and the result is distended veins that bleed easily.

- Bleeding esophageal varices are the most life-threatening complication of cirrhosis.
- Varices rupture and bleed in response to ulceration and irritation. Factors producing ulceration and irritation include alcohol ingestion; swallowing of poorly masticated food; ingestion of coarse food; acid regurgitation from the stomach; and increased intraabdominal pressure caused by nausea, vomiting, straining at stool, coughing, sneezing, or lifting heavy objects.
- Patients may have melena or hematemesis. There may be slow oozing or massive bleeding, which is a medical emergency.

Peripheral edema results from decreased colloidal osmotic pressure from impaired liver synthesis of albumin and increased portocaval pressure from portal hypertension. Peripheral edema occurs as ankle and presacral edema.

Ascites is the accumulation of serous fluid in the peritoneal or abdominal cavity. With portal hypertension, proteins move from the blood vessels by way of larger pores of the sinusoids (capillaries) into the lymph space. When the lymphatic system is unable to carry off excess proteins and water, proteins leak into the peritoneal cavity. A second mechanism is hypoalbuminemia and decreased colloidal oncotic pressure resulting from the inability of the liver to synthesize albumin. A third mechanism is hyperaldosteronism, which results when aldosterone is not metabolized by damaged hepatocytes, causing increased renal reabsorption of sodium and water.

- Ascites is manifested by abdominal distention with weight gain. If ascites is severe, the umbilicus may be everted. Abdominal striae with distended abdominal wall veins may be present.
- The patient has signs of dehydration (e.g., dry tongue and skin, sunken eyeballs, muscle weakness), with a decrease in urinary output.
- Hypokalemia is common and is caused by an excessive loss of potassium from hyperaldosteronism and the use of diuretic therapy to treat ascites.

Hepatic encephalopathy is a neuropsychiatric manifestation of liver disease. It is considered a terminal complication.

Encephalopathy can occur in any condition in which liver damage causes ammonia to enter the systemic circulation without liver detoxification.

- When blood is shunted past the liver by way of collateral anastomoses or the liver is unable to convert ammonia to urea, the levels of ammonia in the systemic circulation rise. Ammonia crosses the blood-brain barrier and produces neurologic manifestations.
- Factors that increase ammonia in the circulation include gastrointestinal (GI) hemorrhage, constipation, infection, hypokalemia, hypovolemia, dehydration, and metabolic alkalosis.
- Hepatic encephalopathy is manifested by changes in neurologic and mental responsiveness, ranging from sleep disturbance to lethargy to deep coma. A characteristic symptom is *asterixis* (flapping tremor), a rapid flexion and extension movement of the hands when the arms and hands are held stretched out.

Hepatorenal syndrome is a serious complication of cirrhosis. It is characterized by functional renal failure with advancing azotemia, oliguria, and intractable ascites.

- There is no structural abnormality of the kidneys. The etiology is complex, but the final common pathway is usually portal hypertension along with liver decompensation that results in splanchnic and systemic vasodilation and decreased arterial blood volume. As a result, renal vasoconstriction occurs and renal failure follows.
- This syndrome frequently follows diuretic therapy, GI hemorrhage, or paracentesis.

Diagnostic Studies

- Liver function studies demonstrate an elevation in alkaline phosphatase, aspartate aminotransferase (AST), alanine aminotransferase (ALT), and γ-glutamyl transferase (GGT).
- Liver biopsy (percutaneous needle) and scan are done.
- Prothrombin time is prolonged.
- Serum albumin and protein levels are decreased, and bilirubin and globulin levels are increased.
- Differential analysis of ascitic fluid may be helpful in establishing a diagnosis.

Collaborative Care

At this time the goal of treatment is to slow the progress of cirrhosis. It has long been thought that rest may promote liver cell regeneration by decreasing metabolic demand on the liver.

Although there is no specific therapy for cirrhosis, certain measures can be taken to promote liver cell regeneration and prevent or treat complications.

Management of ascites is focused on sodium restriction (250 to 500 mg/day for severe ascites), diuretic therapy (e.g., a potassium-sparing diuretic combined with a loop diuretic), and fluid removal (paracentesis) for those patients with impaired respiration or abdominal pain. Peritoneovenous shunt insertion provides for the continuous reinfusion of ascitic fluid into the venous system. Transjugular intrahepatic portosystemic shunt (TIPS) is also used to alleviate ascites. Rifaximin (Xifaxan) may be used to treat hepatic encephalopathy.

The main therapeutic goal related to esophageal varices is avoidance of bleeding and hemorrhage. The patient who has esophageal or gastric varices should avoid ingesting alcohol, aspirin, and irritating foods. Upper respiratory infections should be treated promptly, and coughing should be controlled. For patients who have not bled from esophageal or gastric varices, prophylactic treatment with nonselective β blockers (e.g., propranolol [Inderal]) has been shown to reduce the risk of bleeding.

- When variceal bleeding occurs, the first step is to stabilize the patient and manage the airway. IV therapy is initiated and may include administration of blood products. Drug therapy may include somatostatin analog octreotide (Sandostatin), vasopressin (VP), nitroglycerin (NTG), β-adrenergic blockers, balloon tamponade, sclerotherapy, ligation of varices, and TIPS therapy.
- Supportive measures during an acute variceal bleed include administration of fresh frozen plasma and packed red blood cells (RBCs), vitamin K (AquaMEPHYTON), and histamine blockers such as cimetidine (Tagamet). Neomycin or lactulose (Cephulac) administration may be started to prevent hepatic encephalopathy from the breakdown of blood and the release of ammonia in the intestine.

The goal of management in hepatic encephalopathy is the reduction of ammonia formation. Lactulose (Cephulac) discourages bacterial growth, traps ammonia in the gut, and expels ammonia from the colon. Antibiotics (e.g., neomycin) reduce the bacterial flora of the colon. Bacterial action on protein in the feces results in ammonia production. Cathartics and enemas are also used to decrease bacterial action. Constipation should be prevented.

- Control of hepatic encephalopathy also involves treating GI bleeding and removing blood from the GI tract to decrease protein in the intestine. Electrolyte and acid-base imbalances and infections should also be treated.

Additional Management

A number of medications may be used to treat symptoms and complications of advanced liver disease (see Table 44-15, Lewis et al, *Medical-Surgical Nursing*, ed 8, p. 1080). Specific nutritional therapy varies with the degree of liver damage and the danger of encephalopathy; generally, the diet is high in calories (3000 cal/ day) and carbohydrates with sodium restricted. Protein restriction is rarely justified in patients with persistent hepatic encephalopathy because malnutrition is a more serious clinical problem than hepatic encephalopathy for many of these patients.

Nursing Management

Goals

The patient with cirrhosis will have relief of discomfort, have minimal to no complications (ascites, esophageal varices, hepatic encephalopathy), and return to as normal a lifestyle as possible.

See NCP 44-2 for the patient with cirrhosis, Lewis et al, *Medical-Surgical Nursing*, ed 8, pp. 1082 to 1083.

Nursing Diagnoses/Collaborative Problems

- Imbalanced nutrition: less than body requirement
- Excess fluid volume
- Impaired skin integrity
- Dysfunctional family processes
- Potential complication: hemorrhage
- Potential complication: hepatic encephalopathy

Nursing Interventions

Prevention and early treatment of cirrhosis must focus on reducing or eliminating risk factors.

- Alcoholism must be treated; adequate nutrition, especially for the alcoholic and other individuals at risk for cirrhosis, is essential to promote liver regeneration.
- Identify and treat acute hepatitis early so that it does not progress to chronic hepatitis.
- For those being treated for chronic active hepatitis, encourage compliance with drug regimens.
- Biliary disease must be treated so that stones do not cause obstruction and infection.
- Bariatric surgery for morbidly obese individuals has been shown to reduce liver fibrosis.
- The underlying cause (e.g., chronic lung disease) of right-sided heart failure must be treated so that the heart failure does not lead to cirrhosis.

The focus of nursing care is on conserving the patient's strength. Rest enables the liver to restore itself. Complete bed rest may not always be necessary.

- Anorexia, nausea and vomiting, pressure from ascites, and poor eating habits create problems in maintaining an adequate intake of nutrients. Make between-meal nourishments available so that they can be taken at times when the patient can best tolerate them. Provide food preferences whenever possible.
- The patient's physiologic response to cirrhosis should be assessed, including the presence and progression of jaundice, any pruritus, and urine and stool color.
- Accurate recordings of intake and output, daily weights, and measurements of extremities and abdominal girth help in the ongoing assessment of edema.
- When the patient is taking diuretics, monitor the serum levels of sodium, potassium, chloride, and bicarbonate.
- A semi-Fowler's or Fowler's position allows for maximal respiratory efficiency when dyspnea is a problem. Use pillows to support arms and chest as they will increase patient comfort and ability to breathe.
- Meticulous skin care is essential because edematous tissues are subject to breakdown. Use an alternating air pressure mattress or other special mattress. A turning schedule (minimum of every 2 hours) must be adhered to rigidly. Support the abdomen with pillows.
- When a paracentesis is done, have the patient void immediately before the procedure to prevent puncture of the bladder. After the procedure, monitor for hypovolemia and electrolyte imbalances, and check the dressing for bleeding and leakage.
- If the patient has esophageal and/or gastric varices, monitor for signs of bleeding from varices, such as hematemesis and melena. If hematemesis occurs, assess the patient for hemorrhage, call the physician, and be ready to assist with treatments to control bleeding.
- The focus of care with hepatic encephalopathy is on sustaining life and assisting with measures to reduce the formation of ammonia. Factors known to precipitate encephalopathy should be controlled as much as possible.

▼ **Patient and Caregiver Teaching**
The patient and caregiver need to understand the importance of continuous health care and medical supervision. Teach the patient and caregiver about symptoms of complications and when to seek medical attention.

- Abstinence from alcohol is important and results in improvement in most patients. Provide information regarding community support programs such as Alcoholics Anonymous for help with alcohol abuse.

- Explain both verbally and in writing information about fluid or possible dietary changes to the patient and the caregiver.
- Instruct on the importance of adequate rest periods, skin care, drug therapy precautions, observation for bleeding, and protection from infection.
- Referral to a community or home health nurse may be helpful to ensure adequate patient adherence with prescribed therapy.

COLORECTAL CANCER

Description
Colorectal cancer is the third most common form of cancer and the second leading cause of cancer-related death in the United States. Because symptoms do not appear until the disease is quite advanced, regular screening is necessary to detect precancerous lesions. About 85% of colorectal cancers arise from adenomatous polyps that can be detected and removed from the colon by sigmoidoscopy or colonoscopy.

Pathophysiology
Colorectal cancer may occur at any age but is most prevalent over the age of 50 years. Major risk factors include increasing age, family or personal history of colorectal cancer, colorectal polyps, and inflammatory bowel disease. Certain lifestyle factors are also associated with colorectal cancer including obesity, smoking, alcohol, and a large intake of red meat.

- Physical exercise and a diet with large amounts of fruits, vegetables, and grains may decrease the risk.
- Nonsteroidal antiinflammatory drugs (NSAIDs) (e.g., aspirin) and hormone replacement therapy in women may also decrease the risk.

Adenocarcinoma is the most common type of colorectal cancer. Typically it begins as adenomatous polyps. All tumors tend to spread through the walls of the intestine and into the lymphatic system. Because venous blood leaving the colon and rectum flows through the portal vein and the inferior rectal vein, the liver is a common site of metastasis. The cancer can also spread directly into adjacent structures. Complications include obstruction, bleeding, perforation, peritonitis, and fistula formation.

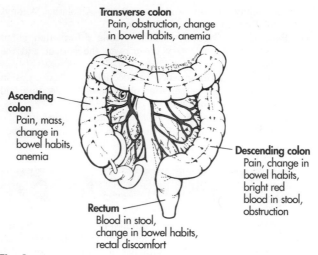

Transverse colon
Pain, obstruction, change
in bowel habits, anemia

**Ascending
colon**
Pain, mass,
change in
bowel habits,
anemia

Descending colon
Pain, change in
bowel habits,
bright red
blood in stool,
obstruction

Rectum
Blood in stool,
change in bowel habits,
rectal discomfort

Fig. 3. Signs and symptoms of colorectal cancer by location of primary tumor.

Clinical Manifestations

Manifestations are usually nonspecific or do not appear until the disease is advanced. Cancer on the right side of the colon has manifestations that differ from those on the left side of the colon (Fig. 3).

- Rectal bleeding, the most common symptom of colorectal cancer, is most often seen with left-sided lesions. Other manifestations of left-sided lesions include alternating constipation and diarrhea, change in stool caliber (narrow, ribbonlike), and sensation of incomplete evacuation. Obstruction symptoms appear earlier with left-sided lesions.
- Cancers on the right side are usually asymptomatic. Vague abdominal discomfort or crampy, colicky abdominal pain may be present. Iron deficiency anemia and occult bleeding lead to weakness and fatigue.

Diagnostic Studies

- Colonoscopy: the screening procedure of choice to examine the entire colon, obtain biopsy specimens, remove polyps, and detect colorectal lesions
- Fecal occult blood tests

- Complete blood count (CBC), coagulation studies, and liver function tests when diagnosis is confirmed by colonoscopy and biopsy
- Computed tomography (CT) scan or magnetic resonance imaging (MRI) of abdomen and pelvis to detect liver metastases
- Carcinoembryonic antigen (CEA) serum test as a baseline to follow progress of patient after surgery or chemotherapy

Collaborative Care

- Prognosis and treatment correlate with the pathologic staging of the disease. The TNM staging system is the most commonly used method to stage the tumor (see p. 799). As with other cancers, prognosis worsens with greater size and depth of tumor, lymph node involvement, and metastasis.

Surgical Therapy

Surgery is the only cure. Surgical goals include complete resection of the tumor with adequate margins of healthy tissue, a thorough exploration of the abdomen to detect spread, removal of all lymph nodes that drain the cancer area, restoration of bowel continuity so that normal bowel function will return, and prevention of surgical complications.

- Polypectomy during colonoscopy can be used to resect colorectal cancer in situ
- The surgical decision involves concerns about the location and staging of the cancer, the restoration of normal bowel function and continence, and preservation of genitourinary function. Most patients need a low anterior resection (LAR) to preserve sphincter function or an abdominal perineal resection (APR).
- When the tumor is not resectable or if metastasis is present, palliative surgery is done to control hemorrhage or relieve an obstruction.

Chemotherapy and Targeted Therapy

Chemotherapy is recommended when the patient has positive lymph nodes at the time of surgery or has metastatic disease. Chemotherapy can be used to shrink the tumor before surgery, as adjuvant therapy following colon resection, and as palliative treatment for nonresectable disease (see Chemotherapy, p. 717). Current chemotherapy protocols include a variety of drugs that are combined with 5-fluorouracil (5-FU) and leucovorin. The combinations are given names such as FOLFOX (5-FU plus leucovorin and oxaliplatin) and FOLFIRI (5FU plus leucovorin and irinotecan). Oxaliplatin (Eloxatin) is also used for metastatic disease.

Bevacizumab (Avastin) prevents the formation of new blood vessels, a process known as *angiogenesis*. It can be used alone or in conjunction with other chemotherapeutic agents. Cetuximab (Erbitux) and panitumumab (Vectibix) block the epidermal growth factor receptor (EGFR). They are used in the treatment of metastatic disease.

Radiation Therapy

Radiation may be used postoperatively as an adjunct to colon resection and chemotherapy or as a palliative measure for patients with advanced lesions. As a palliative measure, it helps to reduce the tumor size and provide symptomatic relief.

Nursing Management

Goals

The patient with colorectal cancer will have normal bowel elimination patterns, quality of life appropriate to disease progression, relief of pain, and feelings of comfort and well-being.

Nursing Diagnoses

- Diarrhea or constipation
- Acute pain
- Fear
- Ineffective coping

Nursing Interventions

Encourage all patients over 50 to have regular colorectal cancer screening. Screening for high-risk patients should begin before age 50, usually beginning with colonoscopy and continuing at more frequent intervals that vary according to risk factors.

Preoperative care. Nursing care for patients with a colon resection is similar to the care of the patient having a laparotomy (see Abdominal Pain, Acute, p. 3). Patients who have an APR will have a permanent ostomy and will consequently need intense emotional support to cope with their prognosis and the change in body appearance and function.

Postoperative care. Many patients will have immediate reanastomosis of bowel and will require general postoperative care. Patients with more extensive surgery (e.g., APR) may have an open wound and drains (e.g., Jackson-Pratt, Hemovac) as well as a permanent stoma.

Postoperative care includes sterile dressing changes, care of drains, and patient and caregiver education about the stoma. A wound and ostomy care nurse should be consulted about care.

- A patient who has open and packed wounds requires meticulous postoperative care. Reinforce dressings and change them frequently during the first several hours postoperatively. Carefully assess all drainage for amount, color, and consistency. Examine the wound regularly and record bleeding, excessive drainage, and unusual odor.

- The patient may experience phantom rectal sensation because the sympathetic nerves responsible for rectal control are not severed during the surgery. Be astute in distinguishing phantom sensations from perineal abscess pain.
- Sexual dysfunction is a possible complication of an abdominal-perineal resection. Although the likelihood of sexual dysfunction depends on the surgical technique used, the surgeon should discuss the possibility with the patient.

▼ **Patient and Caregiver Teaching**

- The patient and caregiver should be aware of community resources and services available for assistance.
- Patients with colostomies will need to know how to care for them.
- Patients and caregivers need to know about diet, incontinence products, and strategies for managing bloating, diarrhea, and bowel evacuation. They may need to experiment with their diets to find the foods that provide the best stool consistency, and will need to find the medications that are best able to control diarrhea and constipation.

CONJUNCTIVITIS

Description

Conjunctivitis is an inflammation or infection of the conjunctiva. Conjunctivitis may be caused by bacteria or viruses, and inflammation can result from exposure to allergens or chemical irritants (including cigarette smoke). The tarsal conjunctiva (lining of the lid's interior surface) may become inflamed as a result of a long-term foreign body in the eye, such as a contact lens or an ocular prosthesis. See Table 28 for a comparison of the clinical manifestations and management of the different types of conjunctivitis.

CONSTIPATION

Description

Constipation is a decrease in the frequency of bowel movements from what is normal for the individual. Constipation also includes hard, difficult-to-pass stool; a decrease in stool volume; and/or retention of feces in the rectum.

- Frequently constipation may result from insufficient dietary fiber, inadequate fluid intake, decreased physical activity,

Table 28 Types of Conjunctivitis

Description	Clinical Manifestations	Management
Bacterial ■ Acute bacterial conjunctivitis (pinkeye) ■ More common in children and most commonly caused by *Staphylococcus aureus*	Irritation, tearing, redness, mucopurulent drainage; rapid spread from one eye to the other	■ Usually self-limiting, but antibiotic drops will shorten course ■ Prevent spread with careful hand washing and use of individual or disposable towels
Viral ■ Caused by many different viruses ■ Adenovirus conjunctivitis contracted by direct contact with infected person and in contaminated swimming pools	Tearing, foreign body sensation, redness, mild photophobia; usually mild and self-limiting but can be severe with increased discomfort and subconjunctival hemorrhaging	■ Treatment usually palliative ■ Topical corticosteroids provide temporary relief if patient is severely symptomatic, but have no benefit in outcome ■ Antiviral drops ineffective ■ Encourage good hygiene practices

C

Chlamydial

- Chlamydia trachomatis (serotypes A–C) causes trachoma, a chronic conjunctivitis that is a major cause of blindness
- Adult inclusion conjunctivitis (AIC) caused by *Chlamydia trachomatis* (serotypes D–K) is increasing with rise in chlamydial infections

Mucopurulent ocular discharge, irritation, redness, lid swelling; AIC does not lead to blindness as does trachoma

- Antibiotic therapy usually effective for both trachoma and AIC
- Patients with AIC have a high risk of concurrent chlamydial genital infection and other sexually transmitted diseases.
- Teach about ocular condition and sexual implications of condition necessary

Allergic

- Conjunctivitis may develop in response to exposure to pollens, animal dander, ocular solutions, contact lenses, or other allergens

Itching (defining symptom), burning, redness, tearing, and white or clear exudate; severe responses cause significant swelling that may cause ballooning of the conjunctiva beyond eyelids

- Artificial tears to dilute allergen and wash from eye
- Effective topical medications include antihistamines and corticosteroids
- Teach to avoid allergen if known

and ignoring the urge to defecate. Many medications, especially opioids, cause constipation. Constipation occurs with many diseases that slow gastrointestinal (GI) transit, such as diabetes mellitus, Parkinson's disease, and multiple sclerosis. Depression and stress can also result in constipation. Long-term laxative use causes *cathartic colon syndrome,* resulting in a dilated and atonic colon that does not empty without a laxative.

Clinical Manifestations

Constipation may vary from a chronic discomfort to an acute event mimicking an acute abdomen. Stools are absent or hard, dry, and difficult to pass. Abdominal distention, bloating, increased flatulence, and increased rectal pressure may also be present.

- Hemorrhoids are the most common complication of chronic constipation. They result from venous engorgement resulting from repeated Valsalva maneuvers (straining) and venous compression from hard impacted stool (see Hemorrhoids, p. 301).
- Diverticulosis is another potential complication of chronic constipation (see Diverticulosis/Diverticulitis, p. 196).
- In the presence of obstipation (fecal impaction secondary to constipation), colonic perforation may occur. Perforation, which is life threatening, causes abdominal pain, nausea, vomiting, fever, and an elevated white blood cell (WBC) count.

Diagnostic Studies

A thorough history and physical examination should be performed so the underlying cause can be identified.

- Abdominal x-rays, barium enema, colonoscopy, sigmoidoscopy, and anorectal manometry may be helpful in the diagnosis.

Collaborative Care

Most cases of constipation can be managed with diet therapy, including fiber and fluids, and an exercise program. Laxatives and enemas may be used to treat acute constipation but are used cautiously because overuse leads to chronic constipation.

- Methylnaltrexone (Relistor) is a peripheral μ-receptor antagonist that reduces constipation caused by opioid use. It is administered subcutaneously.
- Enemas are fast acting and beneficial for immediate treatment of constipation, but should be limited for long-term

treatment. Soapsuds enemas produce inflammation of colon mucosa, tap water enemas can lead to water intoxication, and sodium phosphate enemas may cause electrolyte imbalances in some patients.

- Biofeedback therapy may benefit patients who are constipated as a result of anismus (uncoordinated contraction of the anal sphincter during straining).
- The patient with severe constipation related to a motility or mechanical disorder may require more intensive treatment. In a patient with unrelenting constipation, a subtotal colectomy with ileorectal anastomosis is the procedure of choice.

Many patients experience an improvement in their symptoms when they increase their intake of dietary fiber and fluids. The diet should include fluid intake of at least 2000 mL/day unless contraindicated by cardiac or renal disease.

Nursing Management

Goals
The patient with constipation will increase dietary intake of fiber and fluids; increase physical activity; pass soft, formed stools; and not have any complications, such as bleeding hemorrhoids.

Nursing Diagnosis
- Constipation

Nursing Interventions
Interventions should be based on the assessment and symptoms of the patient.

- Proper position is important when defecating. For a patient in bed, the head of the bed should be elevated as high as the patient can tolerate. For the person who can sit on a toilet, a footstool may be placed in front of the toilet. Placing feet on a footstool promotes flexion of the hips, which assists in defecation.
- Encourage patients to exercise the abdominal muscles and contract the abdominal muscles several times each day. Sit-ups and straight leg raises can also be used to improve abdominal muscle tone.

▼ Patient and Caregiver Teaching
- Teach the patient the importance of dietary measures to prevent constipation. Emphasize the maintenance of a high-fiber diet, increased fluid intake, and a regular exercise program.
- Teach the patient to establish a regular time to defecate and not suppress the urge to defecate.
- Discourage the patient from using laxatives and enemas to achieve fecal elimination.

COR PULMONALE

Description

Cor pulmonale is enlargement of the right ventricle (RV) secondary to diseases of the lung, thorax, or pulmonary circulation. Pulmonary hypertension is usually a preexisting condition in the individual with cor pulmonale. Cor pulmonale may be present with or without overt cardiac failure.

- The most common cause of cor pulmonale is chronic obstructive pulmonary disease (COPD) (see p. 127). Almost any disorder that affects the respiratory system can cause cor pulmonale.

Clinical Manifestations

Manifestations include dyspnea, lethargy, and fatigue.

- Physical signs include evidence of right ventricular hypertrophy on ECG and an increase in intensity of the second heart sound. Chronic hypoxemia leads to polycythemia.
- If heart failure accompanies cor pulmonale, additional manifestations include peripheral edema; weight gain; distended neck veins; full, bounding pulse; and enlarged liver.
- Chest x-ray shows an enlarged RV and pulmonary artery.

Collaborative Care

Management is directed at treating the underlying pulmonary problem. Long-term, low-flow oxygen (O_2) therapy is used to correct hypoxemia and reduce vasoconstriction and pulmonary hypertension.

- If fluid, electrolyte, and acid-base imbalances are present, they must be corrected. Diuretics and a low-sodium diet will help to decrease the plasma volume and the load on the heart.
- Bronchodilator therapy is indicated if the underlying respiratory problem is caused by an obstructive disorder.
- Theophylline may help because of its weak inotropic effect on the heart.
- Other treatments include those for pulmonary hypertension such as vasodilator therapy, calcium channel blockers, and anticoagulants.
- When medical treatment fails, lung transplantation may be an option.

Long-term management of cor pulmonale resulting from COPD is similar to that described for COPD (see p. 127).

CORONARY ARTERY DISEASE

Description

Coronary artery disease (CAD) is a type of blood vessel disorder that is included in the general category of atherosclerosis. Atherosclerosis is derived from two Greek words: *athero,* meaning "fatty mush," and *skleros,* meaning "hard." Atherosclerosis is often referred to as "hardening of the arteries." Although this condition can occur in any artery in the body, the atheromas (fatty deposits) prefer the coronary arteries.

- Arteriosclerotic heart disease, cardiovascular heart disease, ischemic heart disease, coronary heart disease, and CAD are synonymous terms used to describe this disorder.
- Cardiovascular disease is the major cause of death in the United States. CAD is the most common type of cardiovascular disease and accounts for the majority of these deaths.
- Patients with CAD may be asymptomatic or develop *chronic stable angina.*
- More serious manifestations of CAD include *unstable angina (UA)* and *myocardial infarction (MI).* These manifestations are termed *acute coronary syndrome (ACS).*

Figure 1 on p. 6 illustrates the relationship among the clinical manifestations of CAD.

Risk factors for CAD can be categorized as nonmodifiable and modifiable (Table 29).

Pathophysiology

Atherosclerosis is the major cause of CAD. It is characterized by a focal deposit of cholesterol and lipids, primarily within the arterial intimal wall. Plaque formation is the result of complex interactions between components of the blood and the elements forming the vascular wall. Inflammation and endothelial injury play a central role in the development of atherosclerosis.

- The endothelial lining can be injured as a result of tobacco use, hyperlipidemia, hypertension, diabetes, hyperhomocystinemia, and infection (e.g., *Chlamydia pneumoniae,* herpes) causing a local inflammatory response.
- C-reactive protein (CRP) is a nonspecific marker of inflammation. It is increased in many patients with CAD with the level rising when there is systemic inflammation.
- CAD takes many years to develop. When it becomes symptomatic, the disease process is usually well advanced. Stages of development in atherosclerosis are (1) fatty streak,

Table 29	Risk Factors for Coronary Artery Disease

Nonmodifiable Risk Factors	Modifiable Risk Factors
Increasing Age Gender (men > women until 65 yr of age) Ethnicity (whites > African Americans) Genetic predisposition and family history of heart disease	**Major** Serum lipids: ■ Total cholesterol >200 mg/dL ■ Triglycerides ≥150 mg/dL* ■ LDL cholesterol >160 mg/dL ■ HDL cholesterol <40 mg/dL in men or <50 mg/dL in women* Blood pressure: ≥140/90 mm Hg* Diabetes mellitus Tobacco use Physical inactivity Obesity: Waist circumference ≥102 cm (≥40 inches) in men and ≥88 cm (≥35 inches) in women* **Contributing** Fasting blood glucose ≥100 mg/dL* Psychosocial risk factors (e.g., depression, hostility and anger, stress) Elevated homocysteine levels

HDL, High-density lipoprotein; *LDL*, low-density lipoprotein.
*Three or more of these risk factors meet the criteria for metabolic syndrome as defined by the National Cholesterol Education Program Adult Treatment Panel III.

(2) fibrous plaque resulting from smooth muscle cell proliferation, and (3) complicated lesion.

Figure 34-1, Lewis et al., *Medical-Surgical Nursing,* ed 8, p. 762 illustrates the progression of atherosclerosis.

Normally some arterial anastomoses or connections, termed collateral circulation, exist within the coronary circulation.

■ When occlusion of the coronary arteries occurs slowly over a long period, the myocardium may still receive an adequate amount of blood and oxygen. However, with rapid-onset CAD (e.g., familial hypercholesterolemia) or coronary spasm, the time is inadequate for collateral development, and a diminished arterial flow results in a more severe ischemia or infarction.

Clinical Manifestations

CAD is a progressive disease, and patients may be asymptomatic for many years or they may develop chronic stable angina. When the demand for myocardial oxygen exceeds the ability of the coronary arteries to supply the heart with oxygen, myocardial ischemia occurs.

- Angina, or chest pain, is the clinical manifestation of reversible myocardial ischemia. The primary reason for insufficient blood flow is narrowing of coronary arteries by atherosclerosis.

C

- Chronic stable angina refers to chest pain that occurs intermittently over a long period with the same pattern of onset, duration, and intensity of symptoms (see Angina, Chronic Stable, p. 45).
- When ischemia is prolonged and not immediately reversible, acute coronary syndrome (ACS) develops (see Acute Coronary Syndrome, p. 5). ACS encompasses the following spectrum:
  - Unstable angina (UA): chest pain that is new in onset, occurs at rest, or has a worsening pattern. UA represents an emergency
  - Non–ST-segment elevation myocardial infarction (NSTEMI): irreversible myocardial cell death caused by deterioration of an atherosclerotic plaque and lesion *partially* occluded by a thrombus
  - ST-segment elevation myocardial infarction (STEMI): irreversible myocardial cell death caused by deterioration of an atherosclerotic plaque and lesion *totally* occluded by a thrombus

Diagnostic Studies

- Chest x-ray to detect cardiac enlargement, cardiac calcifications, and pulmonary congestion
- 12-lead electrocardiogram (ECG) detect heart rhythm, pacemaker activity, conduction abnormalities, position of heart, size of atria and ventricles, and presence of ischemia/injury/infarction
- Serum lipid levels to screen for positive risk factors
- Exercise or stress testing to detect ST-segment and T-wave changes that indicate ischemia with exercise
- Ambulatory 24- to 48-hour ECG monitoring to identify silent ischemia
- Nuclear imaging studies to determine myocardial perfusion, contractility, and ejection fraction
- Positron emission tomography (PET) to identify and quantify ischemia and infarction

- Angiography studies for visualization of coronary arteries to help determine treatment and prognosis
- Echocardiography with exercise to diagnose coronary artery stenosis

See Chapter 32 and Table 32-6 for a discussion of these studies, including nursing considerations, in Lewis et al., *Medical-Surgical Nursing,* ed 8, pp. 728 to 732.

Collaborative Care

Management of CAD involves modification of risk factors to prevent, modify, or retard disease progression. The risk of CAD can be decreased by maintaining an ideal body weight, getting adequate physical exercise, reducing intake of saturated fats, and avoiding tobacco use. The FITT formula (Frequency, Intensity, Type, and Time) is designed to improve physical fitness, and the Therapeutic Lifestyle Changes Diet is recommended to reduce LDL cholesterol levels and maintain ideal body weight. Specific diet recommendations and plans are presented in Tables 34-4 and 34-5 in Lewis et al., *Medical-Surgical Nursing,* ed 8, p. 768. Drug therapy may be started if diet therapy has not been successful in decreasing serum cholesterol levels.

Drug Therapy
Various drugs are available to treat hyperlipidemia. The statin drugs are the most widely used lipid-lowering drugs. Examples include lovastatin (Mevacor), pravastatin (Pravachol), simvastatin (Zocor), fluvastatin (Lescol), atorvastatin (Lipitor), and rosuvastatin (Crestor). These drugs inhibit the synthesis of cholesterol in the liver by blocking hydroxy-methyl-glutaryl coenzyme A (HMG-CoA) reductase. These drugs primarily lower low-density lipoprotein (LDL) cholesterol and also cause an increase in high-density lipoprotein (HDL). Niacin (Nicobid), a water-soluble B vitamin, also interferes with the synthesis of LDL and triglyceride levels.

Fibric acid derivatives such as gemfibrozil (Lopid) are effective in lowering very-low-density lipoprotein (VLDL) levels and triglycerides, while increasing HDL levels. Drugs that increase lipoprotein removal by increasing conversion of cholesterol to bile acids include cholestyramine (Questran), colestipol (Colestid), and colesevelam (Welchol) and are commonly used. Ezetimibe (Zetia) inhibits the absorption of dietary and biliary cholesterol across the intestinal wall and may be combined with a statin to promote greater reductions in LDL.

- Drug therapy for hyperlipidemia often continues for a lifetime. It is essential that diet modification be used to minimize the need for drug therapy. The patient must fully understand the rationale and goals of treatment as well as drug safety and side effects.

Antiplatelet therapy with low-dose aspirin (e.g., 81 mg) is recommended for most people at risk for CAD unless contraindicated (e.g., history of GI bleeding). For people who are aspirin intolerant, clopidogrel (Plavix) can be considered.

Nursing Management

Regardless of the health care setting, you are well suited to identify the person at risk for CAD. Risk screening involves obtaining personal and family health histories. You should question the patient about a family history of heart disease in parents and siblings. Note the presence of any cardiovascular symptoms.

Assess environmental factors, such as eating habits, type of diet, and level of exercise, to elicit lifestyle patterns. A psychosocial history is included to determine tobacco use, alcohol ingestion, recent life-stressing events (e.g., loss of a spouse), and the presence of any negative psychologic states (e.g., anxiety, depression, anger). Place of work and the type of work provides important information on the kind of activity performed, exposure to pollutants or noxious chemicals, and the degree of emotional stress associated with employment.

- Identify patient attitudes and beliefs about health and illness. This information can give some indication of how disease and lifestyle changes may affect the patient and can reveal possible misconceptions about heart disease.
- Knowledge of the patient's educational background is frequently helpful in deciding at what level to begin teaching.
- If the patient is taking medications, it is important to know the names and dosages, and what the patient's compliance and attitudes are regarding the taking of medications.

CROHN'S DISEASE

Description

Crohn's disease is an autoimmune disorder that, along with ulcerative colitis, is referred to as *inflammatory bowel disease* (IBD). See Inflammatory Bowel Disease, p. 359 for a discussion of the disorder.

CUSHING SYNDROME

Description

Cushing syndrome is a spectrum of clinical abnormalities caused by excess corticosteroids, particularly glucocorticoids. Several conditions can cause Cushing syndrome; the most common cause is iatrogenic administration of exogenous corticosteroids (e.g., prednisone). Approximately 85% of the cases of endogenous Cushing syndrome result from an adrenocorticotropic hormone (ACTH)-secreting pituitary tumor *(Cushing disease)*.

- Other causes of Cushing syndrome include adrenal tumors and ectopic ACTH production by tumors outside the hypothalamic-pituitary-adrenal axis.

Clinical Manifestations

Manifestations can be seen in most body systems and are related to excess levels of corticosteroids (see Table 50-14, Lewis et al., *Medical-Surgical Nursing,* ed 8, p. 1277). Although manifestations of glucocorticoid excess usually predominate, symptoms of mineralocorticoid and androgen excess may also be seen.

- Corticosteroid excess causes pronounced changes in physical appearance. Weight gain, the most common feature, results from accumulation of adipose tissue in the trunk, face, and cervical neck area. Transient weight gain from sodium and water retention may be present because of the mineralocorticoid effects of cortisol. Hyperglycemia occurs because of glucose intolerance (associated with cortisol-induced insulin resistance) and increased gluconeogenesis by the liver.
- Protein wasting is caused by the catabolic effects of cortisol on peripheral tissue. Muscle wasting leads to muscle weakness, especially in the extremities. Loss of bone protein matrix leads to osteoporosis with pathologic fractures (e.g., vertebral compression fractures) and bone and back pain. Loss of collagen makes the skin weaker, thinner, and easier to bruise.
- Mineralocorticoid excess may cause hypertension, whereas adrenal androgen excess may cause pronounced acne, virilization in women, and feminization in men.

Clinical presentation, as revealed by the history and physical examination, is the first indication of Cushing syndrome. Of particular importance are a combination of centripetal obesity; "moon facies" (fullness of face); purplish red striae on abdomen, breast, or buttocks; hypertension; hirsutism and menstrual disorders in women; and unexplained hypokalemia.

Diagnostic Studies

- Plasma cortisol levels may be elevated with loss of diurnal variation.
- Plasma ACTH levels may be low, normal, or elevated, depending on the underlying problem.
- A 24-hour urine collection for free cortisol is done. Urine cortisol levels beyond the normal range of 80 to 120 mcg in 24 hours in adults indicate Cushing syndrome. If these results are borderline, a low-dose dexamethasone suppression test is done.
- Other findings on diagnostic tests associated with, but not diagnostic of, Cushing syndrome include hyperglycemia, hypokalemia, glycosuria, hypercalciuria, and osteoporosis.
- Computed tomography (CT) scan and magnetic resonance imaging (MRI) of the pituitary and adrenal glands may be done.

Collaborative Care

The primary goal is to normalize hormone secretion. The standard treatment for a pituitary adenoma is transsphenoidal hypophysectomy. Radiation to the pituitary adenoma may be necessary if surgical outcomes are not optimal or the patient is not a good surgical candidate. Adrenalectomy is indicated for adrenal tumors or hyperplasia. Patients with ectopic ACTH-secreting tumors (usually lung or pancreas) are managed by treating the neoplasm.

- Drug therapy is used when surgery is contraindicated or as an adjunct to surgery. The goal of drug therapy is inhibition of adrenal function *(medical adrenalectomy)*. Drugs that inhibit corticosteroid synthesis include ketoconazole (Nizoral) and aminoglutethimide (Cytadren).

If Cushing syndrome has developed during the course of prolonged administration of corticosteroids, one or more of the following alternatives may be tried: (1) gradual discontinuance of corticosteroid therapy, (2) reduction of corticosteroid dose, and (3) conversion to an alternate-day regimen.

Nursing Management

Goals

The patient with Cushing syndrome will experience relief of symptoms with no serious complications, maintain a positive self-image, and actively participate in the therapeutic plan.

Nursing Diagnoses

- Risk for infection
- Imbalanced nutrition: more than body requirements

- Chronic low self-esteem
- Impaired skin integrity

Nursing Interventions

Because the therapy for Cushing syndrome has many side effects, the focus of assessment is on the signs and symptoms of hormone and drug toxicity and on complicating conditions (e.g., cardiovascular disease, diabetes mellitus, and infection).

- Assess and monitor vital signs, glucose, and daily weights (gain possibly indicating volume excess)
- Signs and symptoms of inflammation (e.g., fever, redness) may be minimal or absent so assess for pain, loss of function, and purulent drainage.
- Monitor for signs of abnormal thromboembolic phenomena, such as sudden chest pain, dyspnea, and tachypnea

Another important focus of nursing care is emotional support. Changes in appearance, such as centripetal obesity, multiple bruises, hirsutism in females, and gynecomastia in males, can be distressing. You can help by remaining sensitive to the patient's feelings and offering respect and unconditional acceptance. Reassure patient that the physical changes and much of the emotional lability will resolve when hormone levels return to normal.

If treatment involves surgical removal of a pituitary adenoma, an adrenal tumor, or one or both adrenal glands, nursing care will have an additional focus on preoperative and postoperative care.

Preoperative care. Before surgery, hypertension and hyperglycemia need to be controlled, with hypokalemia corrected by diet and potassium supplements; a high-protein meal plan helps correct protein depletion.

Preoperative teaching depends on the type of surgical approach (hypophysectomy or adrenalectomy), but should include information regarding postoperative care the patient should anticipate.

- In the postoperative period (for both open and laparoscopic adrenalectomy), patients may have a nasogastric (NG) tube, urinary catheter, intravenous (IV) therapy, central venous pressure monitoring, and leg sequential compression devices to prevent emboli.

Postoperative care. Because of hormone fluctuations, the patient's blood pressure (BP), fluid balance, and electrolyte levels tend to be unstable after surgery. High doses of corticosteroids (hydrocortisone) are administered IV during surgery and for several days afterward to ensure adequate responses to the stress of the procedure.

- Report any rapid or significant changes in BP, respirations, or heart rate (HR).

- Carefully monitor fluid intake and output and assess for potential imbalance.
- If corticosteroid dosage is tapered too rapidly after surgery, acute adrenal insufficiency may develop. Vomiting, increased weakness, dehydration, and hypotension may indicate hypocortisolism. In addition, the patient may complain of painful joints, pruritus, or peeling skin and may experience severe emotional disturbances.

You must be constantly alert for signs of corticosteroid imbalance. After surgery the patient is usually maintained on bed rest until the BP stabilizes. Also be alert for subtle signs of postoperative infections. Provide meticulous care when changing the dressing and during any other procedures that necessitate access to body cavities, circulation, or areas under skin.

▼ **Patient and Caregiver Teaching**

Discharge instructions are based on the patient's lack of endogenous cortisol and resulting inability to react to stressors physiologically.

- Instruct patients to wear a Medic-Alert bracelet at all times and carry medical identification and instructions in a wallet or purse. Teach the patient to avoid exposure to extremes of temperature, infections, and emotional disturbances as much as possible.
- Stress may produce or precipitate acute adrenal insufficiency because the remaining adrenal tissue cannot meet an increased hormonal demand. Teach patients to adjust their corticosteroid replacement therapy in accordance with stress levels.
- If the patient cannot adjust his or her own medication or if weakness, fainting, fever, or nausea and vomiting occur, the patient should contact the health care provider for a possible adjustment in corticosteroid dosage.

Lifetime replacement therapy is required by many patients, but it may take several months to satisfactorily adjust the hormone dose.

CYSTIC FIBROSIS

Description

Cystic fibrosis (CF) is an autosomal recessive, multisystem disease characterized by altered function of the exocrine glands involving primarily the lungs, pancreas, and sweat glands.

The severity and progression of the disease vary from person to person. With early diagnosis and improvements in therapy, the prognosis has been significantly improved. The median predicted survival in 1970 was 16 years, but has currently increased to more than 37 years.

Pathophysiology

CF results from mutations in a gene located on chromosome 7 that produces a protein called CF transmembrane regulator (CFTR). CFTR regulates sodium and chloride channels in the lining of the exocrine portion of particular organs, such as airways, pancreatic duct, sweat gland duct, and reproductive tract. Mutations in the CFTR gene alter this protein in such a way that the channel is blocked.

- Cells that line the passageways of the lungs, pancreas, and other organs produce abnormally thick, sticky mucus. This mucus plugs up the glands in these organs and causes the glands to atrophy, ultimately resulting in organ failure.
- The hallmark of respiratory involvement is its effect on the airways. The disease progresses from being a disease of the small airways *(chronic bronchiolitis)* to involvement of the larger airways, and finally causes destruction of lung tissue. CF is also characterized by chronic airway infection that is difficult to eradicate. Lung disorders include chronic bronchiolitis and bronchitis that eventually lead to bronchiectasis, blebs, large cysts, and hemoptysis from erosion of pulmonary arteries.
- Pancreatic insufficiency is caused primarily by mucus plugging the pancreatic duct, which results in fibrosis of the acinar glands of the pancreas. Because pancreatic digestive enzymes cannot reach the intestine, malabsorption of fat, protein, and fat-soluble vitamins occurs.
- Fat malabsorption results in steatorrhea, and protein malabsorption results in failure to grow and gain weight.
- Diabetes mellitus may occur if the islets of Langerhans become fibrotic.
- Patients with CF secrete normal volumes of sweat, but are unable to absorb sodium chloride from sweat as it moves through the sweat duct. Therefore they excrete 4 times the normal amount of sodium and chloride in sweat. This abnormality rarely affects the health of the person, but it is useful in diagnosis.

Clinical Manifestations

Manifestations vary depending on the disease severity. Early childhood signs are failure to grow, clubbing, persistent cough with mucous production, tachypnea, and large, frequent bowel movements.

- In the adult, the first symptom is frequent cough that becomes persistent and produces viscous, purulent sputum.
- Over time exacerbations become frequent, bronchiectasis develops, and the recovery of lost lung function is less complete, ultimately leading to respiratory failure.

Pneumothorax is common because of the formation of bullae and blebs. CF-related diabetes, bone disease, and liver disease are also common complications.

Diagnostic Studies

- Sweat chloride test (pilocarpine iontophoresis method) measures sweat production and sodium and chloride concentrations.
- A genetic test is often used if the results from a sweat test are unclear.

Collaborative Care

A multidisciplinary team should be involved in the care of a patient with CF, including a nurse, physician, respiratory and physical therapist, dietitian, pharmacist, and social worker.

- The objectives of therapy are to promote clearance of secretions, control infection in the lungs, and provide adequate nutrition. Management of pulmonary problems is focused on relieving airway obstruction and controlling infection. Drainage of thick bronchial mucus is assisted by aerosol and nebulization treatments that liquefy mucus and facilitate coughing.
- Airway clearance techniques include chest physiotherapy (CPT), positive expiratory pressure (PEP) devices, breathing exercises, and high-frequency chest wall oscillation systems.
- More than 95% of CF patients die of complications resulting from lung infection. Standard treatment includes antibiotics for exacerbations and chronic suppressive therapy. The use of antibiotics should be carefully guided by sputum culture results.

Management of pancreatic insufficiency includes pancreatic enzyme replacement (e.g., lipase, Pancrease, Cotazym-S, Creon) administered before each meal and snack. A high-calorie, high-protein diet and multivitamins are recommended. Fat-soluble vitamins need to be supplemented. Added dietary salt is indicated whenever sweating is excessive, such as during hot weather, in the presence of fever, or from intense physical activity.

- Aerobic exercise also seems to be effective in clearing airways.
- More than 20% of adults with CF have depression, as CF imposes a significant burden on the individual and family. Issues such as fertility, decreased life expectancy, costs of health care, and career choice are but a few of the issues faced.

Nursing Management

Goals

The patient with CF will have adequate airway clearance, reduced risk factors associated with respiratory infections, adequate nutritional support to maintain appropriate body mass index (BMI), the ability to perform activities of daily living (ADLs), recognition and expedient treatment of complications related to CF, and active participation in planning and implementing a therapeutic regimen.

Nursing Diagnoses

- Ineffective airway clearance
- Ineffective breathing pattern
- Impaired gas exchange
- Imbalanced nutrition: less than body requirements
- Ineffective coping

Nursing Interventions

You and other health care professionals can assist young adults to gain independence by helping them assume responsibility for their care and vocational or school goals. For a couple considering children, genetic counseling may be suggested.

▼ **Patient and Caregiver Teaching**

- Sexuality is an important issue that should be discussed with the young adult. Delayed or irregular menstruation is not uncommon. There may also be delayed development of secondary sex characteristics, such as breasts in girls, or prolonged short stature in boys.
- Home management of CF includes an aggressive plan of postural drainage with percussion and vibration, aerosol-nebulization therapy, and breathing retraining.
- Teach the patient huff coughing, pursed lip breathing, and progressive exercise conditioning such as a bicycling program.
- The burden of living with a chronic disease at a young age can be emotionally overwhelming. Community resources are often available to help the family. In addition, the Cystic Fibrosis Foundation can be of assistance.

DIABETES INSIPIDUS

Description

Diabetes insipidus (DI) is associated with a deficiency of production or secretion of antidiuretic hormone (ADH) or a decreased renal response to ADH. The decrease in ADH results in fluid and electrolyte imbalances caused by increased urinary output and increased plasma osmolality. Depending on the cause, DI may be transient or a lifelong condition.

There are several classifications of DI. *Central DI* (also known as *neurogenic DI*) occurs when any organic lesion of the hypothalamus, infundibular stem, or posterior pituitary interferes with ADH synthesis, transport, or release. It is the most common form of DI.

Nephrogenic DI is a condition in which there is adequate ADH, but there is a decreased response to ADH in the kidney. Lithium is one of the most common causes of drug-induced nephrogenic DI.

Psychogenic DI, a less common condition, is associated with excessive water intake. This can be caused by a structural lesion in the thirst center or a psychiatric disorder.

Clinical Manifestations

The primary characteristic of DI is excretion of large quantities of urine (5 to 20 L/day) with a very low specific gravity and urine osmolality. Serum osmolality is elevated as a result of hypernatremia caused by pure water loss in the kidney.

- Most patients compensate for fluid loss by drinking great amounts of water (polydipsia) so that serum osmolality is normal or only moderately elevated. The patient may be fatigued from nocturia and may experience generalized weakness.
- Central DI usually occurs suddenly with excessive fluid loss. Central DI that results from head trauma is usually self-limiting and improves with treatment of the underlying problem. DI following cranial surgery is more likely to be permanent.
- Although the clinical manifestations of nephrogenic DI are similar, the onset and amount of fluid losses are less dramatic than with central DI.
- If oral fluid intake cannot keep up with urinary losses, severe fluid volume deficit results. This is manifested by weight loss, poor tissue turgor, hypotension, tachycardia, constipation, and shock.

- The patient also shows central nervous system (CNS) manifestations ranging from irritability and mental dullness to coma. These symptoms are related to rising serum osmolality and hypernatremia.

Diagnostic Studies

Because DI may be central, nephrogenic, or psychogenic in origin, identification of the cause is the initial step.

- A complete history and physical examination are done. Psychogenic DI is associated with overhydration and hypervolemia, rather than the dehydration and hypovolemia that are often seen in other forms of DI.
- A water restriction test is usually done to confirm the diagnosis of central DI.

Nursing and Collaborative Management

Determining and treating the primary cause is essential. A therapeutic goal is the maintenance of fluid and electrolyte balance.

- In acute DI, hypotonic saline or dextrose 5% in water is administered IV, titrated to replace urinary output.
- In central DI, hormone replacement is necessary; desmopressin (DDAVP), an analog of ADH, is administered orally, IV, or as a nasal spray. Assess the adequacy of treatment by monitoring fluid intake and output and by urine specific gravity. Notify the health care provider immediately if the individual with DI develops increased urine volume with a low specific gravity, because this indicates the need for increased dosing of DDAVP. Teach the patient about the need for close follow-up, including laboratory studies.
- Other drugs available for ADH replacement include aqueous vasopressin (Pitressin), vasopressin tannate, and lysine vasopressin (Diapid). Chlorpropamide (Diabinese) may be used to potentiate the action of ADH and stimulate endogenous ADH release.
- Treatment for nephrogenic DI revolves around dietary measures (low-sodium diet) and thiazide diuretics.

DIABETES MELLITUS

Description

Diabetes mellitus (DM) is a chronic multisystem disease related to abnormal insulin production, impaired insulin use, or both. DM is a serious health problem throughout the world. Diabetes is the leading cause of end-stage renal disease, adult blindness, and nontraumatic lower limb amputations; it is a major contributing factor in heart disease and stroke. Current theories link the causes of diabetes, singly or in combination, to genetic, autoimmune, viral, and environmental factors (e.g., viral, stress). Regardless of its cause, diabetes is primarily a disorder of glucose metabolism related to absent or insufficient insulin supplies or poor use of the insulin that is available.

- The two most common types of diabetes are classified as type 1 or type 2 DM (Table 30).

Type 1 Diabetes Mellitus

Formerly known as "juvenile onset" or "insulin-dependent" diabetes, type 1 DM most often occurs in people who are <40 years old.

Pathophysiology. Type 1 diabetes is an immune-mediated disease. The body's own T cells attack and destroy pancreatic beta (β) cells, which are the source of insulin. In addition, autoantibodies to the islet cells cause a reduction of 80% to 90% of normal β-cell function before hyperglycemia and other manifestations occur.

- A genetic predisposition and exposure to a virus may contribute to the pathogenesis of type 1 diabetes.

Type 1 diabetes is associated with a long preclinical period. Islet cell autoantibodies responsible for β-cell destruction are present for months to years before onset of symptoms. Manifestations develop when the person's pancreas can no longer produce sufficient amounts of glucose to maintain normal glucose. Once this occurs, the onset of symptoms is usually rapid.

- The patient usually has a history of recent and sudden weight loss, as well as the classic symptoms of *polydipsia* (excessive thirst), *polyuria* (frequent urination), and *polyphagia* (excessive hunger).
- The individual with type 1 diabetes requires a supply of insulin from an outside source *(exogenous insulin),* such as an injection, in order to sustain life. Without insulin, the patient develops *diabetic ketoacidosis* (DKA), a life-threatening condition resulting in metabolic acidosis.

Prediabetes

Prediabetes is a condition in which individuals are at an increased risk for developing diabetes. In this condition the blood glucose levels are high but not high enough to meet the diagnostic criteria for diabetes. This group has *impaired fasting glucose* (IFG) or *impaired glucose tolerance* (IGT). IFG is a condition in which blood glucose levels when fasting are 100 mg/dL (5.56 mmol/L) to 125 mg/dL (6.9 mmol/L). With IGT the 2-hour oral glucose tolerance test (OGTT) values are 140 mg/dL (7.8 mmol/l) to

Table 30 Characteristics of Type 1 and Type 2 Diabetes Mellitus

Factor	Type 1 Diabetes Mellitus	Type 2 Diabetes Mellitus
Age at onset	More common in young persons but can occur at any age	Usually age 35 yr or older but can occur at any age Incidence is increasing in children
Type of onset	Signs and symptoms abrupt, but disease process may be present for several years	Insidious, may go undiagnosed for years
Prevalence	Accounts for 5%-10% of all types of diabetes	Accounts for 90%-95% of all types of diabetes
Environmental factors	Virus, toxins	Obesity, lack of exercise
Primary defect	Absent or minimal insulin production	Insulin resistance, decreased insulin production over time, and alterations in production of adipokines
Islet cell antibodies	Often present at onset	Absent
Endogenous insulin	Minimal or absent	Possibly excessive; adequate but delayed secretion or reduced utilization; secretions diminish over time
Nutritional status	Thin, normal, or obese	Obese or normal
Symptoms	Thirst, polyuria, polyphagia, fatigue, weight loss	Frequently none, fatigue, recurrent infections
Ketosis	Prone at onset or during insulin deficiency	Resistant except during infection or stress
Nutritional therapy	Essential	Essential
Insulin	Required for all	Required for some
Vascular and neurologic complications	Frequent	Frequent

199 mg/dL (11.0 mmol/l). A1C in the range of 5.7%-6.4% also indicates that a person is at risk for diabetes.

Most people with prediabetes are at increased risk for developing type 2 diabetes, and if no preventive measures are taken, they will usually develop it within 10 years.

- You are in a good position to recognize patients that are at risk for diabetes and those with prediabetes. Therefore you need to educate patients about risk factors and encourage them to have their glucose levels tested.

Type 2 Diabetes Mellitus

Type 2 DM is the more prevalent type of diabetes, accounting for greater than 90% of patients with diabetes. Type 2 diabetes usually occurs in people older than 35 years, with 80% to 90% of patients being overweight at the time of diagnosis. However, type 2 diabetes is now being seen in children as a result of childhood obesity. Type 2 DM has a tendency to run in families and probably has a genetic basis.

Pathophysiology. In type 2 DM, the pancreas usually continues to produce some endogenous (self-made) insulin. However, the insulin that is produced either is insufficient for the body's needs or is poorly used by the tissues. The presence of endogenous insulin is the major pathophysiologic distinction between type 1 and type 2 diabetes.

- Obesity is believed to be the most powerful risk factor, and genetic mutations that lead to insulin resistance and a higher risk for obesity have been found in many people with type 2 DM.

Four major metabolic abnormalities play a role in the development of type 2 DM.

- The first factor is *insulin resistance,* which is a condition in which body tissues do not respond to the action of insulin. This is caused by insulin receptors that are either unresponsive to the action of insulin or insufficient in number. Entry of glucose into the cell is impeded, resulting in hyperglycemia.
- A second factor is a marked decrease in the ability of the pancreas to produce insulin as the β cells become fatigued from the compensatory overproduction of insulin or when β-cell mass is lost.
- A third factor is inappropriate glucose production by the liver. Instead of properly regulating the release of glucose in response to blood levels, the liver does so in a haphazard way that does not correspond to the body's needs at the time.

- A fourth factor is alteration in the production of hormones and cytokines by adipose tissue (adipokines). Adipokines appear to play a role in glucose and fat metabolism and likely contribute to pathophysiology of type 2 DM.

Another factor related to diabetes is *metabolic syndrome,* a cluster of abnormalities that act synergistically to greatly increase the risk for cardiovascular disease and diabetes. It is characterized by insulin resistance, elevated insulin levels, high levels of triglycerides, decreased levels of high-density lipoproteins (HDLs), increased levels of low-density lipoproteins (LDLs), and hypertension. Risk factors for metabolic syndrome include central obesity, sedentary lifestyle, urbanization, and ethnicities such as Native Americans and Hispanic Americans. See Metabolic Syndrome, p. 426.

Disease onset in type 2 DM is usually gradual. The person may go for many years with undetected hyperglycemia that might produce few, if any, symptoms. If the patient with type 2 DM has marked hyperglycemia (e.g., 500 to 1000 mg/dL [27.6 to 55.1 mmol/L]). A sufficient endogenous insulin supply may prevent DKA from occurring. However, osmotic fluid and electrolyte loss related to hyperglycemia may become severe and lead to hyperosmolar coma.

Clinical Manifestations
Type 1 DM
Because the onset of type 1 DM is rapid, the initial manifestations are usually acute. The osmotic effect of glucose produces the manifestations of polydipsia and polyuria. Polyphagia is a consequence of cellular malnourishment when insulin deficiency prevents use of glucose for energy. Weight loss, weakness, and fatigue may also be experienced.
Type 2 DM
Manifestations of type 2 DM are often nonspecific, including fatigue, recurrent infections, prolonged wound healing, and visual changes.

Acute Complications
A problem that may arise from too much insulin or an excessive dose of an oral antidiabetes agent (OA) is *hypoglycemia* (also referred to as insulin reaction or low blood glucose). It is important for the health care provider to be able to distinguish between hyperglycemia and hypoglycemia, because hypoglycemia can constitute a serious threat and requires immediate attention. Table 31 compares hypoglycemia and hyperglycemia.

Table 31	Comparison of Hyperglycemia and Hypoglycemia

Hyperglycemia	Hypoglycemia
Manifestations* Elevated blood glucose† Increase in urination Increase in appetite followed by lack of appetite Weakness, fatigue Blurred vision Headache Glycosuria Nausea and vomiting Abdominal cramps Progression to DKA or HHS	Blood glucose <70 mg/dL (3.9 mmol/L) Cold, clammy skin Numbness of fingers, toes, mouth Rapid heartbeat Emotional changes Headache Nervousness, tremors Faintness, dizziness Unsteady gait, slurred speech Hunger Changes in vision Seizures, coma
Causes Illness, infection Corticosteroids Too much food Too little or no diabetes medication Inactivity Emotional, physical stress Poor absorption of insulin	Alcohol intake without food Too little food—delayed, omitted, inadequate intake Too much diabetic medication Too much exercise without compensation Diabetes medication or food taken at wrong time Loss of weight without change in medication Use of β-adrenergic blockers interfering with recognition of symptoms
Treatment Get medical care Continue diabetes medication as ordered Check blood glucose frequently and check urine for ketones. Record results Drink fluids at least on an hourly basis	Immediately ingest 15-20 g of simple carbohydrates Ingest another 15-20 g of simple carbohydrates in 15 min if no relief obtained Contact health care provider if no relief obtained Discuss medication dosage with health care provider

Continued

Table 31	Comparison of Hyperglycemia and Hypoglycemia—cont'd

Hyperglycemia	Hypoglycemia
Preventive Measures	
Take prescribed dose of medication at proper time	Take prescribed dose of medication at proper time
Accurately administer insulin/OA	Accurately administer insulin/OA
Maintain diet	Ingest all recommended foods at proper time
Maintain good personal hygiene	Provide compensation for exercise
Adhere to sick-day rules when ill	Recognize and know symptoms and treat them immediately
Check blood for glucose as ordered	Carry simple carbohydrates
Contact health care provider regarding ketonuria	Educate family and caregiver about symptoms and treatment
Wear diabetic identification	Check blood glucose as ordered
	Wear medical alert (diabetic) identification

DKA, Diabetic ketoacidosis; *HHS*, hyperosmolar hyperglycemic syndrome; *OA*, oral agent.
* There is usually a gradual onset of symptoms in hyperglycemia and a rapid onset in hypoglycemia.
† Specific clinical manifestations related to elevated levels of blood glucose vary according to the patient.

Diabetic ketoacidosis. Diabetic ketoacidosis (DKA), also referred to as diabetic acidosis and diabetic coma, is caused by a profound deficiency of insulin and is characterized by hyperglycemia, ketosis, acidosis, and dehydration. Precipitating factors include illness and infection, inadequate insulin dosage, undiagnosed type 1 DM, poor self-management, and neglect.

- DKA is most likely to occur in type 1 diabetes, but may be seen in type 2 in conditions of severe illness or stress when the extra demand for insulin cannot be met by the pancreas.
- Manifestations of DKA include dehydration signs (e.g., poor skin turgor, dry mucous membranes), tachycardia, orthostatic hypotension with a weak and rapid pulse, vomiting, Kussmaul respirations, and a sweet fruity odor of acetone on the breath.

Hyperosmolar hyperglycemic syndrome. Hyperosmolar hyperglycemic syndrome (HHS) is a life-threatening syndrome that can occur in the patient with DM who is able to produce enough insulin to prevent DKA but not enough to prevent severe hyperglycemia, osmotic diuresis, and extracellular fluid depletion. The main difference between HHS and DKA is that the patient with HHS usually has enough circulating insulin so that ketoacidosis does not occur.

- HHS is less common than DKA. It often occurs in patients greater than 60 years of age with type 2 diabetes. Common causes of HHS in a patient with type 2 diabetes are infections of the urinary tract, pneumonia, sepsis, any acute illness, and newly diagnosed type 2 diabetes.

Hypoglycemia. Hypoglycemia, or low blood glucose, occurs when there is too much insulin in proportion to available glucose in the blood. This causes the blood glucose level to drop to <70 mg/dL (<3.9 mmol/L). Manifestations include shakiness, palpitations, nervousness, diaphoresis, anxiety, hunger, and pallor. Untreated hypoglycemia can progress to loss of consciousness, seizures, coma, and death.

Chronic Complications

Chronic complications are primarily those of end-organ disease damage to the large and small blood vessels from chronic hyperglycemia. *Angiopathy,* or blood vessel disease, is estimated to account for the majority of deaths in patients with diabetes. These chronic blood vessel problems are divided into two categories: macrovascular complications and microvascular complications.

Macrovascular complications are diseases of the large- and medium-sized blood vessels that occur with greater frequency and an earlier onset in people with diabetes. Risk factors associated with macrovascular complications—such as obesity, smoking, hypertension, high fat intake, and sedentary lifestyle—can be reduced. Insulin resistance appears to play a role in the development of cardiovascular disease and is implicated in the pathogenesis of essential hypertension and dyslipidemia.

Microvascular complications are specific to diabetes and result from thickening of the vessel membranes in the capillaries and arterioles in response to chronic hyperglycemia. Although microangiopathy can be found throughout the body, the areas most noticeably affected are the eyes (retinopathy), kidneys (nephropathy), and skin (dermopathy).

- *Diabetic retinopathy* is estimated to be the most common cause of new cases of blindness in people ages 20 to 74 years. *Nonproliferative retinopathy* is the most common form and is characterized by capillary microaneurysms, retinal swelling, and hard exudates. Macular edema may result as plasma leaks from macular blood vessels. *Proliferative retinopathy* is more severe and involves the retina and vitreous. When retinal capillaries become occluded, new fragile blood vessels are formed. Eventually light does not reach the retina as vessels tear and bleed. A tear or retinal detachment may then occur. If the macula is involved, vision is lost. Treatment involves laser coagulation.

Diabetic nephropathy is the leading cause of end-stage renal disease in the United States. Tight blood glucose control is critical to the prevention and delay of diabetic nephropathy. In addition, aggressive blood pressure management is indicated for all patients with DM because hypertension significantly accelerates the progression of diabetic nephropathy.

- Patients with diabetes are screened for nephropathy annually with a measurement of the albumin-to-creatinine ratio in a random spot urine collection for albumin. A serum creatinine is also needed.

Neuropathy is nerve damage that occurs because of the metabolic derangements associated with DM and is seen in both type 1 and type 2 diabetes. Two major categories of diabetic neuropathy are *sensory neuropathy,* which affects the peripheral nervous system, and *autonomic neuropathy,* which can affect nearly all body systems.

- The most common form of sensory neuropathy is distal symmetric neuropathy, which affects the hands or feet bilaterally. Characteristics include loss of sensation, abnormal sensations, pain, and paresthesias. The pain, which is often described as burning, cramping, crushing, or tearing, is usually worse at night. The paresthesias may be associated with tingling, burning, and itching.
- Autonomic neuropathy can lead to hypoglycemic unawareness, bowel incontinence and diarrhea, and urinary retention. Delayed gastric emptying (gastroparesis), a complication of autonomic neuropathy, can produce nausea, vomiting, esophageal reflux, and persistent feelings of fullness. Sexual function can be affected, and cardiovascular abnormalities, such as postural hypotension and resting tachycardia, can occur.

Control of blood glucose is the only treatment for diabetic neuropathy. It is effective in many but not all cases. Drug therapy may be used to treat neuropathic symptoms, particularly pain.

Diagnostic Tests

The diagnosis of diabetes can be made through one of four methods. In the absence of unequivocal hyperglycemia, criteria 1 to 3 should be confirmed by repeat testing. These methods and their criteria for diagnosis are as follows:

1. Glycosylated hemoglobin (A1C) ≥6.5%.
2. Fasting plasma glucose (FPG) level ≥126 mg/dL (7.0 mmol/L). *Fasting* is defined as no caloric intake for at least 8 hours.
3. Two-hour plasma glucose level ≥200 mg/dL (11.1 mmol/L) during an oral glucose tolerance test (OGTT), using a glucose load of 75 g.
4. In a patient with classic symptoms of hyperglycemia (polyuria, polydipsia, unexplained weight loss) or hyperglycemic crisis, a random plasma glucose ≥200 mg/dL (11.1 mmol/L).

Collaborative Care

The goals of DM management are to reduce symptoms, promote well-being, prevent acute complications of hyperglycemia, and prevent or delay the onset and progression of long-term complications. Nutrition, drug therapy, exercise, and self-monitoring of blood glucose are the tools used in the management of DM. The two major types of glucose-lowering agents (GLAs) used in the treatment of diabetes are insulin and oral agents (OAs). For the majority of people, drug therapy is necessary.

Drug Therapy: Insulin

Exogenous (injected) insulin is needed when a patient has inadequate insulin to meet specific metabolic needs. People with type 1 diabetes require exogenous insulin to survive. People with type 2 diabetes, who are usually controlled with diet, exercise, and/or OAs, may require exogenous insulin during periods of severe stress, such as illness or surgery. When patients with type 2 diabetes cannot maintain satisfactory blood glucose levels, exogenous insulin is added to the management plan.

Human insulin is prepared through the use of genetic engineering. The insulin is derived from common bacteria (e.g., *Escherichia coli*) or yeast cells using recombinant DNA technology. Insulins differ in regard to onset, peak action, and duration, and are categorized as rapid-acting, short-acting, intermediate-acting, and long-acting insulin (Table 32). The specific properties of each type of insulin are matched with the patient's diet and activity.

Examples of insulin regimens ranging from one to four injections per day are presented in Table 49-4 in Lewis et al.,

| Table 32 | Drug Therapy: Types of Insulin | |

Classification	Examples	Clarity of Solution
Rapid-acting insulin	lispro (Humalog) aspart (NovoLog) glulisine (Apidra)	Clear
Short-acting insulin	regular (Humulin R, Novolin R, ReliOn R)	Clear
Intermediate-acting insulin	NPH (Humulin N, Novolin N, ReliOn N)	Cloudy
Long-acting insulin	glargine (Lantus) detemir (Levemir)	Clear
Combination therapy (premixed)	NPH/regular 70/30* (Humulin 70/30, Novolin 70/30, ReliOn 70/30) NPH/regular 50/50* (Humulin 50/50) lispro protamine/lispro 75/25* (Humalog Mix 75/25) lispro protamine/lispro 50/50* (Humalog Mix 50/50) aspart protamine/aspart 70/30* (NovoLog Mix 70/30)	Cloudy

*These numbers refer to percentages of each type of insulin.

Medical-Surgical Nursing, ed 8, p. 1225. Because insulin is inactivated by gastric juices, it cannot be taken orally.

- The exogenous insulin regimen that most closely mimics endogenous insulin production is a basal-bolus regimen that uses rapid and short-acting (bolus) insulin before meals and long-acting (basal) background insulin once or twice per day.
- In addition to mealtime insulin, people with type 1 diabetes must also use a long-acting basal or intermediate-acting (background) insulin to control blood glucose levels between meals and overnight.
- Combination insulin therapy involves the mixing of short- or rapid-acting insulin with intermediate-acting insulin to provide both mealtime and basal coverage with one

injection. Premixed formulas are available for this regimen, but optimal blood glucose control is not as likely because there is less flexibility in dosing.

Continuous SC insulin infusion can be administered through an insulin pump, a small battery-operated device that resembles a standard paging device in size and appearance. Every 2 or 3 days the insertion site is changed. A major advantage of the pump is the potential for tight glucose control.

Nursing Care Related to Insulin Therapy. Nursing responsibilities for the patient receiving insulin include proper administration, assessment of patient's response to insulin therapy, and education of the patient regarding administration of, adjustment to, and side effects of insulin.

- Assess the patient who is new to insulin and evaluate his or her ability to manage this therapy safely. This includes the ability to understand the interaction of insulin, diet, and activity and to be able to recognize and treat appropriately the symptoms of hypoglycemia.
- The patient or caregiver also must be able to prepare and inject the insulin (see Table 49-5, Lewis et al., *Medical-Surgical Nursing,* ed 8, p. 1226). If the patient or caregiver lacks this ability, additional resources will be needed.
- Follow-up assessment of the patient who has been using insulin therapy includes inspection of insulin sites for lipodystrophy (atrophy of subcutaneous tissue) and other reactions, a review of the insulin preparation and injection technique, a history pertaining to the occurrence of hypoglycemic episodes, and the patient's method for handling hypoglycemic episodes.
- A review of the patient's record of urine and blood glucose tests is also important in assessing overall glycemic control.

Drug Therapy: Oral Agents

OAs are not insulin, but they work on the three defects of type 2 diabetes: insulin resistance, decreased insulin production, and increased hepatic glucose production. OAs may be used in combination with agents from other classes or with insulin to achieve blood glucose targets.

Many classes of oral medications are used in the treatment of type 2 diabetes:

- *Sulfonylureas* increase insulin production from the pancreas and include glipizide (Glucotrol, Glucotrol XL), glyburide (Micronase, DiaBeta, Glynase), and glimepiride (Amaryl).
- *Meglitinides* also increase insulin production from the pancreas, but they are more rapidly absorbed and eliminated than the sulfonylureas, decreasing the potential for

hypoglycemia. Meglitinides include repaglinide (Prandin) and nateglinide (Starlix).

- *Biguanides* primarily reduce glucose production by the liver, but they also enhance insulin sensitivity and improve glucose transport into cells. Metformin (Glucophage) is the first-choice drug for most people with type 2 diabetes.
- *α-Glucosidase inhibitors* slow down the absorption of carbohydrate in the small intestine. Acarbose (Precose) and miglitol (Glyset) are the available drugs in this class.
- *Thiazolidinediones* improve insulin sensitivity, transport, and use at target tissues. These agents include pioglitazone (Actos) and rosiglitazone (Avandia).
- *Dipeptidyl peptidase-4 (DDP) inhibitors* slow the inactivation of incretin hormones. Incretin hormones are released by the intestines throughout the day but levels increase in response to a meal. This class of drugs includes sitagliptin (Januvia) and saxagliptin (Onglyza).

Nursing Care Related to Oral Agents

Your responsibilities for the patient taking OAs are similar to those for the patient taking insulin. Proper administration, assessment of patient's use of and response to OAs, and education of the patient and family are all part of the nurse's role.

- Your assessment can be invaluable in determining the most appropriate OA for a patient. This includes assessing the patient's mental status, eating habits, home environment, attitude toward diabetes, and medication history.
- The patient needs to understand the importance of diet and activity plans.
- In addition, instruct the patient to contact a health care provider if periods of illness or extreme stress occur. During such a period, insulin therapy may be required to prevent or treat hyperglycemic symptoms and avoid a hyperglycemic emergency.

Drug Therapy: Other Agents

Pramlintide (Symlin) is a synthetic analog of human amylin, a hormone secreted by the β cells of the pancreas. When taken concurrently with insulin, it works to control diabetes by slowing gastric emptying, reducing postprandial glucagon secretion, and increasing satiety. It must be administered subcutaneously and cannot be mixed with insulin.

Exenatide (Byetta) and liraglutide (Victoza) are in synthetic peptides that stimulate the release of insulin from the pancreatic β cells. They suppress glucagon secretion from pancreatic β cells, reduce food intake by increasing satiety, and slow gastric emptying. They are used for patients with type 2 diabetes who have not achieved optimal glucose control on OAs. They must be administered subcutaneously.

Nutritional Therapy

Nutritional therapy is the cornerstone of diabetes care. Guidelines from the American Diabetes Association indicate that within the context of an overall healthy eating plan, a person with DM can eat the same foods as a person who does not have diabetes. This means that the same principles of good nutrition that apply to the general population also apply to the person with diabetes. The USDA MyPyramid summarizes and illustrates nutritional guidelines and nutrient needs (see Fig. 40-1 and Table 40-1 in Lewis et al., *Medical-Surgical Nursing,* ed 8, pp. 921 to 922).

- *Type 1 diabetes.* Meal planning should be based on the individual's usual food intake and balanced with insulin and exercise patterns. For patients using conventional, fixed insulin regimens, day-to-day consistency in timing and amount of food eaten is important. Patients using rapid-acting insulin can make adjustments in dosage before meals based on current blood glucose level and the carbohydrate content of the meal. Intensified insulin therapy, such as multiple daily injections or the use of an insulin pump, allows considerable flexibility in food selection and can be adjusted for deviations from usual eating and exercise habits.
- *Type 2 diabetes.* The emphasis for nutritional therapy in type 2 DM should be placed on achieving glucose, lipid, and BP goals. Modest weight loss usually improves glycemic control. Weight loss is best attempted by a moderate decrease in calories and an increase in calorie expenditure (regular exercise).

See Table 49-9, which describes nutritional therapy for patients with diabetes, Lewis et al., *Medical-Surgical Nursing,* ed 8, p. 1231.

Most often, the dietitian initially teaches the principles of the nutrition therapy prescription. Whenever possible, you should be prepared to work with dietitians as part of an interdisciplinary diabetes care team. In some instances, access to a dietitian is not possible for patients with limited insurance coverage or who live in remote areas. In these cases, you often need to assume responsibility for teaching basic dietary management to patients with diabetes.

Management of Acute Complications

Diabetic Ketoacidosis

- Because the fluid imbalance of DKA is potentially life threatening, the initial goal of therapy is to establish IV access and begin fluid and electrolyte replacement.
- Early potassium replacement is essential because hypokalemia is a significant cause of unnecessary and avoidable death during treatment of DKA.
- IV insulin administration is directed toward correcting hyperglycemia and hyperketonemia. Initially a bolus of insulin is delivered, followed by continuous infusion.

Hyperosmolar Hyperglycemic Syndrome

- Laboratory values in HHS include blood glucose >600 mg/dL (>33.33 mmol/L) and a marked increase in serum osmolality. The increased osmolality produces more severe neurologic manifestations, such as somnolence, coma, and seizures.
- HHS constitutes a medical emergency and has a high mortality rate. Therapy is similar to that for DKA except that HHS requires greater fluid replacement.
- Regular insulin is given by IV infusion.
- Electrolytes are monitored and replaced as needed. Assess vital signs, intake and output, tissue turgor, laboratory values, and cardiac monitoring to monitor the efficacy of fluid and electrolyte replacement.

Hypoglycemia

- At the first sign of hypoglycemia, the blood glucose should be checked if possible. If it is <70 mg/dL (3.9 mmol/L), immediately begin treatment for hypoglycemia. If monitoring equipment is not available, hypoglycemia should be assumed and treatment should be initiated.
- Hypoglycemia is treated by ingesting 15 to 20 g of a simple (fast-acting) carbohydrate, such as 4 to 6 ounces of fruit juice or regular soft drink, or 8 ounces of low-fat milk. Treatment with large quantities of quick-acting carbohydrates, such as candy bars, should be avoided so that rapid fluctuation to hyperglycemia does not occur.
- Blood glucose should be checked about 15 minutes following the initial treatment, and treatment should be repeated if the blood glucose remains <70 mg/dL (3.9 mmol/L).
- Once the blood glucose is >70 mg/dL (3.9 mmol/L), the patient should eat a snack to prevent hypoglycemia from recurring. Good snacks include peanut butter and cheese and crackers.
- If there is no significant improvement in the patient's condition after two or three doses of 15 g of simple carbohydrate or if the patient is not alert enough to swallow, 1 mg of glucagon may

be administered by intramuscular (IM) or subcutaneous (SC) injection.

- Once acute hypoglycemia has been reversed, you should explore with the patient the reasons why the situation developed. This assessment may indicate a need for additional education of the patient and caregiver to avoid future episodes of hypoglycemia.

Nursing Management

Goals

The patient with DM will be an active participant in the management of the diabetes regimen; experience few or no episodes of acute hyperglycemic emergencies or hypoglycemia; maintain blood glucose levels at normal or near normal levels; prevent, minimize, or delay the occurrence of chronic complications of diabetes; and adjust lifestyle to accommodate a diabetes regimen with a minimum of stress.

See NCP 49-1 for the patient with diabetes, Lewis et al., *Medical-Surgical Nursing,* ed 8, pp. 1237 to 1238.

Nursing Diagnoses

- Ineffective self-health management
- Imbalanced nutrition: more than body requirements
- Risk for injury
- Risk for peripheral neurovascular dysfunction

Nursing Interventions

Your role in health promotion relates to the identification, monitoring, and education of the patient at risk for the development of DM.

Exercise. Regular, consistent exercise is considered an essential part of diabetes and prediabetes management. Exercise decreases insulin resistance and can have a direct effect on lowering the blood glucose levels. It also contributes to weight loss, which also decreases insulin resistance. Regular exercise may also reduce triglyceride and LDL cholesterol levels, increasing HDL, reducing BP, and improving circulation. Additional information is provided in the patient and caregiver teaching guide (see Table 49-11, Lewis et al., *Medical-Surgical Nursing,* ed 8, p. 1233).

Blood glucose monitoring. Patient self-monitoring of blood glucose (SMBG) enables the patient to make self-management decisions regarding diet, exercise, and medication. SMBG is also important for detecting episodic hyperglycemia and hypoglycemia.

Frequency of monitoring depends on several factors, including the patient's glycemic goals, the type of diabetes that the patient has, medication regimen, the patient's ability to perform the test independently, and the patient's willingness to test. Patients who use multiple insulin injections or insulin pump therapy should monitor their blood sugar three or more times a day. Patients using less frequent insulin injections, noninsulin therapy, or medical nutrition therapy alone must monitor as often as needed to achieve their glycemic goals.

- SMBG is an empowering tool that allows the patient to be an active partner in the treatment of diabetes. Achieving the desired level of patient participation does require time and effort from the health care professional. You should anticipate a close working relationship with patients as they refine their techniques and learn appropriate decision making about managing their diabetes.

Management of acute illness and surgery. Emotional and physical stress can increase blood glucose levels and result in hyperglycemia. Acute illness (even minor), injury, and surgery may evoke a counterregulatory hormone response resulting in hyperglycemia.

- Patients with diabetes who are ill should continue with the regular meal plan while increasing the intake of noncaloric fluids, such as broth, water, diet gelatin, and other decaffeinated beverages. They should also continue taking oral agents and insulin as prescribed and check blood glucose at least every 4 hours. If the glucose is >240 mg/dL (>13.3 mmol/L), urine should be tested for ketones every 3 to 4 hours. Moderate to large ketone levels should be reported to the health care provider.
- If illness causes the patient to eat less than normal, OAs and insulin should be taken as prescribed while supplementing food intake with carbohydrate-containing fluids. The health care provider should be notified promptly if the patient is unable to keep any fluids down.
- Adjustments in the diabetes regimen during the intraoperative period can be planned to ensure glycemic control. The patient is given IV fluids and insulin immediately before, during, and after surgery when there is no oral intake. Patients who are undergoing surgery or any radiologic procedures that involve the use of contrast medium are instructed to temporarily discontinue metformin before surgery or the procedure. They will also be instructed not to resume the metformin until 48 hours after the surgery or the procedure and after their serum creatinine has been checked and is normal.
- When caring for an unconscious surgical patient receiving insulin, you must be alert for hypoglycemic signs, such as

sweating, tachycardia, and tremors. Frequent monitoring of blood glucose will prevent episodes of severe hypoglycemia in this patient.

Ambulatory and home care. Successful management of diabetes requires ongoing interaction among the patient, family, and health care team. It is important that a diabetes nurse educator be involved in the care of the patient and family.

A diagnosis of diabetes affects the patient in many profound ways. Patients with diabetes must continually contend with lifestyle choices that affect the food they eat, the activities they engage in, and demands on their time and energy. In addition, they face the potential of developing the devastating complications of this disease. Careful assessment of what it means to the patient to have diabetes should be the starting point of patient teaching.

The potential for infection requires diligent skin and dental hygiene practices. Routine care includes tooth brushing and flossing and regular bathing, with particular emphasis given to foot care. If cuts, scrapes, or burns occur, they should be treated promptly and monitored carefully. If the injury does not begin to heal within 24 hours or signs of infection develop, the health care provider should be notified immediately.

▼ Patient and Caregiver Teaching

The goals of diabetes self-management education are to enable the patient to become an active participant in his or her care. Patients who actively manage their diabetes care have better outcomes than those who do not. For this reason, an educational approach that facilitates informed decision making on the part of the patient is widely advocated. Guidelines for patient and caregiver teaching for management of diabetes are in Table 33.

Table 33	Patient and Caregiver Teaching Guide: Management of Diabetes Mellitus

When teaching the patient and caregiver management of diabetes mellitus, you should:

Component	What to Teach
Disease process	Include an introduction about the pancreas and the islets of Langerhans. Describe how insulin is made and what affects its production. Discuss the relationship of insulin and glucose.

Continued

Table 33	Patient and Caregiver Teaching Guide: Management of Diabetes Mellitus—cont'd

Component	What to Teach
Physical activity	Discuss the importance of regular exercise on the management of blood glucose, improvement of cardiovascular function, and general health.
Menu planning	Stress the importance of a well-balanced diet as part of a diabetes management plan.
	Explain the impact of carbohydrates on the glycemic index and blood glucose levels.
Medication compliance	Ensure that the patient understands the proper use of insulin (see Table 49-5, Lewis et al., *Medical-Surgical Nursing,* ed. 8, p. 1226) and oral agents.
	Account for a patient's physical limitation or inabilities for self-medication. If necessary, involve the family or caregiver in proper use of medication.
	Discuss all side effects and safety issues regarding medication.
Monitoring blood glucose	Teach correct blood glucose monitoring.
	Include when blood glucose levels should be checked, how to record them, and if necessary, how to adjust insulin levels accordingly.
Risk reduction	Ensure that the patient understands and appropriately responds to the signs and symptoms of hypoglycemia and hyperglycemia (see Table 49-17, Lewis et al., *Medical-Surgical Nursing,* ed. 8, p. 1242).
	Stress the importance of proper foot care (see Table 49-22, Lewis et al., *Medical-Surgical Nursing,* ed. 8, p. 1251), regular eye examinations, and consistent glucose monitoring.
	Inform the patient about the effect that stress can have on blood glucose.
Psychosocial	Advise the patient of resources that are available to facilitate the adjustment and answer questions about living with a chronic condition such as diabetes (see Resources at end of chapter).

You should assess the patient's knowledge base frequently so that gaps in knowledge or incorrect or inaccurate ideas can be quickly corrected.

- Instruct the patient to carry medical identification at all times indicating that he or she has diabetes. An identification card can supply valuable information, such as the name of the health care provider and the type and dose of insulin or OA.
- If the patient is not able to manage the disease, a family member may be able to assume part of this role. If the patient or caregiver cannot make decisions related to diabetes management, you may refer the patient to a social worker or other resources within the community.

D

DIARRHEA

Description
Diarrhea is the passage of at least three loose or liquid stools per day. It may be acute or chronic, and is considered chronic if it lasts longer than four weeks.

Pathophysiology
Infectious organisms attack the intestines in various ways. Some organisms (e.g., *rotavirus, norvirus, Giardia lamblia,* and types of *Escherichia coli [E. coli]*) alter secretion and/or absorption of the enterocytes of the small intestine without causing inflammation. Other organisms (e.g., *Clostridium difficile [C. difficile]*) impair absorption by destroying cells and producing inflammation in the colon.

Clinical Manifestations
Diarrhea may be acute or chronic.

Acute diarrhea most commonly results from infection. Bacteria that attack the cells of the colon cause inflammation and systemic symptoms (e.g., fever, headache, malaise) in addition to nausea, vomiting, abdominal cramping, and diarrhea. Liquid stools also lead to perianal skin irritation. Leukocytes, blood, and mucus may be present in the stool, depending on the causative agent (Table 34).

- Acute diarrhea is often self-limiting in the adult. Keep in mind that people can remain contagious for two weeks or more, even after recovering from a viral infection.
- Severe diarrhea produces life-threatening dehydration, electrolyte disturbances (e.g., hypokalemia), and acid-base

Table 34	Causes of Acute Infectious Diarrhea*

Type of Organism	Symptoms
Viral	
Rotavirus	Fever, vomiting, and profuse watery diarrhea. Lasts 3-8 days.
Norvirus (also called Norwalk-like virus)	Nausea, vomiting, diarrhea, stomach cramping. Rapid onset. Lasts 1-2 days.
Bacterial	
Enterotoxigenic *Escherichia coli*	Watery or bloody diarrhea. Abdominal cramps. Nausea, vomiting, and fever may be present. Mean duration >60 hours.
Enterohemorrhagic *Escherichia coli* (e.g., *E. coli 0157:H7*)	Severe abdominal cramping, bloody diarrhea, and vomiting. Low-grade fever. Usually lasts 5-7 days.
Shigella	Diarrhea (sometimes bloody), fever, and stomach cramps. Usually lasts 5-7 days. Postinfection arthritis may occur.
Salmonella	Diarrhea, fever, and abdominal cramps. Lasts 4-7 days.
Staphylococcal	Nausea, vomiting, abdominal cramps, and diarrhea. Usually mild. May cause illness in as little as 30 minutes. Lasts 1-3 days.
Campylobacter jejuni	Diarrhea, abdominal cramps, and fever. Sometimes nausea and vomiting. Lasts about 7 days.
Clostridium perfringens	Diarrhea, abdominal cramps, nausea, and vomiting. Occurs 6-24 hours after eating contaminated food and lasts approximately 24 hours.
Clostridium difficile	Watery diarrhea, fever, anorexia, nausea, abdominal pain.
Parasitic	
Giardia lamblia	Abdominal cramps, nausea, diarrhea. May interfere with nutrient absorption.

| Table 34 | Causes of Acute Infectious Diarrhea*—cont'd |

Type of Organism	Symptoms
Entamoeba histolytica	Diarrhea, abdominal cramping. Only 10%-20% are ill and symptoms are usually mild.
Cryptosporidium	Watery diarrhea. Lasts about 2 weeks. May also have abdominal cramps, nausea, vomiting, fever, dehydration, and weight loss. Sometimes no symptoms. Long lasting and may be fatal in those who are immunocompromised (e.g., AIDS).

*An expanded version of this table with source of infection and medication treatment is available on the Evolve website.
AIDS, Acquired immunodeficiency syndrome.

imbalances (metabolic acidosis). *C. difficile* causes mild to severe diarrhea, abdominal cramping, and fever.

Chronic diarrhea can result in malabsorption and ultimately malnutrition.

Diagnostic Studies

Accurate diagnosis and management require a thorough history, physical examination, and laboratory testing.

- A history of travel, medication use, diet, previous surgery, and interpersonal contacts, as well as family history, should be obtained.
- Blood tests may identify anemia, elevated white blood cell (WBC) count, iron and folate deficiencies, and abnormal electrolyte levels.
- Increased hemoglobin, hematocrit, and blood urea nitrogen (BUN) levels suggest fluid deficits.
- Stools are examined for blood, mucus, WBCs, and parasites. Stool cultures may help in identifying infectious organisms.
- In a patient with chronic diarrhea, measurement of stool electrolytes, pH, and osmolality may help to determine whether diarrhea is related to decreased fluid absorption or increased fluid secretion (secretory diarrhea).
- Measurement of stool fat and undigested muscle fibers may indicate fat and protein malabsorption conditions, including pancreatic insufficiency.

- Colonoscopy may be used to examine the mucosa and obtain specimens for examination.
- Capsule endoscopy is also used for visualization of the intestinal mucosa.

Collaborative Care

Treatment is based on the cause and is aimed at replacing fluids and electrolytes and resolving the diarrhea. Oral solutions containing glucose and electrolytes (e.g., Gatorade, Pedialyte) may be sufficient to replace losses from mild diarrhea. In severe diarrhea, parenteral administration of fluids, electrolytes, vitamins, and nutrition may be necessary.

Antidiarrheal agents may be given to coat and protect mucous membranes, absorb irritating substances, inhibit gastrointestinal (GI) motility, decrease intestinal secretions, and decrease central nervous system (CNS) stimulation to the GI tract. Antidiarrheal agents are contraindicated in the treatment of infectious diarrhea because they potentially prolong exposure to the infectious organism.

- Antiperistaltic agents are not given to a patient who has infectious diarrheal syndromes because of the potential for prolonging exposure to the infectious agent. Regardless of the cause, antidiarrheal medications should be given only for a short period.
- Antibiotics are rarely used to treat infectious diarrhea.

C. difficile is a particularly challenging hospital-acquired infection. *C. difficile* spores can survive for many days on objects, including commodes, telephones, thermometers, bedside tables, and floors. *C. difficile* can be transmitted from patient to patient by health care workers who do not adhere to infection control precautions.

- The infection may resolve when antibiotic therapy ceases. If not, either metronidazole (Flagyl) or vancomycin (Vancocin) is given to treat the infection.

Nursing Management: Acute Infectious Diarrhea

Goals

The patient with diarrhea will not transmit the microorganism causing the infectious diarrhea, will cease having diarrhea and resume normal bowel patterns, will have normal fluid and electrolyte and acid-base balance, will have a normal nutritional status, and there will be no perianal skin breakdown.

See NCP 43-1 for the patient with acute infectious diarrhea, Lewis et al., *Medical-Surgical Nursing,* ed 8, p. 1010.

Nursing Diagnoses
- Diarrhea
- Deficient fluid volume
- Risk for impaired skin integrity

Nursing Interventions

All cases of acute diarrhea should be considered infectious until the cause is known.

- Strict infection control precautions are necessary to prevent the infection from spreading to others. Wash your hands before and after contact with each patient and when body fluids of any kind are handled.
- Patients with *Clostridium difficile* should be placed in a private room, and gloves and gowns should be worn for visitors and health care providers.

▼ **Patient and Caregiver Teaching**
- Teach the patient and caregiver the principles of hygiene, infection control precautions, and potential dangers of an illness that is infectious to themselves and others.
- Discuss proper food handling, cooking, and storage of food with the patient and caregiver.

DISLOCATION AND SUBLUXATION

Description

A *dislocation* is a severe injury of the ligamentous structures that surround a joint. It results in the complete displacement or separation of joint articular surfaces. A *subluxation* is a partial or incomplete displacement of the joint surface. Manifestations of a subluxation are similar to those of a dislocation but are less severe. Treatment of a subluxation is similar to that of a dislocation, but may require less healing time.

Dislocations characteristically result from forces transmitted to the joint that cause a disruption of the soft tissue support structures surrounding the joint. Joints most frequently dislocated in the upper extremity include the thumb, elbow, and shoulder. In the lower extremity, the hip is vulnerable to dislocation occurring as a result of severe trauma, often associated with motor vehicle collisions.

Clinical Manifestations

The most obvious manifestation of a dislocation is deformity. For example, if a hip is dislocated, the limb can be shorter and is often internally rotated on the affected side.

- Additional manifestations include local pain, tenderness, loss of function of the injured part, and swelling of soft tissues in the region of the joint.

Complications of a dislocated joint are open joint injuries, avascular necrosis (bone cell death as a result of inadequate blood supply), intraarticular fractures, and damage to adjacent neurovascular tissue.

Diagnostic Studies
- X-ray studies determine the extent of displacement of the involved structures.
- Joint aspiration determines the presence of hemarthrosis or fat cells. Fat cells in the aspirate indicate a probable intraarticular fracture.

Collaborative Care
Dislocation requires prompt attention and is considered an orthopedic emergency. The longer the joint remains unreduced, the greater the possibility of avascular necrosis. Compartment syndrome also may occur and is associated with significant vascular injury. The hip joint is particularly susceptible to avascular necrosis.

The first goal of management is to realign the dislocated portion of the joint in its original anatomic position. This can be accomplished by a closed reduction, which may be performed with the patient under local or general anesthesia or intravenous (IV) conscious sedation. In some situations, surgical open reduction may be necessary.

- After reduction, the extremity is usually immobilized by bracing, splinting, taping, or using a sling to allow the torn ligaments and capsular tissue time to heal.

Nursing Management
Nursing care is directed toward relief of pain and support and protection of the injured joint. After the joint has been reduced and immobilized, motion is usually restricted.

- A carefully regulated rehabilitation program can prevent fracture instability and joint dysfunction.
- An exercise program slowly restores the joint to its original range of motion without causing another dislocation.
- Activity restrictions of the affected joint may be imposed to decrease the risk of repeatedly dislocating the joint.

DISSEMINATED INTRAVASCULAR COAGULATION

Description

Disseminated intravascular coagulation (DIC) is a serious bleeding and thrombotic disorder. It results from abnormally initiated and accelerated clotting. Subsequent decreases in clotting factors and platelets may lead to uncontrollable hemorrhage. The term *DIC* can be misleading because it suggests that blood is clotting. The paradox of this condition is that profuse bleeding results from depletion of platelets and clotting factors. DIC is always caused by an underlying disease; the underlying disease must be treated for DIC to resolve.

D

Pathophysiology

DIC is an abnormal response of the normal clotting cascade stimulated by a disease process or disorder. The diseases and disorders known to predispose patients to acute DIC are major physiologic assaults and include shock, septicemia, abruptio placentae, severe head injury, heat stroke, and pulmonary emboli.

- DIC can occur as an acute, catastrophic condition, or it may exist at a subacute or chronic level. Each condition may have one or multiple triggering mechanisms to start the clotting cascade.

Initially in DIC, a stimulus such as an injury or a malignant tumor causes release of tissue factor, and normal coagulation mechanisms are enhanced. Intravascular thrombin is produced, and it catalyzes the conversion of fibrinogen to fibrin and enhances platelet aggregation. There is widespread fibrin and platelet deposition in capillaries and arterioles, resulting in thrombosis. Excessive clotting activates the fibrinolytic system, which in turn breaks down newly formed clots, creating fibrin-split (fibrin-degradation) products (FSPs), which inhibit normal blood clotting. Ultimately the blood loses its ability to form a stable clot at injury sites, which predisposes the patient to hemorrhage.

- Chronic and subacute DIC is most commonly seen in patients with long-standing illnesses such as malignant disorders or autoimmune diseases. In these cases, DIC may be manifested only by laboratory abnormalities.

Clinical Manifestations

There is no well-defined sequence of events in acute DIC. Bleeding in a person with no previous history or obvious cause should be questioned because it may be one of the first manifestations of acute DIC. Other nonspecific manifestations include weakness,

malaise, and fever. There are both bleeding and thrombotic manifestations in DIC (Fig. 4).

- *Bleeding manifestations* are multifactorial and result from
  consumption and depletion of platelets and coagulation
  factors. Manifestations include petechiae, oozing blood,
  tachypnea, hemoptysis, tachycardia, hypotension, bloody
  stools, hematuria, dizziness, headache, changes in mental
  status, and bone and joint pain.
- *Thrombotic manifestations* are a result of fibrin or platelet
  deposition in the microvasculature. Manifestations include
  ischemic tissue necrosis (e.g., gangrene), acute respiratory
  distress syndrome (ARDS), cardiovascular and electrocardiogram (ECG) changes, kidney damage, and paralytic
  ileus.

Diagnostic Studies

- Prolonged prothrombin time and partial thromboplastin time
- Prolonged activated partial thromboplastin time and thrombin
  time
- Reduced fibrinogen, antithrombin III (AT III), and platelets
- Elevated FSPs and elevated D-dimers (cross-linked fibrin
  fragments)
- Reduced levels of factors V, VII, VIII, X, and XIII

Collaborative Care

It is important to diagnose DIC quickly, institute therapy that will
resolve the underlying causative disease or problem, and provide
supportive care. Treatment of DIC remains controversial and under
investigation as researchers determine how to manage this dangerous syndrome. It is imperative that you maintain an ongoing awareness of current modes of therapy. Diagnosing and treating the
primary disease process are essential to the resolution of DIC.
Depending on its severity, a variety of different methods are used
to provide supportive and symptomatic management of DIC.

- If chronic DIC is diagnosed in a patient who is not bleeding,
  no therapy for DIC is necessary. Treatment of the underlying
  disease may be sufficient to reverse DIC (e.g., antineoplastic
  therapy when DIC is caused by malignancy).
- When the patient with DIC is bleeding, therapy is directed
  toward providing support with necessary blood products
  while treating the primary disorder. Blood products are
  administered cautiously on the basis of specific component
  deficiencies to patients who have serious bleeding, are at
  high risk for bleeding (e.g., surgery), or require invasive
  procedures. Platelets are given to correct thrombocytopenia,

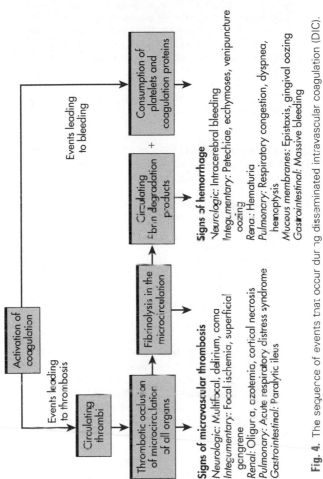

Signs of microvascular thrombosis
Neurologic: Multifocal, delirium, coma
Integumentary: Focal ischemic, superficial gangrene
Renal: Oliguria, azotemia, cortical necrosis
Pulmonary: Acute respiratory distress syndrome
Gastrointestinal: Paralytic ileus

Signs of hemorrhage
Neurologic: Intracerebral bleeding
Integumentary: Petechiae, ecchymoses, venipuncture oozing
Renal: Hematuria
Pulmonary: Respiratory congestion, dyspnea, hemoptysis
Mucous membranes: Epistaxis, gingival oozing
Gastrointestinal: Massive bleeding

Fig. 4. The sequence of events that occur during disseminated intravascular coagulation (DIC).

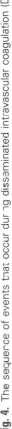

cryoprecipitate replaces factor VIII and fibrinogen, and fresh-frozen plasma (FFP) replaces all clotting factors except platelets and provides a source of antithrombin.

- A patient with manifestations of thrombosis is often treated by anticoagulation with heparin or low-molecular-weight heparin. Use of heparin in the treatment of DIC remains controversial. Antithrombin III (AT III, ATnativ), a cofactor of heparin that becomes depleted during DIC, is sometimes useful in fulminant DIC, although it increases the risk of bleeding.
- A recombinant human activated protein C (drotrecogin alfa [Xigris]) has been shown to have both anticoagulant and antiinflammatory effects and has reduced the relative risk of death from sepsis.

Nursing Management

Nursing Diagnoses
- Ineffective peripheral tissue perfusion
- Acute pain
- Decreased cardiac output
- Anxiety

Nursing Interventions
You must be alert to the possible development of DIC. Remember that because DIC is secondary to an underlying disease, appropriate care for managing the causative problem must be provided while providing supportive care related to the manifestations of DIC.

- Early detection of bleeding, both occult and overt, must be a primary goal. Assess for signs of external bleeding (e.g., petechiae, oozing at intravenous [IV] or injection sites) and signs of internal bleeding (e.g., changes in mental status, increasing abdominal girth, pain) as well as any indications that microthrombi may be causing clinically significant organ damage (e.g., decreased renal output).
- Tissue damage should be minimized and the patient protected from additional foci of bleeding.
- An additional nursing responsibility is to administer blood products correctly.

DIVERTICULOSIS/DIVERTICULITIS

Description
Diverticula are saccular dilations or outpouchings of the mucosa that develop in the colon at points where the vasa recta penetrate the circular muscle layer. In *diverticulosis,* multiple noninflamed

diverticula are present. *Diverticulitis* is inflammation of the diverticula, resulting in perforation into the peritoneum. Clinically diverticular disease covers a spectrum from asymptomatic, uncomplicated diverticulosis to diverticulitis with complications such as perforation, abscess, fistula, and bleeding. Diverticula may occur at any point within the gastrointestinal (GI) tract, but are most commonly found in the sigmoid colon.

- Diverticular disease is a common GI disorder that affects 65% of the population by the age of 80 years. Most cases are asymptomatic.

Pathophysiology

The etiology of diverticulosis of the ascending colon is unknown, but diverticula in the sigmoid colon appear to be associated with high luminal pressures from a deficiency in dietary fiber and perhaps combined with a loss of muscle mass and collagen with the aging process. The disease is more prevalent in Western populations that consume diets low in fiber and high in refined carbohydrates.

- The cause of diverticulosis is unknown; it is thought that diverticula occur because of high interluminal pressure on weakened areas of the bowel wall. Inadequate dietary fiber slows transit time, and more water is absorbed from the stool, making it more difficult to pass through the lumen. Decreased stool size raises intraluminal pressure, which promotes diverticula formation.
- Diverticulitis is characterized by inflamed diverticuli and increased luminal pressures that cause erosion of the bowel wall with microscopic perforation into the peritoneum.

Clinical Manifestations and Complications

A majority of patients with diverticulosis have no symptoms. Those with symptoms typically have abdominal pain or changes in bowel habits but no symptoms of inflammation. Approximately 15% of patients with diverticulosis progress at some point to acute diverticulitis.

In patients with diverticulitis, abdominal pain is localized over the involved area of the colon. The most common symptoms of diverticulitis in the sigmoid colon include left lower quadrant abdominal pain, fever, leukocytosis, and sometimes a palpable abdominal mass. Elderly patients with diverticulitis are frequently afebrile, with little if any abdominal tenderness.

Complications of diverticulitis include perforation with peritonitis, abscess and fistula formation, bowel obstruction, ureteral obstruction, and bleeding. Bleeding can be extensive but usually stops spontaneously. Diverticulitis is the most common cause of lower GI hemorrhage.

Diagnostic Studies

- History and physical examination
- Abdominal and chest x-rays rule out other causes of acute abdominal pain
- Computed tomography (CT) scan with oral contrast confirms the diagnosis

Collaborative Care

Diverticular disease may be prevented by a high-fiber diet composed primarily of fruits and vegetables with a decreased intake of fat and red meat. Risk may also be decreased by high levels of physical activity, and weight reduction is recommended for obese persons. When diverticular disease is present, a high-fiber diet is also recommended, although its benefits are unclear.

In acute diverticulitis, the goal of treatment is to allow the colon to rest and the inflammation to subside. If hospitalized, the patient is kept on nothing by mouth (NPO) status and bed rest and is given parenteral fluids and antibiotics. The white blood cell (WBC) count is monitored, and the patient is observed for signs of peritonitis.

Surgery is reserved for patients with complications, such as an abscess or obstruction, that cannot be managed medically. The usual surgical procedures involve resection of the involved colon with either a primary anastomosis if adequate bowel cleansing is feasible or a temporary diverting colostomy. The colostomy is reanastomosed after the colon is healed.

Nursing Management

Teach patients with diverticular disease to avoid increased intraabdominal pressure because it may precipitate an attack.

- Factors that increase intraabdominal pressure are straining at stool, vomiting, bending, lifting, and tight, restrictive clothing.
- When an acute attack subsides, the patient gradually resumes diet and activity.
- Oral fluids progressing to a semisolid diet are allowed. Ambulation is also permitted.
- If the patient has a bowel resection or colostomy, nursing care is the same as for these procedures.
- Provide the patient with a full explanation of the condition. Patients who understand the disease process well and adhere to the prescribed regimen are less likely to experience an exacerbation of the disease and its complications.

DYSMENORRHEA

Description

Dysmenorrhea is cramping abdominal pain or discomfort associated with menstrual flow. The degree of pain and discomfort varies with the individual. Two types of dysmenorrhea exist: *primary,* in which no pathologic finding exists, and *secondary,* in which a pelvic disease is the underlying cause.

- Approximately 50% of all women experience dysmenorrhea, making it one of the most common gynecologic problems.

Pathophysiology

Primary dysmenorrhea is not a disease; rather it is caused by either an excess of or an increased sensitivity to prostaglandin $F_{2\alpha}$ ($PGF_{2\alpha}$). Primary dysmenorrhea begins in the few years after menarche, typically with the onset of regular ovulatory cycles.

- With the onset of menses, degeneration of the endometrium releases prostaglandin. Prostaglandins increase myometrial contractions and constriction of small endometrial blood vessels, with consequent tissue ischemia and increased sensitization of the pain receptors resulting in menstrual pain.

Secondary dysmenorrhea occurs most commonly in persons in their 30s and 40s. Secondary dysmenorrhea is caused by pelvic diseases such as endometriosis, chronic pelvic inflammatory disease (PID), and uterine leiomyomas (fibroids).

Clinical Manifestations

Primary dysmenorrhea starts 12 to 24 hours before the onset of menses. The pain is most severe the first day of menses and rarely lasts more than 2 days.

- Characteristic manifestations include lower abdominal cramping pain that is colicky in nature, frequently radiating to the lower back and upper thighs. The abdominal pain is often accompanied by nausea, diarrhea, loose stools, fatigue, headache, and light-headedness.

Secondary dysmenorrhea usually occurs after the woman has experienced problem-free periods for some time. The pain, which may be unilateral, is generally more constant in nature and continues for a longer time than primary dysmenorrhea.

- Depending on the cause, symptoms such as *dyspareunia* (painful intercourse), painful defecation, or irregular bleeding may occur at times other than menstruation.

Collaborative Care

Evaluation begins with distinguishing primary from secondary dysmenorrhea. Obtain a complete health history with special attention to menstrual and gynecologic history. A pelvic examination is also done.

- If the pelvic examination is normal and the history reveals an onset shortly after menarche with symptoms only associated with menses, the probable diagnosis is primary dysmenorrhea.
- If any cause or etiology for the pain is evident, the diagnosis is secondary dysmenorrhea.

Treatment for primary dysmenorrhea includes heat applied to the lower abdomen or back, exercise, and drug therapy. Regular exercise is thought to be beneficial because it may reduce endometrial hyperplasia and subsequently reduce prostaglandin production.

Drug therapy involves nonsteroidal antiinflammatory drugs (NSAIDs), such as naproxen (Naprosyn), which have an antiprostaglandin activity. NSAIDs are started at the first sign of menses and continued every 4 to 8 hours for the duration of the usual discomfort.

Oral contraceptives may also be used to decrease dysmenorrhea by reducing endometrial hyperplasia.

Treatment for secondary dysmenorrhea depends on the cause with some of the same approaches being used that are recommended for primary dysmenorrhea.

Nursing Management

- Advise women that during acute pain, relief may be obtained by applying heat to the abdomen or back and taking NSAIDs for analgesia.
- Health care measures that can decrease discomfort include maintenance of proper nutritional habits, avoidance of constipation, maintenance of good body mechanics, and avoidance of stress and overfatigue, particularly during the time preceding menstrual periods.
- Staying active and interested in activities may also help.

DYSRHYTHMIAS

Description

Dysrhythmias are abnormal cardiac rhythms. Prompt assessment of abnormal cardiac rhythms and the patient's response to the rhythm is critical. Dysrhythmias result from disorders of impulse formation, conduction of impulses, or both. A pacemaker from a site other than the sinoatrial (SA) node may be discharged in two ways. If the SA node discharges more slowly than a secondary pacemaker, electrical discharges from the secondary pacemaker may passively "escape" and discharge automatically at its intrinsic rate. Secondary pacemakers can also originate when they discharge more rapidly than the SA node. *Triggered beats* (early or late) may come from an *ectopic focus* (area outside the normal conduction pathway) in the atria, atrioventricular (AV) node, or ventricles. This results in a dysrhythmia, which replaces the normal sinus rhythm.

- Dysrhythmias occur as the result of various abnormalities and disease states. The cause of a dysrhythmia influences the treatment of the patient. Common causes of dysrhythmias are presented in Table 35. Table 36 presents a systematic approach to assessing a cardiac rhythm.

Table 35	Common Causes of Dysrhythmias*

Cardiac Conditions
- Accessory pathways
- Cardiomyopathy
- Conduction defects
- Heart failure
- Myocardial ischemia, infarction
- Valve disease

Other Conditions
- Acid base imbalances
- Alcohol
- Caffeine, tobacco
- Connective tissue disorders
- Drug effects (e.g., antidysrhythmia drugs, stimulants, β-adrenergic blockers) or toxicity
- Electric shock
- Electrolyte imbalances (e.g., hypokalemia, hypocalcemia)
- Emotional crisis
- Herbal supplements (e.g., areca nut, wahoo root bark, yerba mate)
- Hypoxia
- Metabolic conditions (e.g., thyroid dysfunction)
- Near-drowning
- Poisoning
- Sepsis, shock

*List is not all-inclusive.

Table 36	Systematic Approach to Assessing Cardiac Rhythm

When assessing a cardiac rhythm, you should use a systematic approach. One recommended approach includes the following:

1. Look for the presence of the P wave. Is it upright or inverted? Is there one for every QRS complex or more than one? Are there atrial fibrillatory or flutter waves present?
2. Evaluate the atrial rhythm. Is it regular or irregular?
3. Calculate the atrial rate.
4. Measure the duration of the PR interval. Is it normal duration or prolonged?
5. Evaluate the ventricular rhythm. Is it regular or irregular?
6. Calculate the ventricular rate.
7. Measure the duration of the QRS complex. Is it normal duration or prolonged?
8. Assess the ST segment. Is it isoelectric (flat), elevated, or depressed?
9. Measure the duration of the QT interval. Is it normal duration or prolonged?
10. Note the T wave. Is it upright or inverted?

Questions to consider include the following:

1. What is the dominant rhythm and/or dysrhythmia?
2. What is the clinical significance of your findings?
3. What is the treatment for the particular rhythm?

Types of Dysrhythmias

Examples of electrocardiogram (ECG) tracings of common dysrhythmias are presented in Figs. 36-11 to 36-19, Lewis et al., *Medical-Surgical Nursing,* ed 8, pp. 824 to 831. The characteristics of common dysrhythmias are described in the Reference Appendix on pp. 784 to 785.

Sinus Bradycardia

This condition occurs when the SA node discharges at a rate of <60 beats/min. It may be a normal sinus rhythm in aerobically trained athletes or in other individuals during sleep. It also occurs in response to carotid sinus massage, Valsalva maneuver, hypothermia, increased intraocular pressure, vagal stimulation, and the administration of certain drugs (e.g., β-adrenergic blockers, calcium channel blockers). Disease states associated with sinus bradycardia are hypothyroidism, increased intracranial pressure, hypoglycemia, and inferior wall myocardial infarction (MI).

- Clinical significance depends on how the patient tolerates bradycardia hemodynamically. Signs of symptomatic bradycardia include pale, cool skin; hypotension; weakness; angina; dizziness or syncope, confusion, or disorientation; and shortness of breath.

- Treatment consists of administration of atropine for patients with symptoms. Pacemaker therapy may be required. If caused by drugs, these may need to be held or discontinued, or dosages reduced.

Sinus Tachycardia

This dysrhythmia involves a discharge rate of 101 to 200 beats per minute from the SA node as a result of vagal inhibition or sympathetic stimulation. Sinus tachycardia is associated with physiologic and psychologic stressors, such as exercise, fever, pain, hypotension, hypovolemia, anemia, hypoglycemia, myocardial ischemia, heart failure (HF), hyperthyroidism, and anxiety. It can also be an effect of drugs such as epinephrine, norepinephrine, caffeine, theophylline, nifedipine (Procardia), or hydralazine (Apresoline). Pseudoephedrine (Sudafed) found in many over-the-counter cold remedies can also cause tachycardia.

- Clinical significance depends on the patient's tolerance of the increased heart rate (HR). The patient may have symptoms of dizziness, dyspnea, and hypotension. Angina or an increase in infarction size may accompany persistent sinus tachycardia in the patient with an acute MI.
- Treatment is based on the underlying cause. In certain settings, intravenous (IV) adenosine (Adenocard) and β-adrenergic blockers (e.g., metoprolol [Lopressor]) may be used to reduce heart rate and decrease myocardial oxygen (O_2) consumption.

Premature Atrial Contraction (PAC)

PAC occurs as a result of contractions originating from an ectopic focus in the atrium in a location other than the SA node. The impulse originates in the left or right atrium and travels across the atria by an abnormal pathway, creating a distorted P wave. At the AV node it may be stopped (nonconducted PAC), delayed (lengthened PR interval), or conducted normally. If the impulse moves through the AV node, in most cases it is conducted normally through the ventricles. In a normal heart, a PAC can result from emotional stress or physical fatigue or from the use of caffeine, tobacco, or alcohol. A PAC can also result from hypoxia, electrolyte imbalances, and disease states such as hyperthyroidism, chronic obstructive pulmonary disease (COPD), and heart disease, including coronary artery disease (CAD) and valvular disease.

- HR varies with the underlying rate and frequency of PAC, and the rhythm is irregular.

- Isolated PACs are not significant in persons with healthy hearts. In persons with heart disease, PACs may warn of or initiate more serious dysrhythmias (e.g., supraventricular tachycardia).
- Treatment depends on patient symptoms. Withdrawal of sources of stimulation such as caffeine may be warranted. β-Adrenergic blockers may also be used to decrease PACs.

Paroxysmal Supraventricular Tachycardia (PSVT)

PSVT is a dysrhythmia originating in an ectopic focus anywhere above the bifurcation of the bundle of His. Paroxysmal refers to an abrupt onset and termination. Some degree of AV block may be present. In the normal heart PSVT is associated with overexertion, emotional stress, deep inspiration, and stimulants such as caffeine and tobacco. PSVT is also associated with rheumatic heart disease, Wolff-Parkinson-White (WPW) syndrome (conduction by way of accessory pathways), digitalis intoxication, CAD, and cor pulmonale.

- HR is 150 to 220 beats/min, and rhythm is regular.
- Clinical significance depends on symptoms and HR. A prolonged episode and HR >180 beats/min may precipitate a decreased cardiac output (CO), resulting in hypotension, dyspnea, and angina.
- Treatment includes vagal stimulation and drug therapy. Common vagal manuevers include Valsalva and coughing. IV adenosine (Adenocard) is the first drug of choice to convert PSVT to a normal sinus rhythm. IV β-adrenergic blockers (e.g., sotalol [Betapace]), calcium channel blockers (e.g., diltiazem [Cardizem]), and amiodarone (Cordarone) can also be used.

Atrial Flutter

This condition is an atrial tachydysrhythmia identified by recurring, regular, sawtooth-shaped flutter waves that originate from a single ectopic focus in the right atrium. Atrial flutter rarely occurs in a normal heart. It is associated with CAD, hypertension, mitral valve disorders, pulmonary embolus, chronic lung disease, cor pulmonale, cardiomyopathy, hyperthyroidism, and the use of drugs such as digoxin, quinidine, and epinephrine.

- Atrial rate is 250 to 350 beats/min. Ventricular rate varies according to conduction ratio. In 2:1 conduction, ventricular rate is typically about 150 beats/min. Atrial and ventricular rhythms are usually regular.
- High ventricular rates (>100) can decrease CO and cause serious consequences, such as HF.

- Primary treatment goal is to slow ventricular response by increasing AV block. Drugs used to control ventricular rate include calcium channel blockers and β-adrenergic blockers. Antidysrhythmic drugs used to convert atrial flutter to sinus rhythm or maintain sinus rhythm include amiodarone, propafenone (Rythmol), ibutilide (Corvert), and flecainide (Tambocor). Electrical cardioversion may be used to convert atrial flutter to sinus rhythm in an emergency situation. Radiofrequency catheter ablation is the treatment of choice for atrial flutter. Warfarin (Coumadin) is used to prevent stroke from embolization in patients with atrial flutter of greater than 48 hours' duration.

Atrial Fibrillation

This condition is a total disorganization of atrial electrical activity because of multiple ectopic foci. The dysrhythmia may be paroxysmal (i.e., begins and ends spontaneously) or persistent (lasting >7 days). Atrial fibrillation is the most common, clinically significant dysrhythmia with respect to morbidity, mortality, and economic impact. It occurs in about 3% of people over age 65 and its prevalence increases with age. The dysrhythmia usually occurs in the patient with underlying heart disease. It is also associated with thyrotoxicosis, alcohol intoxication, caffeine use, electrolyte disturbances, stress, and cardiac surgery.

- Atrial rate may be as high as 350 to 600 beats/min. Ventricular rate varies and the rhythm is usually irregular.
- Atrial fibrillation results in a decrease in CO because of ineffective atrial contractions and/or rapid ventricular response. Thrombi form in the atria because of blood stasis. An embolized clot may develop and pass to the brain, causing a stroke.
- The goals of treatment include a decrease in ventricular response to <100 beats/min, prevention of cerebral embolic events, and conversion to sinus rhythm, if possible. Drugs used for rate control include calcium channel blockers, β-adrenergic blockers, dronedaron (Multaq), and digoxin. The most common antidysrhythmic drugs used for cardioversion to and maintenance of sinus rhythm include amiodarone and ibutilide. Cardioversion may convert atrial fibrillation to normal sinus rhythm after a period of anticoagulation therapy.

First-Degree AV Block

In this type of AV block every impulse from the atria is conducted to the ventricles, but the duration of AV conduction is prolonged. After the impulse moves through the AV node, it is usually conducted normally through the ventricles. First-degree AV block is associated with MI, CAD, rheumatic fever, hyperthyroidism, vagal stimulation, and drugs such as digoxin, β-adrenergic blockers, calcium channel blockers, and flecainide.

- HR is normal, and rhythm is regular.
- First-degree AV block may be a precursor of higher degrees of AV block.
- There is no treatment for first-degree AV block.

Second-Degree AV Block, Type I (Mobitz I, Wenckebach)

A type I, second-degree AV block is characterized by gradual lengthening of the PR interval. It occurs because of an AV conduction time that is prolonged until an atrial impulse is nonconducted and a QRS complex is blocked (missing). Type I AV block may result from use of digoxin or β-adrenergic blockers. It may be associated with CAD. It is usually the result of myocardial ischemia or infarction. It is usually transient and well tolerated. However, it may be a warning signal of an impending significant AV conduction disturbance.

- The rhythm appears in a pattern of grouped beats.
- If the patient is symptomatic, atropine is used to increase HR or a temporary pacemaker may be needed, especially if the patient has an acute MI.

Second-Degree Heart Block, Type II (Mobitz II)

In this type of heart block, the P wave is nonconducted without progressive PR lengthening; this usually occurs when a bundle branch block is present. On conducted beats, the PR interval is constant. In a second-degree heart block a certain number of impulses from the sinus node are not conducted to the ventricles. This occurs in ratios of 2 : 1, 3 : 1, and so on when there are two P waves to one QRS complex, three P waves to one QRS complex, and so on. It may occur with varying ratios. Type II AV block is associated with rheumatic heart disease, CAD, anterior MI, and drug toxicity.

- Atrial rate is usually normal. Ventricular rate depends on intrinsic rate and degree of AV block. Atrial rhythm is regular, but ventricular rhythm may be irregular.
- Type II AV block often progresses to third-degree AV block and is associated with a poor prognosis.
- Reduced HR may result in decreased CO with subsequent hypotension and myocardial ischemia.
- Type II AV block is an indication for a permanent pacemaker (see Pacemakers, p. 749).

Third-Degree AV Heart Block (Complete Heart Block)

This condition constitutes one form of AV dissociation in which no impulses from the atria are conducted to the ventricles. The atria are stimulated and contract independently of the ventricles. Ventricular rhythm is an escape rhythm, and focus may be above or below the bifurcation of the bundle of His. This rhythm is associated with severe heart disease, including CAD, MI, myocarditis, cardiomyopathy, and some systemic diseases such as amyloidosis and progressive systemic sclerosis (scleroderma). Some medications can also cause third-degree AV block, such as digoxin, β-adrenergic blockers, and calcium channel blockers.

- Atrial rate is usually a sinus rate of 60 to 100 beats/min. Ventricular rate depends on the site of the block. If it is in the AV node, the rate is 40 to 60 beats/min, and if it is in the Purkinje system, it is 20 to 40 beats/min. Atrial and ventricular rhythms are regular but asynchronous.
- Third-degree AV block almost always results in reduced CO with subsequent ischemia and heart failure.
- A temporary transvenous or transcutaneous pacemaker is used until a permanent pacemaker can be inserted. Use of drugs such as atropine, epinephrine, isoproterenol (Isuprel), and dopamine is a temporary measure to increase HR and support blood pressure (BP) before pacemaker insertion (see Pacemakers, p. 749).

Premature Ventricular Contractions (PVCs)

These contractions originate in an ectopic focus in the ventricles. PVCs are a premature occurrence of the QRS complex, which is wide and distorted in shape. PVCs that are initiated from different foci appear different in shape from each other and are termed *multifocal PVCs*. When every other beat is a PVC, it is called *ventricular bigeminy*. When every third beat is a PVC, it is called *ventricular trigeminy*. Two consecutive PVCs are called *couplets*. *Ventricular tachycardia* occurs when there are three or more consecutive PVCs. When a PVC falls on the T wave of a preceding beat, the *R-on-T phenomenon* occurs and is considered to be dangerous because it may precipitate ventricular tachycardia or ventricular fibrillation. PVCs are associated with stimulants such as caffeine, alcohol, nicotine, epinephrine, isoproterenol, and digoxin. They are also associated with electrolyte imbalances, hypoxia, fever, exercise, and emotional stress. Disease states associated with PVCs include MI, mitral valve prolapse, HF, and CAD.

- HR varies according to the intrinsic rate and the number of PVCs. Rhythm is irregular because of premature beats.
- PVCs are usually a benign finding in a patient with a normal heart. In heart disease, PVCs may reduce CO and precipitate angina and HF. PVCs in CAD or acute MI represent ventricular irritability.

- Treatment relates to the cause of the PVCs (e.g., oxygen therapy for hypoxia, electrolyte replacement). Assessing the patient's hemodynamic status is important to determine if drug therapy is indicated. Drugs may include β-adrenergic blockers, procainamide, amiodarone, or lidocaine (Xylocaine).

Ventricular Tachycardia

This dysrhythmia is a run of three or more PVCs that occurs when an ectopic focus or foci fire repetitively and the ventricle takes control as the pacemaker. Different forms of ventricular tachycardia exist. The development of ventricular tachycardia is an ominous sign. It is a life-threatening dysrhythmia because of decreased CO and the possibility of the development of ventricular fibrillation, which is a lethal dysrhythmia. Ventricular tachycardia is associated with MI, CAD, significant electrolyte imbalances, hypoxemia, cardiomyopathy, mitral valve prolapse, long QT syndrome, digitalis toxicity, and central nervous system disorders. The dysrhythmia can be seen in patients who have no evidence of cardiac disease.

- The ventricular rate is 150 to 250 beats/min.
- If the patient is hemodynamically stable and has monomorphic VT (QRS complexes have same shape, size, and direction) with preserved left ventricular function, then IV procainamide, sotalol, amiodarone, or lidocaine is used. If the patient is unstable or has poor left ventricular function, amiodarone or lidocaine is given followed by cardioversion.
- If VT is polymorphic (QRS complexes change from one shape, size, or direction over a series of beats) with normal baseline QT interval, any one of the following medications is used: β-adrenergic blockers, lidocaine, amiodarone, procainamide, or sotalol. Cardioversion is used when drug therapy is ineffective.
- Ventricular tachycardia without a pulse is a lethal dysrhythmia and is treated in the same manner as ventricular fibrillation.

Ventricular Fibrillation

This condition is a severe derangement of the heart rhythm characterized on the ECG by irregular waveforms of varying contour and amplitude. This represents the firing of multiple ectopic foci in the ventricle. Mechanically, the ventricle is simply "quivering," and no effective contraction or CO occurs. This dysrhythmia is lethal. Ventricular fibrillation occurs in acute MI and myocardial ischemia and in chronic diseases such as CAD and cardiomyopathy. It may occur during cardiac pacing or cardiac catheterization procedures because of catheter stimulation of the ventricle. It may also occur with coronary reperfusion after fibrinolytic therapy. Other clinical associations are accidental electrical shock, hyperkalemia, hypoxemia, acidosis, and drug toxicity.

- HR is not measurable. Rhythm is irregular and chaotic.
- Ventricular fibrillation results in an unresponsive, pulseless, and apneic state. If not rapidly treated, the patient will die.
- Treatment consists of cardiopulmonary resuscitation (CPR) and initiation of advanced cardiovascular life support (ACLS) measures with the use of defibrillation and definitive drug therapy with epinephrine and atropine, intubation, and possibly a transcutaneous temporary pacemaker.

ENCEPHALITIS

E

Description
Encephalitis, a serious, sometimes fatal, acute inflammation of the brain, is usually caused by a virus. Many different viruses have been implicated in encephalitis; some of them are associated with certain seasons of the year and are endemic to certain geographic areas. Ticks and mosquitoes transmit epidemic encephalitis, whereas nonepidemic encephalitis may occur as a complication of measles, chickenpox, or mumps.

- Herpes simplex virus (HSV) encephalitis is the most common form of nonepidemic viral encephalitis. Cytomegalovirus encephalitis is one of the common complications in patients with acquired immunodeficiency syndrome (AIDS).

Clinical Manifestations and Diagnostic Studies
The onset of the infection is typically nonspecific, with fever, headache, nausea, and vomiting. It can be acute or subacute. Signs of encephalitis appear on day 2 or 3 and may vary from minimal alterations in mental status to coma.

- Almost any central nervous system (CNS) abnormality can occur, including hemiparesis, tremors, seizures, cranial nerve palsies, personality changes, memory impairment, and amnesia.
- West Nile virus should be strongly considered in adults older than 50 years who develop encephalitis or meningitis in summer or early fall. The best diagnostic test for West Nile virus is a blood test that detects viral RNA.
- Diagnostic findings related to viral encephalitis are shown in Table 37.

Table 37 Comparison of Cerebral Inflammatory Conditions

	Meningitis Bacteria (*Streptococcus pneumoniae, Neisseria meningitidis*, group B streptococcus, viruses, fungi)	Encephalitis Bacteria, Fungi, Parasites, Herpes Simplex Virus (HSV), Other Viruses (e.g., West Nile virus)	Brain Abscess Streptococci, Staphylococci Through Bloodstream
Causative Organisms			
CSF (Reference Interval)			
Pressure (60-150 mm H₂O)	Increased	Normal to slight increase	Increased
WBC count (0-5 cells/μL)	*Bacterial:* >1000/μL (mainly PMN) *Viral:* 25-500/μL (mainly lymphocytes)	500/μL, PMN (early), lymphocytes (later)	25-300/μL (PMN)
Protein (15-45 mg/dL [0.15-0.45 g/Ll)	*Bacterial:* >500 mg/dL *Viral:* 50-500 mg/dL	Slight increase	Normal
Glucose (40-70 mg/dL [2.2-3.9 mmol/L])	*Bacterial:* decreased *Viral:* normal or low	Normal	Low or absent
Appearance	*Bacterial:* turbid, cloudy *Viral:* clear or cloudy	Clear	Clear
Diagnostic Studies	CT scan, Gram stain, smear, culture, PCR*	CT scan, EEG, MRI, PET, PCR, IgM antibodies to virus in serum or CSF	CT scan
Treatment	Antibiotics, dexamethasone, supportive care, prevention of ↑ICP	Supportive care, prevention of ↑ICP, acyclovir (Zovirax) for HSV	Antibiotics, incision and drainage Supportive care

CSF, Cerebrospinal fluid; *CT,* computed tomography; *EEG,* electroencephalogram; *ICP,* intracranial pressure; *MRI,* magnetic resonance imaging; *PCR,* polymerase chain reaction; *PET,* positron emission tomography; *PMN,* polymorphonuclear cells; *WBC,* white blood cell.

*PCR is used to detect viral RNA or DNA.

- Brain imaging techniques include computed tomography (CT), magnetic resonance imaging (MRI), and positron emission tomography (PET).
- Polymerase chain reaction (PCR) tests for early detection of herpes simplex virus (HSV) and West Nile encephalitis.

Collaborative and Nursing Management

Management is symptomatic and supportive. Initially many patients require intensive care. Acyclovir (Zovirax) and vidarabine suspension (Vira-A) are used to treat HSV encephalitis. For maximal benefit, antiviral agents must be started before the onset of coma.

- Prophylactic treatment with antiseizure drugs may be used in severe cases of encephalitis.

E

ENDOCARDITIS, INFECTIVE

Description

Infective endocarditis (IE) is an infection of the endocardial surface of the heart. Inflammation from IE affects the cardiac valves because they are contiguous with the endocardium.

Classification

IE can be classified as subacute or acute.

- The *subacute form* typically affects those with preexisting valve disease and has a clinical course that may extend over months.
- In contrast, the *acute form* typically affects those with healthy valves and presents as a rapidly progressive illness.

IE can also be classified based on the cause (e.g., intravenous drug abuse, fungal endocarditis) or site of involvement (e.g., prosthetic valve endocarditis).

Pathophysiology

The most common causative agents, *Staphylococcus aureus* and *Streptococcus viridans,* are bacterial. Other pathogens include fungi and viruses. Newly identified pathogens that are difficult to cultivate (e.g., *Bartonella, Tropheryma whipplei*) also cause IE.

IE occurs when blood flow turbulence within the heart allows the causative organism to infect previously damaged valves or other endothelial surfaces. This can occur in individuals with a variety of underlying cardiac conditions, including prior endocarditis, prosthetic valves, acquired valve disease, and cardiac lesions. A variety of invasive procedures (e.g., intravenous [IV] drug abuse and renal dialysis) can also allow large numbers of organisms to enter the bloodstream and trigger the infectious process.

Vegetations, the primary lesions of IE, consist of fibrin, leukocytes, platelets, and microbes, which adhere to the valve surface or endocardium. The loss of portions of this vegetation into the circulation results in embolization. Systemic embolization occurs from left-sided heart vegetation, progressing to organ (particularly kidney, spleen, and brain) and limb infarction. Right-sided heart lesions embolize to the lungs.

The infection may spread locally to cause damage to valves or their supporting structures. This results in dysrhythmias, valve incompetence, and eventual invasion of the myocardium leading to heart failure (HF), sepsis, and heart block.

Clinical Manifestations

The clinical manifestations are nonspecific and can involve multiple organ systems. Low-grade fever occurs in more than 90% of patients.

Nonspecific manifestations include chills, weakness, malaise, fatigue, and anorexia. Arthralgias, myalgias, abdominal discomfort, back pain, weight loss, headache, and clubbing of fingers may occur in subacute forms of endocarditis.

Vascular manifestations include splinter hemorrhages (black longitudinal streaks) that may occur in the nail beds. Petechiae, as a result of fragmentation and microembolization of vegetative lesions, are common in the conjunctivae, lips, buccal mucosa, and palate and over the ankles, feet, and antecubital and popliteal areas. *Osler's nodes* (painful, tender, red or purple, pea-size lesions) may be found on the fingertips or toes. *Janeway lesions* (flat, painless, small, red spots) may be found on the palms and soles. Funduscopic examination may reveal hemorrhagic retinal lesions called *Roth's spots.*

- Onset of a new or changing murmur is frequently noted, with the aortic and mitral valves most commonly affected.

Clinical manifestations secondary to embolization in various body organs may also be present: (1) embolization to the spleen may result in sharp, left upper quadrant pain and splenomegaly, local tenderness, and abdominal rigidity; (2) embolization to the kidneys may cause pain in the flank, hematuria, and azotemia; (3) emboli may lodge in the small peripheral blood vessels of the arms and legs and cause gangrene; (4) embolization to the brain may result in hemiplegia, ataxia, aphasia, visual changes, and change in the level of consciousness; and (5) pulmonary emboli may occur in right-sided endocarditis.

Diagnostic Studies

A recent health history should be obtained with inquiry made regarding any recent dental, urologic, surgical, or gynecologic procedures including normal or abnormal obstetric delivery. Document any previous history of heart disease, recent cardiac catheterization, cardiac surgery, intravascular device placement, renal dialysis, and infections (e.g., skin, respiratory, or urinary tract).

- Two blood cultures drawn 30 minutes apart will be positive in more than 90% of patients.
- A mild leukocytosis (white blood cell count ranging from 10,000 to 11,000/μL (10 to 11 × 10^9/L) occurs in acute endocarditis.
- Erythrocyte sedimentation rate (ESR) and C-reactive protein (CRP) levels may be elevated.
- Chest x-ray is used to detect an enlarged heart.
- Electrocardiogram (ECG) may show first- or second-degree heart block because the valves lie in close proximity to the atrioventricular (AV) node.
- Cardiac catheterization may be used to evaluate valve functioning.

Major criteria to diagnose IE include at least two of the following: positive blood cultures, new or changed cardiac murmur, or intracardiac mass or vegetation noted on echocardiography.

Collaborative Care

Prophylactic Treatment

Antibiotic prophylaxis is recommended for high cardiac risk conditions. These include prosthetic heart valves, history of endocarditis, surgically constructed systemic-pulmonary shunts, and pacemakers.

- Specific antibiotic regimens are recommended for dental, respiratory tract, gastrointestinal (GI), and genitourinary (GU) procedures (see Table 37-3 Lewis et al., *Medical-Surgical Nursing,* ed 8, p. 844).

Drug Therapy

Accurate identification of the infecting organism is the key to successful treatment. Complete eradication of the organisms generally takes weeks to achieve, and relapses are common. Initially patients are hospitalized and IV antibiotic therapy is started. Table 37-5 Lewis et al., *Medical-Surgical Nursing,* ed 8, p. 845 outlines specific regimens for outpatient drug therapy.

- Blood cultures are done to evaluate the effectiveness of antibiotic therapy. Blood cultures that remain positive indicate inadequate or inappropriate antibiotic administration,

aortic root or myocardial abscess, or the wrong diagnosis
(e.g., an infection elsewhere).

- Fever may persist for several days after treatment has been
  started and is treated with aspirin, acetaminophen, fluids,
  and rest.
- Complete bed rest is usually not indicated unless the temperature remains elevated or there are signs of heart failure.
- Fungal and prosthetic valve endocarditis responds poorly to
  antibiotic therapy alone. Early valve replacement followed
  by prolonged ($\geq$6 weeks) drug therapy is recommended in
  these situations.

Nursing Management

Goals
The patient with IE will have normal or baseline cardiac function,
perform activities of daily living without fatigue, and understand
the therapeutic regimen to prevent recurrence of endocarditis.

Nursing Diagnoses
- Hyperthermia
- Decreased cardiac output
- Activity intolerance

Nursing Interventions
The incidence of IE can be decreased by identifying individuals
who are at risk for the development of endocarditis. Assessment
of the patient's history and an understanding of the disease process
are crucial for planning and implementing appropriate health maintenance strategies.

IE generally requires treatment with antibiotics for 4 to 6 weeks.
After initial treatment in the hospital, the patient may continue
treatment in the home setting if hemodynamically stable and
compliant.

- Patients who receive outpatient IV antibiotics will require
  vigilant home nursing care. Instruct the patient or caregiver
  about the importance of monitoring body temperature
  because persistent, prolonged temperature elevations may
  mean that the drug therapy is ineffective. Teach patients
  and caregivers to recognize signs and symptoms of these
  complications (e.g., change in mental status, dyspnea,
  chest pain).
- The patient needs adequate periods of physical and emotional rest. Bed rest may be necessary when fever is present
  or there are complications (e.g., heart damage). Otherwise
  the patient may ambulate and perform moderate activity.
- Monitor laboratory data to determine the effectiveness of
  the antibiotic therapy. Assess IV lines for patency, and any

signs of complications (e.g., phlebitis). Administer antibiotics when scheduled and monitor the patient for any adverse reactions to drugs.

- To prevent problems related to decreased mobility, instruct the patient to wear elastic compression gradient stockings; perform range-of-motion (ROM) exercises; and cough and deep breathe every 2 hours.
- The patient may experience anxiety and fear associated with the illness. Recognize this and implement strategies to help the patient cope with the illness.

Patients with active endocarditis are at risk for life-threatening complications such as cerebral emboli and pulmonary edema. Adequacy of the home environment in terms of in-home caregivers and hospital access must be determined for successful management.

- After therapy is completed in either the home or hospital setting, management focuses on teaching the patient about the nature of the disease and reducing the risk of reinfection.

▼ **Patient and Caregiver Teaching**

- Instruct the patient about symptoms that may indicate recurrent infection, such as fever, fatigue, malaise, and chills, and the importance of notifying the health care provider if they occur.
- The patient must be instructed about the need for prophylactic antibiotic therapy before certain invasive procedures.
- Explain to the patient the relationship of follow-up care, good nutrition, and early treatment of common infections (e.g., colds) to maintain good health.

ENDOMETRIAL CANCER

Description

Cancer of the endometrium is the most common gynecologic malignancy. However, it has a relatively low mortality, with a survival rate of 95% if the cancer has not spread at the time of diagnosis.

- The major risk factor for endometrial cancer is estrogen, especially unopposed estrogen. Additional risk factors include increasing age, nulliparity, late menopause, obesity, smoking, and diabetes mellitus (DM). Pregnancy and oral contraceptives are protective factors.

Pathophysiology

This type of cancer arises from the endometrial lining. The precursor may be a hyperplastic state that progresses to invasive carcinoma. Hyperplasia occurs when estrogen is not counteracted by progesterone. The cancer directly extends into the cervix and through the uterine serosa. As invasion of the myometrium occurs, regional lymph nodes, including the paravaginal and paraaortic, become involved. Hematogenous metastases develop concurrently. The usual sites of metastases are the lung, bone, liver, and eventually the brain. Endometrial cancer grows slowly, metastasizes late, and is amenable to therapy if diagnosed early.

Clinical Manifestations

- The first symptom is abnormal uterine bleeding, usually in postmenopausal women. Because perimenopausal women have sporadic periods for a time, it is important that this sign not be ignored or attributed to menopause.
- Pain occurs late in the disease process, and other symptoms that may arise are related to metastasis to other organs.

Diagnostic Studies

Endometrial biopsy is the primary diagnostic procedure for endometrial cancer.

- Occurrence of abnormal or unexpected bleeding in a postmenopausal woman mandates obtaining a tissue sample to exclude endometrial cancer.
- The Pap test is not a reliable diagnostic tool for endometrial cancer, but it can rule out cervical cancer.

Collaborative Care

Treatment is a total hysterectomy and bilateral salpingo-oophorectomy with lymph node biopsies. Most cases of endometrial cancer are diagnosed at an early stage when surgery alone may result in cure. Surgery may be followed by radiation, either to the pelvis or abdomen externally or intravaginally, to decrease local recurrence. Treatment of advanced or recurrent disease is difficult. Progesterone hormonal therapy (e.g., megestrol [Megace]) is the treatment of choice when the progesterone receptor status is positive and the tumor is well differentiated. Tamoxifen (Nolvadex) is also effective in women with advanced or recurrent endometrial cancer. Chemotherapy is considered when progesterone therapy is unsuccessful. Agents used include doxorubicin (Adriamycin), cisplatin (Platinol), 5-fluorouracil (5-FU), carboplatin (Paraplatin), and paclitaxel (Taxol).

Nursing Management: Cancers of the Female Reproductive Tract

See Cervical Cancer, p. 113.

ENDOMETRIOSIS

Description

Endometriosis is the presence of normal endometrial tissue in sites outside the endometrial cavity. The most frequent sites are in or near the ovaries, uterosacral ligaments, and uterovesical peritoneum. However, endometrial tissues can be found in many other locations, such as the stomach, lungs, intestines, and spleen.

- The endometrial tissue responds to hormones of the ovarian cycle and undergoes a mini-menstrual cycle similar to uterine endometrium.
- Endometriosis is one of the most common gynecologic problems.

The etiology of endometriosis is unknown. A widely held view is that retrograde menstrual flow passes through the fallopian tubes, carrying viable endometrial tissues into the pelvis and attaching to various sites.

Clinical Manifestations

A wide range of symptoms and severity exists. The magnitude of a woman's symptoms does not necessarily correlate with the clinical extent of her endometriosis.

- The most common symptoms are secondary dysmenorrhea, infertility, pelvic pain, dyspareunia, and irregular bleeding.
- Less common symptoms include backache, painful bowel movements, and dysuria.
- Symptoms may or may not correspond to the woman's menstrual cycles. With menopause, estrogen is no longer produced in the ovaries, which may lead to the disappearance of symptoms.
- When the ectopic endometrial tissues "menstruate," blood collects in cystlike nodules. When a cyst ruptures, the pain may be acute and the resulting irritation promotes the formation of adhesions, which fix the affected area to another pelvic structure. The adhesions may become severe enough to cause a bowel obstruction or painful micturition.

Diagnostic Studies

Diagnosis is frequently confirmed by patient history and the palpation of firm nodular lumps in the adnexa on bimanual examination. Laparoscopic examination is necessary for a definitive diagnosis.

Collaborative Care

Treatment is influenced by a patient's age, desire for pregnancy, symptom severity, and the extent and location of the disease. When symptoms are not disruptive, a "watch and wait" approach is used.

Drug Therapy

Drug therapy is used to reduce symptoms. Drugs are selected to inhibit estrogen production by the ovary so that the endometrial tissue will shrink. The various drugs used imitate a state of pregnancy or menopause.

- Continuous use (for 9 months) of combined progestin and estrogen causes regression of endometrial tissue. Ovulation is suppressed, and pseudopregnancy (hyperhormonal amenorrhea) is produced by progestin agents such as medroxyprogesterone (Depo-Provera).
- Another approach to hormonal treatment is danazol (Danocrine), a synthetic androgen that inhibits the anterior pituitary. The drug produces a pseudomenopause (ovarian suppression), with atrophy of ectopic endometrial tissue. Subjective relief of symptoms is noted within 6 weeks of danazol use.
- Another class of drugs used is gonadotropin-releasing hormone (GnRH) agonists, such as leuprolide acetate (Lupron) and nafarelin (Synarel). These drugs cause a hypoestrogenic state resulting in amenorrhea.

Surgical Therapy

The only cure for endometriosis is surgical removal of all the endometrial implants. Surgical therapy may be conservative or definitive. *Conservative surgery* to confirm the diagnosis or remove implants involves removal or destruction of endometrial implants and lysing or excision of adhesions by means of laparoscopic laser surgery and laparotomy.

- For women wishing to get pregnant, conservative surgical therapy is used to remove implants that may block the fallopian tube. Adhesions are removed from the tubes, ovaries, and pelvic structures.

Definitive surgery involves removal of the uterus, fallopian tubes, ovaries, and as many endometrial implants as possible. Each woman should be actively involved in making the decision about preserving part or all of her ovaries if surgically possible. Help her to explore her feelings about maintaining her cyclic ovarian function.

Nursing Management

- Teach the patient that a health-threatening situation does not exist that may permit her to accept a conservative and progressive treatment. Assist the patient to understand the drugs ordered to treat the condition.
- Psychologic support may be needed for the patient experiencing severe disabling pain, sexual difficulties secondary to dyspareunia, and infertility.
- If conservative surgery is the treatment selected, nursing care is similar to general preoperative and postoperative care of a patient undergoing laparotomy (see Abdominal Pain, Acute, p. 3).
- If definitive (extensive) surgery is planned, nursing care is similar to the patient undergoing an abdominal hysterectomy. (See NCP 54-1 for the patient undergoing an abdominal hysterectomy, Lewis et al., *Medical-Surgical Nursing,* ed 8, p. 1369.)

ESOPHAGEAL CANCER

Description

Esophageal cancer is uncommon. However, the rates are increasing. Annually in the United States there are approximately 16,500 new cases of esophageal cancer diagnosed and 14,300 deaths from esophageal cancer. The five-year survival remains low at 34%. Incidence of esophageal cancer increases with age.

Risk factors include Barrett's metaplasia, smoking, excessive alcohol intake, central obesity, and diet intake that is low in fruits, vegetables, and vitamins A, B_2, and C. Patients with injury to the esophageal mucosa such as the ingestion of lye are also at greater risk. Occupational exposures to asbestos and cement dust have also been linked to the gender differences in esophageal cancer rates. *Achalasia,* a condition in which there is delayed emptying of the lower esophagus, is associated with squamous cell cancer.

Pathophysiology

Most esophageal cancers are adenocarcinomas, with the remainder being squamous cell. Adenocarcinomas arise from the glands lining the esophagus and resemble cancers of the stomach and small intestine.

- The majority of tumors are located in the middle and lower portions of the esophagus. The tumor may penetrate the muscular layer and extend outside the esophageal wall.
- The malignant tumor usually appears as an ulcerated lesion. It may have advanced to this stage before symptoms appear.

Clinical Manifestations

The onset of symptoms is usually late relative to tumor growth.

- Progressive dysphagia is the most common symptom and may be expressed as a substernal feeling that food is not passing. Initially dysphagia occurs only with meat, then with soft foods, and eventually with liquids.
- Pain develops late and is described as occurring in the substernal, epigastric, or back areas and usually increases with swallowing. The pain may radiate to the neck, jaw, ears, and shoulders.
- If the tumor is in the upper third of the esophagus, symptoms such as sore throat, choking, and hoarseness may occur. Weight loss is fairly common.
- When esophageal stenosis is severe, regurgitation of blood-flecked esophageal contents is common.

Complications may include hemorrhage from cancer eroding through the esophagus and into the aorta. Esophageal perforation into the lung or trachea may also develop. The liver and lung are common metastatic sites.

Diagnostic Studies

- Barium swallow with fluoroscopy may detect esophageal narrowing at the tumor site.
- Esophagoscopy with biopsy is used to make a definitive diagnosis.
- Endoscopic ultrasonography is used for staging.
- Bronchoscopic examination detects involvement of the lung.
- Computed tomography (CT) scan and magnetic resonance imaging (MRI) assess the extent of the disease.

Collaborative Care

Treatment depends on tumor location and whether metastasis has occurred. The best results may be obtained with a combination of surgery, endoscopic ablation, chemotherapy, and radiation.

- The surgical approaches may be open (thoracic, abdominal incision) or laparoscopic. The use of minimally invasive esophagectomy (e.g., laparoscopic vagal nerve sparing surgery) is also being performed.

- Endoscopic approaches using photodynamic and/or laser therapy are used to ablate high grade metaplasia of Barrett's esophagus.

Most patients with newly diagnosed esophageal cancer have local as well as advanced disease. Treatment includes neoadjuvant chemotherapy with or without radiation therapy. Concurrent radiation and chemotherapy are used for palliation of symptoms, especially dysphagia, as well as to increase survival. Palliative therapy consists of restoration of the swallowing function and maintenance of nutrition and hydration. Dilation, stent placement, or both can relieve obstruction.

Nutritional Therapy
After esophageal surgery, parenteral fluids are given. A swallowing study is often given before the patient is allowed to have oral fluids. When fluids are permitted, water (30 to 60 mL) is given hourly, with gradual progression to small, frequent, bland meals. The patient should be in an upright position to prevent fluid regurgitation. Observe the patient for signs of intolerance to the feeding or leakage of the feeding into the mediastinum. Symptoms indicating leakage are pain, increased temperature, and dyspnea. A gastrostomy may be performed for the purpose of feeding the patient.

Nursing Management
Goals
The patient with esophageal cancer will have relief of symptoms, including pain and dysphagia, achieve optimal nutritional intake, understand the prognosis of the disease, and experience a quality of life appropriate to disease progression.

Nursing Diagnoses
- Imbalanced nutrition: less than body requirements
- Chronic pain
- Risk for aspiration
- Deficient fluid volume
- Anxiety
- Grieving

Nursing Interventions
In addition to general preoperative teaching and preparation, pay particular attention to the patient's nutritional needs. Many patients are poorly nourished because of the inability to ingest adequate amounts and fluids. Meticulous oral care is essential. Teaching should include information about chest tubes (if a thoracic approach is used), intravenous (IV) lines, nasogastric (NG) tube, gastrostomy or jejunostomy feeding, turning, coughing, and deep breathing.

Postoperative care should include assessment of drainage; maintenance of the NG tube; oral and nasal care; and prevention of respiratory complications by turning, coughing, and deep breathing, incentive spirometry every 2 hours, and placing the patient in a semi-Fowler's position to prevent gastric reflux and aspiration.

Many patients require long-term follow-up care after surgery for esophageal cancer. The patient may undergo chemotherapy and radiation treatment after surgery. Encourage and assist the patient in maintaining adequate nutrition. A permanent feeding gastrostomy may be needed. The patient usually has fears and anxieties about a diagnosis of cancer.

- Know what the physician has told the patient regarding the prognosis and then provide appropriate counseling.
- Referral to a home health nurse may be necessary for continued care of the patient (e.g., gastrostomy teaching and follow-up wound care).

▼ **Patient and Caregiver Teaching**

- Health promotion includes follow-up evaluation and care for patients diagnosed with GERD, Barrett's esophagus, and hiatal hernia.
- Health counseling should focus on the elimination of smoking and excessive alcohol intake.
- Encourage patients to seek medical attention for any esophageal problems, especially dysphagia.
- Maintenance of good oral hygiene and dietary habits (intake of fresh fruits and vegetables) are important.

FIBROCYSTIC BREAST CHANGES

Description

Fibrocystic changes in the breast constitute the most frequently occurring breast disorder. These benign changes include the development of excess fibrous tissue, hyperplasia of the epithelial lining of the mammary ducts, proliferation of mammary ducts, and cyst formation. Fibrocystic changes occur most frequently in women between 35 and 50 years old, but often begin in women as young as 20 years old. They are not associated with increased breast cancer risk.

Fibrocystic changes most commonly occur in women with premenstrual abnormalities, nulliparous women, women with a history of spontaneous abortion, nonusers of oral contraceptives, and women with early menarche and late menopause.

Pathophysiology

- The cause of fibrocystic changes is thought to be heightened responsiveness of breast tissue to circulating estrogen and progesterone.
- Fibrocystic changes produce pain by nerve irritation from connective tissue edema and fibrosis from nerve pinching.
- Masses or nodularities can appear in both breasts and are often found in the upper, outer quadrants; they usually occur bilaterally.
- Symptoms of fibrocystic changes often are exacerbated in the premenstrual phase and subside after menstruation.

Clinical Manifestations

Manifestations of fibrocystic breast changes include one or more palpable lumps that are usually round, well delineated, and freely movable within the breast. There may be accompanying discomfort ranging from tenderness to pain.

- The lump usually increases in size and perhaps in tenderness before menstruation. Cysts may enlarge or shrink rapidly.
- Nipple discharge associated with fibrocystic breasts is often milky, watery milky, yellow, or green.
- Pain and nodularity often increase over time, but tend to subside after menopause unless high doses of estrogen replacement are used.

Nursing and Collaborative Management

With the initial discovery of a discrete breast mass, aspiration or surgical biopsy may be indicated. A wait of 7 to 10 days may be planned to note any changes related to the menstrual cycle.

- An excisional biopsy should be done if no fluid is found on aspiration, the fluid that is found is hemorrhagic, or a residual mass remains. This surgery is usually performed in an outpatient surgical unit.

Many types of treatment have been suggested for a fibrocystic condition. Some relief may occur if the changes are cyclic with caffeine and coffee and dietary fat reduction, taking vitamins E, A, and B complex and γ-linolenic acid (evening primrose oil); and the continual wearing of a support bra. Drugs might be recommended including oral contraceptives and danazol (Danocrine).

▼ **Patient and Caregiver Teaching**

The role of the nurse in the care of the patient with fibrocystic breast changes is primarily one of teaching. Inform the patient that she may expect recurrences of the cysts in one or both breasts until menopause, and cysts may enlarge or become painful just before menstruation. In addition, offer reassurance that cysts do not "turn into" cancer.

- Encourage the woman with cystic changes to return regularly for follow-up examinations. Also teach her breast self-examination (BSE) to self-monitor the problem. Any new lumps should be evaluated, and changes in symptoms should be reported and investigated.

FIBROMYALGIA SYNDROME

Description

Fibromyalgia syndrome (FMS) is a chronic disorder characterized by widespread, nonarticular musculoskeletal pain and fatigue with multiple tender points. People with FMS also typically experience nonrestorative sleep, morning stiffness, irritable bowel syndrome, and anxiety. Fibromyalgia is a commonly diagnosed musculoskeletal disorder and a major cause of disability. FMS occurs 6 times more frequently in women than men. FMS and chronic fatigue syndrome (CFS) share many commonalities (see Table 25, p. 125).

Pathophysiology

There is general agreement that FMS is a disorder involving neuroendocrine/neurotransmitter dysregulation. The pain amplification experienced by the affected patient is caused by abnormal sensory processing in the central nervous system. Multiple physiologic abnormalities in the FMS patient include increased levels of substance P in the spinal fluid, low levels of blood flow to the thalamus, dysfunction of the hypothalamic pituitary-adrenal (HPA) axis, low levels of serotonin and tryptophan, and abnormalities in cytokine function.

- Serotonin and substance P play a role in mood regulation, sleep, and pain perception. Changes in the HPA axis can lead to depression and a decreased response to stress.
- A recent viral illness or Lyme disease may serve as an infectious trigger in susceptible persons.

Clinical Manifestations

The patient complains of a widespread burning pain that worsens and improves through the course of a day. It is often difficult for the patient to discriminate if pain occurs in the muscles, joints, or soft tissues.

- Head or facial pain often results from stiff or painful neck and shoulder muscles. This pain can accompany temporomandibular joint dysfunction. Nonrestorative sleep and

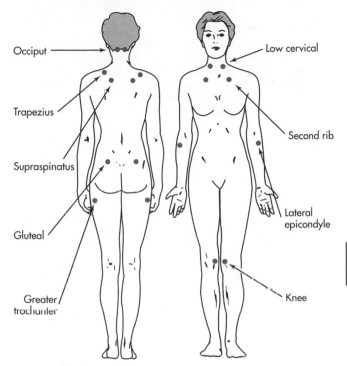

Fig. 5. Tender points in fibromyalgia syndrome.

resulting fatigue are typical. Physical examination characteristically reveals point tenderness at 11 or more of 18 identified sites (Fig. 5).

- Cognitive effects range from difficulty concentrating to memory lapses and a feeling of being overwhelmed when dealing with multiple tasks. Many individuals report migraine headaches, depression, and anxiety.
- Numbness or tingling in the hands or feet (paresthesia) often accompanies FMS. Restless legs syndrome is also common.
- Women with FMS may experience more difficult menstruation, with a worsening of disease symptoms during this time.
- Irritable bowel syndrome with manifestations of diarrhea or constipation, abdominal pain, and bloating can occur, in addition to symptoms of overactive bladder.

Diagnostic Studies

A definitive diagnosis is often difficult to establish. Laboratory results may serve to rule out other suspected disorders based on the patient's history and physical examination.

- Occasionally a low antinuclear antibody (ANA) titer is seen, but it is not considered diagnostic.
- Muscle biopsy may reveal a nonspecific moth-eaten appearance or fiber atrophy.

The American College of Rheumatology classifies an individual as having FMS if two criteria are met: (1) pain is experienced in 11 of the 18 tender points on palpation and (2) a history of widespread pain for at least 3 months.

Collaborative Care

Treatment is symptomatic and requires a high level of patient motivation. You can play a key role in teaching the patient to be an active participant in the therapeutic regimen. Rest can help pain, aching, and tenderness.

In some patients, pain may be managed with OTC analgesics such as acetaminophen (Tylenol), ibuprofen (Motrin, Advil), or naproxen (Aleve).

Drug treatment also may include low doses of tricyclic compounds such as cyclobenzaprine (Flexeril) and amitriptyline (Elavil). Dual reuptake inhibitors (venlafaxine [Effexor], milnacipin [Savella], duloxetine [Cymbalta]), and tramadol (Ultram) work similarly and may be effective for some patients. If amitriptyline is not well tolerated, other similar drugs can be substituted (e.g., doxepin [Sinequan], imipramine [Tofranil], trazodone [Desyrel]). Selective serotonin reuptake inhibitor (SSRI) antidepressants (e.g., sertraline [Zoloft] or paroxetine [Paxil]) tend to be reserved for FMS patients who also have depression.

Zolpidem (Ambien) is sometimes prescribed for patients with severe sleep disturbances. The antiseizure drugs gabapentin (Neurontin) and pregabalin (Lyrica) may reduce pain and fatigue and improve sleep and daily functioning.

Nursing and Collaborative Management

Because of the chronic nature of FMS and the need to maintain an ongoing rehabilitation program, the patient needs consistent support from you and the other health team members. Massage is often combined with ultrasound or the application of alternating heat and cold packs to soothe tense, sore muscles and increase blood circulation.

- Gentle stretching can be performed by a physical therapist or practiced by the patient at home to relieve muscle tension and spasm.
- Dietitians often urge FMS patients to limit their consumption of sugar, caffeine, and alcohol, because these substances have been shown to be muscle irritants.
- Pain and the related symptoms of FMS can cause significant stress. There is also some indication that these patients do not deal with stress. Effective relaxation strategies include biofeedback, guided imagery, and autogenic training. Psychologic counseling (individual or group) may also prove beneficial for the FMS patient.

FLAIL CHEST

Description
Flail chest results from the fracture of two or more ribs, in two or more separate locations, causing an unstable segment.

F

Pathophysiology
The affected (flail) area will move paradoxically with respect to the intact portion of the chest during respiration. During inspiration, the affected portion is sucked in, and during expiration it bulges out. This paradoxic chest movement prevents adequate ventilation of the lung in the injured area and increases the work of breathing.

Clinical Manifestations and Diagnostic Studies
A flail chest is usually apparent on visual examination of the unconscious patient.
- The patient manifests rapid, shallow respirations and tachycardia.
- A flail chest may not be initially apparent in the conscious patient as a result of splinting of the chest wall. The patient moves air poorly and movement of the thorax is asymmetric and uncoordinated.
- Palpation of abnormal respiratory movements, evaluation for crepitus near the rib fractures, chest x-ray, and ABGs all assist in the diagnosis.

Collaborative Care
Initial therapy consists of airway management, adequate ventilation, supplemental oxygen (O_2) therapy, careful administration of

intravenous (IV) solutions, and pain control. Definitive therapy is to reexpand the lung and ensure adequate oxygenation. Although many patients can be managed without the use of mechanical ventilation, a short period of intubation and ventilation may be necessary. Lung parenchyma and fractured ribs will heal with time.

FRACTURE

Description

A fracture is a disruption or break in the continuity of the structure of bone. Traumatic injuries account for the majority of fractures, although some fractures are secondary to a disease process (pathologic fractures from cancer or osteoporosis).

- Fractures can be classified as *open* (formerly called compound) or *closed* (formerly called simple) depending on communication or noncommunication with the external environment. In an open fracture, the skin is broken, exposing the bone and causing soft tissue injury. In a closed fracture the skin has not been ruptured and remains intact.
- Fractures can also be classified as complete or incomplete. Fractures are termed *complete* if the break is completely through the bone and described as *incomplete* if the fracture occurs partly across a bone shaft but the bone is still in one piece. An incomplete fracture is often the result of bending or crushing forces applied to a bone.
- Fractures are also described and classified according to the direction of the fracture line. Types include linear, oblique, transverse, longitudinal, and spiral fractures.
- Fractures can also be classified as *displaced* or *nondisplaced*. In a displaced fracture the two ends of the broken bone are separated from one another and out of their normal positions. Displaced fractures are usually comminuted (more than two fragments) or oblique. In a nondisplaced fracture the periosteum is intact across the fracture and the bone is still in alignment. Nondisplaced fractures are usually transverse, spiral, or greenstick.

Illustrations of the various classifications of fractures can be found in Figs. 63-7, and 63-8 in Lewis et al., *Medical-Surgical Nursing,* ed 8, p. 1590.

Clinical Manifestations

The patient's history indicates a mechanism of injury associated with manifestations including immediate localized pain, decreased function, and inability to bear weight on or use the affected part.

- The patient guards and protects the extremity against movement. Obvious bone deformity may not be present.
- If a fracture is suspected, the extremity is immobilized in the position in which it is found. Unnecessary movement increases soft tissue damage and may convert a closed fracture to an open fracture or create further injury to adjacent neurovascular structures.

Fracture Healing

You need to understand the principles of fracture healing to provide appropriate therapeutic interventions. Bone goes through a remarkable reparative process of self-healing (termed *union*) that occurs in the following stages:

1. *Fracture hematoma.* When a fracture occurs, bleeding creates a hematoma, which surrounds the fragment ends. The hematoma is extravasated blood that changes from a liquid to a semisolid clot. This occurs in the initial 72 hours after injury.
2. *Granulation tissue.* During this stage, active phagocytosis absorbs the products of local necrosis. The hematoma converts to granulation tissue (consisting of new blood vessels, fibroblasts, and osteoblasts), which produces the basis for new bone substance called *osteoid* during days 3 to 14 postinjury.
3. *Callus formation.* As minerals (calcium, phosphorus, and magnesium) and new bone matrix are deposited in the osteoid, an unorganized network of bone is formed that is woven about the fracture parts. It usually appears by the end of the second week after injury. Callus formation can be verified by x-ray.
4. *Ossification.* Ossification of the callus occurs from 3 weeks to 6 months after the fracture and continues until the fracture has healed. Callus ossification is sufficient to prevent movement at the fracture site when bones are gently stressed. However, the fracture is still evident on x-ray. During this stage of *clinical union* the patient may be allowed limited mobility or the cast may be removed.
5. *Consolidation.* As callus continues to develop, the bone fragments eventually close as ossification continues. *Radiologic union* occurs when there is x-ray evidence of complete bony union. This phase can occur up to a year following injury.
6. *Remodeling.* Excess bone tissue is reabsorbed in the final stage of bone healing, and union is completed. Gradual return of the injured bone to its preinjury structural strength and shape occurs. Initially, weight bearing is gradually introduced. New bone is deposited in sites subjected to stress and

F

resorbed at areas where there is little stress. Radiologic union
is present.

Complications

The majority of fractures heal without complications. If death
occurs after a fracture, it is usually the result of damage to underlying
organs and vascular structures or from complications of the
fracture or immobility. For a summary of the complications of
fracture healing, see Table 63-5, Lewis et al., *Medical-Surgical
Nursing,* ed 8, p. 1592.

- Direct complications include problems with bone union,
  avascular necrosis, and bone infection.
- Indirect complications are associated with blood vessel and
  nerve damage resulting in conditions such as compartment
  syndrome, venous thromboembolism, rhabdomyolysis, fat
  embolism, and traumatic or hypovolemic shock. A discussion
  of these complications is in Lewis et al., *Medical-
  Surgical Nursing,* ed 8, pp. 1603 to 1604. Hypovolemic
  shock may also occur (see Shock, p. 572).
- Although most musculoskeletal injuries are not life threatening,
  open fractures or fractures accompanied by severe
  blood loss and fractures that damage vital organs (e.g.,
  lung, heart) are medical emergencies requiring immediate
  attention.

Open fractures and soft tissue injuries have a high incidence
of infection. Devitalized and contaminated tissue is an ideal
medium for many common pathogens, including gas-forming
(anaerobic) bacilli.

Diagnostic Studies

- History and physical examination
- X-ray, examination
- Computed tomography (CT) scan and magnetic resonance
  imaging (MRI)

Collaborative Care

The goals of treatment are anatomic realignment of bone fragments
(reduction), immobilization to maintain realignment, and restoration
of function of the injured part.

Fracture Reduction

Closed reduction is a nonsurgical, manual realignment of bones to
their previous anatomic position. Traction and countertraction are
manually applied to bone fragments to restore position, length, and
alignment.

■ Closed reduction is usually performed with the patient under local or general anesthesia. After reduction, the injured part is immobilized by casting, traction, external fixation, splints, or orthoses (braces) to maintain alignment until healing occurs.

Open reduction is correction of bone alignment through a surgical incision. It may include internal fixation of the fracture with the use of wire, screws, pins, plates, intramedullary rods, or nails.

■ Open reduction with internal fixation (ORIF) facilitates early ambulation, which decreases the risk of complications related to prolonged immobility and promotes fracture healing. If ORIF is used for intraarticular fractures, early initiation of range of motion of the joint is indicated. Machines that provide continuous passive motion (CPM) to various joints are now available.

Traction devices apply a pulling force on the fractured extremity while countertraction pulls in the opposite direction. The two most common types of traction are skin traction and skeletal traction.

■ Skin traction is generally used for short-term treatment (48 to 72 hours) until skeletal traction or surgery is possible. Tape, boots, or slings are applied directly to the skin to maintain alignment, assist in reduction, and help diminish muscle spasms in the injured part.

■ Skeletal traction, generally in place for longer periods, is used to align injured bones and joints or treat joint contractures and congenital hip dysplasia. It provides a long-term pull that keeps injured bones and joints aligned. Skeletal traction requires the insertion of a pin or wire into the bone, to align and immobilize the injured body part. Fracture alignment depends on correct positioning and alignment of the patient, whereas traction forces remain constant. For extremity traction to be effective, forces must be pulling in the opposite direction *(countertraction)*.

■ Countertraction is commonly supplied by the patient's body weight or may be augmented by elevating the end of the bed.

Fracture Immobilization

Casting may occur after closed reduction has been performed. It allows the patient to perform many normal activities of daily living (ADLs) while providing sufficient immobilization to ensure stability.

Immobilization of an acute fracture or soft tissue injury of the upper extremity is often accomplished by use of (1) the sugar-tong splint, (2) the posterior splint, (3) the short arm cast, and (4) the long arm cast. A discussion of these casts is in Lewis et al., *Medical-Surgical Nursing,* ed 8, p. 1593.

An *external fixator* is a metal device composed of metal pins that are inserted into the bone and attached to external rods to stabilize the fracture while it heals. It can be used to apply traction, immobilize reduced fragments when the use of a cast or traction is not appropriate, or compress fracture fragments. The external fixator is attached directly to the bones by percutaneous pins or wires. Assessment for pin loosening and infection is critical. Infection signaled by exudate, redness, tenderness, and pain may require removal of the device.

Internal fixation devices are surgically inserted at the time of realignment. Examples of internal fixation devices include pins, plates, and screws. Biologically inert devices such as titanium, stainless steel, or Vitallium are used to realign and maintain bony fragments. Proper alignment is evaluated by x-ray studies at regular intervals.

Other Therapy
Patients with fractures experience varying degrees of pain associated with muscle spasms.

- Central and peripheral muscle relaxants, such as carisoprodol (Soma), cyclobenzaprine (Flexeril), or methocarbamol (Robaxin), may be prescribed for relief of muscle spasms associated with pain.

Proper nutrition is an essential component of the reparative process in injured tissue.

- The patient's diet must include ample protein (e.g., 1 g/kg body weight), vitamins (especially B, C, and D), and calcium, phosphorus, and magnesium.

Nursing Management
Goals
The patient with a fracture will have physiologic healing with no associated complications, obtain satisfactory pain relief, and achieve maximal rehabilitation potential.

See NCP 63-1 for the patient with a fracture, Lewis et al., *Medical-Surgical Nursing,* ed 8, pp. 1598 to 1599.

Nursing Diagnoses
- Impaired physical mobility
- Risk for peripheral neurovascular dysfunction
- Acute pain
- Ineffective self-health management

Nursing Interventions

Patients with fractures may be treated in an emergency department or physician's office and released to home care, or they may require hospitalization. Specific nursing measures depend on the type of treatment used and setting in which patients are placed.

Preoperative management. If surgical intervention is required to treat the fracture, patients will need preoperative preparation. In addition to the usual preoperative nursing measures, inform patients of the type of immobilization and assistive devices that will be used.

- Proper skin preparation is important. The aim of skin preparation is to clean the skin and remove debris and hair to reduce the possibility of infection.
- Assure patients their needs will be met by the nursing staff until they can again meet their own needs. Knowing that pain medication will be available if needed is often beneficial.

Postoperative management. Frequent neurovascular assessments of the affected extremity are necessary to detect subtle changes. Closely monitor any limitations of movement or activity related to turning, positioning, and extremity support.

- Pain and discomfort can be minimized through proper alignment and positioning.
- Carefully observe dressings or casts for any overt signs of bleeding or drainage. Report a significant increase in the size of the drainage area.
- If a wound drainage system is in place, regularly assess the patency of the system and the volume of drainage. Whenever the contents of a drainage system are measured or emptied, use sterile technique to avoid contamination.

If the patient is immobilized as a result of the fracture, plan your care to prevent complications of immobility. Prevent constipation by increased activity, maintenance of a high fluid intake, and a diet high in bulk and roughage. If these measures are not effective in maintaining the patient's normal bowel pattern, stool softeners, laxatives, or suppositories may be necessary. Maintain a regular time for elimination to promote regularity.

- Renal calculi can develop as a result of bone demineralization. Unless contraindicated, a fluid intake of 2500 mL/day is recommended. Cranberry juice or ascorbic acid (500 mg/day) may be recommended to acidify the urine and prevent calcium precipitation.
- Rapid deconditioning of the circulatory system can occur as a result of prolonged bed rest, resulting in

Table 38	Patient and Caregiver Teaching Guide: Cast Care

You should include the following instructions when teaching the patient with a cast:

Do Not
Get cast wet.
Remove any padding.
Insert any objects inside cast.
Bear weight on new cast for 48 hr (not all casts are made for weight-bearing; check with health care provider when unsure).
Cover cast with plastic for prolonged periods.

Do
Apply ice directly over fracture site for first 24 hr (avoid getting cast wet by keeping ice in plastic bag and protecting cast with cloth).
Check with health care provider before getting fiberglass cast wet.
Dry cast thoroughly after exposure to water.
Blot dry with towel.
Use hair dryer on low setting until cast is thoroughly dry.
Elevate extremity above level of heart for first 48 hr.
Move joints above and below cast regularly.
Use hair dryer on cool setting for itching.
Report signs of possible problems to health care provider.
    Increasing pain
    Swelling associated with pain and discoloration of toes or fingers
    Pain during movement
    Burning or tingling under cast
    Sores or foul odor under the cast
Keep appointment to have fracture and cast checked.

---

orthostatic hypotension and decreased lung capacity. Unless contraindicated, these effects can be diminished by having the patient sit on the side of the bed, allowing the patient's lower limbs to dangle over the bedside, and having the patient perform standing transfers.

■ Also assess patients for deep vein thrombosis (DVT) and pulmonary emboli.

▼ **Patient and Caregiver Teaching**

Because many fractures are treated in an outpatient setting, the patient often requires only a short hospitalization or none at all. Therefore patient and caregiver teaching is important to prevent complications. In addition to specific instructions for cast care (Table 38) and recognition of complications, encourage the patient to contact the health care provider if questions arise. Validate the patient's and caregiver's understanding of these instructions before discharge.

For further information on rehabilitation management of fractures, including the use of assistive devices such as walkers and crutches, see Lewis et al., *Medical-Surgical Nursing,* ed 8, p. 1602, and also the specific types of fractures discussed in this *Companion.*

FRACTURE, HIP

Description

Hip fractures are common in older adults, with 90% of these fractures caused by a fall. In adults older than 65 years, hip fractures occur more often in women than men because of osteoporosis. An estimated 30% of patients who experience a hip fracture will die within 1 year of the injury because of medical complications caused by the fracture or resulting immobility. Many older adults with a hip fracture develop disabilities necessitating long-term care.

A fracture of the hip refers to a fracture of the proximal third of the femur, which extends up to 5 cm below the lesser trochanter.

- Fractures that occur within the hip joint capsule are called *intracapsular fractures.* Intracapsular fractures (femoral neck) are further identified by their specific locations: capital, subcapital, and transcervical. These fractures are often associated with osteoporosis and minor trauma.

- *Extracapsular fractures* occur outside the joint capsule. They are termed *intertrochanteric* if they occur in a region between the greater and lesser trochanter or *subtrochanteric* if they occur in the region below the lesser trochanter. Extracapsular fractures are usually caused by severe direct trauma or a fall.

Clinical Manifestations

Manifestations of a hip fracture are external rotation, muscle spasm, shortening of the affected extremity, and severe pain and tenderness in the region of the fracture site. Displaced femoral neck fractures cause serious disruption of the blood supply to the femoral head, which can result in avascular necrosis.

Collaborative Care

Surgical repair is the preferred method of managing intracapsular and extracapsular hip fractures. Surgical treatment permits early mobilization of the patient and decreases the risk of major complications. Initially the affected extremity may be temporarily immobilized by Buck's traction until the patient's physical condition is stabilized and surgery can be performed. Buck's traction relieves painful muscle spasms.

- Intracapsular fractures may also be repaired with the use of an endoprosthesis to replace the femoral head (hemiarthroplasty). Extracapsular fractures are repaired using fixed nail plates, sliding nail plates, intramedullary devices, and replacement prostheses. The principles of patient care for these procedures are similar. Internal fixation devices for a hip fracture can be seen in Fig. 63-18 in Lewis et al., *Medical-Surgical Nursing,* ed 8, p. 1606.

Nursing Management

Preoperative management. Because older adults are most prone to hip fractures, chronic health problems (e.g., diabetes mellitus, hypertension, arthritis) must often be considered when planning treatment. Surgery may be delayed for a brief time until the patient's general health is stabilized.

- Before surgery, severe muscle spasms can increase pain. Appropriate analgesics or muscle relaxants, comfortable positioning unless contraindicated, and properly adjusted traction can help manage spasms.
- When possible, teach the patient the method and frequency for exercising the unaffected leg and both arms. Encourage the patient to use the overhead trapeze bar and opposite side rail to assist in changing positions. A physical therapist can begin to teach out-of-bed and chair transfers.
- Inform the caregiver about the patient's weight-bearing status after surgery. Plans for discharge begin as the patient enters the hospital, because the length of postoperative stay is only a few days.

Postoperative management. Initial management of a patient after open reduction and internal fixation (ORIF) of a hip fracture is similar to that for any older surgical patient. Monitor vital signs and intake and output, supervise respiratory activities such as deep breathing and coughing, give pain medication cautiously, and observe the dressing and incision for signs of bleeding and infection. Specific nursing interventions for the orthopedic surgical patient are presented in NCP 63-2, Lewis et al., *Medical-Surgical Nursing,* ed 8, p. 1600.

In the early postoperative period there is potential for neurovascular impairment. Assess the patient's extremity for motor function, temperature and color, sensation, distal pulses, capillary refill, edema, and pain.

- Edema is alleviated by elevation of the leg whenever the patient is in a chair.
- Pain resulting from poor alignment of the affected extremity can be prevented by keeping pillows (or an abductor splint) between the knees when the patient is turning to either side. Sandbags and pillows are also used to prevent external rotation.
- If an endoprosthesis was placed, the patient is at risk for hip dislocation. Hip precautions must be demonstrated and explained to the patient.

Ambulation usually begins the first or second postoperative day. In collaboration with the physical therapist, monitor the patient's ambulation status for proper crutch walking or use of the walker. For the patient to be discharged home, have the patient demonstrate the proper use of crutches or a walker, the ability to transfer into and from a chair and bed, and the ability to ascend and descend stairs.

If the hip fracture has been treated by insertion of a femoral-head prosthesis with a *posterior approach* (hip joint is accessed from the back), measures to prevent dislocation must always be used (Table 39). If the hip fracture is treated by pinning, dislocation precautions are not necessary.

- The patient and caregiver must be fully aware of positions and activities that predispose the patient to dislocation (>90 degrees of flexion, abduction, or internal rotation). Many daily activities may reproduce these positions including putting on shoes and socks, crossing legs or feet while seated, assuming the side-lying position incorrectly, standing up or sitting down while the body is flexed >90 degrees relative to the chair, sitting on low seats, especially low toilet seats.
- Until the soft tissue capsule surrounding the hip has healed sufficiently to stabilize the prosthesis, teach the patient to avoid these activities, usually for at least 6 weeks.
- Sudden severe pain, a lump in the buttock, limb shortening, and extreme external rotation indicate prosthesis dislocation. This requires a closed reduction or open reduction to realign the femoral head in the acetabulum.

When the hip fracture is accessed during surgery with an *anterior approach* (joint reached from front of body), the hip muscles are left intact. This approach generally results in a more stable hip

F

Table 39	Patient and Caregiver Teaching Guide: Femoral Head Prosthesis*

You should include the following instructions when teaching a patient with a femoral head prosthesis:

Do Not
- Force hip into greater than 90 degrees of flexion (e.g., sitting in low chairs or toilet seats).
- Force hip into adduction.
- Force hip into internal rotation.
- Cross legs at knees.
- Put on own shoes or stockings until 6 weeks after surgery without adaptive device (e.g., long-handled shoehorn or stocking-helper).
- Sit on chairs without arms to aid rising to a standing position.

Do
- Use an elevated toilet seat.
- Place chair inside shower or tub and remain seated while washing.
- Use pillow between legs for first 6 weeks after surgery when lying on nonoperative side or when supine.
- Keep hip in neutral, straight position when sitting, walking, or lying.
- Notify surgeon if severe pain, deformity, or loss of function occurs.
- Inform dentist of presence of prosthesis before dental work so that prophylactic antibiotics can be given if indicated.

*For patients having surgery by a posterior approach.

in the postoperative period with a lower rate of complications. Patient precautions related to motion and weight-bearing are few and may include instructions to avoid hyperextension.

In addition to teaching the patient and caregiver how to prevent prosthesis dislocation you should also place a large pillow between the patient's legs when turning, avoid extreme hip flexion, and avoid turning the patient on the affected side until it is approved by the surgeon. Some health care providers prefer that the patient keep leg abductor splints on except when bathing.

Assist both the patient and family in adjusting to the restrictions and dependence imposed by the hip fracture. Depression can easily occur, but creative nursing care and awareness of the problem can do much to prevent it.

- Assist both the patient and the caregiver in adjusting to the restrictions and dependence imposed by the hip fracture.
- The patient and caregiver may need to be informed about community referral services that can assist in the postdischarge rehabilitation phase.
- Hospitalization averages 4 days. Patients frequently require care in a subacute unit, skilled nursing facility, or rehabilitation facility for a few weeks before returning home.

FRACTURE, HUMERUS

Fractures involving the shaft of the humerus are a common injury among young and middle-aged adults. Clinical manifestations are an obvious displacement of the humeral shaft, shortened extremity, abnormal mobility, and pain.

- Major complications are radial nerve injury and vascular injury to the brachial artery as a result of laceration, transection, or muscle spasm.

Treatment for a fracture of the humerus depends on the location and displacement of the fracture.

- Nonoperative treatment may include a hanging arm cast, shoulder immobilizer, or the sling and swathe, which is a type of immobilization that prevents glenohumeral movement.

When these devices are used, elevate the head of the bed to assist gravity in reducing the fracture. Allow the arm to hang freely when the patient is sitting and standing.

Include measures in your care to protect the axilla and prevent skin maceration. Carefully place lightly powdered absorption pads in the axilla and change them twice daily or as needed.

- Skin or skeletal traction may be used for purposes of reduction and immobilization.
- During the rehabilitative phase an exercise program geared toward improving strength and motion of the injured extremity is extremely important. This program should include assisted motion of the hands and fingers. The shoulder can also be exercised to prevent stiffness if the fracture is stable.

FRACTURE, MANDIBLE

A fracture of the mandible may result from trauma to the face or jaws and may be simple, with no bone displacement, or it may involve loss of tissue and bone. Mandibular fracture may also be therapeutically performed to correct an underlying malocclusion problem that cannot be corrected by orthodontic procedures alone. In these conditions, the mandible is resected during surgery and manipulated forward or backward depending on the occlusion problem.

Surgery consists of immobilization, usually by wiring the lower jaw to the upper jaw with wires or rubber bands (intermaxillary fixation). When teeth are missing or if there is bone displacement, other forms of fixation, such as metal arch bars in the mouth or insertion of a pin in the bone, may be needed.

Postoperative care should focus on a patent airway, oral hygiene, communication, pain management, and adequate nutrition. Two major potential problems in the immediate postoperative period are airway obstruction and aspiration of vomitus.

- Tape a wire cutter or scissors (for rubber bands) to the head of the bed and send them with the patient on all appointments and examinations away from the bedside. Once the patient is awake, the wires should be cut only in the case of cardiac arrest or respiratory distress requiring access to the pharynx or lungs.
- If the patient begins to vomit or choke, try to clear the mouth and airway, suctioning may be necessary. A nasogastric tube may help prevent aspiration and vomiting and may be used later as a feeding tube.

Oral hygiene is an extremely important part of nursing care.

- The mouth should be rinsed after each meal and snack with warm normal saline solution or water or alkaline mouthwashes. Inspect the mouth several times per day with a flashlight and tongue depressor.

Ingestion of sufficient nutrients is a challenge because the diet must be liquid. Liquid protein supplements may be helpful for improving nutritional status.

- The low-bulk, high-carbohydrate diet and the intake of air through the straw create a problem with constipation and flatus. Ambulation, prune juice, and bulk-forming laxatives may help to relieve these problems.

The patient is usually discharged with the wires in place. Discharge teaching should include oral care, techniques of handling secretions, diet, how and when to use wire cutters, and when to notify the health care provider for concerns and problems.

FRACTURE, PELVIS

Although only a small percentage of all fractures are pelvic fractures, this type of injury is associated with the highest mortality rate. Preoccupation with more obvious injuries at the time of a traumatic event may result in an oversight of pelvic injuries. Pelvic fractures range from benign to life threatening, depending on the mechanism of injury and associated vascular insult.

- Pelvic fractures may cause serious intraabdominal injury, such as paralytic ileus, hemorrhage, and laceration of the urethra, bladder, or colon. Patients may survive the initial pelvic injury, only to die from complications such as sepsis, fat embolism syndrome, or thromboembolism.
- Pelvic fractures are diagnosed by x-ray and computed tomography (CT) scan.
- They can range in severity from benign to life threatening, depending on the mechanism of injury and associated vascular insult.
- Physical examination demonstrates local swelling, tenderness, deformity, unusual pelvic movement, and ecchymosis on the abdomen.

Treatment depends on the severity of the injury. Bed rest for stable pelvic fractures is maintained from a few days to 6 weeks. More complex fractures may be treated with pelvic sling traction, skeletal traction, hip spica casts, external fixation, open reduction, or a combination of these methods. Open reduction and internal fixation of a pelvic fracture may be necessary if the fracture is displaced.

- Extreme care in handling or moving the patient is important to prevent serious injury from a displaced fracture fragment. Only turn the patient when ordered by the health care provider. Because a pelvic fracture can damage other organs, assess bowel and urinary tract function and assessment of distal neurovascular status.
- Provide back care while the patient is raised from the bed, with either independent use of the trapeze or adequate assistance.

GASTRITIS

Description

Gastritis, an inflammation of the gastric mucosa, is one of the most common problems affecting the stomach. Gastritis may be acute or chronic and may be diffuse or localized.

Pathophysiology

Gastritis is the result of a breakdown in the normal gastric mucosal barrier. The mucosal barrier normally protects the stomach tissue from autodigestion by hydrochloric (HCl) acid and the enzyme pepsin. When the barrier is broken, HCl acid diffuses back into the mucosa. This back diffusion results in tissue edema, disruption of capillary walls with plasma lost into the gastric lumen, and possible hemorrhage.

Risk factors for gastritis are ulcerogenic drugs (especially nonsteroidal antiinflammatory drugs [NSAIDs]), repeated use of alcohol, *Helicobacter pylori* infection, and an autoimmune condition.

Corticosteroids and NSAIDs inhibit the synthesis of prostaglandins that are protective to the gastric mucosa. This leaves the mucosa more susceptible to injury. Risk factors for NSAID-induced gastritis include being female, being greater than age 60, having a history of ulcer disease, concomitant use of anticoagulants, use of other NSAIDs including low-dose aspirin, taking other ulcerogenic drugs (including corticosteroids) and the presence of a chronic debilitating disorder such as cardiovascular disease.

Alcohol can cause acute damage to the gastric mucosa. Eating large quantities of spicy, irritating foods and metabolic conditions such as renal failure can also cause acute gastritis.

H. pylori is capable of promoting the breakdown of the gastric mucosal barrier, given certain "triggers" or conditions. The role of *H. pylori* in ulcer development is discussed in greater detail under Peptic Ulcer Disease p. 493.

Autoimmune metaplastic atrophic gastritis is a form of chronic gastritis that affects both the fundus and the body of the stomach and is associated with an increased risk of gastric cancer.

Clinical Manifestations

- Symptoms of *acute gastritis* include anorexia, nausea and vomiting, epigastric tenderness, and a feeling of fullness. Hemorrhage is commonly associated with alcohol abuse and at times may be the only manifestation. Acute gastritis is self-limiting, lasting from a few hours to a few days, with complete healing of mucosa expected.

- Manifestations of chronic gastritis are similar to those of acute gastritis. Some patients have no symptoms directly associated with the gastric lesion. However, when the parietal cells are lost as a result of atrophy, the source of intrinsic factor is lost and cobalamin (vitamin B_{12}) cannot be absorbed in the ileum, ultimately resulting in pernicious anemia.

Diagnostic Studies

Diagnosis of acute gastritis is most often based on a history of drug and alcohol use.

- Endoscopic examination with biopsy to obtain a definitive diagnosis
- Breath, urine, serum, stool, or gastric tissue biopsy tests are available for determination of *H. pylori*
- Complete blood count (CBC) may demonstrate anemia from blood loss or lack of intrinsic factor
- Stools tested for occult blood
- Serum tests for antibodies to parietal cells and intrinsic factor

Collaborative Care

Eliminating the cause and preventing or avoiding it in the future are generally all that are needed to treat acute gastritis. The plan of care is supportive and similar to that described for nausea and vomiting.

- If vomiting accompanies acute gastritis, rest, NPO status, and IV fluids may be prescribed. Antiemetics are given for nausea and vomiting. In severe cases, a nasogastric (NG) tube may be used to observe for bleeding, lavage of the precipitating agent from the stomach, or to keep the stomach empty and free of noxious stimuli.
- Clear liquids are resumed when acute symptoms have subsided, with gradual reintroduction of solid, bland foods.
- Antacids are used for relief of abdominal discomfort, and H_2-histamine receptor (H_2R) blockers (e.g., ranitidine [Zantac], cimetidine [Tagamet]) or proton pump inhibitors (PPIs) (e.g., omeprazole [Prilosec], lansoprazole [Prevacid]) reduce gastric HCl acid secretion.

Treatment of chronic gastritis focuses on evaluating and eliminating the specific cause.

- Currently antibiotic combinations are used to eradicate infection with *H. pylori*.

- For the patient with pernicious anemia, lifelong administration of cobalamin is needed. It can be given IM or intranasally.
- High-dose oral cobalamin and sublingual cobalamin are also available for those in which GI absorption is intact.

The patient undergoing treatment for chronic gastritis may have to adapt to lifestyle changes and strictly adhere to a drug regimen. An interdisciplinary team approach in which the physician, nurse, dietitian, and pharmacist provide consistent information and support may increase patient success in making these alterations.

GASTROESOPHAGEAL REFLUX DISEASE

Description

Gastroesophageal reflux disease (GERD) is not a disease but a syndrome produced by conditions that result in the reflux of acidic gastric contents into the lower esophagus. GERD is the most common upper gastrointestinal (GI) problem in adults.

Predisposing conditions include hiatal hernia, incompetent lower esophageal sphincter (LES), decreased esophageal clearance, and decreased gastric emptying.

Pathophysiology

Gastric hydrochloric (HCl) acid and pepsin secretions that reflux up into the lower esophagus result in esophageal irritation and inflammation (esophagitis). If the refluxate contains intestinal proteolytic enzymes (e.g., trypsin) and bile, this further irritates the esophageal mucosa. The degree of inflammation depends on the amount and composition of gastric reflux and the ability of the esophagus to clear the acidic contents.

Clinical Manifestations

- Heartburn (pyrosis), caused by irritation of the esophagus by secretions, is the most common clinical manifestation. Heartburn is a burning, tight sensation that is felt intermittently beneath the lower sternum and spreads upward to the throat or jaw.
- Patients may also complain of dyspepsia, which is pain or discomfort centered in the upper abdomen (mainly in or around the midline as opposed to the right or left hypochondrium).
- Regurgitation (the effortless return of material from the stomach into the esophagus or mouth) is another common

manifestation. It is often described as hot, bitter, or sour liquid coming into the throat or mouth.

- GERD-related chest pain can mimic angina. It is described as burning or squeezing and can radiate to the back, neck, jaw, or arms. Unlike angina, GERD-related chest pain is relieved with antacids.

Complications

Complications are related to the effects of gastric acid secretion on the esophageal mucosa. Esophagitis (inflammation of the esophagus) is a common complication of GERD. Repeated esophagitis may cause scar tissue formation and decreased distensibility, which may result in dysphagia.

Barrett's esophagus, a precancerous lesion that increases the patient's risk for esophageal cancer, may also occur.

- The potential for pulmonary complications (especially pneumonia) exists secondary to aspiration of gastric contents into the pulmonary system. Other respiratory complications include cough, bronchospasm, laryngospasm, asthma, and chronic bronchitis.
- Dental erosion may result from acid reflux into the mouth.

Diagnostic Studies

Diagnostic studies help determine the cause of the GERD.

- Barium swallow determines if there is protrusion of the upper part of the stomach into the esophagus.
- Endoscopy is useful in assessing LES competence and extent of inflammation (if present), potential scarring, and strictures.
- Biopsy and cytologic specimens can be taken to differentiate stomach and esophageal cancer from Barrett's esophagus (see Esophageal Cancer, p. 219).

Collaborative Care

Teach the patient to avoid those factors that aggravate symptoms. Give particular attention to diet and other medications that may affect the LES, acid secretion, or gastric emptying. Patients who smoke are encouraged to stop.

Food can aggravate symptoms. No specific diet is necessary, but food causing reflux should be avoided. High-fat foods decrease the rate of gastric emptying. Foods that decrease LES pressure, such as chocolate, coffee, and tea, should be avoided because they predispose to reflux. Small, frequent meals are advised. Fluids should be taken between rather than with meals to reduce gastric distention. Late evening meals and nocturnal snacking should be avoided. Weight reduction is recommended if the patient is obese.

Drug therapy focuses on improving LES function, increasing esophageal clearance, decreasing volume and acidity of reflux, and protecting esophageal mucosa. Proton pump inhibitors (PPIs) and histamine-2-receptor (H_2R) blockers are the most common and effective treatments for symptomatic GERD. The goal of hydrochloric (HCl) acid suppression treatment is to reduce the acidity of the gastric refluxate. Patients who are symptomatic with GERD but do not have evidence of esophagitis achieve symptom relief with PPI and H_2R agents. The PPIs are more effective in healing esophagitis than H_2Rs.

- PPIs such as omeprazole (Prilosec), esomeprazole (Nexium), lansoprazole (Prevacid), and rabeprazole (AcipHex) promote esophageal healing in approximately 80% to 90% of patients.
- In prescription doses, H_2R blockers such as cimetidine (Tagamet), ranitidine (Zantac), famotidine (Pepcid), and nizatidine (Axid) reduce symptoms and promote esophageal healing in approximately 50% of patients.

Antacids with or without alginic acid (e.g., Gaviscon) may be useful in patients with mild, intermittent heartburn.

Surgical therapy is reserved for patients with complications of reflux, including esophagitis, intolerance of medications, stricture, Barrett's metaplasia, and persistence of severe symptoms. Most surgical procedures are performed laparoscopically. The objective of surgery is to restore gastroesophageal integrity. In these procedures the fundus of the stomach is wrapped around the lower portion of the esophagus to reinforce and repair the defective barrier.

Alternatives to surgical therapy include endoscopic mucosal resection, photodynamic therapy, cryotherapy, and radiofrequency ablation (image-guided technique that kills cells by heating and destroying them).

Nursing Management

Nursing care for the patient who is having acute symptoms consists mainly of teaching and encouraging the patient to follow the necessary regimen found in the teaching guide provided in Table 40.

Postoperative care focuses on concerns related to prevention of respiratory complications, maintenance of fluid and electrolyte balance, and prevention of infection. Laparoscopic procedures reduce the risk of respiratory complications. Only fluids are given initially, and solids are added gradually so that the stomach is not overdistended.

Table 40	Patient and Caregiver Teaching Guide: Gastroesophageal Reflux Disease (GERD)

When teaching the patient and/or caregiver management of GERD, you should:

1. Explain the rationale for a high-protein, low-fat diet.
2. Encourage the patient to eat small, frequent meals to prevent gastric distention.
3. Explain the rationale for avoiding alcohol, smoking (causes an almost immediate, marked decrease in LES pressure), and beverages that contain caffeine.
4. Advise the patient not to lie down for 2 to 3 hr after eating, wear tight clothing around the waist, or bend over (especially after eating).
5. Have the patient avoid eating within 3 hr of bedtime.
6. Encourage the patient to sleep with head of bed elevated on 4- to 6-in blocks (gravity fosters esophageal emptying).
7. Provide information regarding drugs, including rationale for their use and common side effects.
8. Discuss strategies for weight reduction if appropriate.
9. Encourage patient and caregiver to share concerns about lifestyle changes and living with a chronic problem.

LES, Lower esophageal sphincter.

G

GASTROINTESTINAL BLEEDING, UPPER

Description

In the United States there are approximately 225,000 hospital admissions each year for nonvariceal upper GI bleeding. Many of these are adults greater than age 65. Despite advances in the drug management of predisposing conditions, identification of risk factors, intensive care, hemodynamic monitoring, and endoscopy, there has been little change in the mortality rate for upper gastrointestinal (GI) bleeding, which has remained at approximately 6% to 10%.

Pathophysiology

Although the most serious loss of blood from the upper GI tract is characterized by a sudden onset, insidious occult bleeding can also be a major problem. Bleeding severity depends on whether the origin is venous, capillary, or arterial. Bleeding from an arterial source is profuse, and the blood is bright red. In contrast, "coffee ground" vomitus indicates that the blood has been in the stomach

Table 41	Common Causes of Upper Gastrointestinal Bleeding

Drug Induced
- Corticosteroids
- Nonsteroidal antiinflammatory drugs (NSAIDs)
- Salicylates

Esophagus
- Esophageal varices
- Esophagitis
- Mallory-Weiss tear

Stomach and Duodenum
- Gastric cancer
- Hemorrhagic gastritis
- Peptic ulcer disease
- Polyps
- Stress-related mucosal disease

Systemic Diseases
- Blood dyscrasias (e.g., leukemia, aplastic anemia)
- Renal failure

for some time. *Melena* (black, tarry stools) indicates slow bleeding from an upper GI source.

A variety of areas in the GI tract may be involved. Table 41 lists the common causes of upper GI bleeding. The most common sites are the esophagus, stomach, and duodenum.

- Bleeding from the esophagus is most likely caused by chronic esophagitis, Mallory-Weiss tear, or esophageal varices. A *Mallory-Weiss tear* occurs in the mucosa near the esophagogastric junction and is often related to severe retching and vomiting. Esophageal varices most often occur secondary to cirrhosis of the liver (see Cirrhosis, p. 138).
- Bleeding peptic ulcers account for 50% of the cases of upper GI bleeding. Drugs, either prescribed by the health care provider or OTC, are a major cause of upper GI bleeding.
- Stress-related mucosal disease, also called *physiologic stress ulcers,* occurs in patients who have sustained severe burns or trauma or had major surgery.
- Less common causes of upper GI bleeding include tumors and vascular lesions. Stomach cancer causes steady blood loss as it grows and ulcerates through the mucosa and blood vessels located in its path.

Complications

Although approximately 80% to 85% of patients who have massive hemorrhage spontaneously stop bleeding, the cause must be identified and treatment initiated immediately.

The immediate physical examination includes a systemic evaluation of the patient's condition with emphasis on BP, rate and character of pulse, peripheral perfusion with capillary refill, and observation for the presence or absence of neck vein distention. Monitor vital signs every 15 to 30 minutes. Assess signs and symptoms of shock. Treatment is started as soon as possible.

- Laboratory studies include a complete blood count (CBC), blood urea nitrogen (BUN), serum electrolytes, blood glucose, prothrombin time, liver enzymes, arterial blood gases (ABGs), and a type and cross-match for possible blood transfusions. Test all vomitus and stools for gross and occult blood. Urinalysis including specific gravity provides information on hydration status.
- IV lines, preferably two, with a 16- or 18-gauge needle are placed for fluid and blood replacement. A central venous pressure line may be inserted for fluid volume status assessment. An indwelling urinary catheter may also be inserted so that output can be accurately assessed hourly.
- The use of supplemental oxygen delivered by face mask or nasal cannula may help increase blood oxygen saturation.

Diagnostic Studies

- Endoscopy is the primary tool for diagnosing the source (e.g., esophageal or gastric varices, gastritis) of upper GI bleeding.
- Angiography is used in diagnosing upper GI bleeding when endoscopy cannot be done or when bleeding persists following endoscopic therapy.

Collaborative Care

Endoscopy performed within the first 24 hours of bleeding is important for diagnosis as well as the determination of the need for surgical intervention. Endoscopic therapy can be useful to stop bleeding in patients with severe gastritis, Mallory-Weiss tear, esophageal and gastric varices, bleeding peptic ulcers, and polyps. Multipolar electrocoagulation and thermal probe are the two most commonly used procedures.

Surgical intervention is indicated when bleeding continues regardless of the therapy provided and when the site of the bleeding has been identified. The site of the hemorrhage determines the choice of operation.

During the acute phase, drugs are used to decrease bleeding, decrease HCl acid secretion, and neutralize the HCl acid that is present. Injection therapy with epinephrine (1:10,000 dilution) during endoscopy is effective for acute hemostasis. To prevent rebleeding, injection therapy is combined with other therapies (e.g., thermocoagulation or laser treatment).

- Efforts are made to reduce acid secretion because the acidic environment can alter platelet function, as well as interfere with clot stabilization. PPIs (e.g., pantoprazole [Protonix]) or H_2R blockers (e.g., [Tagamet]) are administered IV to decrease acid secretion (see Table 42-14 Lewis et al., *Medical-Surgical Nursing,* ed 8, p. 983).

Nursing Management

Goals
The patient with upper GI bleeding will have no further GI bleeding, have the cause of the bleeding identified and treated, experience a return to a normal hemodynamic state, and have minimal or no symptoms of pain or anxiety.

Nursing Diagnoses
- Risk for aspiration
- Decreased cardiac output
- Deficient fluid volume
- Ineffective peripheral tissue perfusion
- Anxiety

Nursing Interventions
Consider the patient with a history of chronic gastritis or peptic ulcer disease at high risk for upper GI bleeding because of the increased incidence of bleeding associated with chronic irritation. Instruct the at-risk patient to avoid gastric irritants such as alcohol and smoking, prevent or decrease stress-inducing situations at home or at work, and take only prescribed medications.

When working with the patient who has a history of liver cirrhosis with esophageal varices, instructions must be specific regarding the importance of avoiding known irritants, such as alcohol and smoking.

A majority of upper GI bleeding episodes cease spontaneously, even without intervention. Although the use of room temperature, cool, or iced gastric lavage is used in some institutions, its effectiveness as a treatment for upper GI bleeding is questionable. When lavage is used, approximately 50 to 100 mL of fluid is instilled at a time into the stomach.

- Monitor vital signs, especially in patients with cardiovascular disease because dysrhythmias may occur. Keep the head of the bed elevated to provide comfort and prevent possible aspiration.

- Assess stools for blood. Black, tarry stools are not usually associated with a brisk hemorrhage but are indicative of the presence of bleeding of prolonged duration. Bright red or maroon-colored (hematochezia) stools are usually from a source in the lower bowel.
- Monitor the patient's laboratory studies to estimate the effectiveness of therapy. The hemoglobin and hematocrit are usually evaluated about every 4 to 6 hours if the patient is actively bleeding.
- When oral nourishment starts, observe the patient for symptoms of nausea and vomiting and a recurrence of bleeding. Feedings initially consist of clear fluids and are given hourly until tolerance is determined. Gradual introduction of foods follows if the patient exhibits no signs of discomfort.
- When the hemorrhage is the result of chronic alcohol abuse, closely observe the patient for delirium tremens as withdrawal from alcohol takes place.

▼ **Patient and Caregiver Teaching**
- Teach the patient and caregiver how to avoid future bleeding episodes.
- Ulcer disease, drug or alcohol abuse, and liver and respiratory diseases can all result in upper GI bleeding.
- Help the patient and caregiver be aware of the consequences of noncompliance with drug therapy.
- Emphasize that no drugs (especially aspirin, NSAIDs) other than those prescribed by the health care provider should be taken.
- Smoking and alcohol should be eliminated because they are sources of irritation and interfere with tissue repair.
- The need for long-term follow-up care may be necessary because of possible recurrence.

GLAUCOMA

Description

Glaucoma is a group of disorders characterized by increased intraocular pressure (IOP) and the consequences of elevated pressure, optic nerve atrophy, and peripheral visual field loss. At least 2 million persons have glaucoma, of these, more than 50% are unaware of their condition.

- Glaucoma is the second leading cause of permanent blindness in the United States and the leading cause of blindness among African Americans.

Pathophysiology

The etiology of glaucoma is related to the consequences of elevated IOP. Increased IOP results when the rate of aqueous production (inflow) is greater than aqueous reabsorption (outflow). If the pressure remains elevated, permanent visual damage may begin. Outflow of aqueous humor can be decreased by several mechanisms.

- Primary open-angle glaucoma (POAG) represents 90% of the cases of primary glaucoma. In POAG, the aqueous outflow is decreased in the trabecular meshwork. The drainage channels become clogged, like a clogged kitchen sink. Damage to the optic nerve can then result.
- In primary angle-closure glaucoma (PACG), the mechanism reducing the outflow of aqueous humor is angle closure. The lens usually bulges forward because of age-related changes, blocking aqueous outflow. Angle closure may also occur as a result of pupil dilation in the patient with anatomically narrow angles. An acute attack may occur because of drug-induced mydriasis, emotional excitement, or darkness. Check drug records and documentation before administering medications to the patient with angle-closure glaucoma and instruct the patient not to take any mydriatic-producing medications.
- In secondary glaucoma, increased IOP results from other ocular or systemic conditions that may block the outflow channels in some way, such as trauma and ocular tumors.

Clinical Manifestations

- PAOG develops slowly with no symptoms of pain or pressure. The patient usually does not notice gradual visual field loss until peripheral vision is severely compromised (tunnel vision).
- Acute angle-closure glaucoma causes symptoms of sudden, excruciating pain in or around the eye that is often accompanied by nausea and vomiting. Visual symptoms include seeing colored halos around lights, blurred vision, and ocular redness. The acute pressure rise may cause corneal edema, giving the cornea a frosted appearance.
- Manifestations of subacute or chronic angle-closure glaucoma appear gradually. The patient who has had a previous unrecognized episode of subacute angle-closure glaucoma might report

a history of blurred vision, colored halos around lights, ocular redness, or eye or brow pain.

Diagnostic Studies

- IOP with tonometry
- Visual acuity measurement and visual field perimetry
- Slit-lamp microscopy
- Gonioscopy
- Ophthalmoscopy (direct and indirect)

Collaborative Care

The primary focus of therapy is to keep the IOP low enough to prevent the patient from developing optic nerve damage leading to severe and permanent visual loss. Specific therapies vary with the type of glaucoma.

- In chronic open-angle glaucoma, initial drug therapy can include β-adrenergic receptor blocking agents, α-adrenergic agents, cholinergic agents (miotics), and carbonic anhydrase inhibitors (hyperosmotic agents).
- When medications are not effective or are not used as prescribed, surgical options include argon laser trabeculoplasty (ALT), trabeculectomy, or surgical placement of a tube to shunt aqueous humor from the anterior chamber.
- Acute angle-closure glaucoma is an ocular emergency that requires immediate interventions, including miotics and oral or intravenous (IV) hyperosmotic agents. Laser peripheral iridotomy or surgical iridectomy is necessary for long-term treatment and prevention of subsequent episodes.
- Secondary glaucoma is managed by treating the underlying problem and using antiglaucoma drugs.

Nursing Management

Nursing management focuses on the chronicity of this disease and the fact that visual impairment is preventable in most patients with proper therapeutic management.

Goals

The patient with glaucoma will have no progression of visual impairment, understand the disease process and rationale for therapy, comply with all aspects of therapy (including medication administration and follow-up care), and have no postoperative complications

Nursing Diagnoses

- Acute pain
- Self-care deficits

- Noncompliance
- Risk for injury

Nursing Interventions

- The patient with acute angle-closure glaucoma requires immediate medication to lower the IOP. This patient may be uncomfortable, and nursing comfort interventions may include darkening the environment, applying cool compresses to the patient's forehead, and providing a quiet and private space. Most surgical procedures for glaucoma are outpatient procedures.
- The patient needs encouragement to follow therapy recommendations, including information about the disease processes, normal course of the condition, and treatment options that include the rationale underlying each option.

▼ **Patient and Caregiving Teaching**

See Table 22, Patient and Caregiver Teaching Guide: After Eye Surgery, p. 110.

- Because loss of vision from glaucoma is preventable, it is important to teach patients about risk factors of glaucoma and stress the importance of its early detection and treatment.
- The patient should know that the incidence of glaucoma increases with age and that a comprehensive ophthalmologic examination is invaluable in identifying persons with glaucoma or at risk for developing glaucoma.
- All persons between the ages of 40 and 64 years should be instructed to have an ophthalmologic examination every 2 to 4 years and every 1 to 2 years for persons age 65 years or older. African Americans should have examinations more often because of the increased incidence and more aggressive course of glaucoma.
- The patient with glaucoma should be provided with information about prescribed antiglaucoma drugs. Encourage compliance by helping the patient identify the most convenient and appropriate times for medication administration. Advocate a change in therapy if the patient reports unacceptable side effects.

GLOMERULONEPHRITIS

Glomerulonephritis is an inflammation of renal glomeruli caused by immunologic processes. It affects both kidneys equally and is the third leading cause of renal failure in the United States.

Two types of antibody-induced injury can initiate glomerular damage.

- In the first type, antibodies have specificity for antigens within the glomerular basement membrane (GBM). The mechanism that causes a person to develop autoantibodies against its GBM is not known.
- In the second type of immune process, antibodies react with circulating nonglomerular antigens and are randomly deposited as immune complexes along the GBM. Bacterial products appear to be important in poststreptococcal glomerulonephritis. Viral agents have been recognized in rare cases of glomerulonephritis that develop after hepatitis B or C and rubella (measles).
- All forms of immune complex disease are characterized by an accumulation of antigen, antibody, and complement in the glomeruli. Immune complexes activate complement; complement activation results in release of chemotactic factors that attract inflammatory mediators; and glomerular injury results.

Clinical manifestations of glomerulonephritis include varying degrees of hematuria (ranging from microscopic to gross) and urinary excretion of various formed elements, including red blood cells (RBCs), white blood cells (WBCs), and casts. Proteinuria and elevated blood urea nitrogen (BUN) and serum creatinine levels are other manifestations.

In most cases, recovery from the acute illness is complete. If progressive involvement occurs, the result is destruction of renal tissue and marked renal insufficiency.

- The patient's history provides important information related to glomerulonephritis. It is necessary to assess exposure to drugs, immunizations, microbial infections, and viral infections such as hepatitis.
- It is also important to evaluate the patient for more generalized conditions involving immune disorders, such as systemic lupus erythematosus and systemic sclerosis.

GLOMERULONEPHRITIS, ACUTE POSTSTREPTOCOCCAL

Description

Acute poststreptococcal glomerulonephritis (APSGN) is most common in children and young adults, but all age-groups can be affected. It develops 5 to 21 days after an infection of the tonsils, pharynx, or skin (e.g., streptococcal sore throat, impetigo) by certain nephrotoxic strains of group A β-hemolytic streptococci. Antibodies are produced to the streptococcal antigen, and tissue injury occurs as the antigen-antibody complexes are deposited in the glomeruli and complement is activated.

Greater than 95% of patients with APSGN recover completely or improve rapidly with conservative management. Chronic glomerulonephritis develops in 5% to 15% of affected persons, and irreversible renal failure occurs in <1% of patients.

Clinical Manifestations

Manifestations appear as a variety of signs and symptoms, which may include generalized body edema, hypertension, oliguria, hematuria with a smoky or rusty appearance, and proteinuria. Fluid retention occurs as a result of decreased glomerular filtration.

- Edema initially appears in low-pressure tissues, such as the eyes (periorbital edema), but later progresses to involve the total body as ascites or peripheral edema in the legs.
- Smoky urine indicates bleeding in the upper urinary tract. The degree of proteinuria varies with the severity of the glomerulonephropathy.
- Hypertension mainly results from increased extracellular fluid volume.
- The patient may have abdominal or flank pain. At times the patient has no symptoms, with the problem found on routine urinalysis.

Diagnostic Studies

- Laboratory studies determine the presence or history of a group A β-hemolytic streptococcus in a throat or skin lesion.
- Urinalysis reveals significant numbers of erythrocytes. Erythrocyte casts are highly suggestive of acute glomerulonephritis. Proteinuria may be mild to severe.
- Complete blood count (CBC), blood urea nitrogen (BUN), serum creatinine, and albumin assess extent of renal impairment.
- Decreased complement levels indicate an immune-mediated response.
- Antistreptolysin O (ASO) titers demonstrate an immune response to *Streptococcus*.
- Renal biopsy may be performed to confirm the diagnosis.

Collaborative Care

Management focuses on symptomatic relief. Rest is recommended until the signs of glomerular inflammation (proteinuria, hematuria) and hypertension subside. Edema is treated by restricting sodium and fluid intake and administering diuretics.

- Severe hypertension is treated with antihypertensive drugs.
- Dietary protein intake may be restricted if there is evidence of an increase in nitrogenous wastes (e.g., elevated BUN).
- Antibiotics should be given only if streptococcal infection is still present. Corticosteroids and cytotoxic drugs have not been shown to be of value.

Nursing Management

One of the most important ways to prevent the development of APSGN is to encourage early diagnosis and treatment of sore throats and skin lesions. If streptococci are found in the culture, treatment with appropriate antibiotic therapy (usually penicillin) is essential. The patient must be encouraged to take the full course of antibiotics to ensure that the bacteria have been eradicated

- Good personal hygiene is an important factor in preventing the spread of cutaneous streptococcal infections.

G

GLOMERULONEPHRITIS, CHRONIC

Chronic glomerulonephritis is a syndrome that reflects the end stage of glomerular inflammatory disease. Most types of glomerulonephritis and nephrotic syndrome can eventually lead to chronic glomerulonephritis.

The syndrome is characterized by proteinuria, hematuria, and the slow development of the uremic syndrome as a result of decreasing renal function. Chronic glomerulonephritis progresses insidiously toward renal failure over a few years to as many as 30 years.

- Chronic glomerulonephritis is often found coincidentally when an abnormality on a urinalysis or elevated blood pressure (BP) is detected. It is common to find that the patient has no recollection or history of acute nephritis or any renal problems. A renal biopsy may be performed to determine the exact cause and nature of the glomerulonephritis. Ultrasound and computed tomography (CT) scan are preferred diagnostic measures.

Treatment is supportive and symptomatic. Hypertension and urinary tract infections (UTIs) should be treated vigorously. Protein and phosphate restrictions may slow the rate of progression of renal failure (see Kidney Disease, Chronic, p. 381).

GONORRHEA

Description
Gonorrhea is the second most frequently occurring sexually transmitted disease (STD) in the United States. Overall cases of gonorrhea had stabilized from 1997 to 2005. However, since 2006 the national gonorrhoea rate has increased and today >700,000 new cases are diagnosed yearly.
- Gonorrhea rates are highest in adolescents of all racial and ethnic groups and among African Americans.
- Most states have enacted laws that permit examination and treatment of minors without parental consent.

Pathophysiology
Gonorrhea is caused by *Neisseria gonorrhoeae,* a gram-negative diplococcus. Mucosa with columnar epithelium is susceptible to gonococcal infection. This tissue is present in the genitalia (urethra in men, cervix in women), rectum, and oropharynx.
- The disease is spread by direct physical contact with an infected host, usually during sexual activity (vaginal, oral, or anal).
- Neonates can develop a gonococcal infection during delivery from an infected mother.
- Indirect transmission by instruments or linens is rare because the delicate gonococcus is easily killed by drying, heating, or washing with an antiseptic.
- Incubation period is 3 to 8 days. The disease confers no immunity to subsequent reinfection.
- Gonococcal infection elicits an inflammatory response, which, if left untreated, leads to formation of fibrous tissue and adhesions. This fibrous scarring is subsequently responsible for many complications such as strictures and tubal abnormalities, which can lead to tubal pregnancy, chronic pelvic pain, and infertility.

Clinical Manifestations
Men. The initial site of infection in men is usually the urethra.
- Symptoms of urethritis consist of dysuria and profuse, purulent urethral discharge developing 2 to 5 days after infection. Painful or swollen testicles may also occur.

- Men generally seek medical evaluation early in the disease because symptoms are usually obvious and distressing. It is unusual for men with gonorrhea to be asymptomatic.

Women. Many women who contract gonorrhea are asymptomatic or have minor symptoms that are often overlooked, making it possible for them to remain a source of infection.

- A few women may complain of vaginal discharge, dysuria, or frequency of urination. Changes in menstruation may be a symptom, but these changes are often disregarded by the woman.
- After the incubation period, redness and swelling occur at the site of contact, which is usually the cervix or urethra. A greenish-yellow purulent exudate often develops with a potential for abscess formation.
- The disease may remain local or can spread by direct tissue extension to the uterus, fallopian tubes, and ovaries. Although the vulva and vagina are uncommon sites for a gonorrheal infection, they may become involved when little or no estrogen is present, such as in prepubertal girls and postmenopausal women.

General. Anorectal gonorrhea may be present and is usually caused by anal intercourse. Symptoms may include soreness, itching, and discharge.

- Most patients with rectal infections and infections in the throat have few symptoms. A small percentage of individuals develop gonococcal pharyngitis resulting from orogenital sexual contact. When the gonococcus can be demonstrated by culture, individuals of either gender are infectious to their sexual partners.

Complications

Because men often seek treatment early in the course of the disease, they are less likely to develop complications. Complications that do occur in men are prostatitis, urethral strictures, and sterility from orchitis or epididymitis.

Because women who are asymptomatic seldom seek treatment, complications are more common and usually are the reason for seeking medical attention. Pelvic inflammatory disease (PID), Bartholin's abscess, ectopic pregnancy, and infertility are the main complications in women.

- A small percentage of infected persons, mainly women, may develop a disseminated gonococcal infection (DGI). In DGI the appearance of skin lesions, fever, arthralgia, arthritis, or endocarditis usually causes the patient to seek medical help.

Diagnostic Studies

- For men, a presumptive diagnosis of gonorrhea is made if there is a history of sexual contact with an infected individual followed within a few days by a urethral discharge. Typical clinical manifestations combined with a positive finding in a gram-stained smear of discharge from the penis gives an almost certain diagnosis.
- A culture is indicated for men whose smears are negative in the presence of strong clinical evidence. Cultures of the discharge or secretion can provide definitive diagnosis after incubation for 24 to 48 hours.
- Making a diagnosis in women is difficult because most women are symptom free. A culture must be performed to confirm the diagnosis.
- The nucleic acid amplification test (NAAT) is a nonculture test with sensitivity similar to culture tests for *N. gonorrhoeae*. It can be done on a wide variety of samples, including vaginal, endocervical, urethral, and urine specimens. Other nonculture testing procedures include enzyme immunoassays (EIAs) and direct fluorescent antibody (DFA) tests.

Collaborative Care

Because of a short incubation period and high infectivity, treatment is instituted without awaiting culture results, even in the absence of signs or symptoms.

Treatment of gonorrhea in the early stage is curative with the most common treatment being a single oral or intramuscular (IM) dose of ceftriaxone (Rocephin). The high frequency (up to 20% in men and 40% in women) of coexisting chlamydial and gonococcal infections has led to the addition of azithromycin (Zithromax) or doxycycline (Vibramycin) to the treatment regimen. Patients with coexisting syphilis are likely to be treated by the same drugs used for gonorrhea.

- All sexual contacts of patients with gonorrhea must be treated to prevent reinfection after resumption of sexual relations. The "ping-pong" effect of reexposure, treatment, and reinfection can cease only when infected partners are treated simultaneously.
- The patient should be counseled to abstain from sexual intercourse and alcohol during treatment. Sexual intercourse allows the infection to spread and can retard complete

healing as a result of vascular congestion. Alcohol has an irritating effect on the healing urethral walls.

- Men should be cautioned against squeezing the penis to look for further discharge.
- Reinfection, rather than treatment failure, is the main cause of infections identified after treatment has ended.

Nursing Management
See Nursing Management: Sexually Transmitted Diseases, p. 570.

GOUT

Description
Gout is caused by an increase in uric acid production, underexcretion of uric acid by the kidneys, or increased intake of foods containing purines, which are metabolized to uric acid by the body. Characteristic deposits of monosodium urate crystals occur in articular, periarticular, and subcutaneous tissues. Joint involvement includes recurrent attacks of acute arthritis.

Gout may be classified as primary or secondary. In *primary gout,* a hereditary error of purine metabolism leads to overproduction or retention of uric acid. Primary gout (90% of cases) occurs predominantly in middle-aged men and is very rare in premenopausal women. *Secondary gout* may be related to another acquired disorder, or may be the result of medications known to inhibit uric acid excretion. Secondary gout may also be caused by drugs that increase the rate of cell death, such as the chemotherapeutic agents used in treating leukemia.

Pathophysiology
Uric acid is the major end product of purine catabolism and is primarily excreted by the kidneys. Hyperuricemia may be the result of increased purine synthesis, decreased renal excretion, or both.

- A high dietary intake of purine alone has little effect on uric acid levels. Hyperuricemia may result from prolonged fasting or excessive drinking because of increased production of ketoacids, which then inhibit uric acid excretion.

Clinical Manifestations
In the acute phase, gouty arthritis may occur in one or more joints. Affected joints may appear dusky or cyanotic and are extremely tender. Inflammation of the great toe *(podagra)* is the most common

initial problem. Other joints affected are the midtarsal area of the foot, ankle, knee, wrist, and the olecranon bursa.

- Acute gouty arthritis is usually precipitated by events such as trauma, surgery, alcohol ingestion, or systemic infection. Onset of symptoms is usually rapid, with swelling and pain peaking within several hours, often accompanied by a low-grade fever.
- Individual attacks usually subside, treated or untreated, in 2 to 10 days. The affected joint returns entirely to normal, and patients are often free of symptoms between attacks.

Chronic gout is characterized by multiple joint involvement and deposits of sodium urate crystals *(tophi)*. These are typically seen in the synovium, subchondral bone, olecranon bursa, and vertebrae; along tendons; and in the skin and cartilage. Tophi are generally noted many years after the onset of the disease.

Chronic inflammation may result in joint deformity, and cartilage destruction may predispose the joint to secondary osteoarthritis. Large and unsightly tophaceous deposits may perforate overlying skin, producing draining sinuses that often become infected. Excessive uric acid excretion may lead to urinary tract stone formation. Pyelonephritis associated with intrarenal sodium urate deposits and obstruction may contribute to renal disease.

The severity of gouty arthritis is variable. The clinical course may consist of infrequent mild attacks or multiple severe episodes associated with a slowly progressive disability.

Diagnostic Studies

- Serum uric acid levels are usually elevated >6 mg/dL.
- Specimens for 24-hour urine uric acid levels may be obtained to determine if the disease is caused by decreased renal excretion or overproduction of uric acid.
- X-rays appear normal in the early stages of gout, with tophi, an indicator of chronic disease, appearing as eroded areas in the bone.
- Synovial fluid aspiration helps distinguish gout from septic arthritis and *pseudogout* (calcium phosphate crystals are formed). Affected fluid characteristically contains needlelike crystals of sodium urate.

Collaborative Care

Goals for care include termination of an acute attack through the use of an antiinflammatory agent such as colchicine, with nonsteroidal antiinflammatory drugs (NSAIDs) for pain management.

Future attacks are prevented by a maintenance dose of allopurinol (Zyloprim), weight reduction if necessary, and possible avoidance of alcohol and high-purine foods (red and organ meats). Treatment is also aimed at preventing formation of uric acid kidney stones and other associated conditions, such as hypertriglyceridemia and hypertension.

Drug Therapy

Acute gouty arthritis is treated with colchicine and NSAIDs. Recurrent gout may be prevented by combining colchicine with a xanthine oxidase inhibitor such as allopurinol or a uricosuric drug such as probenecid (Benemid). Febuxostat (Uloric), a selective inhibitor of xanthine oxidase, is given for long-term management of hyperuricemia in persons with chronic gout.

- Corticosteroids, either orally or by intraarticular injection, can be helpful in treating acute attacks.
- Aspirin inactivates the effect of uricosurics, resulting in urate retention, and should be avoided while patients are taking uricosuric drugs (e.g., probenecid [Benemid]). Acetaminophen can be used safely if analgesia is required.
- Adequate urine volume must be maintained to prevent precipitation of uric acid in the renal tubules. Allopurinol, which blocks production of uric acid, is particularly useful in patients with uric acid stones or renal impairment, in whom uricosuric drugs may be ineffective or dangerous.

Regardless of which drugs are used to treat gout, serum uric acid levels must be checked regularly to monitor treatment effectiveness.

Nutritional Therapy

Dietary restrictions may include limiting the use of alcohol and foods high in purine. However, drugs can generally control gout without necessitating these changes. Obese patients should be instructed in a weight-reduction program.

Nursing Management

Nursing intervention is directed at supportive care of the inflamed joints.

- Bed rest may be appropriate, with affected joints properly immobilized. Involvement of a lower extremity may require use of a cradle or footboard to protect the painful area from the weight of bed clothes.
- Assess the limitation of motion and degree of pain and document treatment effectiveness.

▼ **Patient and Caregiver Teaching**

Help the patient and caregiver to understand that hyperuricemia and gouty arthritis are chronic problems that can be controlled with careful adherence to a treatment program.

- Offer explanations concerning the importance of drug therapy and the need for periodic determination of serum uric acid levels.
- Help the patient understand precipitating factors that may cause an attack, including overindulgence in purine-containing foods and alcohol, starvation (fasting), medication use (e.g., aspirin, diuretics), and major medical events (e.g., surgery, myocardial infarction).

GUILLAIN-BARRÉ SYNDROME

Description

Guillain-Barré syndrome is an acute, rapidly progressing, and potentially fatal form of polyneuritis. It is also called *postinfectious polyneuropathy* and *ascending polyneuropathic paralysis*. It is characterized by ascending, symmetric paralysis that usually affects cranial nerves and the peripheral nervous system. With adequate supportive care, 85% to 95% of these patients recover completely.

Pathophysiology

The etiology is unknown. Both cellular and humoral immune mechanisms play a role in the immune reaction directed at the nerves. The result is a loss of myelin (a segmental demyelination) and edema and inflammation of the affected nerves. As demyelination occurs, the transmission of nerve impulses is stopped or slowed down. The muscles innervated by the damaged peripheral nerves undergo denervation and atrophy. In the recovery phase, remyelination occurs slowly and returns in a proximal-to-distal pattern.

- The syndrome is often preceded by immune system stimulation from a viral infection, trauma, surgery, viral immunizations, or human immunodeficiency virus (HIV). *Campylobacter jejuni* is the most recognized organism associated with Guillain-Barré syndrome. *C. jejuni* gastroenteritis is thought to precede Guillain-Barré syndrome in approximately 30% of cases. Other potential pathogens include *Mycoplasma pneumoniae,* cytomegalovirus, Epstein-Barr virus, varicella-zoster virus, and vaccines (rabies, swine influenza).

Clinical Manifestations

Guillain-Barré syndrome is a heterogeneous condition with symptoms ranging from mild to severe. Symptoms usually develop 1 to 3 weeks after an upper respiratory or gastrointestinal (GI) infection.

- Weakness of the lower extremities (evolving more or less symmetrically) occurs over hours to days to weeks, usually peaking about day 14. Distal muscles are more severely affected.
- Paresthesia (numbness and tingling) is frequent, and paralysis usually follows in the extremities. Hypotonia and areflexia are common, persistent symptoms. Sensory loss is variable, with deep sensation more affected than superficial sensations.
- Autonomic nervous system dysfunction is usually seen in patients with severe muscle involvement and respiratory muscle paralysis. The most dangerous autonomic dysfunctions include orthostatic hypotension, hypertension, and abnormal vagal responses (bradycardia, heart block, and asystole).
- Other autonomic dysfunctions include bowel and bladder dysfunction, facial flushing, and diaphoresis.
- Patients may also have the syndrome of inappropriate antidiuretic hormone (SIADH) secretion (see Syndrome of Inappropriate Antidiuretic Hormone, p. 620).
- Progression of Guillain-Barré syndrome to include the lower brainstem involves the facial, abducens, oculomotor, hypoglossal, trigeminal, and vagus cranial nerves. This involvement manifests itself through facial weakness, extraocular eye movement difficulties, dysphagia, and facial paresthesia.
- Pain is a common finding; the pain can be categorized as paresthesias, muscular aches and cramps, and hyperesthesias. Pain appears to be worse at night. Opioids may be indicated for those experiencing severe pain. Pain may lead to a decrease in appetite and interfere with sleep.

The most serious complication is respiratory failure, which occurs as paralysis progresses to the nerves that innervate the thoracic area. Respiratory infections or urinary tract infections (UTIs) may occur. Fever is generally the first sign of infection, and treatment is directed at the infecting organism. Immobility from the paralysis can cause problems such as paralytic ileus, muscle atrophy, deep vein thrombosis, pulmonary emboli, skin breakdown, and orthostatic hypotension.

G

Diagnostic Studies

Diagnosis is based primarily on patient history and clinical signs.
- Cerebrospinal fluid is normal or has a low protein content initially, but after 7 to 10 days it shows a greatly elevated protein level (700 mg/dL [7 g/L]).
- Electromyographic (EMG) and nerve conduction studies are markedly abnormal (showing reduced nerve conduction velocity) in affected extremities.

Collaborative Care

Management is aimed at supportive care, particularly ventilatory support, during the acute phase.
- Plasmapheresis is used in the first 2 weeks. In patients with severe disease treated within 2 weeks of onset, there is a distinct reduction in length of stay, length of time on ventilator, and time required to resume walking.
- Intravenous (IV) administration of high-dose immunoglobulin (Sandoglobulin) has been as effective as plasmapheresis and has the advantage of immediate availability and increased safety. After 3 weeks past disease onset, plasmapheresis and immunoglobin therapies have little value.
- Corticosteroids appear to have little effect on the disease prognosis or duration.

Nursing Management

Goals

The patient with Guillain-Barré syndrome will maintain adequate ventilation, be free from aspiration, be free of pain or have pain controlled, maintain an acceptable method of communication, maintain adequate nutritional intake, and return to usual physical functioning.

Nursing Diagnoses

- Impaired spontaneous ventilation
- Risk for aspiration
- Acute pain
- Impaired verbal communication
- Fear
- Self-care deficits

Nursing Interventions

The objective of care is to support the body systems until the patient recovers. Respiratory failure and infection are serious threats.

- Monitoring vital capacity and arterial blood gases (ABGs) is essential. A tracheostomy or endotracheal intubation may be done so that the patient can be mechanically ventilated (see Tracheostomy, p. 754, and Artificial Airways: Endotracheal Tubes, p. 699).

- Whether the patient has an endotracheal tube or tracheostomy, meticulous suctioning technique is needed to prevent infection. Thorough bronchial hygiene and chest physiotherapy help clear secretions and prevent respiratory deterioration.

- If fever develops, obtain sputum cultures to identify the pathogen. Appropriate antibiotic therapy is then initiated.

A communication system must be established with the use of the patient's available abilities. This is extremely difficult if the disease progresses to involvement of cranial nerves; at the peak of a severe episode the patient may be incapable of communicating.

- The nurse must explain all procedures before doing them and reassure the patient that muscle function will probably return.

Urinary retention is common for a few days. Intermittent catheterization is preferred to an indwelling catheter to avoid UTIs. However, for the acutely ill patient receiving a large volume of fluids (>2.5 L/day), indwelling catheterization may be safer to reduce overdistention of a temporarily flaccid bladder and to prevent vesicoureteral reflux.

Physical therapy is indicated early to help prevent problems related to immobility. Range-of-motion (ROM) exercises and attention to body position help maintain function and prevent contractures.

Nutritional needs must be met in spite of possible problems associated with gastric dilation, paralytic ileus, and aspiration potential if the gag reflex is lost.

- Note drooling and other difficulties with secretions, which may indicate an inadequate gag reflex.

- Initially enteral feedings or parenteral nutrition may be used to ensure adequate caloric intake. Monitor fluid and electrolyte therapy to prevent electrolyte imbalances.

HEAD INJURY

Description

Head injury is a broad classification that includes any trauma to the scalp, skull, or brain. A serious form of head injury is traumatic brain injury (TBI). The term *head trauma* refers primarily to

craniocerebral trauma, which includes an alteration in consciousness no matter how brief.

- Motor vehicle crashes and falls are the most common causes
  of head injury. Other causes of head injury include firearms,
  assaults, sports-related trauma, recreational injuries, and
  war-related injuries.
- Males are twice as likely to sustain a TBI as females.

Deaths from head trauma occur at three time points after injury:
immediately after injury, within 2 hours of injury, and approximately 3 weeks after injury. The majority of deaths occur immediately after the injury, either from the direct head trauma or
massive hemorrhage and shock. Deaths occurring within a few
hours of the trauma are caused by progressive worsening of the
head injury or internal bleeding. Recognizing changes in neurologic status and surgical intervention are critical in the prevention
of deaths at this point. Deaths occurring 3 weeks or more after the
injury result from multisystem failure.

Types of Head Injuries

Scalp lacerations. Because the scalp contains many blood vessels
with poor constrictive abilities, even relatively small lacerations
can bleed profusely. The major complications of scalp lesions are
blood loss and infection.

Skull fractures. Fractures frequently occur with head trauma.
Fractures may be closed or open, depending on the presence of a
scalp laceration or extension of the fracture into the air sinuses or
dura.

- Type and severity of a skull fracture depend on the velocity,
  momentum, and direction of the injuring agent, and the site
  of impact. Specific manifestations of a skull fracture are
  generally associated with the location of the injury (see
  Table 57-7, Lewis et al., *Medical-Surgical Nursing,* ed. 8,
  p. 1439).

Major potential complications of skull fracture are intracranial
infections and hematoma, as well as meningeal and brain tissue
damage.

Head trauma. Brain injuries are categorized as *diffuse* (generalized) or *focal* (localized). In diffuse injury (i.e., concussion, diffuse
axonal) damage to the brain cannot be localized to one particular
area of the brain, whereas a focal injury (e.g., contusion, hematoma) can be localized to a specific area of the brain.

Diffuse injury. *Concussion* is a minor, sudden, transient, and
diffuse head injury associated with a disruption in neural activity
and a change in the level of consciousness (LOC). The patient may
not lose total consciousness. Signs include a brief disruption in

LOC, amnesia for the event (retrograde amnesia), and headache. Manifestations are generally of short duration.

- Postconcussion syndrome may develop in some patients and is usually seen anywhere from 2 weeks to 2 months after the concussion. Symptoms include persistent headache, lethargy, behavior changes, decreased short-term memory, and changes in intellectual ability.

Although concussion is generally considered benign and usually resolves spontaneously, the symptoms may be the beginning of a more serious, progressive problem. At the time of discharge it is important to give the patient and caregiver instructions for observation and accurate reporting of symptoms or changes in neurologic status.

Diffuse axonal injury. Diffuse axonal injury (DAI) is widespread axonal damage occurring after a mild, moderate, or severe TBI.

- Clinical signs of DAI include decreased LOC, increased ICP, decortication or decerebration, and global cerebral edema. Approximately 90% of patients with DAI remain in a persistent vegetative state.
- Patients who survive the initial event are rapidly triaged to an ICU where they will be vigilantly watched for signs of increased ICP and treated for increased ICP (see Increased Intracranial Pressure, p. 352).

Focal injury. Focal injury can be minor to severe, and can be localized to an area of injury. Focal injury consists of lacerations, contusions, hematomas, and cranial nerve injuries.

Lacerations involve actual tearing of brain tissue and often occur with compound fractures and penetrating injuries. Tissue damage is severe, and surgical repair of the laceration is impossible because of the nature of brain tissue. If bleeding is deep into the brain parenchyma, focal and generalized signs are noted.

- Prognosis is generally poor for the patient with a large intracerebral hemorrhage.

A *contusion* is the bruising of brain tissue within a focal area. It is usually associated with a closed head injury. A contusion may contain areas of hemorrhage, infarction, necrosis, and edema, and frequently occurs at a fracture site.

- Contusions or lacerations may occur both at the site of the direct impact of the brain on the skull *(coup)* and at a secondary area of damage on the opposite side away from injury *(contrecoup)*, leading to multiple contused areas.
- Patient prognosis depends on the amount of bleeding around the contusion site. Neurologic assessment may demonstrate focal findings as well as generalized findings. Seizures are a common complication.

When major head trauma occurs, many delayed responses are seen, including hemorrhage, hematoma formation, seizures, and cerebral edema. Intracerebral hemorrhage is generally associated with cerebral laceration (see Increased Intracranial Pressure, p. 352, and Seizure Disorders, p. 562).

Complications

Epidural hematoma. An epidural hematoma results from bleeding between the dura and inner surface of the skull. An epidural hematoma is a neurologic emergency and is usually associated with a linear fracture crossing a major artery in the dura, causing a tear. It can have a venous or an arterial origin.

- Venous epidural hematomas are associated with a tear of the dural venous sinus and develop slowly.
- With arterial hematomas, the middle meningeal artery lying under the temporal bone is frequently torn. Because this is an arterial hemorrhage, the hematoma develops rapidly.

Manifestations typically include an initial period of unconsciousness at the scene, with a brief lucid interval followed by a decrease in LOC. Other symptoms may be headache, nausea and vomiting, or focal findings. Rapid surgical intervention to evacuate the hematoma and prevent cerebral herniation, along with medical management for increasing ICP, can dramatically improve outcomes.

Subdural hematoma. A subdural hematoma occurs from bleeding between the dura mater and the arachnoid layer of the meningeal covering of the brain. A subdural hematoma usually results from injury to the brain tissue and its blood vessels. A subdural hematoma is usually venous in origin, with slow development of the hematoma, but rapid development can occur if the hematoma is of arterial origin. Subdural hematomas may be acute, subacute, or chronic (Table 42).

- An *acute subdural hematoma* manifests signs within 24 to 48 hours of the injury. Manifestations are similar to those associated with brain tissue compression in increased intracranial pressure (ICP) (see Increased Intracranial Pressure, p. 352). The patient's appearance may range from drowsy and confused to unconscious. The ipsilateral pupil dilates and becomes fixed if ICP is significantly increased.
- A *subacute subdural hematoma* usually occurs within 2 to 14 days of the injury. After the initial bleeding, a subdural hematoma may appear to enlarge over time as the breakdown products of the blood draw fluid into the subdural space.

Table 42 Types of Subdural Hematomas

Type	Occurrence After Injury	Progression of Symptoms	Treatment
Acute	24-48 hr after severe trauma	Immediate deterioration	Craniotomy, evacuation, and decompression
Subacute	48 hr to 2 wk after severe trauma	Alteration in mental status as hematoma develops; progression dependent on size and location of hematoma	Evacuation and decompression
Chronic	Weeks, months, usually >20 days after injury; often injury seemed trivial or was forgotten by patient	Nonspecific, nonlocalizing progression; progressive alteration in LOC	Evacuation and decompression, membranectomy

LOC, Level of consciousness.

H

- A *chronic subdural hematoma* develops over weeks or months after a seemingly minor head injury. Chronic subdural hematomas are more common in older adults because of a potentially larger subdural space as a result of brain atrophy. The presenting complaints are focal symptoms, rather than signs of increased ICP.

Intracerebral hematoma. An *intracerebral hematoma* occurs from bleeding within the brain tissue. It usually occurs within the frontal and temporal lobes, possibly from the rupture of intracerebral vessels at the time of injury.

Diagnostic Studies

- Computed tomography (CT) scan is the best diagnostic test to evaluate for craniocerebral trauma.
- Magnetic resonance imaging (MRI), positron emission therapy (PET), and evoked potential studies assist in diagnosis and differentiation of head injuries.
- Transcranial Doppler studies are used to measure cerebral blood flow velocity.
- Cervical spine x-ray series or CT scan of the spine may be done.

Collaborative Care

Emergency management of the patient with head injury includes measures to prevent secondary injury by treating cerebral edema and managing increased ICP (see Table 57-9, Lewis et al., *Medical-Surgical Nursing,* ed. 8, p. 1442). The principal treatment of head injuries is timely diagnosis and surgery if necessary. For the patient with a concussion or contusion, observation and management of increased ICP are primary management strategies.

- The treatment of skull fractures is usually conservative. For depressed fractures and fractures with loose fragments, a craniotomy is necessary to elevate depressed bone and remove free fragments. If large amounts of bone are destroyed, the bone may be removed (craniectomy) and a cranioplasty will be needed at a later time (see the section on cranial surgery, Lewis et al., *Medical-Surgical Nursing,* ed. 8, pp. 1449 to 1451).
- In cases of large acute subdural and epidural hematomas or those associated with significant neurologic impairment, the blood must be removed. A craniotomy is generally performed to visualize the bleeding vessels so that bleeding can be controlled. Burr-hole openings may be used in an extreme emergency for more rapid decompression, followed by a craniotomy. A drain is generally placed postoperatively for several days to prevent any reaccumulation of blood.

Nursing Management

Goals

The patient with an acute head injury will maintain adequate cerebral oxygenation and perfusion; remain normothermic; achieve control of pain and discomfort; be free from infection; and attain maximal cognitive, motor, and sensory function.

Nursing Diagnoses/Collaborative Problems

- Risk for ineffective cerebral tissue perfusion
- Hyperthermia
- Acute pain (headache)
- Impaired physical mobility
- Anxiety
- Potential complication: increased ICP

Nursing Interventions

One of the best ways to prevent head injuries is to prevent car and motorcycle accidents

- You can be active in campaigns that promote driving safety and can speak to driver education classes regarding the dangers of unsafe driving and driving after drinking alcohol and using drugs
- The use of seat belts in cars and the use of helmets for riding on motorcycles are the most effective measures in increasing survival after accidents

The general goal of nursing management of the head-injured patient is to maintain cerebral oxygenation and perfusion and prevent secondary cerebral ischemia. Surveillance or monitoring for changes in neurologic status is critically important because the patient's condition may deteriorate rapidly, necessitating emergency surgery

- Explain the need for frequent neurologic assessments to both the patient and family
- Behavioral manifestations associated with head injury can result in a frightened, disoriented patient who is combative and resists help.

The Glasgow Coma Scale (GCS) is useful in assessing the LOC (see Glasgow Coma Scale, p. 789). Indications of a deteriorating neurologic state, such as a decreasing LOC or lessening of motor strength, should be reported to the health care provider and the patient's condition should be closely monitored. .

The major focus of nursing care for the brain-injured patient relates to increased ICP (see Increased Intracranial Pressure: Nursing Management, p. 357).

- Loss of the corneal reflex may necessitate administering lubricating eye drops or taping the eyes shut to prevent abrasion.

- Periorbital ecchymosis and edema disappear spontaneously, but cold and, later, warm compresses provide comfort and hasten the process.
- Diplopia can be relieved by use of an eye patch.
- Hyperthermia can result in increased metabolism, cerebral blood flow, cerebral blood volume, and ICP. Increased metabolic waste also produces further cerebral vasodilation. Avoid hyperthermia with a goal of 36° C to 37° C as the standard of care.
- If cerebrospinal fluid (CSF) rhinorrhea or otorrhea occurs, inform the physician immediately and elevate the head of the bed to decrease the CSF pressure. A loose collection pad may be placed under the nose or over the ear. Instruct the patient not to sneeze or blow the nose.
- Nausea and vomiting may be a problem and can be alleviated by antiemetic drugs.
- Headache can usually be controlled with acetaminophen or small doses of codeine.

If the patient's condition deteriorates, intracranial surgery may be necessary. A burr-hole opening or craniotomy may be indicated, depending on the underlying injury. The patient is often unconscious before surgery, making it necessary for a family member to sign the consent form for surgery. This is a difficult and frightening time for the patient's caregiver and family and requires sensitive nursing management. Suddenness of the situation makes it especially difficult for the family to cope.

Once the condition has stabilized, the patient is usually transferred for acute rehabilitation management. There may be chronic problems related to motor and sensory deficits, communication, memory, and intellectual functioning.

- The patient's outward appearance is not a good indicator of how well the patient will function in the home or work environment given recovery time and rehabilitation.

Progressive recovery may continue for 6 months or more before a plateau is reached and a prognosis for recovery can be made. Specific nursing management depends on residual deficits. In all cases the caregiver and family must be given special consideration. They need to understand what is happening and be taught appropriate interaction patterns.

- The family often has unrealistic expectations of the patient as the coma begins to recede. The family expects full return to pretrauma status. In reality, the patient usually experiences a reduced awareness and ability to interpret environmental stimuli.

- Prepare the family for the emergence of the patient from coma and explain that the process of awakening often takes several weeks. Arrange for social work and chaplain consultations for the family in addition to providing open-visitation and frequent status updates.
- Family members, particularly spouses, go through role transition as the role changes from one of spouse to that of caregiver.

HEAD AND NECK CANCER

Description
Head and neck cancer arises from mucosal surfaces and includes tumors of the paranasal sinuses, oral cavity, nasopharynx, oropharynx, and larynx. Most people present with locally advanced disease. Disability is great because of the potential loss of voice, disfigurement, and social consequences. Most head and neck cancers occur at age 50 years or older after prolonged use of tobacco and alcohol. Other risk factors include consumption of a diet poor in fruits and vegetables and infection by the human papillomavirus (HPV). Men are affected two to five times greater than women.

Clinical Manifestations
Early signs of head and neck cancer vary with tumor location. Cancer of the oral cavity may be a painless growth in the mouth, an ulcer that does not heal, or a change in the fit of dentures. Pain is a late symptom that may be aggravated by acidic food.

Cancers of the oropharynx, hypopharynx, and supraglottic larynx are almost always squamous cell carcinomas, rarely produce early symptoms, and are usually diagnosed in later stages.

- The patient may complain of persistent unilateral sore throat or otalgia (ear pain). Hoarseness may be a symptom of early laryngeal cancer. Some patients experience a change in voice quality or what may feel like a lump in the throat.
- Oral leukoplakia (white patch) or erythroplakia (red patch) may be seen and should be noted for later biopsy. Both leukoplakia and carcinoma in situ (localized to a defined area) may precede invasive carcinoma by many years.
- There may be thickening of the normally soft and pliable oral mucosa.
- Late stages of head and neck cancer have easily detectable signs and symptoms, including pain, dysphagia, decreased

mobility of the tongue, airway obstruction, and cranial neuropathies.

Diagnostic Studies

- If lesions are suspected, upper airways may be examined using an indirect laryngoscopy or a flexible nasopharyngoscope. The larynx and vocal cords are visually inspected for lesions and tissue mobility.
- A computed tomography (CT) scan or magnetic resonance imaging (MRI) may be performed to detect local and regional spread.
- Multiple biopsy specimens are obtained to determine the extent of the disease.

Collaborative Care

The stage of the disease is determined based on tumor size (T), number and location of involved nodes (N), and extent of metastasis (M). TNM staging classifies the disease as stage I to stage IV and guides treatment (see p. 799).

- Patients in stage I or II at diagnosis can undergo radiation therapy or surgery with the goal of cure. Nearly all patients with advanced disease will require radiation, either preoperatively or postoperatively. In addition, brachytherapy is sometimes used to treat head and neck cancer.
- Advanced lesions of the larynx are treated by a total laryngectomy in which the entire larynx and preepiglottic region are removed and a permanent tracheostomy is performed (see Tracheostomy, p. 754). Radical neck dissection frequently accompanies total laryngectomy. Depending on the extent of involvement, extensive dissection and reconstruction may be performed.
- Some patients refuse surgical intervention for advanced lesions because of the extent of the procedure and the potential risk to the patient. In this situation, external radiation therapy is used as the sole treatment or in combination with chemotherapy.
- Chemotherapy (e.g., cisplatin [Platinol] and cetuximab [Erbitux]), a targeted therapy, are used in combination with radiation therapy for patients with unresectable cancers.

Nutritional Therapy

After radical neck surgery, the patient may be unable to take in nutrients through the normal route of ingestion. Parenteral fluids are given for the first 24 to 48 hours.

- Because of swelling and difficulty swallowing postoperatively, tube feedings are usually given through a nasogastric, nasointestinal, or gastrostomy tube that was placed during surgery.

When the patient can swallow, small amounts of water are given with the patient in high Fowler's position. Close observation for choking is essential. Suctioning may be necessary to prevent aspiration.

- You should anticipate swallowing problems when the patient resumes eating. Using a commercially available thickening agent (Thick It) to thicken liquids will enhance swallowing.
- If radiation therapy is used, good nutrition is important to provide calories and protein for tissue repair.

Nursing Management
Goals
The patient with head or neck cancer will have a patent airway, no complications related to therapy, adequate nutritional intake, minimal to no pain, the ability to communicate, and an acceptable body image.

See NCP 27-2 for the patient having total laryngectomy or radical neck surgery, Lewis et al., *Medical-Surgical Nursing,* ed. 8, pp. 539 to 540.

Nursing Diagnoses
- Anxiety
- Ineffective airway clearance
- Imbalanced nutrition: less than body requirements
- Impaired verbal communication
- Disturbed body image
- Acute pain

Nursing Interventions
Provide information about the risk factors of prolonged tobacco and alcohol use in your health teaching. If cancer has been diagnosed, smoking cessation is still important because the patient who continues to smoke during radiation therapy has a lower rate of response and survival.

- Radiation therapy may be used in the treatment of early tumors. Suggest interventions to reduce the side effects of radiation therapy to the head and neck.

Preoperative care for radical neck surgery should include explanations of postoperative measures relating to communication and feeding. For procedures that involve a laryngectomy, teaching should include information about expected changes in speech. The nurse or speech pathologist should demonstrate means of communicating without speech.

After surgery, maintenance of a patent airway is essential and a laryngectomy (tracheostomy) tube will be in place. The patient will be in a semi-Fowler's position to decrease edema and tension on the suture lines. Monitor vital signs frequently because of the risk of hemorrhage and respiratory compromise. Immediately after surgery the postlaryngectomy patient requires frequent suctioning by way of the laryngectomy tube.

- Monitor patency of wound drainage tubes every 4 hours for 24 hours to ensure that they are properly removing serous drainage. After drainage tubes are removed, closely monitor the area to detect any swelling. If fluid continues to accumulate, aspiration may be necessary.
- Depression and changes in sexuality patterns because of altered body image are common in the patient who has had radical neck dissection. Expect to help the patient regain an acceptable self-concept.
- A speech therapist should meet with the patient to discuss voice restoration. Options available include voice prosthesis, esophageal speech, and an electrolarynx.

▼ **Patient and Caregiver Teaching**

- Instruct patient and caregiver about the feeding and laryngectomy tubes and stoma care, allowing them to perform care repeatedly in the hospital to ensure correct performance of technique.
- Teach the patient to cover the stoma before performing activities such as shaving and the application of makeup to avoid inhalation of foreign materials.
- Encourage the patient to report changes, such as stoma narrowing, difficulty swallowing, and a lump in the throat. These changes may indicate tumor recurrence or tracheal stenosis.
- Address measures to provide adequate humidity at home using a bedside humidifier.
- Changes following a total laryngectomy include loss of speech, loss of the ability to taste and smell, inability to produce audible sounds (including laughing and crying), and a permanent tracheal stoma. Ensure the patient receives a referral for a home health care nurse to provide ongoing assistance and support.

HEADACHE

Description

Headache is probably the most common type of pain experienced by humans. The majority of people have functional headaches, such as migraine or tension type; the remainder have organic headaches caused by intracranial or extracranial disease.

- Primary headache classifications include tension-type, migraine, and cluster headaches. Secondary headaches include headaches caused by conditions such as sinus infection, neck injury, and stroke. Characteristics of primary headaches are shown in Table 43.

Tension-Type Headache

Tension-type headache is the most common type of headache and is characterized by its bilateral location and pressing/tightening quality. It is usually of mild or moderate intensity and is not aggravated by physical activity. It is likely that neurovascular factors similar to those involved in migraine headaches play a role in the development of tension-type headaches.

Clinical manifestations. There is no prodrome (early manifestation of impending disease) in tension-type headache. The headache does not involve nausea or vomiting but may involve sensitivity to light *(photophobia)* or sound *(phonophobia)*.

- Headaches may occur intermittently for weeks, months, or years. Many patients can have a combination of migraine and tension-type headaches with features of both headaches occurring simultaneously.

Diagnostic studies. Careful history taking is the most important diagnostic tool. Electromyography (EMG) may or may not reveal sustained contraction of the neck, scalp, or facial muscles. If tension-type headache is present during physical examination, increased resistance to passive movement of the head and tenderness of head and neck may be present.

Migraine Headache

Migraine headache is a recurring headache characterized by unilateral or bilateral throbbing pain, a triggering event or factor, strong family history, and manifestations associated with neurologic and autonomic nervous system dysfunction. By the late teens, females are about twice as likely to suffer from migraine headaches as males.

Pathophysiology. The current theory is that a complex series neurovascular events initiates a migraine headache. People wh have migraines have a state of neuronal hyperexcitability in the cerebral cortex, especially in the occipital cortex. Approximately

H

Table 43 Comparison of Tension-Type, Migraine, and Cluster Headaches

Pattern	Tension-Type Headache	Migraine Headache	Cluster Headache
Site*	Bilateral, bandlike pressure at base of skull	Unilateral (in 60%), may switch sides, commonly anterior	Unilateral, radiating up or down from one eye
Quality	Constant, squeezing tightness	Throbbing, synchronous with pulse	Severe, bone-crushing
Frequency	Cycles for many years	Periodic; cycles of several months to years	May have months or years between attacks
			Attacks occur in clusters over a period of 2-12 wk
Duration	30 min to 7 days	4-72 hr	5-180 min
Time and mode of onset	Not related to time	May be preceded by prodrome	Nocturnal; commonly awakens patient from sleep
		Onset after awakening; gets better with sleep	
Associated symptoms	Palpable neck and shoulder muscles, stiff neck, tenderness	Nausea, vomiting, irritability, sweating, Photophobia	Facial flushing or pallor
		Phonophobia; Prodrome of sensory, motor, or psychic phenomena	Unilateral lacrimation, ptosis, and rhinitis
		Family history (in 65%)	

* See Fig. 59-1, Lewis et al., *Medical-Surgical Nursing*, ed. 8, p. 1486.

70% of those with migraine have a first degree relative who also had migraine headaches.

Migraines can be preceded by prodrome and aura. The prodrome may precede the headache by several hours or several days.

- An *aura* is a complex of neurologic symptoms characterized by visual (e.g., bright lights, scotomas (patchy blindness), visual distortions, zig zag lines), sensory (hearing voices or sounds that do not exist, strange smells), and/or motor (e.g., weakness, paralysis, feeling that limbs are moving) phenomena.

In many cases, migraine headaches have no known precipitating events. However, for other patients, the headache may be precipitated or triggered by foods, hormonal fluctuation, head trauma, physical exertion, fatigue, stress, and drugs.

Clinical manifestations. *Migraine without aura* is the most common type of migraine headache. *Migraine with aura* occurs in only 10% of migraine headache episodes.

The headache may last 4 to 72 hours. During the headache phase, some patients may tend to "hibernate"; that is, they seek shelter from noise, light, odors, people, and problems. The headache is described as a steady, throbbing pain that is synchronous with the pulse. Although the headache is usually unilateral, it may switch to the opposite side in another episode. In some patients, the symptoms of the migraine headaches may become progressively worse over time.

Diagnostic studies. There are no specific laboratory or radiologic tests for migraine headache. The diagnosis is usually made from the history. Neurologic and other diagnostic examinations are often normal.

Cluster Headache

Cluster headaches, a rare form of headache, involve repeated headaches that can occur for weeks to months at a time, followed by periods of remission.

Pathophysiology. Neither the cause nor pathophysiology of cluster headache is fully known. The vasodilation that occurs in the affected part of the face is extracranial with the trigeminal nerve implicated in the production of pain. Cluster headaches also involve dysfunction of intracranial blood vessels, the sympathetic nervous system, and pain modulation systems. Because of the circadian rhythmicity of the headaches, the hypothalamus is believed to play a role.

Clinical manifestations. The pain of cluster headache is sharp and stabbing. It is one of the most severe forms of headache, with intense pain typically lasting from a few minutes to 3 hours.

H

- The pain is generally located around the eye, radiating to the temple, forehead, cheek, nose, or gums.
- Other manifestations include swelling around the eye, lacrimation (tearing), facial flushing or pallor, rhinitis, and constriction of the pupil.
- The patient with a cluster headache is often agitated and restless, unable to sit still or relax.

Diagnostic studies. Diagnosis is primarily based on the history. However, a computed tomography (CT) scan, magnetic resonance imaging (MRI), or cerebral angiography may be done.

Collaborative Care

If no systemic underlying disease is found, therapy is directed toward the functional type of headache. Table 59-3, Lewis et al., *Medical-Surgical Nursing,* ed. 8, p. 1489 summarizes current therapies for prophylaxis and symptomatic relief of headaches. These therapies can include drugs, meditation, yoga, biofeedback, cognitive-behavioral therapy, and relaxation training.

Drug Therapy

Tension-type headache. Drug treatment usually involves a non-opioid analgesic (e.g., aspirin, acetaminophen) used alone or in combination with a sedative, muscle relaxant, tranquilizer, or codeine. Many of these drugs have serious side effects.

Migraine headache. Drug treatment is aimed at terminating or decreasing the symptoms of the acute attack. Many people with mild or moderate migraine can obtain relief with aspirin or acetaminophen. For moderate to severe headaches, the triptans have become the first line of therapy.

- Triptans affect selected serotonin receptors, reducing the neurogenic inflammation of the cerebral blood vessels and producing vasoconstriction. They include sumatriptan (Imitrex), naratriptan (Amerge), rizatriptan (Maxalt), almotriptan (Axert), frovatriptan (Frova), zolmitriptan (Zomig), and eletriptan (Relpax). Because these drugs cause constriction of coronary arteries, they are avoided in patients with heart disease. Triptan medications should be taken at the first symptom of migraine headache.
- Topiramate (Topamax), taken daily, has been shown to be an effective therapy for migraine prevention in adults. It must be used for 2 to 3 months to determine its effectiveness. Other preventive drugs for migraine headaches can include β-adrenergic blockers (e.g., propranolol [Inderal], atenolol [Tenormin]), tricyclic antidepressants (e.g., amitriptyline [Elavil]), selective serotonin reuptake inhibitors (e.g., fluoxetine [Prozac]), calcium channel blockers (e.g.,

verapamil [Isoptin]), divalproex (Depakote), clonidine (Catapres), and thiazides.

- Botulinum toxin A (Botox) is being successfully used in the prophylactic treatment of chronic daily headaches and migraines with minimal side effects.

Cluster headache. Because these headaches occur suddenly, often at night, and are not long lasting, drug therapy is not as useful as it is for other types of headache. Prophylactic medications may include verapamil (Isoptin), lithium, ergotamine, divalproex (Depakote), or nonsteroidal antiinflammatory drugs (NSAIDs). Acute treatment of cluster headache is inhalation of 100% oxygen (O_2) delivered at a rate of 7 to 9 L/min for 15 to 20 minutes, which may relieve headache by causing vasoconstriction. Methysergide may be used prophylactically when the cluster headache recurs at a known time. Intranasal administration of lidocaine has also been shown to abort cluster headaches.

Nursing Management

Goals

The patient with a headache will have reduced or no pain, experience increased comfort and decreased anxiety, demonstrate an understanding of triggering events and treatment strategies, use positive coping strategies to deal with chronic pain, and experience increased quality of life and decreased disability.

See NCP 59-1 for the patient with headache, Lewis et al., *Medical-Surgical Nursing,* ed. 8, p. 1491.

Nursing Diagnoses

- Acute pain

Nursing Interventions

Headaches may result from an inability to cope with daily stresses. The most effective therapy may be to help patients examine their lifestyle, recognize stressful situations, and learn to cope with them more appropriately. Help the patient identify precipitating factors and ways of avoiding them can be developed. Encourage daily exercise, relaxation periods, and socializing because each can help decrease the recurrence of headache.

- Suggest alternative ways of handling the pain of headache through techniques such as relaxation, meditation, yoga, and self-hypnosis. Massage and moist hot packs to the neck and head can help a patient with tension-type headaches.
- The patient should learn about drugs prescribed for prophylactic and symptomatic treatment of headache and should be able to describe the purpose, action, dosage, and side effects.
- For the patient whose headaches are triggered by food, dietary counseling may be provided. The patient is

encouraged to eliminate foods that may provoke headaches (e.g., chocolate, alcohol, excessive caffeine, cheese, fermented foods, monosodium glutamate).

▼ **Patient and Caregiver Teaching**

A teaching guide for the patient with a headache is provided in Table 44.

Table 44	Patient and Caregiver Teaching Guide: Headaches

You should include the following instructions when teaching the patient and/or caregiver management of headaches:

1. Keep a diary or calendar of headaches and possible precipitating events.
2. Avoid factors that can trigger a headache:
   - Foods containing amines (cheese, chocolate), nitrites (meats such as hot dogs), vinegar, onions, monosodium glutamate
   - Fermented or marinated foods
   - Caffeine
   - Oranges
   - Tomatoes
   - Onions
   - Aspartame
   - Nicotine
   - Ice cream
   - Alcohol (particularly red wine)
   - Emotional stress
   - Fatigue
   - Drugs such as ergot-containing preparations and monoamine oxidase inhibitors
3. Learn the purpose, action, dosage, and side effects of drugs taken.
4. Self-administer sumatriptan (Imitrex) subcutaneously if prescribed.
5. Use stress reduction techniques such as relaxation.
6. Participate in regular exercise.
7. Contact health care provider if the following occur:
   - Symptoms become more severe, last longer than usual, or are resistant to medication
   - Nausea and vomiting (if severe or not typical), change in vision, or fever occurs with the headache
   - Problems with drugs

HEART FAILURE

Description

Heart failure (HF) is an abnormal clinical syndrome involving impaired cardiac pumping and/or filling. HF, formerly called congestive HF, is the terminology preferred today because not all patients will have pulmonary congestion or volume overload. HF is associated with numerous types of cardiovascular diseases, particularly long-standing hypertension, coronary artery disease (CAD), and myocardial infarction (MI).

- HF is a major health problem in the United States. In contrast to other cardiovascular diseases, HF is increasing in incidence and prevalence. This is because of improved survival after cardiovascular events and the increased aging population. HF is associated with high rates of morbidity and mortality.
- CAD and advancing age are the primary risk factors for HF. Other factors, including hypertension, diabetes, cigarette smoking, obesity, and high serum cholesterol, contribute to the development of HF.

Pathophysiology

HF may be caused by any interference with the normal mechanisms regulating cardiac output (CO). CO depends on (1) preload, (2) afterload, (3) myocardial contractility, and (4) heart rate (HR). Any alteration in these factors can lead to decreased ventricular function and subsequent HF.

- Major causes of HF may be divided into two subgroups: (1) primary causes, consisting of underlying cardiac diseases, such as CAD and cardiomyopathy, and (2) precipitating causes, such as anemia, pulmonary disease, and hypervolemia (see the complete listing of causes in Tables 35-1 and 35-2, Lewis et al., *Medical-Surgical Nursing*, ed 8, p. 798).

Heart failure is classified as systolic or diastolic failure. *Systolic failure* results from an inability of the heart to pump effectively. It is caused by impaired contractile function (e.g., myocardial infarction [MI]), increased afterload (e.g., hypertension), cardiomyopathy, and mechanical abnormalities (e.g., valvular heart disease). The hallmark of systolic dysfunction is a decrease in the left ventricular ejection fraction (EF).

Diastolic failure is the inability of the ventricles to relax and fill during diastole. Decreased filling results in decreased stroke volume and CO and venous engorgement in both the pulmonary and systemic vascular systems. The diagnosis of diastolic failure is based on the presence of pulmonary congestion, pulmonary hypertension, ventricular hypertrophy, and a normal EF. Diastolic failure is usually the result of left ventricular hypertrophy from chronic hypertension, aortic stenosis, or hypertrophic cardiomyopathy.

Mixed systolic and diastolic failure is seen in disease states such as dilated cardiomyopathy, in which poor systolic function (weakened muscle function) is further compromised by dilated left ventricular walls that are unable to relax.

The patient with ventricular failure of any type has low systemic arterial blood pressure (BP), low CO, and poor renal perfusion. Whether a patient arrives at this point acutely (from an MI) or chronically (from worsening cardiomyopathy or hypertension), the body's response to this low CO is to mobilize compensatory mechanisms to maintain CO and BP. The main compensatory mechanisms include (1) sympathetic nervous system activation, (2) neurohormonal responses, (3) ventricular dilation, and (4) ventricular hypertrophy.

HF is usually manifested by biventricular failure, although one ventricle may precede the other in dysfunction.

- The most common form of initial heart failure is left-sided failure. Left-sided failure causes blood to back up through the left atrium and into the pulmonary veins. The increased pulmonary pressure causes fluid extravasation from the pulmonary capillary bed into the interstitium and then the alveoli, which is manifested as pulmonary congestion and edema.

- Right-sided failure causes backward blood flow to the right atrium and venous circulation. Venous congestion in the systemic circulation results in peripheral edema, hepatomegaly, and jugular venous distention. The primary cause of right-sided failure is left-sided failure. *Cor pulmonale* (right ventricular dilation and hypertrophy caused by pulmonary pathologic conditions) can also cause right-sided failure (See Cor Pulmonale, p. 154).

Manifestations of Acute Decompensated Heart Failure

Regardless of etiology, acute decompensated heart failure (ADHF) manifests as *pulmonary edema*. This is an acute, life-threatening situation in which the lung alveoli become filled with serosanguineous fluid. The most common cause of pulmonary edema is acute left ventricle (LV) failure secondary to CAD.

- Manifestations of pulmonary edema are distinctive: the patient is usually anxious, pale, and possibly cyanotic, with clammy and cold skin.
- The patient has severe dyspnea, as evidenced by the use of respiratory accessory muscles, respiratory rate >30 breaths/min, and orthopnea. Wheezing and coughing with production of frothy, blood-tinged sputum may also occur.
- Auscultation of the lungs may reveal bubbling crackles, wheezes, and rhonchi. The patient's HR is rapid, and BP may be elevated or decreased depending on the severity of the HF.

Manifestations of Chronic Heart Failure

Manifestations of chronic HF depend on the patient's age, underlying type and extent of heart disease, and which ventricle is failing to pump effectively. Table 45 lists manifestations of left-sided and right-sided failure. The patient with chronic HF will probably have manifestations of biventricular failure.

- Fatigue after usual activities is one of the earliest symptoms.
- Dyspnea is a common sign. Shortness of breath occurs when the patient is in the recumbent position (orthopnea).
- Paroxysmal nocturnal dyspnea (PND) occurs when the patient is asleep. The patient awakens in a panic, has feelings of suffocation, and has a strong desire to seek relief by sitting up.
- Other common signs include tachycardia; edema in the legs, liver, abdominal cavity, and lungs; nocturia; cool and dusky skin; restlessness and confusion; angina-type chest pain; and weight changes.

Complications

Pleural effusion results from increasing pressure in the pleural capillaries. Enlargement of the heart chambers in chronic HF can cause atrial fibrillation. Patients also have a high risk of fatal dysrhythmias.

Left ventricular thrombus may occur with ADHF or chronic HF in which the enlarged LV and decreased CO combine to increase the chance of thrombus formation in the LV. This places the patient at risk for stroke

Hepatomegaly may result as liver lobules become congested with venous blood. Hepatic congestion leads to impaired liver function; eventually liver cells die, and cirrhosis can develop.

Table 45	Clinical Manifestations of Heart Failure

Right-Sided Heart Failure	Left-Sided Heart Failure
Signs	
▪ RV heaves	▪ LV heaves
▪ Murmurs	▪ Pulsus alternans (alternating
▪ Jugular venous distention	pulses: strong, weak)
▪ Edema (e.g., pedal,	▪ ↑ HR
scrotum, sacrum)	▪ PMI displaced interiorly and
▪ Weight gain	posteriorly (LV hypertrophy)
▪ ↑ HR	▪ ↓ PaO_2, slight ↑ $PaCO_2$ (poor
▪ Ascites	O_2 exchange)
▪ Anasarca (massive	▪ Crackles (pulmonary edema)
generalized body edema)	▪ S_3 and S_4 heart sounds
▪ Hepatomegaly (liver	▪ Pleural effusion
enlargement)	▪ Changes in mental status
	▪ Restlessness, confusion
Symptoms	
▪ Fatigue	▪ Weakness, fatigue
▪ Anxiety, depression	▪ Anxiety, depression
▪ Dependent, bilateral edema	▪ Dyspnea
▪ Right upper quadrant pain	▪ Shallow respirations up to
▪ Anorexia and GI bloating	32-40/min
▪ Nausea	▪ Paroxysmal nocturnal
	dyspnea
	▪ Orthopnea (shortness of
	breath in recumbent position)
	▪ Dry, hacking cough
	▪ Nocturia
	▪ Frothy, pink-tinged sputum
	(advanced pulmonary edema)

GI, Gastrointestinal; *HR,* heart rate; *LV,* left ventricle; *PaO_2,* partial pressure of oxygen in arterial blood; *$PaCO_2$,* partial pressure of carbon dioxide in arterial blood; *PMI,* point of maximal impulse; *RV,* right ventricle.

Diagnostic Studies

Diagnosing HF is often difficult because neither patient signs nor symptoms are highly specific, and both may mimic many other medical conditions (e.g., anemia, lung disease). Diagnostic tests for acute decompensated and chronic heart failure are presented in Table 46.

A primary diagnostic goal is to determine the underlying etiology. An endomyocardial biopsy (EMB) may be done in patients

Table 46 Collaborative Care: Heart Failure

Both ADHF and Chronic HF	ADHF	Chronic HF
Diagnostic		
History and physical examination	ABGs	Exercise stress testing
Determination of underlying cause	Thyroid function tests	
Serum chemistries, cardiac enzymes, BNP level, liver function tests	CBC	
	Endomyocardial biopsy	
Chest x-ray		
12-lead ECG		
Hemodynamic monitoring		
Echocardiogram		
Nuclear imaging studies (see Table 32-6, Lewis et al., *Medical-Surgical Nursing*, ed. 8, p. 728)		
Cardiac catheterization		

Continued

H

Table 46   Collaborative Care: Heart Failure—cont'd

Both ADHF and Chronic HF	ADHF	Chronic HF
Collaborative Therapy Treatment of underlying cause Circulatory assist devices (e.g., intraaortic balloon pump, ventricular assist device) Daily weights Sodium and, possibly, fluid-restricted diet	High Fowler's position O₂ by mask or nasal catheter BiPAP Endotracheal intubation and mechanical ventilation Vital signs, urinary output at least q 1 hr Continuous ECG and pulse oximetry monitoring Hemodynamic monitoring (e.g., intraarterial BP, PAWP, CO) Drug therapy (see Table 35-8, Lewis et al., *Medical-Surgical Nursing*, ed. 8, p. 805) Possible cardioversion (e.g., atrial fibrillation) Ultrafiltration	Oxygen therapy at 2-6 L/min by nasal cannula Rest-activity periods Cardiac rehabilitation Home health nursing care (e.g., telehealth monitoring) Drug therapy (see Table 35-8, Lewis et al., *Medical-Surgical Nursing*, ed. 8, p. 805) Cardiac resynchronization therapy with internal cardioverter-defibrillator Cardiac transplantation Palliative and end-of-life care

ABGs, Arterial blood gases; *ADHF,* acute decompensated heart failure; *BiPAP,* bilevel positive airway pressure; *BNP,* b-type natriuretic peptide; *BP,* blood pressure; *CBC,* complete blood count; *CO,* cardiac output; *ECG,* electrocardiogram; *PAWP,* pulmonary artery wedge pressure.

who develop unexplained, new-onset HF that is unresponsive to usual care. EF can be used to differentiate systolic and diastolic HF. In general, b-type natriuretic peptide (BNP) levels correlate positively with the degree of left ventricular dysfunction.

Nursing and Collaborative Management: Acute Decompensated Heart Failure

With the addition of new drugs and device therapies, the management of HF has dramatically changed in the past few years. Table 46 lists collaborative therapy for the patient with ADHF.

Place the patient in a high Fowler's position with the feet horizontal in the bed or dangling at the bedside. This position helps decrease venous return because of the pooling of blood in the extremities. Supplemental oxygen helps increase the percentage of oxygen in inspired air. In severe pulmonary edema the patient may need noninvasive ventilatory support or intubation and mechanical ventilation

The ADHF patient needs continuous monitoring and assessment, which is usually done in an ICU setting. Monitor ECG and oxygen saturation. Vital signs and urinary output are assessed often. The patient may have continuous hemodynamic monitoring.

- Ultrafiltration is an option for the patient with volume overload. It rapidly removes extracellular and intravascular fluid volume. Volume is removed similar to hemodialysis but without hemodynamic instability.
- Circulatory assist devices are used to manage patients with deteriorating HF. The intraaortic balloon pump (IABP) increases coronary blood flow to the heart muscle and decreases the heart's workload. Ventricular assist devices can be used to maintain the pumping ability of a heart.
- Assess patients with HF for depression and anxiety, and treatment plans should be initiated if appropriate.

Drug therapy. Drug therapy is essential in treating acute heart failure.

- Diuretics: Decreasing venous return (preload) reduces the amount of volume returned to the LV during diastole. Decreasing intravascular volume with the use of loop diuretics (e.g., furosemide [Lasix], bumetanide [Bumex]) reduces venous return.
- Vasodilators: IV nitroglycerin reduces preload, slightly reduces afterload (in high doses), and increases myocardial oxygen supply. Sodium nitroprusside (Nipride) reduces both preload and afterload, thus improving myocardial contraction, increasing CO, and reducing pulmonary congestion. IV

nesiritide (Natrecor), a recombinant form of BNP, causes both arterial and venous dilation.

- Morphine: Morphine sulfate reduces preload and afterload and is used in the treatment of ADHF and pulmonary edema. It dilates the pulmonary and systemic blood vessels, thereby decreasing pulmonary pressures and improving gas exchange.

- Positive inotropics: Inotropic therapy increases myocardial contractility. Currently, inotropic therapy is only recommended for use in the short-term management of patients with ADHF who have not responded to conventional pharmacotherapy (e.g., diuretics, vasodilators, morphine).

  - Digitalis is a positive inotrope that improves contractility but also increases myocardial oxygen consumption. It has a slow onset of action and thus is not a first line drug to treat ADHF. Other positive inotropes include β-adrenergic agonists.

  - β-adrenergic agonists are positive inotropes (e.g., dopamine [Intropin], dobutamine (Dobutrex), epinephrine, norepinephrine [Levophed]) currently recommended for use in the short-term management of patients with ADHF who have not responded to conventional pharmacotherapy (e.g., diuretics, vasodilators, morphine).

Collaborative Care: Chronic Heart Failure

The main goal in the treatment of chronic HF is to treat the underlying cause and contributing factors, maximize CO, provide treatment to alleviate symptoms, improve ventricular function, improve quality of life, preserve target organ function, and improve mortality and morbidity. The treatment of causes such as dysrhythmias, hypertension, valvular disorders, and CAD are discussed elsewhere in this book.

Nondrug Therapy

- Administration of O_2 improves saturation and assists in meeting tissue oxygen needs, thereby helping to relieve dyspnea and fatigue.

- Physical and emotional rest conserves energy and decreases the need for additional O_2. A patient with severe HF may be on bed rest with limited activity. A patient with mild to moderate HF can be ambulatory with a restriction of strenuous activity.

Cardiac resynchronization therapy (CRT), unlike traditional pacing, coordinates right and left ventricular contractility through biventricular pacing. The ability to have normal simultaneous electrical conduction (synchrony) within the right and left ventricles increases left ventricular function and CO.

Mechanical options such as the intraaortic balloon pump (IABP) and ventricular assist devices (VADs) are available for patients with deteriorating conditions, especially those awaiting cardiac transplantation. Limitations of bed rest, infection, and vascular complications preclude long-term use of IABP. VADs provide highly effective long-term support for up to 2 years.

Drug Therapy

- Diuretics mobilize edematous fluid, reduce pulmonary venous pressure, and reduce preload.
    - Thiazide diuretics (e.g., hydrochlorothiazide [Hydrodiuril]) may be the first choice because of their convenience, safety, low cost, and effectiveness.
    - Loop diuretics such as furosemide (Lasix), bumetanide (Bumex), and torsemide (Demadex) are potent but can cause hypokalemia and ototoxicity.
- Angiotensin-converting enzyme (ACE) inhibitors (e.g., captopril [Capoten], enalapril [Vasotec]) are the primary drugs of choice for blocking the renin-angiotensin-aldosterone system in HF patients with systolic dysfunction. A reduction in SVR with the use of ACE inhibitors produces a significant increase in CO. Although BP decreases, tissue perfusion is maintained or increased as a result of improved CO, and diuresis is enhanced by the suppression of aldosterone.
- Nitrates (e.g., nitroglycerin) cause vasodilation by acting directly on the smooth muscle of the vessel wall. Nitrates are of particular benefit in the management of myocardial ischemia related to HF because they promote vasodilation of the coronary arteries.
- A combination drug containing isosorbide dinitrate and hydralazine (BiDil) is used for the treatment of HF in African Americans who are already being treated with standard therapy.
- β-Adrenergic blockers, especially carvedilol (Coreg) and metoprolol (Toprol-XL), contribute to marked improvement in patient survival in chronic HF. These agents directly block the negative effects of the sympathetic nervous system on the failing heart.
- Positive inotropes are used to improve cardiac contractility.
    - Digitalis preparations (e.g., digoxin [Lanoxin]) increase the force of cardiac contraction *(inotropic action)*. They also decrease conduction speed within the myocardium and slow the HR *(chronotropic action)*. This allows for more complete emptying of the ventricles, thus

H

diminishing the volume remaining in the ventricles during diastole. CO increases because of increased stroke volume from improved contractility.

- Other inotropic agents include β-adrenergic agonists (dobutamine [Dobutex]) and phosphodiesterase inhibitors (milrinone [Primacor]).

Nutritional Therapy

Diet education and weight management are critical to the control of chronic HF. You or a dietitian should obtain a detailed diet history to determine not only what foods the patient eats but also when, where, and how often they dine out.

The edema of chronic HF is often treated by dietary restriction of sodium. Teach the patient what foods are low and high in sodium and ways to enhance food flavors without the use of salt (e.g., substituting lemon juice and various spices). The degree of sodium restriction depends on the severity of the HF and the effectiveness of diuretic therapy.

- A commonly prescribed diet for a patient with mild HF is a 2.5 g sodium diet. All foods high in sodium should be eliminated. For more severe HF, sodium intake is restricted to 500 to 1000 mg (For sample menu plans for sodium restricted diets see Table 35-10, Lewis et al., *Medical-Surgical Nursing,* ed. 8, p. 809).

Fluid restrictions are not commonly prescribed for mild to moderate HF. Diuretic therapy, ACE inhibitors, and digitalis preparations act as effective diuretics to promote fluid excretion. However, in moderate to severe HF, fluid restrictions are usually implemented.

- Instruct patients to weigh themselves at the same time each day, preferably before breakfast, while wearing the same type of clothing. For a weight gain of 3 lb (1.4 kg) over 2 days or a 5 lb (2.3 kg) gain over 1 week the primary health care provider should be called.

Nursing Management: Chronic Heart Failure

Goals

The patient with HF will have a decrease in symptoms (e.g., shortness of breath, fatigue), decreased peripheral edema, increased exercise tolerance, adherence with medical regimen, and no complications related to HF.

See NCP 35-1 for the patient with HF, Lewis et al., *Medical-Surgical Nursing,* ed. 8, pp. 810 to 811.

Nursing Diagnoses

- Activity intolerance
- Excess fluid volume

- Decreased cardiac output
- Impaired gas exchange
- Deficient knowledge

Nursing Interventions

Health promotion. An important measure used to prevent HF is the treatment or control of underlying heart disease. For example, patients with valvular disease should have valve replacement long before lung congestion develops and coronary revascularization procedures should be performed in patients with CAD.

- When a patient is diagnosed with HF, preventive care should focus on slowing the progression of the disease. Knowing the importance of following the medication, diet, and exercise regimen is essential.

Acute intervention. Many persons with HF will experience one or more episodes of ADHF. When they do, they are usually managed in an intensive care unit, an intermediate care unit with continuous cardiac monitoring capability, or a specialized HF unit.

Ambulatory and home care. HF is a chronic illness for most persons. Important nursing responsibilities are (1) teach the patient about physiologic changes that have occurred, (2) assist the patient to adapt to both physiologic and psychologic changes, and (3) integrate the patient and the patient's caregiver in the overall care plan.

A patient and caregiver teaching guide for HF is presented in Table 47.

Table 47	**Patient and Caregiver Teaching Guide: Heart Failure**

You should include the following instructions when teaching the patient and/or caregiver management of heart failure:

Health Promotion
1. Obtain annual flu vaccination.
2. Obtain pneumococcal vaccine (e.g., Pneumovax) and revaccination after 5 yr (for people at high risk of infection or serious disease).
3. Continue to address risk factors (e.g., blood pressure control, smoking cessation, weight reduction).

Rest
1. Plan a regular daily rest and activity program.
2. After exertion, such as exercise and ADLs, plan a rest period.
3. Shorten working hours or schedule rest period during working hours.
4. Avoid emotional upsets. Verbalize any concerns, fears, feelings of depression, etc. to health care provider.

Continued

Table 47	Patient and Caregiver Teaching Guide: Heart Failure—cont'd

Drug Therapy
1. Take each drug as prescribed.
2. Develop a system (e.g., daily chart, weekly pill box) to ensure medications have been taken.
3. Take pulse rate each day before taking medications (if appropriate). Know the parameters that your health care provider wants for your heart rate.
4. Take BP at determined intervals (if appropriate). Know your target BP limits.
5. Know signs and symptoms of orthostatic hypotension and how to prevent them (see Table 33-14, Lewis et al., *Medical-Surgical Nursing,* ed. 8, p. 755).
6. Know signs and symptoms of internal bleeding (bleeding gums, increased bruises, blood in stool or urine) and what to do if on anticoagulants.
7. Know own INR if taking warfarin (Coumadin) and how often to have blood monitored.

Dietary Therapy
1. Consult the written diet plan and list of permitted and restricted foods.
2. Examine labels to determine sodium content. Also examine the labels of over-the-counter drugs such as laxatives, cough medicines, and antacids.
3. Avoid using salt when preparing foods, or adding salt to foods.
4. Weigh yourself the same time each day, using the same scale and wearing the same or similar clothes.
5. Eat smaller, more frequent meals.

Activity Program
1. Increase walking and other activities gradually, provided they do not cause fatigue or dyspnea. Consider a cardiac rehabilitation program.
2. Avoid extremes of heat and cold.

Ongoing Monitoring
1. Know the signs and symptoms of recurring or progressing heart failure (e.g., FACES: **f**atigue, limitation of **a**ctivities, chest **c**ongestion/cough, **e**dema, **s**hortness of breath).
2. Recall the symptoms experienced when illness began; reappearance of previous symptoms may indicate a recurrence.

Table 47	Patient and Caregiver Teaching Guide: Heart Failure—cont'd

3. Report immediately to health care provider any of the following:
   - Weight gain of 3 lb (1.4 kg) in 2 days, or 3 to 5 lb (2.3 kg) in a week
   - Difficulty breathing, especially with exertion or when lying flat
   - Waking up breathless at night
   - Frequent dry, hacking cough, especially when lying down
   - Fatigue, weakness
   - Swelling of ankles, feet, or abdomen; swelling of face or difficulty breathing (if taking ACE inhibitors)
   - Nausea with abdominal swelling, pain, and tenderness
   - Dizziness or fainting
4. Follow up with health care provider on regular basis.
5. Consider joining a local support group with your family members and/or caregiver(s).

ACE, Angiotensin-converting enzyme; *ADLs*, activities of daily living; *BP*, blood pressure; *INR*, international normalized ratio.

HEMOPHILIA

Description

Hemophilia is an X-linked recessive genetic disorder caused by defective or deficient coagulation factor. The two major forms of hemophilia that can occur in mild to severe forms are *hemophilia A* (classic hemophilia, factor VIII deficiency) and *hemophilia B* (Christmas disease, factor IX deficiency). *von Willebrand's disease* is a related disorder involving a deficiency of the von Willebrand's coagulation protein.

Hemophilia A is the most common form of hemophilia, accounting for about 80% of all cases. Von Willebrand's disease is considered the most common congenital bleeding disorder in humans, with estimates as high as 1 in 100 persons.

Deficiency and inheritance patterns of these three forms of inherited coagulopathies are compared in Table 48.

Clinical Manifestations and Complications

Clinical manifestations and complications related to hemophilia include (1) slow, persistent, prolonged bleeding from minor trauma and small cuts; (2) delayed bleeding after minor injuries (the delay may be several hours or days); (3) uncontrollable

Table 48   Comparison of Types of Hemophilia

Disorder	Deficiency	Laboratory Results*	Inheritance Pattern
Hemophilia A	Factor VIII	Bleeding time normal; prolonged partial thromboplastin time because of deficiency of coagulation factor	Recessive sex-linked (transmitted by female carriers, displayed almost exclusively in men)
Hemophilia B	Factor IX	Bleeding time normal; prolonged partial thromboplastin time because of deficiency of coagulation factor	Recessive sex-linked (transmitted by female carriers, displayed almost exclusively in men)
von Willebrand's disease	vWF, variable factor VIII deficiencies and platelet destruction	Prolonged bleeding time because of defective platelets; prolonged partial thromboplastin time because of deficiency of coagulation factor	Autosomal dominant, seen in both genders Recessive (in severe forms of the disease)

vWF, von Willebrand factor.
*Prothrombin time, thrombin time, and platelet count normal in hemophilia.

hemorrhage after dental extractions or irritation of the gingiva with a hard-bristle toothbrush; (4) epistaxis, especially after a blow to the face; (5) GI bleeding from ulcers and gastritis; (6) hematuria from genitourinary (GU) trauma and splenic rupture resulting from falls or abdominal trauma; (7) ecchymoses and subcutaneous hematomas; (8) neurologic signs, such as pain, anesthesia, and paralysis, that may develop from nerve compression caused by hematoma formation; and (9) hemarthrosis (bleeding into the joints), which may lead to joint deformity severe enough to cause crippling (commonly in knees, elbows, shoulders, hips, and ankles).

- All manifestations relate to bleeding. Any bleeding episode in persons with hemophilia may lead to life-threatening hemorrhage.
- The contamination of blood products with the human immunodeficiency virus (HIV) in the 1980s caused the majority of hemophilia deaths in the late 1980s. However, survival of up to 72 years old is now being observed because of improved preparation of replacement products, improved screening of blood donors, and use of recombinant replacement factors.
- Hepatitis C antibody screening is now routinely done on all donated blood and blood products to prevent hepatitis C transmission.

Diagnostic Studies
Laboratory studies affected by the deficient factor within the intrinsic system will yield the results presented in Table 48.

Collaborative Care
The goal of care is to prevent and treat bleeding. Persons with hemophilia or von Willebrand's disease require preventive care, the use of replacement therapy during acute bleeding episodes and as prophylaxis, and treatment of complications of the disease and its therapy.

- Replacement of deficient clotting factors is the primary means of supporting patients with hemophilia. In addition to treating acute crises, replacement therapy may be given before surgery and dental care as a prophylactic measure.
- For mild hemophilia A or certain subtypes of von Willebrand's disease, desmopressin acetate (DDAVP), a synthetic analog of vasopressin, may be used to stimulate an increase in factor VIII and von Willebrand's factor (vWF).

Complications of treatment of hemophilia include development of inhibitors to factors VIII or IX, transfusion-transmitted infectious disorders, allergic reactions, and thrombotic complications with the use of factor IX because it contains activated coagulation factors.

The most common difficulty with acute management is starting factor replacement therapy too late and stopping it too soon. Generally, minor bleeding episodes should be treated for at least 72 hours. Surgery and traumatic injuries may need more prolonged support. Chronically, the development of inhibitors to the factor products has occurred and requires individualized expert patient management.

Nursing Management

Because of the hereditary nature of hemophilia, referral for genetic counseling is essential when considering preventive measures. Counseling is especially important because persons with hemophilia are living into adulthood.

Interventions are related primarily to controlling the bleeding and include the following:

1. Stop the topical bleeding as quickly as possible by applying direct pressure or ice, packing the area with Gelfoam or fibrin foam, and applying topical hemostatic agents, such as thrombin.

2. Administer the specific coagulation factor concentrate as ordered. Monitor the patient for signs and symptoms such as hypersensitivity.

3. When joint bleeding occurs, it is important to totally rest the involved joint to prevent crippling deformities from hemarthrosis. Pack the joint in ice. Give analgesics (e.g., acetaminophen, codeine) to reduce severe pain; aspirin and aspirin-containing compounds should never be used. As soon as bleeding ceases, encourage mobilization of the affected area through range-of-motion (ROM) exercises and physical therapy. Weight bearing is avoided until all swelling has resolved and muscle strength has returned.

4. Manage life-threatening complications that may develop as a result of hemorrhage. Examples include prevention or treatment of airway obstruction from hemorrhage into the neck and pharynx, as well as early assessment and treatment of intracranial bleeding.

▼ Patient and Caregiver Teaching

Quality and length of life may be significantly affected by the patient's knowledge of the illness and how to live with it. Provide ongoing assessment of the patient's adaptation to the illness.

- Teach the patient with hemophilia that immediate medical attention is required for severe pain or swelling of a muscle or joint that restricts movement or inhibits sleep and for a head injury, swelling in the neck or mouth, abdominal pain, hematuria, melena, and skin wounds in need of suturing.

- Daily oral hygiene must be performed without causing trauma.
- Instruct the patient how to prevent injuries. The patient can learn to participate in noncontact sports (e.g., golf) and wear gloves when doing household chores to prevent cuts or abrasions from knives, hammers, and other tools.
- The patient should wear a Medic-Alert tag to ensure that health care providers know about the hemophilia in case of an accident.
- The patient needs information about routine follow-up care, and compliance with scheduled visits must be assessed.
- A reliable person can be taught to self-administer some of the factor replacement therapies at home.

HEMORRHOIDS

Description
Hemorrhoids are dilated hemorrhoidal veins that may be internal (occurring above the internal sphincter) or external (occurring outside the external sphincter).

Pathophysiology

H

Hemorrhoids are thought to develop as a result of increased anal pressure and weakened connective tissue that normally support the hemorrhoidal veins. When supporting tissues in the anal canal weaken, usually as a result of straining at defecation, venules become dilated. In addition, blood flow through the veins of the hemorrhoidal plexus is impaired. An intravascular clot in the venule results in a thrombosed external hemorrhoid.

Hemorrhoids are the most common reason for bleeding with defecation. Hemorrhoids may be precipitated by many factors, including pregnancy, prolonged constipation, straining in an effort to defecate, heavy lifting, prolonged standing and sitting, and portal hypertension (as found in cirrhosis).

Clinical Manifestations
Classic symptoms of hemorrhoids include bleeding, anal pruritus, prolapse, and pain.

- *Internal hemorrhoids* may be asymptomatic, but when they become constricted, pain occurs. Internal hemorrhoids can bleed, resulting in blood on toilet paper after defecation or

blood on the outside of the stool. The patient may report a
chronic, dull aching discomfort, particularly when hemorrhoids have prolapsed.

■ *External hemorrhoids* are reddish blue and seldom bleed or
cause pain unless a vein ruptures. Blood clots in external
hemorrhoids cause pain and inflammation and are described
as thrombosed. External hemorrhoids cause intermittent
pain, pain on palpation, itching, and burning. Patients also
report bleeding associated with defecation. Constipation or
diarrhea can aggravate these symptoms.

Diagnostic Studies

■ *Internal hemorrhoids* are diagnosed by digital examination,
anoscopy, and sigmoidoscopy.

■ *External hemorrhoids* can be diagnosed by visual inspection
and digital examination.

Collaborative Care

Therapy is directed toward the causes of the condition and the
patient's symptoms. A high-fiber diet and increased fluid intake
prevent constipation and reduce straining. Ointments, creams, suppositories, and impregnated pads that contain antiinflammatory
agents (e.g., hydrocortisone) or astringents and anesthetics (e.g.,
witch hazel, benzocaine, pramoxine) may be used to shrink mucous
membranes and relieve discomfort. The use of topical corticosteroids such as hydrocortisone agents should be limited to 1 week or
less to prevent side effects such as contact dermatitis and mucosal
atrophy. Stool softeners may keep stools soft, and sitz baths help
relieve pain.

External hemorrhoids are usually managed by conservative
therapy unless they become thrombosed. For internal hemorrhoids,
nonsurgical approaches (band ligation, infrared coagulation, cryotherapy, laser treatment) can be used. A hemorrhoidectomy (surgical excision of hemorrhoids) is indicated when there is prolapse,
excessive pain or bleeding, or large hemorrhoids. Surgical removal
may be done by cautery, clamp, or excision.

■ Hemorrhoids may recur. Occasionally anal strictures
develop and dilation is necessary.

Nursing Management

Nursing care includes teaching measures to prevent constipation,
avoidance of prolonged standing or sitting, proper use of over-the-
counter medications available for hemorrhoidal symptoms, and
instructions on when to seek medical care for symptoms (e.g.,
excessive pain and bleeding, prolapsed hemorrhoids).

- Pain is a common problem after a hemorrhoidectomy. Although the procedure is minor, the pain is severe, and opioids are usually given initially. Topical nitroglycerin preparations may be used postoperatively to decrease pain and subsequent opioid use.
- Sitz baths are started 1 or 2 days after surgery. A sponge ring in the sitz bath helps relieve pressure on the area. Initially the patient should not be left alone because of the possibility of weakness or fainting.
- Packing may be inserted into the rectum to absorb drainage. A T-binder may hold the dressing in place. If packing is inserted, it usually is removed the first or second postoperative day. Assess for rectal bleeding. The patient may be embarrassed when the dressing is changed, and privacy should be provided.
- A stool softener such as docusate sodium (Colace) is usually ordered the first few postoperative days. If the patient does not have a bowel movement within 2 or 3 days, an oil retention enema is given.
- The patient usually dreads the first bowel movement and often resists the urge to defecate. Pain medication may be given before the bowel movement to reduce discomfort.

▼ **Patient and Caregiver Teaching**
- Teach the importance of diet, care of the anal area, symptoms of complications (especially bleeding), and avoidance of constipation and straining.
- Sitz baths are recommended for 1 to 2 weeks
- The health care provider may order a stool softener to be taken for a time.
- Regular checkups are important in the prevention of any further problems.

H

HEPATITIS, VIRAL

Description

Hepatitis is an inflammation of the liver. Viral hepatitis is the most common cause of hepatitis. The types of viral hepatitis are A, B, C, D, E, and G. Approximately 1.4 million cases of infection with hepatitis A virus (HAV) occur worldwide annually, and nearly 2 billion people are infected with hepatitis B virus (HBV).

- Worldwide approximately 170 million people are infected with hepatitis C virus (HCV). Approximately 20% of patients with chronic HCV progress to cirrhosis within 20 to 30 years. Chronic HBV and HCV account for 80% of liver cancer cases today.

- Approximately 30% to 40% of HIV-infected patients also have HCV. This high rate of co-infection is primarily related to intravenous (IV) drug use. Co-infection with HIV and HCV places the patient at greater risk for more serious liver disease.

Etiology

Viral hepatitis can be caused by one of six viruses: A, B, C, D, E, and G. Other viruses known to damage the liver include cytomegalovirus, Epstein-Barr virus, herpes virus, coxsackievirus, and rubella virus.

- The only definitive way to distinguish the various forms of viral hepatitis is by the presence of the antigens and the subsequent development of antibodies to them. Outbreaks of hepatitis are generally caused by hepatitis A virus (HAV) and hepatitis B virus (HBV).
- Approximately 44% of viral hepatitis cases in adults in the United States are hepatitis B, 19% are hepatitis C, and 37% are hepatitis A. Table 49 lists characteristics of hepatitis viruses.
- Infection with HAV or HBV provides immunity to that virus (homologous immunity). However, the patient can still develop another type of viral hepatitis, and patients with hepatitis C can be reinfected with another strain of hepatitis C. For a more complete description of each hepatitis virus, see Lewis et al., *Medical-Surgical Nursing,* ed. 8, pp. 1059 to 1062.

Pathophysiology

The pathophysiologic changes in the various types of viral hepatitis are similar. Hepatitis involves widespread inflammation of liver tissue.

- During acute infection, liver damage is mediated by cytotoxic cytokines and natural killer cells that cause lysis of infected hepatocytes. Liver damage results in hepatic cell necrosis. Inflammation of the periportal areas may interrupt bile flow (cholestasis).
- Liver cells can regenerate in an orderly manner, and if no complications occur, they should resume their normal appearance and function.
- Antigen-antibody complexes between the virus and its corresponding antibody form a circulating immune complex in the early phases of hepatitis. These circulating complexes

Table 49   Characteristics of Hepatitis Viruses

Type of Virus	Incubation Period/Mode of Transmission	Sources of Infection/Spread of Disease	Infectivity
Hepatitis A virus (HAV)	15-50 days (average 28) Fecal-oral (primarily fecal contamination and oral ingestion)	Crowded conditions (e.g., day care); poor personal hygiene; poor sanitation; contaminated food, milk, water, and shellfish; persons with subclinical infections; infected food handlers; sexual contact; IV drug users	Most infectious during 2 wk before onset of symptoms; infectious until 1-2 wk after the start of symptoms
Hepatitis B virus (HBV)	45-180 days (average 56-96) Percutaneous (parenteral)/permucosal exposure to blood or blood products Sexual contact Perinatal transmission	Contaminated needles, syringes, and blood products; sexual activity with infected partners asymptomatic carriers Tattoo/body piercing with contaminated needles; bites	Before and after symptoms appear; infectious for 4-6 mo; in carriers continues for patient's lifetime

Continued

H

Table 49 Characteristics of Hepatitis Viruses—cont'd

Type of Virus	Incubation Period/Mode of Transmission	Sources of Infection/Spread of Disease	Infectivity
Hepatitis C virus (HCV)	14-180 days (average 56) Percutaneous (parenteral)/ mucosal exposure to blood or blood products High-risk sexual contact Perinatal contact	Blood and blood products, needles and syringes, sexual activity with infected partners	1-2 wk before symptoms appear; continues during clinical course; 75%-85% go on to develop chronic hepatitis
Hepatitis D virus (HDV)	2-26 wk; HBV must precede HDV; chronic carriers of HBV are always at risk Can cause infection only when HBV is present; routes of transmission same as for HBV	Same as HBV	Blood is infectious at all stages of HDV infection
Hepatitis E virus (HEV)	15-64 days (average 26-42 days) Fecal-oral Outbreaks associated with contaminated water supply in developing countries	Contaminated water; poor sanitation; found in Asia, Africa, and Mexico; not common in United States	Not known; may be similar to HAV

IV, Intravenous.

activate the complement system. Manifestations of this activation are rash, angioedema, arthritis, fever, and malaise.

Clinical Manifestations

A large number of patients with acute hepatitis have no symptoms. Manifestations of viral hepatitis may be classified into acute and chronic phases.

- The acute phase usually lasts 1 to 4 months. During the incubation period, symptoms may include malaise, anorexia, fatigue, nausea, occasional vomiting, and right upper quadrant abdominal discomfort. The anorexia can be severe, and other symptoms may include headache, low-grade fever, arthralgias, and skin rashes. Physical examination may reveal hepatomegaly, lymphadenopathy, and sometimes splenomegaly. This is the period of maximal infectivity for hepatitis A.

- The acute phase may be *icteric* (symptomatic, including jaundice) or anicteric. Jaundice results when bilirubin diffuses into the tissues. The urine may darken because of excess bilirubin being excreted by the kidneys. If conjugated bilirubin cannot flow out of the liver because of bile duct obstruction, stools will be light or clay colored. Pruritus, caused by bile salts beneath the skin, may result if cholestasis is present.

- When jaundice occurs, the fever usually subsides, but the gastrointestinal (GI) symptoms usually remain and fatigue may continue.

- The convalescence following the acute phase begins as jaundice is disappearing and lasts weeks to months, with an average of 2 to 4 months. During this period the patient's major complaints are malaise and easy fatigability. Hepatomegaly remains for several weeks. Relapses may occur, and the disappearance of jaundice does not mean the patient has totally recovered.

Additional considerations include:

- Many HBV infections and the majority of HCV infections result in chronic (lifelong) viral infection. Some patients may be asymptomatic, but others may have intermittent or ongoing malaise, fatigue, myalgias, arthralgias, and hepatomegaly.

- Not all patients with viral hepatitis have jaundice. This is referred to as *anicteric hepatitis*. A high percentage of persons with HAV are anicteric and do not have symptoms.

- There is slight variation in manifestations between the types of hepatitis. In hepatitis A the onset is more acute and the symptoms are usually mild and flulike. In hepatitis B the onset is more insidious and the symptoms are usually more severe. In hepatitis C the majority of cases are mild or asymptomatic, but HCV has a high rate of persistence.

Complications

Most patients with acute viral hepatitis recover completely with no complications. The overall mortality rate is less than 1%.

Complications include fulminant hepatic failure, chronic hepatitis, cirrhosis of the liver (see Cirrhosis, p. 138), and hepatocellular carcinoma (see Liver Cancer, p. 402).

- *Fulminant viral hepatitis* results in severe impairment or necrosis of liver cells and potential liver failure.
- Fulminant viral hepatitis develops in a small percentage of patients. The disorder may occur as a complication of hepatitis B or C, particularly hepatitis B accompanied by infection with hepatitis D virus (HDV). Toxic reactions to drugs and congenital metabolic disorders may also cause fulminant hepatitis and liver failure. Hepatocellular failure with death usually occurs unless liver transplant surgery is performed.

Diagnostic Studies

- Many of the liver function tests show significant abnormalities.
- Physical assessment may reveal hepatic tenderness, hepatomegaly, and splenomegaly.
- Liver biopsy allows for histologic examination of liver cells in chronic hepatitis.
- Table 50 presents the serologic tests for the different types of viral hepatitis.
- Newer techniques (sonograms [Fibroscan]) may provide information about the degree of liver fibrosis or scarring.

Collaborative Care

There is no specific treatment for acute viral hepatitis. Most patients can be managed at home. Emphasis is on measures to rest the body and assist the liver in regenerating. Adequate nutrients and rest seem to be most beneficial for healing and liver cell regeneration. The degree of rest ordered depends on symptom severity; usually alternating periods of activity with rest is adequate.

Table 50	Tests for Viral Hepatitis	

Virus	Tests	Significance
A	Anti-HAV IgM	Acute infection
	Anti-HAV IgG	Previous infection and long-term immunity or immunization
B	HBsAg (hepatitis B surface antigen)	Current infection (but not necessarily acute)*
		Positive in chronic carriers
	Anti-HBs (antibody to surface antigen)	Indicates previous infection with hepatitis B or immunization
		Marker of response to vaccine
	HBeAg (hepatitis B e antigen)	Indicates high infectivity; present in acute, active infection
	Anti-HBe (antibody to e antigen)	Indicates previous infection
	HBcAg (hepatitis B core antigen)	Ongoing infection with hepatitis B
	Anti-HBc IgM (antibody to hepatitis B core antigen)	Acute infection*
	Anti-HBc IgG	Indicates previous infection or ongoing infection with hepatitis B
		Does not appear after vaccination
	HBV DNA	Indicates active ongoing viral replication
		Best indicator of viral replication and effectiveness of therapy in patient with chronic hepatitis B
	HBV genotyping	Indicates the genotype of HBV virus

H

Continued

Table 50	Tests for Viral Hepatitis—cont'd	

Virus	Tests	Significance
C	Anti-HCV (antibody to hepatitis C)	Marker for acute or chronic infection with HCV
	Enzyme immunoassay (EIA)	Used in initial screening for HCV
	Recombinant immunoblot assay (RIBA)	More sensitive antibody test
	HCV RNA	Indicates active ongoing viral replication
	HCV genotyping	Indicates the genotype of HCV virus
D	Anti-HDV	Present in past or current infection with hepatitis D
	HDV Ag (hepatitis D antigen)	Present within a few days after infection

A, Hepatitis A virus (HAV); *B*, hepatitis B virus (HBV); *C*, hepatitis C virus (HCV); *D*, hepatitis D virus (HDV); *DNA*, deoxyribonucleic acid; *RNA*, ribonucleic acid.
*If positive HBsAg and anti-HBc IgM, it indicates the presence of acute infection.

Drug Therapy

There are no specific drug therapies for the treatment of acute viral hepatitis. Supportive drug therapy may include antiemetics, such as dimenhydrinate (Dramamine) or trimethobenzamide (Tigan).

Drug therapy for chronic HBV is focused on decreasing the viral load, serum levels of aspartate aminotransferase (AST) and alanine aminotransferase (ALT), the rate of disease progression, and the rate of drug-resistant HBV.

- α-Interferon interferes with viral replication and is available in long-acting preparations (Pegasys, PEG-Intron). The long-acting preparations are administered subcutaneously once per week and are preferred to conventional α-interferon that must be injected more frequently. One third of the patients receiving α-interferon will have a significant reduction of serum HBV DNA levels, normalization of ALT levels, and loss of HBV e antigen (HBeAg).
- Nucleoside and nucleotide analogs suppress HBV replication by inhibiting viral DNA synthesis. The drugs used in the treatment of chronic HBV when there is evidence of active viral replication include lamivudine (Epivir), adefovir

(Hepsera), entecavir (Baraclude), and telbivudine (Tyzeka). These drugs can reduce viral load and liver damage.

Drug therapy for hepatitis C is directed at eradicating the virus, reducing the viral load, and decreasing progression of the disease. Treatment for HCV includes a combination of ribavirin (Rebetol, Copegus) and long-acting α-interferon (PEG-Intron, Pegasys).

Prevention

Drug therapy is also used for prevention of HAV and HBV infection.

Both hepatitis A vaccine and immune globulin (IG) are used for prevention of hepatitis A. The vaccine is used for preexposure prophylaxis, and IG can be used either before or after exposure.

- IG provides temporary (1 to 2 months) passive immunity and is effective for preventing hepatitis A if given within 2 weeks after exposure.
- IG is recommended for persons who do not have anti-HAV antibodies and are exposed because of close contact with persons who have HAV.
- Although IG may not prevent infection in all persons, it may modify the illness to a subclinical infection.
- Twinrix, a combined HAV and HBV vaccine, is available for persons over the age of 18 years.
- Immunization with hepatitis B vaccine is the most effective method of preventing HBV infection.
- For postexposure prophylaxis, the vaccine and hepatitis B immune globulin (HBIG) are used. HBIG contains anti-bodies to HBV and confers temporary passive immunity. HBIG is recommended for postexposure prophylaxis in cases of needle stick, mucous membrane contact, or sexual exposure and for infants born to mothers who are positive for HBsAg.

Nutritional Therapy

An important measure in assisting hepatocytes to regenerate is adequate nutrition. No special diet is required. However, a diet high in carbohydrates and proteins with a low fat content is usually recommended.

Nursing Management

Goals

The patient with viral hepatitis will have relief of discomfort, be able to resume normal activities, and return to normal liver function without complications.

See NCP 44-1 for the patient with viral hepatitis, Lewis et al., *Medical-Surgical Nursing*, ed. 8, p. 1068.

Nursing Diagnoses
- Imbalanced nutrition: less than body requirements
- Activity intolerance
- Risk for impaired liver function
- Ineffective self-health management

Nursing Interventions
Viral hepatitis is a community health problem. Your role is important in the prevention and control of this disease.

Hepatitis A. Vaccination is the best protection against HAV. Preventive measures include personal and environmental hygiene and health education to promote good sanitation.

Hand washing is essential and is probably the most important precaution. Health teaching should include careful hand washing after bowel movements and before eating.

Hepatitis B. The HBV vaccine is the best means of protection. Control and prevention of hepatitis B focus on the identification of possible exposure through percutaneous and sexual transmission.

- Good hygienic practices, including hand washing and the use of gloves when expecting contact with blood, are important. A condom is advised for sexual intercourse, and the partner should be vaccinated. Razors, toothbrushes, and other personal items should not be shared. Close contacts of the patient with hepatitis B who are HBsAg negative and antibody negative should be vaccinated.

Hepatitis C. There currently is no vaccine available. Primary measures to prevent HCV transmission are similar to those of HBV, including the screening of blood, organ, and tissue donors; use of infection control measures; and modification of high-risk sexual behavior.

During acute intervention, assess for the degree of jaundice. Comfort measures to relieve pruritus (if present), headache, and arthralgias are helpful.

- Ensuring that the patient receives adequate nutrition is not always easy. Small, frequent meals may be preferable to three large ones and may also help prevent nausea. Consider measures to stimulate the appetite, such as mouth care, antiemetics, and attractively served meals in pleasant surroundings.
- Assess the patient's response to the rest and activity plan and modify accordingly. If the patient is on bed rest, initiate measures to prevent skin, respiratory, and circulatory complications.
- Psychologic and emotional rest is as essential as physical rest. Bed rest may produce anxiety and extreme restlessness

in some patients. Diversional activities, such as reading and hobbies, may help the patient.

▼ **Patient and Caregiver Teaching**

- Teach the patient and caregiver how to prevent transmission to other family members. The patient should know what symptoms need to be reported to the health care provider.

- Assess the patient for manifestations of complications. Bleeding tendencies with increasing prothrombin time values, symptoms of encephalopathy, or elevated liver function tests indicate problems.

- Stress the importance of regular follow-up visits for at least 1 year after the diagnosis of hepatitis. Because relapses are fairly common with hepatitis B and C, the patient should be instructed about the symptoms of recurrence. Alcohol should be avoided in patients with chronic hepatitis B and C.

- The patient who is receiving α-interferon for the treatment of hepatitis B or C requires education regarding this drug.

HERNIA

Description

A hernia is a protrusion of a viscus through an abnormal opening or a weakened area in the wall of the cavity in which it is normally contained. A hernia may occur in any part of the body, but it usually occurs within the abdominal cavity.

- Hernias that easily return to the abdominal cavity are called *reducible*. The hernia can be reduced manually or may reduce spontaneously when the person lies down.

- If the hernia cannot be placed back into the abdominal cavity, it is known as *irreducible* or *incarcerated*. In this situation intestinal flow may be obstructed. When the hernia is irreducible and intestinal flow and blood supply are obstructed, the hernia is *strangulated*. The result is an acute intestinal obstruction.

Types

Types of hernias include inguinal, femoral, umbilical, and ventral (incisional).

- *Inguinal hernia* is the most common type of hernia and occurs at the point of weakness in the abdominal wall where the spermatic cord in men and the round ligament in women emerge. When the protrusion escapes through the inguinal ring and follows the spermatic cord or round ligament, it is termed an indirect hernia. When it escapes through the posterior inguinal wall, it is a direct hernia. An inguinal hernia is more common in men.

- *Femoral hernia* occurs when there is a protrusion through the femoral ring into the femoral canal. It becomes strangulated easily and occurs more frequently in women.
- *Umbilical hernia* occurs when the rectus muscle is weak (as with obesity) or the umbilical opening fails to close after birth.
- *Ventral* or *incisional hernia* is caused by a weakness of the abdominal wall at the site of a previous incision. It occurs most commonly in patients who are obese, who have had multiple surgical procedures in the same area, or who have had inadequate wound healing because of poor nutrition or infection.

Clinical Manifestations

A hernia may be readily visible, especially when the person tenses the abdominal muscles. Discomfort may result from tension. If the hernia becomes strangulated, the patient will experience severe pain and symptoms of a bowel obstruction, such as vomiting, cramping abdominal pain, and distention.

Diagnosis is based on history and physical examination findings.

Collaborative Care

Surgery is the treatment of choice for hernias and prevents strangulation. Surgical repair of a hernia is known as a *herniorrhaphy*. Repairs are by laparoscopic surgery and are usually an outpatient procedure. The reinforcement of the weakened area with wire, fascia, or mesh is known as a *hernioplasty*. Strangulated hernias are treated immediately with resection of the involved area or a temporary colostomy so that necrosis and gangrene do not occur.

Nursing Management

Some patients with hernias may wear a truss, which is a pad placed over the hernia and held in place with a belt. The truss is worn to keep the hernia from protruding. If a patient wears a truss, check for skin irritation caused by continual rubbing of the truss.

After a hernia repair, the patient may have difficulty voiding. You should observe for a distended bladder.

- Scrotal edema is a painful complication after inguinal hernia repair. A scrotal support with application of an ice bag may help relieve pain and edema.

- Coughing is not encouraged, but deep breathing and turning should be done. If the patient needs to cough or sneeze, the incision should be splinted during coughing, and sneezing should be done with mouth open.
- After discharge the patient may be restricted from heavy lifting or physical activities for 6 to 8 weeks.

HERPES, GENITAL

Description
Two different strains of herpes simplex virus (HSV) cause infection.

- HSV type 1 (HSV-1) generally causes infection above the waist, involving the gingivae, dermis, upper respiratory tract, and central nervous system (CNS).
- HSV type 2 (HSV-2) most frequently involves the genital tract and perineum (i.e., locations below the waist).

However, either strain can cause disease on the mouth or genitals. When a person is infected with HSV, the virus usually persists within the individual for life. It is estimated that more than 45 million people have had a genital HSV infection. Many people infected with HSV are asymptomatic or unaware of their infection.

Pathophysiology
The HSV enters through the mucous membranes or breaks in the skin during contact with an infected person. HSV then reproduces inside the cell and spreads to surrounding cells. It next enters the peripheral or autonomic nerve endings and ascends to the sensory or autonomic nerve ganglion, where it often becomes dormant. Viral reactivation (recurrence) may occur when the virus travels down to the initial site of infection.

Clinical Manifestations
In the *primary (initial) episode* of genital herpes the patient initially may complain of burning, itching, or tingling at the site of inoculation. Multiple, small vesicular lesions may occur on the penis, scrotum, vulva, perineum, perianal region, vagina, or cervix, and contain large quantities of infectious viral particles. The lesions rupture and form shallow, moist ulcerations. Finally, crusting and epithelialization of the erosions occur.

- Primary infections tend to be associated with local inflammation and pain accompanied by systemic

H

manifestations of fever, headache, malaise, myalgia, and regional lymphadenopathy.

- Urination may be painful from urine touching active lesions. Urinary retention may occur as a result of HSV urethritis or cystitis. A purulent vaginal discharge may develop with HSV cervicitis.
- Primary lesions are generally present for 17 to 20 days, but new lesions sometimes continue to develop for 6 weeks.
- The lesions heal spontaneously unless secondary infection occurs.

Recurrent genital herpes occurs in about 50% to 80% of individuals during the year following the primary episode. Stress, fatigue, sunburn, general illness, immunosuppression, and menses are noted trigger factors.

- Many patients can predict a recurrence by noticing early prodromal symptoms of tingling, burning, and itching at the site where lesions will eventually appear. Symptoms of recurrent episodes are less severe, and the lesions usually heal within 8 to 12 days. With time the recurrent lesions will generally occur less frequently.
- Women with recurrent symptomatic genital herpes can shed the virus up to 1% of the time with no visible lesions present.
- Barrier forms of contraception, especially condoms, used during asymptomatic periods may decrease transmission of the virus. When lesions are present, the patient should avoid sexual activity altogether because even barrier protection is not satisfactory in eliminating disease transmission.

Complications

Although most infections are relatively benign, complications of genital herpes may involve the CNS, causing aseptic meningitis and lower motor neuron damage.

- Autoinoculation of the virus to extragenital sites such as the fingers and lips ("cold sores") may occur.
- Neuron damage may result in atonic bladder, impotence, and constipation.

Diagnostic Studies

- Diagnosis is usually based on the patient's symptoms and history.
- Isolation of the virus by tissue culture from active lesions confirms diagnosis. Viral cultures may result in a false-negative result. Therefore it is recommended that a serologic test for HSV-2 be done in addition to a viral culture.

- Type-specific immunoassays for HSV infection test for the presence of antibodies to HSV and determine the presence of a chronic HSV infection.

Collaborative Care

Encourage good genital hygiene and the wearing of loose-fitting cotton undergarments. The lesions should be kept clean and dry. To ensure complete drying of the perineal area, women may use a hair dryer set on a cool setting. Drying agents such as colloidal oatmeal (Aveeno) and aluminum salts (Burow's solution) may provide relief from the burning and itching.

- Frequent sitz baths may soothe the area and reduce inflammation. Pain may require a local anesthetic, such as lidocaine (Xylocaine), or systemic analgesics, such as codeine and aspirin.
- Barrier forms of contraception, especially condoms, used during asymptomatic periods, decrease the transmission of the disease. When lesions are present, the patient should avoid sexual activity altogether because even barrier protection is not satisfactory in eliminating disease transmission.

Drug Therapy

Three antiviral agents are available for the treatment of HSV: acyclovir (Zovirax), valacyclovir (Valtrex), and famciclovir (Famvir). These drugs inhibit herpetic viral replication and are prescribed for primary and recurrent infections. Although not a cure, these drugs shorten the duration of viral shedding and healing time of genital lesions and reduce outbreaks by 75%. Continued use of oral acyclovir for up to 5 years is safe and effective. Acyclovir ointment appears to have no clinical benefit in the treatment of recurrent lesions, either in speed of healing or in resolution of pain. Intravenous (IV) acyclovir is reserved for severe or life-threatening infections.

Nursing Management: Genital Herpes

See Sexually Transmitted Diseases, p. 569.

HIATAL HERNIA

Description

Hiatal hernia is herniation of a portion of the stomach into the esophagus through an opening (or hiatus) in the diaphragm. It is also referred to as diaphragmatic hernia or esophageal hernia. Hiatal hernias are common in older adults and occur more frequently in women than men. Hiatal hernias are classified into two types (Fig. 6).

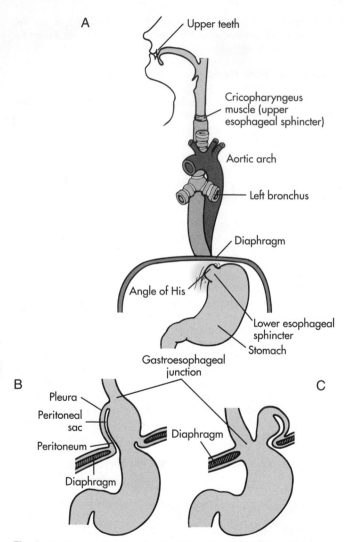

Fig. 6. A, Normal esophagus. **B,** Sliding hiatal hernia. **C,** Rolling or paraesophageal hernia.

- A *sliding hernia* is the most common type. It occurs at the junction of the stomach and esophagus located above the hiatus of the diaphragm. A part of the stomach "slides" through the hiatal opening in the diaphragm. This occurs when the patient is supine and usually goes back into the abdominal cavity when the patient is standing upright.
- A *paraesophageal* or *rolling hernia* occurs at the esophagogastric junction where the fundus and greater curvature of the stomach roll up through the diaphragm to form a pocket alongside the esophagus.

Pathophysiology

Many factors contribute to the development of hiatal hernia, including structural changes, such as weakening of the muscles in the diaphragm around the esophagogastric opening. Factors that increase intraabdominal pressure, including obesity, pregnancy, ascites, intense physical exertion, and heavy lifting on a continual basis may also contribute to the development of a hiatal hernia.

Clinical Manifestations

When present, signs and symptoms of hiatal hernia are similar to those described for gastroesophageal reflux disease (GERD).
- Heartburn, especially after a meal or after lying supine, is a common symptom. Bending over may cause a severe burning pain, which is usually relieved by sitting or standing. Large meals, alcohol, and smoking may precipitate pain.
- Nocturnal attacks are common, especially if the person has eaten before lying down.

Complications may include GERD, esophagitis, hemorrhage from erosion, stenosis, ulcerations of the herniated portion of the stomach, strangulation of the hernia, and regurgitation with tracheal aspiration.

Diagnostic Studies

- Barium swallow may show gastric mucosa protrusion through the esophageal hiatus.
- Upper gastrointestinal (GI) endoscopy with biopsy and cytologic analysis determines if lower esophageal sphincter (LES) is incompetent and gastric reflux is present.
- Esophageal motility (manometry) studies determine pressure gradients.

Nursing and Collaborative Management

Conservative therapy is similar to that described under GERD, including lifestyle modifications (elimination of constricting garments, avoidance of lifting and straining, elevating the head of the bed, and elimination of alcohol and smoking), reducing body weight if overweight, and the administration of antacids and antisecretory agents (see Gastroesophageal Reflux Disease, p. 244).

Surgical approaches include reduction of the herniated stomach into the abdomen, *herniotomy* (excision of the hernia sac), *herniorrhaphy* (closure of the hiatal defect), an antireflux procedure, and *gastropexy* (attachment of the stomach subdiaphragmatically to prevent reherniation).

- Laparoscopically performed Nissen and Toupet fundoplication techniques are the standard antireflux surgeries for hiatal hernia.

HODGKIN'S LYMPHOMA

Description

Hodgkin's lymphoma, also called Hodgkin's disease, is a malignant condition characterized by proliferation of abnormal, giant, multinucleated cells called *Reed-Sternberg cells,* which are located in lymph nodes. The disease makes up 11% of all lymphomas and has a bimodal age-specific incidence, occurring most frequently in persons from 15 to 35 years old and above 50 years old. In adults it is twice as prevalent in men as in women, and its prevalence is increased among patients with human immunodeficiency virus infection.

Pathophysiology

Although the cause of Hodgkin's lymphoma remains unknown, several key factors are thought to play a role in its development. The main interacting factors include infection with the Epstein-Barr virus, genetic predisposition, and exposure to occupational toxins.

In Hodgkin's lymphoma the normal structure of the lymph nodes is destroyed by hyperplasia of monocytes and macrophages. The disease is believed to arise in a single location (it originates in the lymph nodes in 90% of patients) and then spread along adjacent lymphatics. It eventually infiltrates other organs, especially the lungs, spleen, and liver. In about two thirds of patients the cervical lymph nodes are the first to be affected.

Clinical Manifestations

The initial sign is most often an enlargement of the cervical, axillary, or inguinal lymph nodes. The enlarged nodes are not painful unless pressure is exerted on adjacent nerves.

- The patient may note weight loss, fatigue, weakness, fever, chills, tachycardia, or night sweats. A group of initial findings, including fever, night sweats, and weight loss (referred to as *B symptoms*), correlates with a worse prognosis.
- Generalized pruritus without skin lesions may develop. Cough, dyspnea, stridor, and dysphagia may all reflect mediastinal node involvement.
- In more advanced disease there may be hepatomegaly and splenomegaly. Anemia results from increased destruction as well as decreased production of erythrocytes. Intrathoracic involvement may lead to superior vena cava syndrome. Enlarged retroperitoneal nodes may cause palpable abdominal masses or interfere with renal function
- Jaundice may result from liver involvement.
- Spinal cord compression leading to paraplegia may occur with extradural involvement

Diagnostic Studies

- Peripheral blood analysis often reveals microcytic hypochromic anemia; neutrophilic leukocytosis (15,000 to 28,000/μL [15 to 28×10^9/L]), which may be associated with lymphopenia; and an increased platelet count
- Other blood studies may show hypoferremia caused by excessive iron uptake by the liver and spleen, elevated alkaline phosphatase from liver and bone involvement, hypercalcemia from bone involvement, and hypoalbuminemia from liver involvement.
- Computed tomography (CT) or magnetic resonance imaging (MRI) scans are used as clinical staging tools. Positron emission tomography (PET) scans may show increased uptake of carbohydrate by cancer cells, and concurrent CT scans may identify masses such as mediastinal lymphadenopathy, renal displacement caused by retroperitoneal node enlargement, abdominal lymph node enlargement, and liver, spleen, bone, and brain infiltration.

Collaborative Care

Treatment decisions are made based on the clinical stage of the disease. The standard for chemotherapy is the ABVD regimen: doxorubicin (Adriamycin), bleomycin, vinblastine, and dacarbazine given for two to eight cycles of treatment depending on disease stage and prognosis. The role of radiation as a supplement to chemotherapy varies depending on site of disease and the presence of resistant disease after chemotherapy.

Intensive chemotherapy with or without the use of autologous or allogeneic hematopoietic stem cell transplantation (HSCT) and hematopoietic growth factors is the treatment of choice for advanced, refractory, or relapsed Hodgkin's lymphoma.

Nursing Management

Nursing care for Hodgkin's lymphoma is largely based on managing problems related to the disease, such as pain, and side effects of therapy, such as pancytopenia.

- Because the survival of patients with Hodgkin's lymphoma depends on their response to treatment, supporting the patient through the consequences of treatment is extremely important.
- Psychosocial considerations are just as important as they are with leukemia (see Leukemia, p. 396). Although the prognosis for Hodgkin's lymphoma is better than that for many forms of cancer or leukemia, patients must still be helped to deal with the physical, psychologic, social, and spiritual consequences of their disease.
- Evaluation of patients for long-term effects of therapy is important because delayed consequences of the disease and treatment, such as secondary malignancies and long-term endocrine, cardiac, and pulmonary toxicities, may not be apparent for many years.

HUMAN IMMUNODEFICIENCY VIRUS INFECTION

Description

Over one million people are living with HIV in the United States, with an estimated 56,000 new infections each year. In North America the epidemic is growing at faster rates among women, people of color, people who live in poverty, and adolescents. In addition, treatment has provided major advances in the ability to keep HIV-infected people healthy for longer periods of time, and the death rate has fallen dramatically.

Pathophysiology

HIV is a ribonucleic acid (RNA) virus. Like all viruses, HIV cannot replicate unless it is in a living cell. HIV infects human cells that have CD4+ receptors on their surfaces. These include lymphocytes, monocytes/macrophages, astrocytes, and oligodendrocytes. Immune dysfunction in HIV disease is caused predominantly by destruction of CD4+ T cells (also known as T-helper cells or CD4+ lymphocytes). The major concern related to immune suppression is the development of opportunistic diseases (infections and cancers that occur in immunosuppressed patients that can lead to disability, disease, and death).

HIV is a fragile virus. It can be transmitted under specific conditions that allow contact with infected blood, semen, vaginal secretions, and breast milk. An HIV-infected individual can transmit HIV to others within a few days of becoming infected. The ability to transmit HIV is lifelong.

Clinical Manifestations

The typical course of untreated HIV infection follows the pattern shown in Fig. 7. It is important to remember that disease progression is highly individualized and that treatment can significantly alter the pattern.

Acute infection. During acute HIV infection, HIV-specific antibodies are produced (seroconversion) and a mononucleosis-like syndrome of fever, lymphadenopathy, pharyngitis, headache, malaise, nausea, and/or a diffuse rash may occur.

- Symptoms generally occur 2 to 4 weeks after initial infection and last for 1 to 2 weeks.
- During this time a high viral load is noted and CD4+ T-cell counts fall temporarily but quickly return to baseline. In

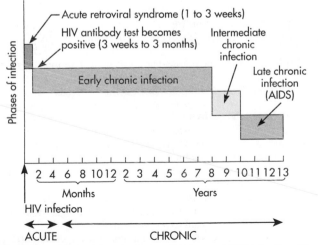

Fig. 7. Timeline for the spectrum of untreated HIV infection. The timeline represents the course of untreated illness from the time of infection to clinical manifestations of disease.

most people these symptoms are mild and are mistaken for a bad case of the flu.

Early chronic infection. The median interval between untreated HIV infection and a diagnosis of AIDS is about 11 years. During this time CD4$^+$ lymphocyte counts remain above 500 cells/μL (normal or slightly decreased) and the viral load in the blood is low. This phase has been referred to as asymptomatic disease, but fatigue, headache, low-grade fever, night sweats, persistent generalized lymphadenopathy (PGL), and other symptoms often occur.

Intermediate chronic infection. When the CD4$^+$ T-cell count drops below 200 to 500 cells/μL and the viral load increases, HIV advances to a more active stage.

- Symptoms include persistent fever, frequent drenching night sweats, chronic diarrhea, headaches, and fatigue. Other problems that may occur include localized infections, lymphadenopathy, and nervous system manifestations.

Late chronic infection. A diagnosis of acquired immunodeficiency syndrome (AIDS) cannot be made until the HIV-infected patient meets the criteria established by the Centers for Disease Control and Prevention (CDC), which include the development of at least one of these conditions:

1. CD4$^+$ lymphocyte count <200/μL
2. Development of an opportunistic infection (see Tables 15-9 and 15-10, Lewis et al., *Medical-Surgical Nursing,* ed. 8, p. 245)
3. Development of an opportunistic cancer (e.g., Kaposi sarcoma)
4. Wasting syndrome (defined as a loss of 10% or more of ideal body mass)
5. Development of AIDS dementia complex (ADC)

Diagnostic Studies

The most useful screening tests are those that detect HIV-specific antibodies. A major problem is that there is a median delay of 2 months after infection before antibodies can be detected. This creates a period during which an infected individual may not test positive for HIV antibody.

Diagnosis of HIV infection

- Highly sensitive enzyme immunoassay (EIA) detects serum antibodies that bind to HIV antigens.
- Western blot (WB) or immunofluorescence assay (IFA) more specifically confirms HIV if a repeat EIA indicates the blood is HIV antibody positive.

- Rapid HIV-antibody testing provides highly accurate screening results within 20 minutes. Positive results are then confirmed by WB or IFA.

Progression of HIV infection

- $CD4^+$ T-cell count and viral load monitor the progression of the infection.
- White blood cell (WBC) count, red blood cell (RBC) count, and platelets decrease with progression of HIV.

Collaborative Care

Treatment focuses on (1) monitoring the disease progression and immune function; (2) initiating and monitoring antiretroviral therapy (ART); (3) preventing, detecting, and treating opportunistic diseases; (4) managing symptoms; (5) preventing or decreasing the complications of treatment; and (6) preventing further transmission of HIV.

Drug Therapy

The goals of drug therapy in HIV infection are to decrease the viral load, maintain or raise $CD4^+$ T-cell counts, and delay the development of HIV-related symptoms and opportunistic diseases.

The most effective means to suppress HIV replication is using at least three effective antiretroviral drugs from at least two different drug classes in optimum schedules and at full dosages (Table 51). Indications for initiation of ART in the chronically infected patient are described in Table 15-12, Lewis et al., *Medical-Surgical Nursing,* ed 8, p. 247.

- Combination ART limits the potential for resistance, which is the major factor limiting treatment effect.
- Many antiretroviral agents cause dangerous and potentially lethal interactions when used in combination with other commonly used drugs, including over-the-counter drugs and herbal therapies.

Opportunistic diseases associated with HIV can be delayed or prevented through prophylactic interventions, including (1) pneumococcal, influenza, and hepatitis B vaccines; (2) trimethoprim-sulfamethoxazole (TMP-SMX) inhalation for *Pneumocystis jiroveci* and toxoplasma; and (3) rifabutin (Mycobutin) for *Mycobacterium avium* complex. See Table 15-10, Lewis et al., *Medical-Surgical Nursing,* ed. 8, p. 245 for a complete description.

Nursing Management

Goals

The patient with HIV infection will adhere to drug regimens; promote a healthy lifestyle that includes avoiding exposure to additional sexual and blood-borne diseases; protect others from HIV;

Table 51	Antiretroviral Agents Used to Treat HIV
Mechanism of Action	**Examples of Drugs**
Nucleoside Reverse Transcriptase Inhibitors (NRTIs)	
Insert a piece of DNA into developing HIV DNA chain, blocking further development of the chain	zidovudine (AZT, ZDV, Retrovir) lamivudine (3TC, Epivir) abacavir (Ziagen)
Nonnucleoside Reverse Transcriptase Inhibitors (NNRTIs)	
Inhibit the action of reverse transcriptase	nevirapine (Viramune) delavirdine (Rescriptor) efavirenz (Sustiva)
Nucleotide Reverse Transcriptase Inhibitors (NtRTIs)	
Combine with reverse transcriptase to block the process needed to convert HIV RNA to DNA	tenofovir DF (Viread) Truvada (tenofir and emtricitabine combination)
Protease Inhibitors (PIs)	
Prevents protease enzyme from cutting HIV proteins into the proper lengths needed to allow viable virions to assemble and bud out from the cell membrane	saquinavir (Fortovase, Invirase) indinavir (Crixivan) ritonavir (Norvir) nelfinavir (Viracept) Kaletra (lopinavir and ritonavir combination)
Integrase Inhibitors	
Binds with the integrase enzyme and prevents HIV from incorporating its genetic material into the host cell	raltegravir (Isentress)
Entry Inhibitors	
Prevent binding of HIV to cells, thus preventing replication of HIV in these cells	enfuvirtide (Fuzeon) maraviroc (Selzentry)

maintain or develop healthy and supportive relationships; maintain activities and productivity; explore spiritual issues; come to terms with issues related to disease, disability, and death; and cope with the frequent symptoms caused by HIV and its treatments. Goals are individualized and change as new treatment protocols develop and/or as HIV disease progresses.

Nursing Diagnoses
- Acute pain
- Anxiety
- Fear
- Imbalanced nutrition: less than body requirements
- Disturbed body image
- Ineffective coping
- Diarrhea

Nursing Interventions

HIV infection is preventable. Avoiding and/or modifying risky behaviors are the most effective prevention tools. All patients should be provided with education and behavior change counseling specific to the patient's need, culturally sensitive, language appropriate, and age specific.

- Any individual who is at risk for HIV should be encouraged to be tested. HIV testing should be accompanied by pretest and posttest counseling.
- Early intervention after detection of HIV infection can promote health and limit disability. It should focus on early detection of symptoms, opportunistic diseases, and psychosocial problems.

Useful interventions for HIV-infected patients include nutritional support; moderation or elimination of alcohol, tobacco, and drug use; keeping recommended vaccines up to date; adequate rest, exercise, and stress reduction; avoiding exposure to new infectious agents; mental health counseling; and getting involved in support groups and community activities.

- Teach patients to recognize symptoms that may indicate disease progression and/or drug side effects so that prompt medical care can be initiated.
- During acute exacerbations of opportunistic diseases or adverse effects of treatment, symptomatic care may include education and treatment for diarrhea, pneumonia, fatigue, wasting syndrome, and AIDS-dementia complex.
- The focus of terminal care is patient comfort, facilitation of emotional and spiritual issues, and helping significant others deal with grief and loss.

▼ Patient and Caregiver Teaching

HIV education emphasizes prevention and risk-reducing activities. Teaching that outlines the proper use of male and female condoms and the proper use of drug-using equipment promotes risk reduction. For an infected patient, teaching is directed toward health promotion, managing the problems caused by HIV infection, and maximizing the patient's quality of life.

- Teach advantages and disadvantages of new treatments, including drug therapy, dangers of nonadherence to therapeutic regimens, how and when to take each medication, drug interactions to avoid, and side effects that need to be reported to the primary care provider. Tables 15-17, 15-18 and 15-19, Lewis et al., *Medical-Surgical Nursing*, ed. 8, pp. 253 and 254 provide guidance for patient teaching in these areas.

- Teach energy conservation measures and the use of assistive devices to increase safety and decrease fatigue.
- Discuss infection control measures with the patient, caregiver, family, and visitors.
- Provide information about support groups and community resources.

HUNTINGTON'S DISEASE

Huntington's disease (HD) is a genetically transmitted, autosomal dominant disorder that affects both men and women of all races. Offspring of a person with this disease have a 50% risk of inheriting it. The onset of HD is usually between 30 and 50 years of age. About 30,000 Americans are symptomatic, and 150,000 are at risk.

Like Parkinson's disease, the pathologic process of HD involves the basal ganglia and the extrapyramidal motor system. However, instead of a deficiency of DA, HD involves a deficiency of the neurotransmitters ACh and γ-aminobutyric acid (GABA). The net effect is an excess of DA, which leads to symptoms that are the opposite of those of parkinsonism.

Clinical manifestations are characterized by abnormal and excessive involuntary movements (chorea). These are writhing, twisting movements of the face, limbs, and body that get worse as the disease progresses.

- Facial movements involving speech, chewing, and swallowing are affected; this may cause aspiration and malnutrition. The gait deteriorates, and ambulation eventually becomes impossible.
- Cognitive deterioration involves perception, memory, attention, and learning. A combination of the motor and cognitive disorders eventually results in complete loss of speech capacity.
- Depression is very common. Other psychiatric symptoms include irritability, anxiety, agitation, impulsivity, apathy, social withdrawal, and obsessiveness.

- Death usually occurs 10 to 20 years after the onset of symptoms.

Diagnosis in the past was based on family history and clinical symptoms. However, since the gene for HD has been discovered, one can now be tested for the presence of the gene.

Because there is no cure, collaborative care is palliative. The first drug approved specifically for HD is tetrabenazine (Xenazine). It is used to treat the chorea, and works to decrease the amount of dopamine available at synapses in the brain and thus decreases the involuntary movements of chorea.

- Other medications may include neuroleptics such as haloperidol [Haldol]) and risperidone (Risperdal), benzodiazepines such as diazepam (Valium) and clonazepam (Klonopin), and dopamine depleting agents such as reserpine and tetrabenazine.
- Cognitive disorders are treated with nondrug therapies (e.g., counseling, memory books). The psychiatric disorders can be treated with selective serotonin uptake inhibitors such as sertraline (Zoloft) and paroxetine (Paxil). Antipsychotic medication may also be needed, such as haloperidol (Haldol) or risperidone (Risperdal).

The goal of nursing management is to provide the most comfortable environment possible for the patient and caregiver by maintaining physical safety, treating physical symptoms, and providing emotional and psychologic support.

- Because of the choreic movements, caloric requirements are high. Patients may require as many as 4000 to 5000 kcal/day to maintain body weight. As the disease progresses, meeting caloric needs becomes a greater challenge when the patient has difficulty swallowing and holding the head still. Depression and mental deterioration can also compromise nutritional intake.
- End-of-life issues need to be discussed with the patient and caregiver. These include care in the home or long-term care facility, artificial methods of feeding, advance directives and CPR, use of antibiotics to treat infections, and guardianship.

H

HYPERPARATHYROIDISM

Description

Hyperparathyroidism is a condition involving increased secretion of parathyroid hormone (PTH). PTH helps regulate calcium and phosphate levels by stimulating bone resorption, renal tubular reabsorption of calcium, and activation of vitamin D. Thus over-secretion of PTH is associated with increased serum calcium levels.

Hyperparathyroidism is classified as primary, secondary, or tertiary.

- *Primary hyperparathyroidism* is caused by an increased secretion of PTH leading to disorders of calcium, phosphate, and bone metabolism. The most common cause is a benign adenoma in the parathyroid gland. Previous head and neck radiation may be a predisposing factor for a parathyroid adenoma.

- *Secondary hyperparathyroidism* is a compensatory response to conditions that induce or cause hypocalcemia, the main stimulus of PTH secretion. These conditions include vitamin D deficiencies, malabsorption, chronic kidney disease, and hyperphosphatemia.

- *Tertiary hyperparathyroidism* occurs when there is hyperplasia of the parathyroid glands and a loss of negative feedback from circulating calcium levels. This causes autonomous secretion of PTH even with normal calcium levels. It is observed in the patient who has had a kidney transplant after a long period of dialysis treatment for chronic kidney disease.

Pathophysiology

Excessive levels of circulating PTH usually lead to hypercalcemia and hypophosphatemia, creating a multisystem effect (see Table 50-12, et al., *Medical-Surgical Nursing,* ed. 8, p. 1274).

- In the bones, decreased bone density, cyst formation, and general weakness can occur as a result of the effect of PTH on osteoclastic (bone resorption) and osteoblastic (bone formation) activity.

- In the kidneys, excess calcium cannot be reabsorbed, which leads to hypercalciuria. This urinary calcium, along with a large amount of urinary phosphate, can lead to calculi formation. In addition, PTH stimulates the synthesis of a form of vitamin D, which increases gastrointestinal (GI) absorption of calcium and leads to high serum calcium levels.

Clinical Manifestations

Hyperparathyroidism has varying symptoms, including weakness, loss of appetite, emotional disorders, constipation, increased need for sleep, and shortened attention span.

- Major signs include loss of calcium from the bones (osteoporosis), fractures, and kidney stones (nephrolithiasis). Neuromuscular abnormalities are characterized by muscle weakness, particularly in proximal muscles of the lower extremities.

Complications include renal failure; pancreatitis; cardiac changes; and long bone, rib, and vertebral fractures.

Diagnostic Studies

- PTH levels are elevated.
- Serum calcium levels are elevated with decreased phosphorous levels.
- Urine calcium, serum chloride, serum uric acid, and serum creatinine are elevated.
- Serum amylase (if pancreatitis present) and alkaline phosphatase (if bone disease present) are both elevated.
- Bone density tests are used to detect bone loss.
- Magnetic resonance imaging (MRI), computed tomography (CT) scan, and ultrasound can be used to localize adenoma.

Collaborative Care

Treatment objectives are to relieve the symptoms and prevent complications caused by excess PTH. The choice of therapy depends on the urgency of the clinical situation, the degree of hypercalcemia, and the underlying cause of the disorder.

- The most effective treatment of primary and secondary hyperparathyroidism is partial or complete surgical removal of the parathyroid glands. The procedure most commonly used involves the use of an endoscope on an outpatient basis. Autotransplantation of normal parathyroid tissue in the forearm or near the sternocleidomastoid muscle is usually done, allowing PTH secretion to continue with normalization of calcium levels.
- If the patient does not meet surgical criteria or if the patient is elderly or at increased surgical risk from other health problems, a conservative management approach is used. This includes an annual examination with tests for serum PTH, calcium, phosphorous, and alkaline phosphatase levels and renal function; x-rays to assess for metabolic bone disease; and measurement of urinary calcium excretion.

Additional measures include maintenance of a high fluid intake, a moderate calcium intake, and phosphorous supplementation, unless contraindicated by an increased risk for urinary calculi formation.

- Bisphosphonates (e.g., alendronate [Fosamax]) inhibit osteoclastic bone resorption and rapidly normalize serum calcium levels. Oral phosphate may be used to inhibit the calcium-absorbing effects of vitamin D in the intestine.

H

- Calcimimetic agents (e.g., cinacalcet [Sensipar]) are a class of drugs that increase the sensitivity of the calcium receptor on the parathyroid gland, resulting in decreased PTH secretions and calcium blood levels, thus sparing calcium stores in the bone.
- Diuretics may be given to increase urinary excretion of calcium.

Nursing Management

Nursing care after surgery is similar to that for the patient after thyroidectomy (see Hyperthyroidism, p. 339). The major postoperative complications are hemorrhage and fluid and electrolyte disturbances. Tetany is usually apparent early in the postoperative period but may develop over several days. Mild tetany, characterized by an unpleasant tingling of the hands and around the mouth, may be present but should resolve without problems. Intravenous calcium should be readily available for use if tetany becomes more severe (e.g., muscular spasms or laryngospasms develop).

- Monitor intake and output to evaluate fluid status.
- Assess calcium, potassium, phosphate, and magnesium levels frequently.
- Encourage mobility to promote bone calcification.
- If surgery is not performed, treatment to relieve symptoms and prevent complications is initiated.

▼ **Patient and Caregiver Teaching**
- Assist the patient with hyperparathyroidism to adapt the meal plan to his or her lifestyle. A referral to a dietitian may be useful.
- Because immobility can aggravate bone loss, stress the importance of an exercise program.
- Encourage the patient to keep annual appointments. Instruct the patient regarding the symptoms of hypocalcemia or hypercalcemia and to report them when they occur.

HYPERTENSION

Description

One in three adults in the United States has hypertension or high BP. An additional 28% are at high risk of developing hypertension. The overall risk for hypertension increases with age. An elevated systolic BP (SBP) is a more important risk factor for developing hypertension than an elevated diastolic BP (DBP) in individuals older than age 50.

Table 52	Classification of Hypertension	
Category	**SBP (mm Hg)**	**DBP (mm Hg)**
Normal	<120 and	<80
Prehypertension	120-139 or	80-89
Hypertension, Stage 1	140-159 or	90-99
Hypertension, Stage 2	≥160 or	≥100

From the National Institutes of Health: *Seventh Report of the Joint National Committee on Prevention, Detection, Evaluation, and Treatment of High Blood Pressure*, Washington, DC, 2003, U.S. Department of Health and Human Services.
DBP, Diastolic blood pressure; *SBP*, systolic blood pressure.

- There is a direct relationship between hypertension and cardiovascular disease (CVD), and a proportional increase in the risk of myocardial infarction (MI), heart failure, stroke, and renal disease with higher BP.
- Most people with hypertension are aware that they have high BP and nearly two thirds of these individuals control their BP with treatment. People who remain undiagnosed and untreated for hypertension present the greatest challenge and opportunity for health care providers.

Hypertension is defined as a persistent SBP ≥ 140 mm Hg, DBP ≥ 90 mm Hg, or current use of antihypertensive medication. *Prehypertension* is defined as SBP 120 to 139 mm Hg or DBP 80 to 89 mm Hg. Classification of hypertension for adults according to stages is described in Table 52.

- Two subtypes of hypertension include *isolated systolic hypertension (ISH)* and *pseudohypertension.* ISH is an average SBP ≥ 140 mm Hg coupled with an average DBP < 90 mm Hg and is associated with loss of elasticity in larger arteries from atherosclerosis in older adults. Pseudohypertension, or false hypertension, can occur with advanced atherosclerosis. This results in much higher cuff pressures than are actually present within the vessels. The only way to accurately measure BP in pseudohypertension is with an intraarterial catheter.

The etiology of hypertension can be classified as primary (essential or idiopathic) or secondary. *Primary hypertension* accounts for up to 90% of all cases of hypertension. Although the exact cause of primary hypertension is unknown, several contributing factors, including greater than ideal body weight, diabetes mellitus (DM), increased sympathetic nervous system (SNS) activity, increased sodium intake, and excessive alcohol intake have been identified.

H

Secondary hypertension is elevated BP with a specific cause that often can be identified and corrected. This type of hypertension accounts for 5% to 10% of hypertension in adults. Causes of secondary hypertension include coarctation or congenital narrowing of the aorta, renal artery stenosis, endocrine disorders such as Cushing syndrome, cirrhosis, neurologic disorders such as brain tumors and head injury, sleep apnea, and pregnancy-induced hypertension. Treatment of secondary hypertension is directed at eliminating the underlying cause.

Pathophysiology of Primary Hypertension

The hemodynamic hallmark of hypertension is persistently increased systemic vascular resistance (SVR). Table 53 presents factors that relate to the development of primary hypertension or contribute to its consequences.

Clinical Manifestations

Hypertension is often called the "silent killer" because it is frequently asymptomatic until it becomes severe and target organ disease has occurred. A patient with severe hypertension may

Table 53	Risk Factors for Primary Hypertension
Risk Factor	**Description**
Age	SBP rises progressively with increasing age.
	After age 50, SBP >140 mm Hg is a more important cardiovascular risk factor than DBP.
Alcohol	Excessive alcohol intake is strongly associated with hypertension.
	Patients with hypertension should limit their daily intake to 1 oz of alcohol.
Cigarette smoking	Smoking greatly ↑ risk of cardiovascular disease.
	People with hypertension who smoke are at even greater risk for cardiovascular disease.
Diabetes mellitus	Hypertension is more common in diabetics.
	When hypertension and diabetes coexist, complications (e.g., target organ disease) are more severe.

Table 53	Risk Factors for Primary Hypertension—cont'd
Risk Factor	**Description**
Elevated serum lipids	↑ Levels of cholesterol and triglycerides are primary risk factors in atherosclerosis. Hyperlipidemia is more common in people with hypertension.
Excess dietary sodium	High sodium intake can contribute to hypertension in some patients, and decrease the effectiveness of certain antihypertensive medications.
Gender	Hypertension is more prevalent in men in young adulthood and early middle age (<55 yr of age). After age 55, hypertension is more prevalent in women.
Family history	History of a close blood relative (e.g., parents, sibling) with hypertension is associated with an ↑ risk for developing hypertension.
Obesity	Weight gain is associated with increased frequency of hypertension. The risk is greatest with central abdominal obesity.
Ethnicity	Incidence of hypertension is 2x high in African Americans as in whites.
Sedentary lifestyle	Regular physical activity can help control weight and reduce cardiovascular risk. Physical activity may ↓ BP.
Socioeconomic status	Hypertension is more prevalent in lower socioeconomic groups and among the less educated.
Stress	People exposed to repeated stress may develop hypertension more frequently than others. People who develop hypertension may respond differently to stress than those who do not develop hypertension.

H

DBP, Diastolic blood pressure; *SBP*, systolic blood pressure.

experience a variety of symptoms secondary to effects on blood vessels in the various organs and tissues or to the increased workload of the heart. These secondary symptoms include fatigue, reduced activity tolerance, dizziness, palpitations, angina, and dyspnea.

The most common complications of hypertension are target organ diseases, including the heart (hypertensive heart disease), brain (cerebrovascular disease), peripheral vasculature (peripheral vascular disease), kidney (nephrosclerosis), and eyes (retinal damage).

Hypertensive heart disease. Hypertension is a major risk factor for coronary artery disease (CAD). The mechanisms by which hypertension contributes to the development of atherosclerosis are not fully known. Injury to the coronary artery endothelium causes arteriolar changes that result in the high incidence of CAD. Sustained high BP also increases the cardiac workload and produces left ventricular hypertrophy (LVH). Progressive LVH, especially in association with CAD, is associated with the development of heart failure.

Heart failure occurs when the heart's compensatory adaptations are overwhelmed and the heart can no longer pump enough blood to meet the metabolic needs of the body.

- The patient may complain of shortness of breath on exertion, paroxysmal nocturnal dyspnea, and fatigue. Signs of an enlarged heart may be present on x-ray, and an electrocardiogram (ECG) may show electrical changes indicative of LVH.

Cerebrovascular disease. Hypertension is a major risk factor for stroke and cerebral atherosclerosis. Atherosclerotic plaques are commonly distributed at the bifurcation of the common carotid artery. Portions of the atherosclerotic plaque, or the blood clot that forms on the plaque, may break off and travel to intracerebral vessels, producing a thromboembolism. The patient may experience transient ischemic attacks or a stroke.

Peripheral vascular disease. Hypertension speeds up the process of atherosclerosis in peripheral blood vessels, leading to the development of aortic aneurysm, aortic dissection, and peripheral vascular disease. *Intermittent claudication* (ischemic muscle pain precipitated by activity and relieved with rest) is a classic symptom of peripheral arterial disease involving the arteries in the legs.

Nephrosclerosis. Hypertension is one of the leading risk factors for end-stage renal disease, especially among African Americans. Some degree of renal dysfunction is usually present in the hypertensive patient, even one with a minimally elevated BP. This disorder is the result of ischemia caused by the narrowed lumen of intrarenal blood vessels. Gradual narrowing of arteries and arterioles leads to the destruction of glomeruli, atrophy of tubules, and eventual death of nephrons. These changes may eventually lead to renal failure. The earliest symptom of renal dysfunction is usually nocturia.

Retinal damage. The appearance of the retina provides important information about the severity and duration of the hypertensive process. The blood vessels of the retina can be directly visualized with an ophthalmoscope. Damage to the retinal vessels provides an indication of concurrent vessel damage in the heart, brain, and kidneys. Manifestations of severe retinal damage include blurring of vision, retinal hemorrhage, and loss of vision.

Diagnostic Studies
Initially take the BP at least twice in each arm, at least 1 minute apart. Record the average pressure as the value for that visit. Document any differences between arms and use the arm with the higher reading for all future BP measurements.

Basic laboratory studies are performed to evaluate target organ disease, determine overall cardiovascular risk, or establish baseline levels before initiating therapy.

- Routine urinalysis, blood urea nitrogen (BUN), and serum creatinine levels to screen for renal involvement.
- Serum electrolytes, especially potassium (K^+) levels, to detect hyperaldosteronism.
- Blood glucose level to assess for diabetes mellitus.
- Lipid profile to assess for atherosclerosis risk factors.
- ECG for baseline cardiac status.

Collaborative Care
Treatment goals include achieving and maintaining goal BP, and reducing cardiovascular risk and target organ disease. Lifestyle modifications are indicated for all patients with prehypertension and hypertension. These modification measures include weight reduction, Dietary Approaches to Stop Hypertension (DASH) eating plan, dietary sodium reduction, regular aerobic physical activity, moderation of alcohol consumption, management of psychosocial risk factors, and avoidance of tobacco use.

- Dietary therapy consists of restricting sodium intake to less than 2.3 g/day and following the DASH eating plan, which is rich in vegetables, fruit, and nonfat dairy products. (See Table 33-7, Lewis et al., *Medical-Surgical Nursing,* ed. 8, p. 745 for a description of the DASH diet.) Men should limit their intake of alcohol to no more than two drinks per day and women and lighter men to no more than one drink per day.

- Adults should perform moderate-intensity aerobic physical activity for at least 30 minutes most days of the week or vigorous-intensity aerobic activity for at least 20 minutes three days a week. The 30-minute goal can be accomplished by performing shorter periods of exercise that last at least 10 minutes or more. Muscle-strengthening activities should also be performed using the major muscles of the body at least twice a week. Flexibility and balance exercises are recommended at least twice a week for older adults, especially for those at risk for falls. Individuals with CVD or other serious health problems need a thorough examination and possibly a stress test before beginning an exercise program.
- Psychosocial risk factors (e.g., depression, social isolation, low socioeconomic status) can contribute to the risk of developing CVD, and to a poorer prognosis and clinical course in patients with CVD. Screening for these factors is important. Make appropriate referrals (e.g., counseling) when indicated.
- Nicotine contained in tobacco causes vasoconstriction and increases BP in hypertensive people. Strongly encourage everyone, especially a hypertensive patient, to avoid tobacco use.

Drug Therapy

The goal for treating primary hypertension is a BP of <140/90 mm Hg. A lower goal of <130/80 mm Hg is recommended for patients at high risk of CAD (e.g., patients with diabetes mellitus and chronic kidney disease) as well as for patients with pre-existing CAD (e.g., stable angina, heart failure, MI). The drugs currently available for treating hypertension have two main actions: reducing SVR and decreasing the volume of circulating blood.

- Drugs used in treatment of hypertension include diuretics, adrenergic (SNS) inhibitors, direct vasodilators, angiotensin inhibitors, and calcium channel blockers. (See Table 33-8, Lewis et al., *Medical-Surgical Nursing*, ed. 8, pp. 748 to 751 for a description of antihypertensive drug therapy.)
- Most patients who are hypertensive will require two or more antihypertensive medications to achieve their goal BP.
- Once antihypertensive therapy is started, most patients should return for follow-up and adjustment of medications at monthly intervals until the goal BP is reached.

Nursing Management

Goals

The patient with hypertension will achieve and maintain goal BP; understand, accept, and implement the therapeutic plan; experience minimal or no unpleasant side effects of therapy; and be confident of ability to manage and cope with this condition.

Nursing Diagnoses/Collaborative Problems

- Ineffective self- health management
- Anxiety
- Potential complication: stroke
- Potential complication: hypertensive crisis

Nursing Interventions

You are in an ideal position to assess for the presence of hypertension, identify risk factors for hypertension and CAD, and teach the patient about these conditions.

- Effort and resources should be focused on controlling BP in persons already identified as having hypertension; identifying and controlling BP in high-risk groups such as African Americans, obese persons, and relatives of people with hypertension; and screening those with limited access to the health care system.

Your primary nursing responsibilities for long-term management of hypertension are to assist the patient in reducing BP and adhere to the treatment plan. Nursing actions include patient and caregiver teaching, detection and reporting of adverse treatment effects, assessment of adherence and evaluation of therapeutic effectiveness.

▼ **Patient and Caregiver Teaching**

Patient and caregiver education includes nutritional therapy, drug therapy, physical activity, and, if appropriate, home BP monitoring and tobacco cessation (Table 54).

HYPERTHYROIDISM

Description

Hyperthyroidism is hyperactivity of the thyroid gland with a sustained increase in synthesis and release of thyroid hormones. The most common form of hyperthyroidism is Graves' disease. Other causes include toxic nodular goiter, thyroiditis, pituitary tumors, and thyroid cancer. *Thyrotoxicosis* is hypermetabolism that results from excess circulating levels of thyroxine (T_4), triiodothyronine (T_3), or both. Hyperthyroidism and thyrotoxicosis usually occur together as in Graves' disease, but in some cases thyrotoxicosis

Table 54	Patient and Caregiver Teaching Guide: Hypertension

When teaching the patient and/or caregiver about hypertension, you should:

General Instructions

1. Provide the numeric value of the patient's BP and explain what it means (e.g., high, low, normal, borderline). Encourage patient to monitor BP at home and instruct the patient to call health care provider if BP exceeds high or low limits set by health care provider.
2. Inform the patient that hypertension is usually asymptomatic and symptoms do not reliably indicate BP levels.
3. Explain that hypertension means high blood pressure and does not relate to a "hyper" personality.
4. Explain that long-term therapy and follow-up care are necessary to treat hypertension. Therapy involves lifestyle changes (e.g., weight management, sodium reduction, smoking cessation, regular physical activity) and, in most cases, medications.
5. Explain that therapy will not cure, but should control hypertension.
6. Tell patient that controlled hypertension is usually compatible with an excellent prognosis and a normal lifestyle.
7. Explain the potential dangers of uncontrolled hypertension.

Instructions Related to Medications

1. Be specific about the names, actions, dosages, and side effects of prescribed medications.
2. Assist the patient to plan regular and convenient times for taking medications and measuring BP.
3. Caution the patient not to stop drugs abruptly because withdrawal may cause a severe hypertensive reaction.
4. Tell the patient not to double up on doses when a dose is missed.
5. Inform the patient that, if BP increases, the patient should not take an increased medication dosage before consulting with the health care provider.
6. Tell the patient not to take a medication belonging to someone else.
7. Tell the patient to supplement diet with foods high in potassium (e.g., citrus fruits and green leafy vegetables) if taking potassium-wasting diuretics.

Table 54	Patient and Caregiver Teaching Guide: Hypertension—cont'd

8. Tell the patient to avoid hot baths, excessive amounts of alcohol, and strenuous exercise within 3 hours of taking medications that promote vasodilation.

9. Many medications cause orthostatic hypotension. Explain that the effects of orthostatic hypotension can be reduced by instructing the patient to rise slowly from bed, sit on the side of the bed for a few minutes, stand slowly, and begin moving if no symptoms develop (e.g., dizziness, lightheadedness). Remind the patient not to stand still for prolonged periods of time, to do leg exercises to increase venous return, sleep with the head of the bed raised or on pillows, and lie or sit down when dizziness occurs.

10. Many medications cause sexual problems (e.g., erectile dysfunction, decreased libido). Encourage the patient to consult with the health care provider about changing drugs or dosages if sexual problems develop.

11. Inform the patient that the side effects of medication(s) may diminish with time.

12. Caution about potentially high-risk over-the-counter medications, such as high-sodium antacids, appetite suppressants, and cold and sinus medications. Advise patient to read warning labels and to consult with a pharmacist.

BP, Blood pressure.

H

may occur without hyperthyroidism. Graves' disease accounts for 75% of the cases of hyperthyroidism.

- The incidence of hyperthyroidism is greater in women, with the highest frequency in persons 20 to 40 years old.

Pathophysiology

Graves' disease is an autoimmune disease of unknown etiology marked by diffuse thyroid enlargement and excessive thyroid hormone secretion. The patient develops antibodies to the thyroid-stimulating hormone (TSH) receptor. These antibodies attach to receptors and stimulate the thyroid gland to release T_3, T_4, or both. The excessive release of thyroid hormones leads to the clinical manifestations associated with thyrotoxicosis.

- The disease is characterized by remissions and exacerbations, with or without treatment. It may progress to destruction of thyroid tissue, causing hypothyroidism.

- Precipitating factors, such as insufficient iodine supply, infections, and emotions, may interact with genetic factors to cause Graves' disease.

Nodular goiters are characterized by nodules that secrete thyroid hormone independent of TSH stimulation. If associated with hyperthyroidism, a nodule is termed *toxic.* There may be multiple nodules or a single nodule. The frequency of toxic multinodular goiter is highest in people over 40 years of age.

Clinical Manifestations

The manifestations of hyperthyroidism are related to the effects of excess thyroid hormones. Manifestations are numerous and include hypertension, palpitations, dysrhythmias, angina, fatigue, nervousness, insomnia, weight loss, increased appetite, diarrhea, diaphoresis, intolerance to heat, menstrual irregularities in women, and impotence in men.

- When the thyroid gland is excessively large, a goiter may be palpated and noted on inspection.
- *Exophthalmos,* a protrusion of the eyeballs from the orbits, is caused by impaired venous drainage from the orbit leading to increased deposits of fat and fluid (edema) in the retroorbital tissues. This sign is seen in 20% to 40% of patients with Graves' disease. When the eyelids do not close completely, exposed corneal surfaces become dry and irritated. Serious consequences, such as corneal ulcers and eventual loss of vision, can occur.
- A patient with advanced disease may exhibit many symptoms, whereas a patient in the early stages of hyperthyroidism may only exhibit weight loss and increased nervousness. Table 50-5, Lewis et al., *Medical-Surgical Nursing,* ed. 8, p. 1264 compares features of hyperthyroidism in younger and older adult patients.

Complications

Thyrotoxic crisis (thyroid storm) is an acute, rare condition in which all hyperthyroid manifestations are heightened. Although considered a life-threatening emergency, death is rare when treatment is initiated early. Thyrotoxic crisis is thought to result from stressors (e.g., infection, trauma, surgery) in a patient with preexisting hyperthyroidism, either diagnosed or undiagnosed.

- Manifestations include severe tachycardia, heart failure, shock, hyperthermia (up to 105.3° F [40.7° C]), restlessness, agitation, abdominal pain, nausea, vomiting, diarrhea, delirium, and coma.

- Treatment is aimed at reducing circulating thyroid hormone levels by appropriate drug therapy, fever reduction, fluid replacement, and elimination or management of the initiating stressor or stressors.

Diagnostic Studies

- Diagnosis is confirmed with findings of decreased serum TSH levels and elevated free T_4 levels.
- Total T_3 and T_4 may be assessed.
- Radioactive iodine uptake (RAIU) differentiates Graves' disease from other forms of thyroiditis.

Collaborative Care

The therapeutic goals are to block the adverse effects of thyroid hormones and stop their oversecretion. Three primary treatment options are antithyroid medications, radioactive iodine therapy, and subtotal thyroidectomy. Generally the treatment of choice in nonpregnant adults is radioactive iodine therapy. If surgery is to be performed, the patient is usually given antithyroid drugs and iodine to produce a euthyroid state. Drugs used in the treatment of hyperthyroidism are useful in controlling symptoms in thyrotoxic states, but they are not curative.

Drug Therapy

Antithyroid drugs. The first-line antithyroid drugs commonly used are propylthiouracil (PTU) and methimazole (Tapazole). These drugs inhibit the synthesis of thyroid hormones; PTU also blocks the peripheral conversion of T_4 to T_3. Indications for their use include Graves' disease in the young patient, hyperthyroidism during pregnancy, and the need to achieve a euthyroid state before surgery or radiation therapy.

Iodine. In large doses, iodine (e.g., Lugol's solution, saturated solution of potassium iodide [SSKI]) inhibits the synthesis of T_3 and T_4 and blocks the release of these hormones into circulation. Iodine decreases thyroid vascularity, making surgery safer and easier. The maximal effect is usually seen within 1 to 2 weeks.

β-Adrenergic blockers. Propranolol (Inderal) is a frequently used β-adrenergic blocker. It relieves the symptoms of thyrotoxicosis that result from increased β-adrenergic receptor stimulation caused by excess thyroid hormones.

Radioactive iodine. Radioactive iodine limits thyroid hormone secretion by damaging or destroying thyroid tissue. Because of a delayed response, the maximum effect may not be seen for 2 to 3 months, and other drug therapy may be used until the effects of irradiation become apparent. This treatment is effective but often results in hypothyroidism.

Surgical Therapy

Thyroidectomy is indicated for individuals who have been unresponsive to antithyroid therapy, for individuals with very large goiters causing tracheal compression, and for individuals with a possible malignancy.

For subtotal thyroidectomy to be effective, approximately 90% of the thyroid tissue must be removed. If too much tissue is taken, the gland will not regenerate after surgery and hypothyroidism will develop.

Endoscopic thyroidectomy is a minimally invasive procedure. It is performed for patients with small nodules (<3 cm) where there is no evidence of malignancy.

Postoperative complications include hypothyroidism, damage or inadvertent removal of the parathyroid glands, hemorrhage, injury to the recurrent or superior laryngeal nerve, thyrotoxic crisis, and infection.

Nutritional Therapy

The potential for nutritional deficits is high when an increased metabolic rate is present. A high-calorie diet (4000 to 5000 kcal/day) may be ordered to satisfy hunger and prevent tissue breakdown. This is accomplished with six full meals each day and snacks high in protein, carbohydrates, minerals, and vitamins, particularly vitamin A, thiamine, vitamin B_6, and vitamin C.

- Teach the patient to avoid highly seasoned and high-fiber foods because these foods can further stimulate the already hyperactive GI tract. Provide substitutes for caffeine-containing liquids such as coffee, tea, and cola because the stimulating effects of these fluids increase restlessness and sleep disturbances.
- Consult a dietitian for guidance in meeting the nutritional needs of a patient with hyperthyroidism.

Nursing Management

Goals

The patient with hyperthyroidism will experience relief of symptoms, have no serious complications related to the disease or treatment, maintain nutritional balance, and cooperate with the therapeutic plan.

See NCP 50-1 for the patient with hyperthyroidism, Lewis et al., *Medical-Surgical Nursing,* ed. 8, p. 1268.

Nursing Diagnoses

- Activity intolerance
- Imbalanced nutrition: less than body requirements

Nursing Interventions

Acute thyrotoxicosis requires aggressive treatment, often in an intensive care unit. Administer medications (previously discussed) that block thyroid hormone production and the sympathetic nervous system.

Provide supportive therapy to the patient. This includes monitoring for cardiac dysrhythmias and decompensation, ensuring adequate oxygenation, and administering IV fluids to replace fluid and electrolyte losses. This is especially important in the patient who experiences fluid losses because of vomiting and diarrhea.

A restful, calm, quiet room should be provided because increased metabolism causes sleep disturbances. Provision of adequate rest may be a challenge because of the patient's irritability and restlessness.

- Interventions may include placing the patient in a cool room away from very ill patients and noisy, high-traffic areas; using light bed coverings and changing the linen frequently if the patient is diaphoretic; encouraging and assisting with exercise involving large muscle groups (tremors can interfere with small-muscle coordination) to allow the release of nervous tension and restlessness; and establishing a supportive, trusting relationship to help the patient cope with aggravating events and lessen anxiety.

If exophthalmos is present, there is a potential for corneal injury. The patient may also have orbital pain. Interventions to relieve eye discomfort and prevent corneal ulceration include applying artificial tears to soothe and moisten conjunctival membranes, restricting salt, elevating the patient's head to reduce periorbital edema, and providing dark glasses to reduce glare and prevent irritation from smoke, air currents, dust, and dirt. If the eyelids cannot be closed, they should be lightly taped shut for sleep.

- To maintain flexibility, the patient should be taught to exercise intraocular muscles several times each day by turning the eyes in the complete range of motion.

Nursing Management: Patient Having Thyroid Surgery

When subtotal thyroidectomy is the treatment of choice, the patient must be adequately prepared to avoid postoperative complications.

- Preoperative teaching should include comfort and safety measures in which the patient can participate and practice the importance of deep breathing and leg exercises. The patient should also be taught how to support the head manually while turning in bed to minimize stress on the surgery suture line. Range-of-motion (ROM) exercises of the neck should be practiced, and the patient should be told that talking is likely to be difficult for a short time after surgery.

- Recurrent laryngeal nerve damage leads to vocal cord paralysis. If there is paralysis of both cords, spastic airway obstruction will occur, requiring an immediate tracheostomy.
- Respiration may become difficult because of excess swelling of the neck tissue, hemorrhage, and hematoma formation.
- Laryngeal stridor (harsh, vibratory sound) may occur during respiration as a result of edema of the laryngeal nerve or because of tetany, which occurs if the parathyroid glands are removed or damaged during surgery. To treat tetany, IV calcium salts such as calcium gluconate or gluceptate should be available.

After a thyroidectomy, do the following:

- Assess the patient every 2 hours for 24 hours for signs of hemorrhage or tracheal compression, such as irregular breathing, neck swelling, frequent swallowing, sensations of fullness at the incision site, choking, and blood on anterior or posterior dressings.
- Place the patient in a semi-Fowler's position, and support the head with pillows, avoiding flexion of the neck and any tension on the suture lines.
- Monitor vital signs. Check for signs of tetany secondary to hypoparathyroidism (e.g., tingling of toes, fingers, or around the mouth; muscular twitching; apprehension) and by evaluating any difficulty in speaking and hoarseness.
- Control postoperative pain by giving medication.

▼ **Patient and Caregiver Teaching**

Follow-up care is important for the patient who has undergone thyroid surgery.

- Hormone balance should be monitored periodically to ensure normal function has returned.
- Caloric intake must be reduced substantially below the amount that was required before surgery to prevent weight gain.
- Adequate iodine is necessary to promote thyroid function, but excesses inhibit the thyroid. Seafood once or twice per week or the normal use of iodized salt should provide sufficient intake.
- Encourage regular exercise to help stimulate the thyroid.
- Teach the patient to avoid high environmental temperatures because they inhibit thyroid regeneration.

If a complete thyroidectomy has been performed, instruct the patient about the need for lifelong thyroid replacement therapy. Teach the patient the signs and symptoms of progressive thyroid failure and instruct him or her to seek medical care if these develop. Hypothyroidism is relatively easy to manage with oral administration of thyroid replacement.

HYPOPARATHYROIDISM

Description
Hypoparathyroidism is an uncommon condition characterized by inadequate circulating parathyroid hormone (PTH) that results in hypocalcemia. PTH resistance at the cellular level may also occur. This is caused by a genetic defect resulting in hypocalcemia in spite of normal or high PTH levels and is often associated with hypothyroidism and hypogonadism.

Pathophysiology
The most common cause of hypoparathyroidism is the accidental removal of parathyroids or damage to the vascular supply of the glands during neck surgery (e.g., thyroidectomy, radical neck surgery).

- Idiopathic hypoparathyroidism resulting from absence, fatty replacement, or atrophy of the glands is a rare disease that usually occurs early in life and may be associated with other endocrine disorders. Affected patients may have antiparathyroid antibodies.
- Severe hypomagnesemia also leads to suppression of PTH secretion.

Clinical Manifestations
Clinical features of acute hypoparathyroidism are caused by hypocalcemia (see Table 50-12, Lewis et al., *Medical-Surgical Nursing*, ed. 8, p. 1274).

Sudden decreases in calcium concentration cause tetany, characterized by lip tingling and extremity stiffness. Painful tonic spasms of smooth and skeletal muscles can cause dysphagia, a constricted feeling in the throat, and laryngospasms that can compromise breathing.

Abnormal laboratory findings include decreased serum calcium and PTH levels and increased serum phosphate levels. Other causes of chronic hypocalcemia include chronic kidney disease, vitamin D deficiency, and hypomagnesemia.

Collaborative Care

The primary objectives for a patient with hypoparathyroidism are to treat acute complications such as tetany, maintain normal serum calcium levels, and prevent long-term complications. Emergency treatment of tetany requires the administration of IV calcium.

- Give IV calcium chloride, calcium gluconate, or calcium gluceptate slowly. ECG monitoring needs to be used during calcium administration because high serum calcium blood levels can cause hypotension, serious cardiac dysrhythmias, or cardiac arrest.

Nursing Management

- Rebreathing may partially alleviate acute neuromuscular symptoms associated with hypocalcemia such as generalized muscle cramps or mild tetany. Instruct the patients (if cooperative) to breathe in and out of a paper bag or breathing mask.

▼ **Patient and Caregiver Teaching**

The patient with hypoparathyroidism needs instruction in the management of long-term nutrition and drug therapy.

- A high-calcium meal plan includes foods such as dark green vegetables, soybeans, and tofu. Tell the patient that foods containing oxalic acid (e.g., spinach, rhubarb), phytic acid (e.g., bran, whole grains), and phosphorus reduce calcium absorption.
- Instruct the patient about the need for lifelong treatment and follow-up care including the monitoring of calcium levels three to four times a year.

HYPOTHYROIDISM

Description

Hypothyroidism results from insufficient circulating thyroid hormone as a result of a variety of abnormalities. Hypothyroidism can be *primary* (related to destruction of thyroid tissue or defective hormone synthesis) or *secondary* (related to pituitary disease with decreased thyroid-stimulating hormone [TSH] secretion or hypothalamic dysfunction with decreased thyrotropin-releasing hormone [TRH] secretion). It may also be transient related to a thyroiditis or discontinuance of thyroid hormone therapy.

- Hypothyroidism is one of the most common medical disorders in the United States, affecting approximately 1 in 50 women and 1 in 300 men.

- The most common cause of primary hypothyroidism in adults is atrophy of the thyroid gland as the result of Hashimoto's thyroiditis and Graves' disease. These autoimmune diseases destroy the thyroid gland.
- Hypothyroidism that develops in infancy *(cretinism)* is caused by thyroid hormone deficiencies during fetal or early neonatal life.

Clinical Manifestations

All hypothyroid states have certain features in common, regardless of the cause. Manifestations vary depending on severity and duration of thyroid deficiency, as well as the patient's age at onset of the deficiency.

Hypothyroidism has systemic effects characterized by an insidious and nonspecific slowing of body processes. Clinical presentation can range from a patient with no symptoms to a patient with classic symptoms and physical changes easily detected on examination.

- The adult with hypothyroidism often is fatigued and lethargic and experiences personality and mental changes including impaired memory, slowed speech, decreased initiative, and somnolence.
- Hypothyroidism is associated with decreased cardiac output and decreased cardiac contractility. Anemia is a common feature. Increased serum cholesterol and triglyceride levels and the accumulation of mucopolysaccharides in the intima of small blood vessels can result in coronary atherosclerosis.
- Gastrointestinal (GI) motility is decreased in hypothyroidism, and *achlorhydria* (absence or decreased secretion of hydrochloric acid) is common. Constipation, which is a common complaint, may progress to obstipation and, rarely, to intestinal obstruction.
- Other physical changes include cold intolerance, hair loss, dry and coarse skin, brittle nails, hoarseness, muscle weakness and swelling, and weight gain.

Those with severe long-standing hypothyroidism may display *myxedema,* the accumulation of hydrophilic mucopolysaccharides in the dermis and other tissues. This mucinous edema causes the characteristic facies of hypothyroidism (i.e., puffiness, periorbital edema, and masklike affect).

Complications

The mental sluggishness, drowsiness, and lethargy of hypothyroidism may progress gradually or suddenly to a notable impairment of consciousness or coma. This situation, termed *myxedema coma,* constitutes a medical emergency.

- Myxedema coma can be precipitated by infection, drugs (especially opioids, tranquilizers, and barbiturates), exposure to cold, and trauma. It is characterized by subnormal temperature, hypotension, and hypoventilation.
- For the patient to survive, vital functions must be supported, and IV thyroid hormone replacement must be administered.

Diagnostic Studies

- Serum TSH and free thyroxine (FT_4) are the most reliable indicators of thyroid function.
- Serum TSH levels help determine the cause of hypothyroidism. If high, the defect is in the thyroid; if low, it is in the pituitary or hypothalamus.
- TRH stimulation test shows an increase in TSH if the problem is hypothalamic dysfunction; no change in TSH suggests anterior pituitary dysfunction.
- Serum cholesterol and triglycerides are increased.

Collaborative Care

Overall treatment in a patient with hypothyroidism is the restoration of the euthyroid state as safely and rapidly as possible with hormone replacement therapy.

Levothyroxine (Synthroid) is the drug of choice to treat hypothyroidism. In the young, otherwise healthy patient, the maintenance replacement dose is adjusted according to the patient's response and laboratory findings. In the older adult patient and the person with compromised cardiac status, a small or initial dose is recommended because the usual dose may increase myocardial oxygen (O_2) consumption. Any chest pain experienced by a patient starting thyroid replacement should be reported immediately, and electrocardiogram (ECG) and serum cardiac enzyme tests must be performed. In the patient without side effects the dose is increased at 4- to 6-week intervals.

It is important that the patient take replacement medication regularly. Lifelong thyroid replacement therapy is usually required.

Nursing Management
Goals
The patient with hypothyroidism will experience relief of symptoms, maintain a euthyroid state, maintain a positive self-image, and comply with lifelong thyroid replacement therapy.

See NCP 50-2 for the patient with hypothyroidism, Lewis et al., *Medical-Surgical Nursing,* ed. 8, pp. 1272 to 1273.

Nursing Diagnoses
- Imbalanced nutrition: more than body requirements
- Constipation
- Fatigue
- Impaired memory

Nursing Interventions

Most individuals with hypothyroidism are managed on an outpatient basis. The patient who develops myxedema coma requires acute nursing care, often in an intensive care setting. Mechanical respiratory support is frequently necessary, and the patient will require cardiac monitoring. Administer thyroid hormone replacement therapy and all other medications IV because paralytic ileus may be present in the patient with myxedema coma. If the patient is hyponatremic, hypertonic saline may be administered until the serum sodium reaches at least 130 mEq/L (130 mmol/L). Monitor core temperature because the patient with myxedema coma is often hypothermic.

- Monitor the patient's progress, vital signs, body weight, fluid intake and output, and visible edema. Cardiac assessment is especially important because the cardiovascular response to the hormone determines the medication regimen.
- Note energy level and mental alertness. These should increase within 2 to 14 days and continue to rise steadily to normal levels.

▼ **Patient and Caregiver Teaching**

Initially the hypothyroid patient needs more time than usual to comprehend all the necessary information. It is important to provide written instructions, repeat the information often, and assess the patient's comprehension level.

- Stress the need for lifelong drug therapy. Signs and symptoms of hypothyroidism or hyperthyroidism that indicate hormone imbalance should be included in the teaching plan. Toxic symptoms should be clearly defined.
- Teach the patient to contact a health care provider immediately if signs of overdose appear, such as orthopnea, dyspnea, rapid pulse, palpitations, nervousness, or insomnia.
- The patient with diabetes mellitus (DM) should test his or her capillary blood glucose at least daily because a return to the euthyroid state frequently increases insulin requirements.
- In addition, thyroid preparations potentiate the effects of other common drugs, such as anticoagulants,

antidepressants, and digitalis compounds. Instruct the patient on the toxic signs and symptoms of these medications and the need to remain under close medical observation until stable.

INCREASED INTRACRANIAL PRESSURE

Description
Increased intracranial pressure (ICP) is a life-threatening situation that results from an increase in any or all of the three components of the skull: brain tissue, blood, and cerebrospinal fluid (CSF). Cerebral edema is an important factor contributing to increased ICP. Regardless of the cause (Table 55), cerebral edema results in an increase in tissue volume that has the potential for increased ICP. The extent and severity of the original insult are factors that determine the degree of cerebral edema.

Three types of cerebral edema—vasogenic, cytotoxic, and interstitial—have been identified. More than one type may occur in the same patient.

Table 55	Causes of Cerebral Edema

Mass Lesions
- Brain abscess
- Brain tumor (primary or metastatic)
- Hematoma (intracerebral, subdural, epidural)
- Hemorrhage (intracerebral, cerebellar, brainstem)

Head Injuries and Brain Surgery
- Contusion
- Hemorrhage
- Posttraumatic brain swelling

Cerebral Infections
- Meningitis
- Encephalitis

Vascular Insult
- Anoxic and ischemic episodes
- Cerebral infarction (thrombotic or embolic)
- Venous sinus thrombosis

Toxic or Metabolic Encephalopathic Conditions
- Lead or arsenic intoxication
- Hepatic encephalopathy
- Uremia

- *Vasogenic cerebral edema* is the most common type of edema. It occurs mainly in the white matter and is attributed to changes in the endothelial lining of the cerebral capillaries. These changes result in the flow of fluid from the intravascular to the extravascular space.
- *Cytotoxic cerebral edema* results from local disruption of the functional or morphologic integrity of the cell membranes and occurs most often in the gray matter. This type of edema develops from destructive lesions or trauma to brain tissue.
- *Interstitial cerebral edema* is the result of rupture of the CSF brain barrier and is usually a result of obstructive or uncontrolled hydrocephalus. It can also be caused by enlargement of the extracellular space as a result of systemic water excess (e.g., water intoxication, hyponatremia).

Pathophysiology

Increased ICP can be caused by many factors, including a mass lesion (e.g., hematoma), cerebral edema associated with brain tumors, head injury, or brain inflammation, or by metabolic insult. These insults may result in hypercapnia, cerebral acidosis, impaired autoregulation, and systemic hypertension, which promote the formation and spread of cerebral edema. This edema distorts brain tissue, further increasing ICP, which leads to more tissue hypoxia and acidosis. Figure 8 illustrates the progression of increased ICP.

Sustained increases in ICP result in brainstem compression and herniation of the brain from one compartment to another. With brain displacement and herniation, ischemia and edema are further increased. Fig. 57-4, Lewis et al., *Medical-Surgical Nursing*, ed. 8, p. 1428 illustrates herniation.

- Herniations force the cerebellum and brainstem downward through the foramen magnum. If compression of the brainstem is unrelieved, respiratory arrest will occur.

Clinical Manifestations

Manifestations of increased ICP can take many forms, depending on the cause, location, and rate at which the pressure increase occurs. The earlier the condition is recognized and treated, the better the prognosis.

- *Change in the level of consciousness (LOC).* LOC is the sensitive and important indicator of the patient's neurologic status. The change in consciousness may be dramatic, as in coma, or subtle, such as a change in orientation or a decrease in the level of attention.

PATHOPHYSIOLOGY MAP

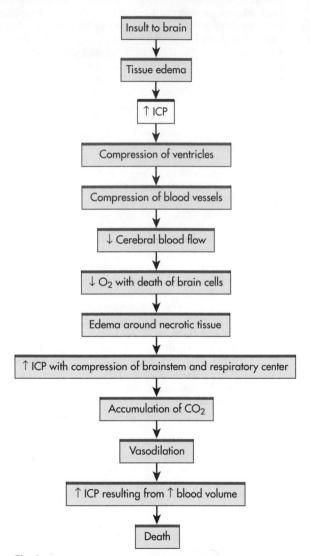

Fig. 8. **Progression of increased intracranial pressure (ICP).**

- *Changes in vital signs.* Manifestations such as Cushing triad consisting of increasing systolic pressure (widening pulse pressure), bradycardia with a full and bounding pulse, and irregular respirations may be present but often do not appear until ICP has been increased for some time or markedly increased suddenly (e.g., head trauma). The effect of increased ICP on the hypothalamus can cause a change in body temperature.
- *Ocular signs.* Compression of the oculomotor nerve (CN III) results in dilation of the pupil ipsilateral to the mass, sluggish or no response to light, an inability to move the eye upward, and ptosis of the eyelid. A fixed, unilaterally dilated pupil is a neurologic emergency that indicates brain herniation. Other cranial nerves may also be affected, with signs of blurred vision, diplopia, and changes in extraocular eye movements. Papilledema, a nonspecific sign that is associated with persistent increases in ICP, is also seen.
- *Decrease in motor function.* As ICP continues to rise, the patient manifests changes in motor ability. A contralateral hemiparesis or hemiplegia may be seen. If painful stimuli are used to elicit a motor response, the patient may exhibit localization to the stimuli or a withdrawal from it. Decorticate (flexor) and decerebrate (extensor) posturing may also be elicited by noxious stimuli (see Fig. 57-5, Lewis et al., *Medical-Surgical Nursing,* ed. 8, p. 1429).
- *Headache.* Although the brain itself is insensitive to pain, compression of other intracranial structures, such as the walls of arteries and veins and the cranial nerves, can produce headache. The headache is often continuous but is worse in the morning. Straining or movement may accentuate the pain.
- *Vomiting.* Vomiting, usually not preceded by nausea, is often a nonspecific sign of increased ICP.

Diagnostic Studies

- Magnetic resonance imaging (MRI) and computed tomography (CT) scan are used to detect the cause of increased ICP.
- Other tests that may include cerebral angiography, EEG, ICP measurement, brain tissue oxygenation measurement via the LICOX catheter, transcranial Doppler studies, and evoked potential studies.
- Positron emission tomography (PET) is also used to diagnose the cause of increased ICP.

Collaborative Care

The goals of management are to identify and treat the underlying cause of increased ICP and to support brain function. A careful history is an important diagnostic aid that can direct the search for the underlying cause.

Ensuring adequate oxygenation to support brain function is important. ABG analysis guides the oxygen therapy. To meet the goal of maintaining the partial pressure of oxygen in arterial blood (PaO_2) at 100 mm Hg or greater, an endotracheal tube or tracheostomy and mechanical ventilation may be necessary.

- If the condition is caused by a mass lesion, such as a tumor or hematoma, surgical removal of the mass is the best management (see Brain Tumors, p. 79).
- Nonsurgical intervention for the reduction of tissue volume related to cerebral tissue swelling and edema includes the use of diuretics and corticosteroids.

Drug Therapy

Drug therapy plays an important part in the management of increased ICP.

- IV mannitol (Osmitrol) is an osmotic diuretic that decreases ICP in two ways: plasma expansion and osmotic effect. The plasma expansion effect reduces the hematocrit and blood viscosity, thereby increasing cerebral blood flow and cerebral oxygenation. The osmotic effect causes fluid to move from the tissue into the blood vessels, resulting in a decrease in total brain fluid content.
- Corticosteroids (e.g., dexamethasone [Decadron]) are used to treat vasogenic edema surrounding tumors and abscesses but are not recommended in the management of head-injured patients. It is theorized that they act by stabilizing the cell membrane and by inhibiting the synthesis of prostaglandins. They are also thought to improve cerebral blood flow and restore autoregulation.
- Metabolic demands such as fever ($>38°$ C), agitation/shivering, pain, and seizures can also increase ICP. The health care team should plan to reduce these metabolic demands in order to lower the intracranial pressure in the at risk patient.
- High-dose barbiturates (e.g., pentobarbital [Nembutal] and thiopental [Pentothal]) are used in patients with an increased ICP refractory to treatment. These drugs produce a decrease in cerebral metabolism and a subsequent decrease in increased ICP.

Nutritional Therapy

The patient with increased ICP is in a hypermetabolic and hypercatabolic state that increases the need for glucose to provide the necessary fuel for metabolism of the injured brain. Because malnutrition promotes continued cerebral edema, maintenance of optimal nutrition is imperative. If the patient cannot maintain an adequate oral intake, other means of meeting the nutritional requirements, such as enteral or parenteral nutrition, should be started. Current fluid therapy is directed at keeping patients normovolemic.

Nursing Management

Goals

The overall goals are that the patient with increased ICP will have ICP within normal limits, maintain a patent airway, demonstrate normal fluid and electrolyte balance, and have no complications secondary to immobility and decreased LOC.

See NCP 57-1 for the patient with increased intracranial pressure, Lewis et al., *Medical-Surgical Nursing,* ed. 8, pp. 1436 to 1437.

Nursing Diagnoses

- Risk for ineffective cerebral tissue perfusion
- Decreased intracranial adaptive capacity
- Risk for disuse syndrome

Nursing Intervention

Respiratory function. Maintenance of a patent airway is critical with increased ICP and is a primary nursing responsibility. As the LOC decreases, the patient is at increased risk of airway obstruction.

- Be alert to altered breathing patterns and keep the patient lying on one side (with frequent position changes) to maintain airway patency. Snoring sounds indicate obstruction and require immediate intervention. An oral airway facilitates breathing and provides an easier suctioning route in the comatose patient.
- You need to prevent hypoxia and hypercapnia. Proper positioning of the head is important.
- Elevation of the head of the bed by 30 degrees enhances respiratory exchange and aids in decreasing cerebral edema.
- Suctioning and coughing can cause transient increases in ICP and decreases in PaO_2. Suctioning should be kept to a minimum.
- Try to prevent abdominal distention as it can interfere with respiratory function. Insertion of a nasogastric tube to aspirate the stomach contents can prevent distention, vomiting, and possible aspiration. In patients with facial and skull fractures, a nasogastric tube is contraindicated, and oral insertion of a gastric tube is preferred.

- ABGs should be measured and evaluated regularly. The appropriate ventilatory support can be ordered on the basis of the PaO_2 and $PaCO_2$ values.

Fluid and electrolyte balance. Fluid and electrolyte disturbances can have an adverse effect on ICP. Closely monitor IV fluids. Intake and output, with insensible losses and daily weights taken into account, are important parameters in the assessment of fluid balance.

- Electrolyte determinations should be made daily. It is especially important to monitor serum glucose, sodium (Na^+), potassium (K^+), and osmolality. Assess urinary output for problems related to diabetes insipidus (DI) and syndrome of inappropriate antidiuretic hormone (SIADH) (see Diabetes Insipidus, p. 167, and Syndrome of Inappropriate Antidiuretic Hormone, p. 620).

Monitoring intracranial pressure. ICP monitoring is used in combination with other physiologic parameters to guide the care of the patient and assess the patient's response to routine care. Valsalva maneuver, coughing, sneezing, hypoxemia, and arousal from sleep are factors that can increase ICP. Methods of monitoring ICP are discussed in detail in Chapter 57, Lewis et al., *Medical-Surgical Nursing*, ed. 8.

Body position. Maintain the patient with increased ICP in the head-up position. Take care to prevent extreme neck flexion, which can cause venous obstruction and contribute to elevated ICP. Adjust the body position to decrease the ICP maximally and to improve cerebral perfusion pressure (CPP).

- Take care to turn the patient with slow, gentle movements because rapid changes in position may increase ICP. Prevent discomfort in turning and positioning the patient because pain or agitation also increases pressure. Increased intrathoracic pressure contributes to increased ICP by impeding venous return. Thus coughing, straining, and the Valsalva maneuver should be avoided. Avoid extreme hip flexion to decrease the risk of raising the intraabdominal pressure, which increases ICP.

Protection from injury. The patient with increased ICP and a decreased LOC needs protection from self-injury. Confusion, agitation, and the possibility of seizures can put the patient at risk of injury. Use restraints judiciously in the agitated patient. The patient can benefit from a quiet, nonstimulating environment and the presence of a family member. Touching and talking to the patient, even one who is in coma, are always an appropriate approach.

Psychologic considerations. Anxiety over the diagnosis and prognosis for the patient with neurologic problems can be distressing to the patient, caregiver, family, and nursing staff. Short, simple explanations are appropriate and allow the patient and family to acquire the amount of information they desire. There is a need for support, information, and education of both patients and families.

Assess the family members' desire and need to assist in providing care for the patient and allow for their participation as appropriate.

INFLAMMATORY BOWEL DISEASE

Description

Inflammatory bowel disease (IBD) is a poorly understood, chronic inflammation of the gastrointestinal (GI) tract, characterized by periods of remission interspersed with periods of exacerbation. The cause is unknown and there is no cure. IBD is classified as either *Crohn's disease or ulcerative colitis* based on clinical symptoms (Table 56), although in some cases the disease does not clearly fit either category. Because the cause is unknown, treatment relies on medications to treat the acute inflammation and maintain a remission. Surgery is reserved for patients who are unresponsive to medications or who develop life-threatening complications.

Table 56	Comparison of Ulcerative Colitis and Crohn's Disease	
Characteristic	**Ulcerative Colitis**	**Crohn's Disease**
Clinical		
Usual age at onset	Teens to mid-30s*	Teens to mid-30s*
Diarrhea	Common	Common
Abdominal cramping pain	Common	Common
Fever (intermittent)	During acute attacks	Common
Weight loss	Rare	Common, may be severe
Rectal bleeding	Common	Infrequent
Tenesmus	Common	Rare
Malabsorption and nutritional deficiencies	Minimal incidence	Common

Continued

Table 56	Comparison of Ulcerative Colitis and Crohn's Disease—cont'd	
Characteristic	**Ulcerative Colitis**	**Crohn's Disease**
Pathologic		
Location	Usually starts in rectum and spreads in a continuous pattern up the colon	Occurs anywhere along GI tract in characteristic skip lesions; most frequent site is terminal ileum
Distribution	Continuous areas of inflammation	Healthy tissue is interspersed with areas of inflammation (skip lesions)
Depth of involvement	Mucosa and submucosa	Entire thickness of bowel wall (transmural)
Granulomas (noted on biopsy)	Occasional	Common
Cobblestoning of mucosa	Rare	Common
Pseudopolyps	Common	Rare
Small bowel involvement	Minimal, only backwash into ileum	Common
Complications		
Fistulas	Rare	Common
Strictures	Occasional	Common
Anal abscesses	Rare	Common
Perforation	Common (because of toxic megacolon)	Common (because inflammation involves entire bowel wall)
Toxic megacolon	Relatively more common	Rare
Carcinoma	Increased incidence after 10 yr of disease	Small intestine, increased; colon, increased but not as much as with ulcerative colitis
Recurrence after surgery	Cure with colectomy	Common at site of anastomosis

*Second peak in incidence after age 60.

IBD is an autoimmune disease. Although an antigen probably initiates the inflammation, the actual tissue damage is caused by an overactive, inappropriate, and sustained inflammatory response. Multiple factors are likely involved in the etiology of IBD. Both ulcerative colitis and Crohn's disease commonly occur during the teenage years and early adulthood, but both have a second peak in the sixth decade.

Over 30 susceptibility genes have been linked to IBD. This suggests IBD is a group of diseases (not just two) with multiple causes that produce similar types of destruction to the mucosa and thus present with similar symptoms. A treatment may or may not be effective depending on whether or not it is appropriate for the underlying genetic variation in a particular patient.

Pathophysiology

The pattern of inflammation differs between Crohn's disease and ulcerative colitis.

Crohn's Disease

- The inflammation in Crohn's disease involves all layers of the bowel wall and can occur anywhere in the GI tract from the mouth to the anus. It most commonly occurs in the terminal ileum and colon. Segments of normal bowel can occur between diseased portions, often called *skip lesions*.
- Typically, ulcerations are deep and longitudinal and penetrate between islands of inflamed edematous mucosa, causing the classic cobblestone appearance.
- Strictures at the areas of inflammation may cause bowel obstruction.
- Because the inflammation goes through the entire bowel wall, microscopic leaks can allow bowel contents to enter the peritoneal cavity and form abscesses or peritonitis.

Ulcerative Colitis

- Ulcerative colitis usually starts in the rectum and moves in a continual fashion toward the cecum.
- Inflammation and ulcerations occur in the mucosal layer, the innermost layer of the bowel wall. Fistulas and abscesses are rare because the disease process does not extend through the bowel wall.
- Areas of inflamed mucosa form pseudopolyps, tongue-like projections into the bowel lumen.

Clinical Manifestations

Symptoms are often the same (diarrhea, bloody stools, weight loss, abdominal pain, fever, and fatigue) in both conditions. Both forms of IBD are chronic disorders with mild to severe acute exacerbations that occur at unpredictable intervals over many years.

Crohn's Disease

- Diarrhea and colicky abdominal pain are common symptoms of Crohn's disease.
- If the small intestine is involved, weight loss occurs from malabsorption and a mass is sometimes felt in the right iliac fossa.
- Rectal bleeding sometimes occurs with Crohn's disease although not as often as with ulcerative colitis.

Ulcerative Colitis

- The primary symptoms of ulcerative colitis are bloody diarrhea and abdominal pain. Pain may vary from the mild, lower abdominal cramping associated with diarrhea to the severe, constant abdominal pain associated with acute perforations.
- With mild disease, diarrhea may consist of one or two semi-formed stools daily that contain small amounts of blood. The patient may have no other systemic manifestations.
- In moderate disease there is increased stool output (four or five stools/day), increased bleeding, and systemic symptoms (fever, malaise, and anorexia).
- In severe disease, diarrhea is bloody, contains mucus, and occurs 10 to 20 times a day. In addition, fever, weight loss (10% of total body weight), anemia, tachycardia, and dehydration are present.

Complications

Patients with IBD experience both gastrointestinal (GI) and systemic complications.

- GI tract complications include hemorrhage, strictures, perforation, fistulas, and colonic dilation (toxic megacolon).
- Toxic megacolon is more common with ulcerative colitis, whereas abscesses and perianal fistulas occur more often with Crohn's disease.
- Hemorrhage and malabsorption lead to anemia, fluid and electrolyte imbalances, and nutritional deficiencies.
- Ulcerative colitis increases the risk for colorectal cancer, whereas Crohn's disease increases the risk for small intestine cancer.
- Arthritis, ankylosing spondylitis, eye inflammation, and skin lesions such as erythema nodosum and pyoderma gangrenosum are systemic manifestations that may occur.
- Thromboembolism, primary sclerosing cholangitis, gallstones, and kidney stones are additional complications of IBD.

Diagnostic Studies

Diagnosis of IBD includes ruling out other diseases with similar symptoms and then determining whether the patient has Crohn's disease or ulcerative colitis.

- Stool is examined for blood, pus, and mucus and cultured to rule out infectious diarrhea.
- Laboratory studies may indicate electrolyte disturbances, anemia, leukocytosis, hypoalbuminemia, and an elevated erythrocyte sedimentation rate.
- Sigmoidoscopy and colonoscopy directly examine large intestine mucosa for inflammation, ulcerations, pseudopolyps, and strictures.
- Biopsies may be taken using a sigmoidoscope or colonoscope.
- Double-contrast barium enema may show areas of granular inflammation with ulcerations.

Collaborative Care

The goals of treatment are to rest the bowel, control inflammation, correct malnutrition, alleviate stress, provide symptomatic relief, and improve quality of life.

A variety of medications are available to treat IBD and are the preferred treatment in Crohn's disease because there is a high recurrence rate following surgical treatment. Hospitalization is indicated if the patient does not respond to drug therapy, if the disease is severe, or if complications are suspected.

Drug Therapy

Drugs are used to induce and maintain a remission of IBD in order to improve quality of life. Medications are chosen based on the location and severity of inflammation. Five major classes of medications are used to treat IBD: aminosalicylates antimicrobials, corticosteroids, immunosuppressants, and biologic and targeted therapy (Table 57).

- *Aminosalicylates* are combination drugs that contain 5-aminosalicylic acid (5-ASA) and an agent that delivers 5-ASA to the colon when it is taken orally. 5-ASA suppresses proinflammatory cytokines and other inflammatory mediators when applied to the intestinal mucosa. Sulfasalazine (Azulfidine) contains 5-ASA and sulfapyridine, but newer agents that are better tolerated include olsalazine (Dipentum), mesalamine (Pentasa), and balsalazide (Colazal). Preparations with 5-ASA can be administered orally or rectally as suppositories, enemas, and foams. They are first-line therapies for mild to moderate Crohn's

Table 57 Drug Therapy: Inflammatory Bowel Disease

Category	Action	Examples
5-Aminosalicylates (5-ASA)	Decrease GI inflammation through direct contact with bowel mucosa	*Systemic* sulfasalazine (Azulfidine) mesalamine (Asacol, Pentasa) olsalazine (Dipentum) balsalazide (Colazal) *Topical* 5-ASA enema (Rowasa) mesalamine suppositories (Canasa)
Antimicrobials	Prevent or treat secondary infection	metronidazole (Flagyl) ciprofloxacin (Cipro) clarithromycin (Biaxin)
Corticosteroids	Decrease inflammation	*Systemic:* corticosteroids (prednisone, budesonide [Entocort] (oral); hydrocortisone or methylprednisolone (IV for severe IBD) *Topical:* hydrocortisone suppository or foam (Cortifoam) or enema (Cortenema)

Immunosuppressants	Suppress immune response	azathioprine (Imuran), 6-mercaptopurine (6-MP), methotrexate, cyclosporine
Biologic and Targeted Therapy (Immunomodulators)	Inhibits the cytokine tumor necrosis factor (TNF)	infliximab (Remicade) adalimumab (Humira) certolizumab (Cimzia)
	Prevents migration of leukocytes from bloodstream to inflamed tissue	natalizumab (Tysabri)
Antidiarrheals	Decrease GI motility*	diphenoxylate with atropine (Lomotil) loperamide (Imodium)
Hematinics and Vitamins	Correct iron deficiency anemia and promote healing	oral ferrous sulfate, ferrous gluconate; iron dextran injection (Imferon) cobalamin, zinc, folate

GI, Gastrointestinal; *IBC*, inflammatory bowel disease; *IV*, intravenous.
*Used with caution during severe disease because of potential to produce toxic megacolon.

disease, especially when the colon is involved, but are more effective for ulcerative colitis.

- *Antimicrobials* are used to treat IBD although no specific infectious agent has been identified. Metronidazole (Flagyl), ciprofloxacin (Cipro), and clarithromycin (Biaxin) are used to treat IBD.
- *Corticosteroids* such as prednisone are used to achieve remission in IBD but are not effective for maintaining the remission. When the disease affects the left colon, sigmoid, and rectum, corticosteroid suppositories, enemas, and foams can be used to deliver the drug directly to inflamed tissue with minimal systemic effects. Oral prednisone is given to patients who do not respond to either 5-ASA or topical corticosteroids. IV corticosteroids are reserved for those with severe inflammation.
- *Immunosuppressants* (azathioprine [Imuran] and 6-mercaptopurine [Purinethol]) are given to maintain remission after corticosteroid induction therapy. Methotrexate has also been found to be effective for Crohn's disease.
- *Biologic and targeted drug therapy* includes anti-tumor necrosis factor (TNF) agents (infliximab [Remicade], adalimumab [Humira], and certolizumab pegol [Cimzia]). Natalizumab [Tysabri] inhibits leukocyte adhesion and movement into inflamed tissue.

Surgical Therapy

Many patients with Crohn's disease will eventually require surgery for emergency situations, such as excessive bleeding, obstruction, or peritonitis, or when medical treatment has failed.

- The main surgical treatment for Crohn's disease is stricture-plasty to widen areas of narrowed bowel.
- If diseased bowel is resected with an anastomosis of bowel ends, the disease commonly recurs at the area of anastomosis.

In the patient with ulcerative colitis, surgery is indicated if the patient fails to respond to conservative treatment; if exacerbations are frequent and debilitating; or if massive hemorrhage, perforation, strictures, intestinal obstruction, dysplasia, or carcinoma develops. Because ulcerative colitis affects only the colon, a total proctocolectomy is curative.

- Surgical procedures include total colectomy with rectal mucosal stripping and ileoanal reservoir, total proctocolectomy with permanent ileostomy, and total proctocolectomy with continent ileostomy.

For descriptions of these procedures, see Lewis et al., *Medical-Surgical Nursing,* ed. 8, pp. 1027 to 1028, 1039 to 1041, and NCP 43-3 for the patient with a colostomy or ileostomy, p. 1043.

Nutritional Therapy

Diet is an important component in the treatment of IBD. A dietitian should be consulted regarding dietary recommendations.

- The goals of diet management are to provide adequate nutrition without exacerbating symptoms, correct and prevent malnutrition, replace fluid and electrolyte losses, and prevent weight loss. Parenteral nutrition may be necessary to provide positive nitrogen balance while resting the bowel, but enteral feedings are preferred because of their effects on the colonic microflora.
- There are no universal food triggers for IBD, but individuals may find that certain foods initiate diarrhea. A food diary helps to identify problem foods to avoid.

Nursing Management

Goals

The patient with IBD will experience a decrease in the number and severity of acute exacerbations, maintain normal fluid and electrolyte balance, be free from pain or discomfort, comply with medical regimens, maintain nutritional balance, and have improved quality of life.

See NCP 43-2 for the patient with inflammatory bowel disease, Lewis et al., *Medical-Surgical Nursing,* ed 8, pp. 1030 to 1031.

Nursing Diagnoses

- Diarrhea
- Impaired skin integrity
- Anxiety
- Imbalanced nutrition: less than body requirements
- Ineffective coping
- Ineffective self-health management

Nursing Interventions

During the acute phase, attention is focused on hemodynamic stability, pain control, fluid and electrolyte balance, and nutritional support. Maintain accurate intake and output records and monitor the number and appearance of stools. Direct your care toward an intensive therapeutic and supportive program.

- It is important that you establish rapport and encourage the patient to talk about self-care strategies. An explanation of all procedures and treatment will help to build trust and allay apprehension.

- Psychotherapy may be indicated if the patient has emotional problems, but any person who has 10 to 20 bowel movements each day, rectal discomfort, and an unpredictable disease may be anxious, frustrated, discouraged, and depressed. You and other team members can assist patients to learn strategies to cope with the chronicity of IBD.
- Severe fatigue limits the patient's energy for physical activity. Nutritional deficiencies and anemia may leave the patient feeling weak and listless. Rest is important because patients may lose sleep because of frequent episodes of diarrhea and abdominal pain. Schedule activities around rest periods.
- Until diarrhea is controlled, the patient must be kept clean, dry, and free of odor. Place a deodorizer in the room, and patients must have ready access to a toilet. Meticulous perianal skin care using plain water (no harsh soap) is necessary to treat and prevent skin breakdown. Sitz baths, dibucaine (Nupercainal), witch hazel, or other soothing compresses or prescribed ointments may reduce irritation and relieve anal discomfort.

▼ **Patient and Caregiver Teaching**

The patient and caregiver may need help in setting realistic short- and long-term goals.

- Your teaching should include: (1) the importance of rest and diet management, (2) perianal care, (3) action and side effects of medications, (4) symptoms of disease recurrence, (5) when to seek medical care, and (6) the use of diversional activities to reduce stress.
- Excellent teaching resources are available from the Crohn's and Colitis Foundation of America (www.ccfa.org).

INTERSTITIAL CYSTITIS/PAINFUL BLADDER SYNDROME

Description

Interstitial cystitis (IC) is a chronic, painful inflammatory disease of the bladder characterized by symptoms of urgency/frequency and pain in the bladder and/or pelvis. *Painful bladder syndrome* (PBS) is suprapubic pain related to bladder filling, accompanied by other symptoms such as frequency, in the absence of urinary tract infection (UTI) or other obvious pathology. The average age at onset is 40 years, and the ratio of women to men with IC/PBS is 10:1 to 12:1.

Although the etiology of IC remains unknown, probable contributing factors include chronic inflammation with mast cell invasion of the bladder wall (possibly resulting from an infection or autoimmune disorder), defects of the glycosaminoglycan layer that protects bladder mucosa from the irritating effects of urine exposure, abnormal constituents in the urine, dysfunction of the sympathetic innervation of the lower urinary tract, and reflex sympathetic dystrophy.

Clinical Manifestations

Two primary clinical manifestations of IC include pain and bothersome lower urinary tract symptoms (e.g., frequency, urgency).

- The pain is usually located in the suprapubic area but may involve the vagina, labia, or entire perineal region. It varies from moderate to severe in intensity and is exacerbated by bladder filling, postponing urination, physical exertion, pressure against the suprapubic area, dietary intake of certain foods, or emotional distress. The pain is transiently relieved by urination.
- Bothersome lower urinary tract symptoms are very similar to a UTI, and the condition is frequently misdiagnosed as a recurring or chronic UTI or, in men, chronic prostatitis.
- Women report that pain occurs premenstrually and is aggravated by sexual intercourse and/or emotional stress. Some patients experience an onset of symptoms that disappears altogether after a period of weeks to months, whereas others have persistent symptoms over a period of months to years.

Diagnostic Studies

IC/PBS is a diagnosis of exclusion. The condition is suspected whenever a patient experiences symptoms of a UTI despite the absence of bacteriuria, pyuria, or a positive urine culture.

- History and physical examination are necessary to exclude other disorders that produce somewhat similar symptoms, such as UTI or endometriosis.
- In IC, cystoscopic examination may reveal a small bladder capacity and superficial ulceration with bladder filling.

Collaborative Care

No single treatment has been identified that consistently reverses or relieves symptoms. Dietary and lifestyle alterations are used to relieve pain and diminish voiding frequency and nocturia. Dietary alterations include elimination of foods and beverages likely to exacerbate the symptoms. A diet low in acidic foods and avoiding beverages such as coffee, tea, and carbonated or alcoholic drinks may be helpful.

- Advise patients that an over-the-counter (OTC) dietary supplement, calcium glycerophosphate (Prelief), alkalinizes the urine and can provide relief from the irritating effects of certain foods.
- Because stress can exacerbate IC/PBS, basic relaxation techniques (e.g., sitz baths, application of heat or cold to perineum or bladder, stress reduction tapes) may be helpful.
- Use of lubrication or altering positions may decrease pain associated with sexual intercourse.

Two tricyclic antidepressants, amitriptyline (Elavil) and nortriptyline (Aventyl), are used to reduce the burning pain and urinary frequency. In IC, pentosan (Elmiron) is used to enhance the protective effects of the glycosaminoglycan layer of the bladder.

- Although these drugs are effective over time (weeks to months), they do not provide the immediate relief that may be needed with an acute exacerbation of symptoms. In this case, a short course of opioid analgesics may be given.

Several agents may be instilled directly into the bladder through a small catheter.

- Dimethyl sulfoxide (DMSO) acts by desensitizing pain receptors in the bladder wall.
- Heparin and hyaluronic acid also may be instilled into the bladder to enhance the protective properties of the glycosaminoglycan layer of the bladder and relieve symptoms.
- Bacille Calmette-Guérin (BCG), an attenuated form of the *Mycobacterium bovis,* administered intravesically is a common treatment for IC. Its mechanism of action is unclear, but it may alleviate inflammation induced by a possible autoimmune reaction.

Distention of the bladder during endoscopic examination relieves IC/PBS-related pain, urgency, and voiding frequency, probably by temporarily disrupting sensory nerve endings in the bladder wall. Several surgical procedures, such as urinary diversion, can be used in an attempt to relieve severe, debilitating pain.

Nursing Management

Reassurance that IC is a real condition experienced by others and that it can be effectively treated may relieve the anxiety, anger, guilt, and frustration related to experiences of chronic pain and voiding dysfunction in the absence of a definitive diagnosis and treatment strategy.

Provide the patient with instruction about the need to maintain good nutrition, particularly in light of the dietary restrictions often necessary to control IC-related pain.

- Elimination of a variety of foods and beverages from the diet likely to irritate the bladder typically provides modest to profound relief from symptoms. Teach the patient to self-use Prelief.
- Advise the patient to avoid clothing that creates suprapubic pressure, including pants with tight belts or restrictive waistlines.
- Written educational materials concerning diet, coping with the need for frequent urination, and strategies for coping with the emotional burden of IC are available from the Interstitial Cystitis Association (www.ichelp.com).

INTERVERTEBRAL LUMBAR DISK DAMAGE

Pathophysiology

An intervertebral disk is interposed between the vertebrae from the cervical axis to the sacrum. Structural degeneration of both lumbar and cervical disks is often caused by *degenerative disk disease* (DDD) (Fig. 9). This progressive degeneration is a normal process

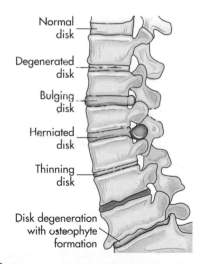

Normal disk

Degenerated disk

Bulging disk

Herniated disk

Thinning disk

Disk degeneration with osteophyte formation

Fig. 9. Common causes of degenerative disk damage.

of aging and results in the intervertebral disks losing their elasticity, flexibility, and shock-absorbing capabilities.

An acute *herniated intervertebral disk* (slipped disk) can be the result of natural degeneration with age or repeated stress and trauma to the spine. The nucleus pulposus (gelatinous center of the disk) may first bulge and then it can herniate, placing pressure on nearby nerves. The most common sites of rupture are the lumbosacral disks, specifically L4-5 and L5-S1.

- Disk herniation may be the result of spinal stenosis, in which narrowing of the spinal canal creates a bulging of the intervertebral disk.

Clinical Manifestations

The most common feature of lumbar disk damage is low back pain. Radicular pain that radiates down the buttock and below the knee along the distribution of the sciatic nerve generally indicates disk herniation. The straight-leg raise test may be positive indicating nerve root irritation. Back or leg pain may be reproduced by raising the leg and flexing the foot at 90 degrees.

Reflexes may be depressed or absent, depending on the spinal nerve root involved. The patient may report paresthesia or muscle weakness in the legs, feet, or toes. Multiple nerve root (cauda equina) compression may be manifested as bowel or bladder incontinence or impotence. This condition is a medical emergency.

In cervical disk damage, there is often radicular pain radiating into the arms and hands, following the pattern of the nerve involved. As in lumbar disk damage, reflexes may or may not be present, and there is often weakness of the hand grips.

Diagnostic Studies

- X-rays are done to note structural defects.
- A myelogram, magnetic resonance imaging (MRI), or computed tomography (CT) scan is helpful in localizing the herniation site.
- An epidural venogram or diskogram may be necessary if other methods of diagnosis are unsuccessful.
- An electromyogram (EMG) of the extremities can be performed to determine severity of nerve irritation or to rule out other pathologic conditions, such as peripheral neuropathy.

Collaborative Care

Conservative Therapy

The patient with suspected disk damage is usually managed first with conservative therapy. This includes limitation of extremes of spinal movement (brace/corset/belt), local heat or ice, ultrasound and massage, traction, and transcutaneous electrical nerve stimulation (TENS). Drug therapy includes nonsteroidal antiinflammatory drugs (NSAIDs), short-term opioids, and muscle relaxants. Epidural corticosteroid injections may be effective in reducing inflammation and relieving acute pain. Conservative treatment can result in a healing over of the damaged area if not caused by DDD, with a concomitant decrease in pain.

Once symptoms subside, back-strengthening exercises are begun twice per day and are encouraged for a lifetime. Teach the patient the principles of good body mechanics. Extremes of flexion and torsion are strongly discouraged.

Most patients initially recover with a conservative treatment plan. If the radiculopathy *(nerve root pain)* becomes progressively worse or there is a loss of bowel or bladder control, surgery may be indicated.

Surgical Therapy

Surgery for a damaged disk is generally indicated when diagnostic tests indicate that the problem is not responding to conservative treatment and the patient is in consistent pain and/or has a persistent neurologic deficit.

- The traditional and most common procedure for lumbar disk disease is a *laminectomy*. It involves the surgical excision of part of the posterior arch of the vertebra (referred to as the lamina) to gain access to part or all of the entire protruding disk to remove it. A minimal hospital stay is usually required.

- A *diskectomy* is another common type of surgical procedure that may be performed to decompress the nerve root. Microsurgical diskectomy is a version of the standard diskectomy in which the surgeon uses a microscope to allow better visualization of the disk to aid in the removal of the damaged portion.

- A *percutaneous laser diskectomy* is an outpatient surgical procedure that is done by using fluoroscopy and passing a tube through retroperitoneal soft tissues to the lateral border of the disk. A laser is then used on the damaged portion of the disk.

- An *intradiskal electrothermoplasty* is a minimally invasive outpatient procedure that may help in treating back and sciatica pain. It involves the insertion of a needle into the affected disk with the guidance of an x-ray. The wire is heated, which denervates the small nerve fibers that have grown into the cracks and invaded the degenerating disk.

- A similar outpatient technique is *radiofrequency diskal nucleoplasty,* in which a special radiofrequency probe is inserted into the disk and generates energy that breaks up the molecular bonds of the gel in the nucleus.

- Another procedure uses an *interspinous process decompression system* (X stop) that fits onto a mount that is placed on vertebrae in the lower back. The device works by pushing open the spinal cord by pressing against parts of either side of the vertebrae. The effect is similar to and less invasive than a laminectomy.

Artificial disk replacement surgery for patients with DDD include the use of the Charité disk for lower disk damage and the Prestige cervical disk system.

A *spinal fusion* may be performed if an unstable bony mechanism is present. The spine is stabilized by creating an ankylosis (fusion) of contiguous vertebrae with a bone graft from the patient's fibula or iliac crest or from donated cadaver bone. Metal fixation with rods, plates, or screws may be implanted. A posterior lumbar interbody fusion may be performed to provide extra support for bone grafting or a prosthetic device.

Nursing Management: Spinal Surgery

Postoperative care focuses on maintaining proper spine alignment at all times until healing has occurred. Depending on the type and extent of surgery and the surgeon's preference, the patient may be able to dangle the legs at the side of the bed, stand, or even ambulate the first day after surgery. Know the specific orders related to activity for any patient. Place pillows under the thighs of each leg when supine and between the legs when in the side-lying position to provide comfort and ensure alignment.

The patient often fears turning or any movement that increases pain. Offer reassurance to the patient that the proper technique is being used to maintain body alignment.

Most patients require the postoperative use of opioids, such as morphine, intravenously for 24 to 48 hours. Patient-controlled analgesia (PCA) allows for optimal analgesic levels and is the preferred method of continued pain management during this time.

- Once fluids are being taken, the patient may be switched to oral drugs such as acetaminophen with codeine, hydrocodone (Vicodin), or oxycodone (Percocet). Diazepam (Valium) may be prescribed for muscle relaxation.
- Because the spinal canal may be entered during the surgical procedure, there is potential for cerebrospinal fluid (CSF) leakage. Severe headache or leakage of CSF on the dressing should be reported immediately.
- Frequently monitor the peripheral neurologic signs of the patient after spinal surgery. Movement of arms and legs and

assessment of sensation should be unchanged when compared with preoperative status. Paresthesias, such as numbness and tingling, may not be relieved immediately after surgery. Any new muscle weakness or paresthesias should be documented and reported immediately.

- Paralytic ileus and interference with bowel function may occur for several days and may manifest as nausea, abdominal distention, and constipation. Assess whether the patient is passing flatus, has bowel sounds in all quadrants, and has a flat, soft abdomen. Stool softeners (e.g., docusate sodium [Colace]) may aid in relieving and preventing constipation.

- Adequate bladder emptying may be altered because of activity restrictions, opioids, or anesthesia. Patients should use the commode or ambulate to the bathroom when allowed to promote adequate emptying of the bladder. Intermittent catheterization or an indwelling catheter may be necessary for patients who have difficulty urinating.

Additional nursing responsibilities are required if the patient has also had a spinal fusion. Because a bone graft is usually involved, the postoperative healing time is prolonged compared with that for a laminectomy. Limited activity over an extended time may be necessary. A rigid orthosis (thoracic-lumbar-sacral orthosis or chair-back brace) is often used during this period.

If surgery is done on the cervical spine, be alert for symptoms of spinal cord edema such as respiratory distress and a worsening neurologic status of the upper extremities. After surgery, the patient's neck is immobilized in either a soft or hard cervical collar.

In addition to the primary surgical site, the donor site for the bone graft must be regularly assessed. The donor site usually causes greater postoperative pain than the fused area. A pressure dressing is applied to the donor site to prevent excessive bleeding. If the donor site is the fibula, neurovascular extremity assessments are a postoperative nursing responsibility.

- Instruct the patient to avoid sitting or standing for prolonged periods. Encourage activities that include walking, lying down, and shifting weight from one foot to the other when standing.

- The patient should learn to think through an activity before starting any potentially injurious task, such as bending, or stooping. Any twisting movement of the spine is contraindicated. The thighs and knees, rather than the back, should be used to absorb the shock of activity and movement.

- A firm mattress or bed board is essential.

INTESTINAL OBSTRUCTION

Description

Intestinal obstruction occurs when intestinal contents cannot pass through the gastrointestinal (GI) tract. The obstruction may occur in the small intestine or colon and can be partial or complete. Causes of intestinal obstruction can be classified as mechanical or nonmechanical.

- Mechanical obstruction is a detectable occlusion of the intestinal lumen that mainly occurs in the small intestine. Surgical adhesion is the most common cause of small bowel obstructions and can occur within days of surgery or several years later. Hernias and tumors are the next most common causes. Carcinoma is the most common cause of large bowel obstruction, followed by volvulus and diverticular disease.
- Nonmechanical obstruction may result from a neuromuscular or vascular disorder. *Paralytic (adynamic) ileus* (lack of intestinal peristalsis and the presence of no bowel sounds) is the most common form of nonmechanical obstruction. It occurs to some degree after any abdominal surgery. Other causes of paralytic ileus include inflammatory reactions (e.g., acute pancreatitis, acute appendicitis), electrolyte abnormalities (especially hypokalemia), and thoracic or lumbar spinal fractures. Vascular obstructions are rare and are caused by an interference with the blood supply to a portion of the bowel. The most common causes of vascular bowel obstructions are emboli and atherosclerosis of the mesenteric arteries.

Pathophysiology

When fluid, gas, and intestinal contents accumulate proximal to the intestinal obstruction, distention occurs, and the distal bowel may collapse. As the proximal bowel becomes increasingly distended, the intraluminal bowel pressure rises. The increased pressure leads to an increase in capillary permeability and extravasation of fluids and electrolytes into the peritoneal cavity. Retention of fluid in the intestine and peritoneal cavity can lead to a severe reduction in circulating blood volume and result in hypotension and hypovolemic shock.

- In the most dangerous situation the bowel becomes so distended that the blood flow is arrested, causing edema, cyanosis, and gangrene of bowel segment. This is called intestinal strangulation. If not corrected quickly, the bowel will become necrotic and rupture, leading to massive infection and death.

- The location of the obstruction determines the extent of fluid, electrolyte, and acid-base imbalances. With a high obstruction, metabolic alkalosis may result from the loss of gastric hydrochloric (HCl) acid through vomiting or nasogastric (NG) intubation. When the obstruction is in the small bowel, dehydration occurs rapidly. If the obstruction is below the proximal colon, solid fecal material accumulates until symptoms of discomfort appear.

Clinical Manifestations

Manifestations vary, depending on the location of the obstruction, and include nausea, vomiting, abdominal pain, distention, inability to pass flatus, and obstipation.

- An obstruction in the proximal small intestine produces rapid-onset, sometimes projectile vomiting with bile-containing vomitus. Vomiting from more distal obstructions of the small intestine is more gradual in onset. Vomitus may be orange-brown and fecal smelling.
- Vomiting usually relieves abdominal pain in proximal intestinal obstructions. Persistent, colicky abdominal pain is seen with lower intestinal obstruction. A characteristic sign of mechanical obstruction is pain that comes and goes in waves. This is because of intestinal peristalsis trying to move bowel contents past the obstructed area. In contrast, paralytic ileus produces a more constant generalized discomfort. Strangulation causes severe, constant pain that is rapid in onset.
- Abdominal distention is usually absent or minimally noticeable in proximal small intestine obstructions and markedly increased in lower intestinal obstructions. Abdominal tenderness and rigidity are usually absent unless strangulation or peritonitis has occurred.
- Auscultation of bowel sounds reveals high-pitched sounds above the area of obstruction. Bowel sounds may also be absent. Borborygmi (audible abdominal sounds caused by hyperactive intestinal motility) are often noted by the patient. The patient's temperature rarely rises above 100° F (37.8° C) unless strangulation or peritonitis has occurred.

Diagnostic Studies

- Upright and lateral abdominal x-rays show the presence of gas and fluid in the intestines. The presence of intraperitoneal air indicates perforation.

- Sigmoidoscopy or colonoscopy may provide direct visualization of an obstruction in the colon.
- Computed tomography (CT) scans may also be used in diagnosis.
- An elevated white blood cell (WBC) count may indicate strangulation or perforation; elevated hematocrit (Hct) values may reflect hemoconcentration; decreased hemoglobin and Hct values may indicate bleeding from a neoplasm or strangulation with necrosis.
- Serum electrolytes, BUN, and creatinine are monitored frequently to assess the degree of dehydration.
- Check stool for occult blood.

Collaborative Care
Emergency surgery is indicated if the bowel is strangulated, but many obstructions resolve with conservative treatment.

Initial treatment of bowel obstruction caused by adhesions includes placing the patient on NPO status, insertion of an NG tube, IV fluid resuscitation with either normal saline or Lactated Ringer's (because fluid losses from the gut are isotonic), addition of potassium to IV fluids after renal function is verified, and analgesics for pain control.

If the obstruction does not improve within 24 hours or if the patient's condition deteriorates, surgery is performed to relieve the obstruction.

- Surgery may involve simply resecting the obstructed segment of bowel and anastomosing the remaining healthy bowel back together. Partial or total colectomy, colostomy, or ileostomy may be required when extensive obstruction or necrosis is present.
- Occasionally obstructions can be removed nonsurgically. A colonoscope can be used to remove polyps, dilate strictures, and remove and destroy tumors with a laser.

Nursing Management
Goals
The patient with an intestinal obstruction will have relief from the obstruction and a return to normal bowel function, minimal to no discomfort, and normal fluid and electrolyte status.
Nursing Diagnoses
- Acute pain
- Deficient fluid volume
- Imbalanced nutrition: less than body requirements

Nursing Interventions
The patient should be monitored closely for signs of dehydration and electrolyte imbalance.

- Maintain a strict intake and output record that includes all emesis and tube drainage. IV fluids should be administered as ordered.
- Serum electrolyte levels should be monitored closely. A patient with a high obstruction is more likely to have metabolic alkalosis; a patient with a low obstruction is at greater risk of metabolic acidosis.
- The patient is often restless and constantly changes position to relieve the pain.
- Provide comfort measures, promote a restful environment, and keep distractions and visitors to a minimum.
- Nursing care of the patient after surgery for an intestinal obstruction is similar to the care of the patient after a laparotomy (see Abdominal Pain, Acute, p. 3).

IRRITABLE BOWEL SYNDROME

Description
Irritable bowel syndrome (IBS) is a chronic functional disorder characterized by intermittent and recurrent abdominal pain and stool pattern irregularities (diarrhea, constipation, or both). IBS affects approximately 10% to 15% of Western populations and about twice as many women as men.

The cause of IBS is unknown, but altered bowel motility, heightened visceral sensitivity, inflammation, and psychologic distress are likely to be involved. For some patients, psychologic factors such as depression, anxiety, and posttraumatic stress disorder play a role in the pathophysiology of IBS.

- In addition to abdominal pain and diarrhea or constipation, patients commonly experience additional GI symptoms, including abdominal distention, excessive flatulence, bloating, urgency, and sensation of incomplete evacuation, and non-GI symptoms, mainly fatigue and sleep disturbances.
- Stress, psychologic factors, prior gastroenteritis, and specific food intolerances have been identified as major factors that precipitate IBS symptoms.

There are no specific physical findings with IBS. The key to accurate diagnosis is a thorough history and physical examination. Diagnostic tests are selectively used to rule out more serious disorders with symptoms similar to those of IBS, such as colorectal cancer, inflammatory bowel disease, and malabsorption disorders (e.g., celiac disease).

Symptom-based criteria for IBS are referred to as the Rome criteria which include the following: abdominal discomfort or pain for at least 3 months, with onset at least 6 months before that and has at least two of the following characteristics: (1) relieved with defecation; (2) onset associated with a change in stool frequency; and (3) onset associated with a change in stool appearance.

Treatment is directed at psychologic and dietary factors as well as medications to regulate stool output. Patients are more likely to improve with treatment if they have a trusting relationship with their health care provider. Encourage the patient to verbalize concerns. No single therapy has been found to be effective for all patients with IBS.

- Because treatment is often focused on symptoms, patients may benefit from keeping a diary of symptoms, diet, and episodes of stress to help identify factors that seem to trigger the IBS symptoms.
- Encourage the patient to increase dietary intake of fiber to at least 20 g per day or use a bulking agent such as Metamucil. Increases in dietary fiber should be instituted gradually to avoid bloating and intestinal gas pains.
- Advise the patient whose primary symptoms are abdominal distention and increased flatulence to eliminate common gas-producing foods (e.g., broccoli, cabbage) from the diet and to substitute yogurt for milk products to help determine if there is lactose intolerance.

Drug therapy includes loperamide (Imodium), a synthetic opioid which decreases intestinal transit and enhances intestinal water absorption and sphincter tone for use in IBS patients with diarrhea. Alosetron (Lotronex), a serotonergic, is prescribed only for women with severe IBS and diarrhea because of a risk of serious side effects (e.g., severe constipation, ischemic colitis). Lubiprostone (Amitiza) is approved for the treatment of women with IBS-constipation.

Psychologic therapies include cognitive-behavioral therapy, stress management techniques, acupuncture, and hypnosis.

KIDNEY CANCER

Kidney cancers arise from the cortex or pelvis. Adenocarcinoma (renal cell carcinoma) is the most common type and is twice as frequent in men as in women. It is typically discovered when the person is 50 to 70 years old. The most significant risk factor is cigarette smoking. Other risk factors include family history (first-degree relatives), obesity, hypertension, and exposure to cadmium, asbestos, and gasoline.

There are no characteristic early symptoms. The most common manifestations are hematuria, flank pain, and a palpable mass in the flank or abdomen. Other symptoms include weight loss, fever, hypertension, and anemia. Local extension of kidney cancer into the renal vein and vena cava is common. The most common sites of metastases include the lungs, liver, and long bones.

Diagnosis is based on computerized tomography (CT) scan, and ultrasound which differentiates between a solid mass tumor and a cyst. Angiography, percutaneous needle aspiration, MRI (magnetic resonance imaging), and IVP may also be used in diagnosis. Radio-nuclide isotope scanning is used to detect metastases.

Treatment for patients with stage I or II tumors and selected stage III tumors is usually a radical nephrectomy, which is removal of the kidney, adrenal gland, surrounding fascia, part of the ureter, and draining lymph nodes.

Radiation therapy is used palliatively in inoperable cases and when there are metastases to the bone or lungs. Chemotherapy, which is used as a treatment in metastatic disease, includes 5-fluorouracil (5-FU), floxuridine (FUDR), and gemcitabine (Gemzar). However, renal cell carcinoma is refractory to most chemotherapy drugs. Biologic therapy, including α-interferon and interleukin-2 (IL-2), is another treatment in metastatic disease. Targeted therapy is also used to treat metastatic kidney cancer and includes sunitinib (Sutent), sorafenib (Nexavar), temsirolimus (Torisel), everolimus (Afinitor), ofatumumab (Arzerra), bevaci-zumab (Avastin), and pazopanib (Votrient).

KIDNEY DISEASE, CHRONIC

Description

K

Chronic kidney disease (CKD) involves progressive, irreversible loss of kidney function. CKD can be defined as either the presence of kidney damage or a decreased GFR <60 mL/min/1.73m^2 for >3 months. The classification of CKD is presented in Table 58. The last stage of kidney failure (*end-stage kidney [renal] disease* [ESRD]) occurs when the GFR is <15 mL/min. At this point, renal replacement therapy (dialysis or transplantation) is required.

Although there are many different causes of CKD, the leading causes of CKD are diabetes mellitus (DM) and hypertension.

Table 58	Stages of Chronic Kidney Disease		
Stage	Description	GFR (mL/min/1.73 m^2)	Clinical Action Plan
1	Kidney damage with normal or ↑ GFR	≥90	Diagnosis and treatment CVD risk reduction Slow progression
2	Kidney damage with mild ↓ GFR	60-89	Estimating progression
3	Moderate ↓ GFR	30-59	Evaluating and treating complications
4	Severe ↓ GFR	15-29	Preparation for kidney replacement therapy
5	Kidney failure	<15 (or dialysis)	Kidney replacement (if uremia present and patient desires treatment)

Source: National Kidney Foundation.
CKD, Chronic kidney disease; *CVD*, cardiovascular disease; *GFR*, glomerular filtration rate.

Because the kidneys are highly adaptive, kidney disease is often not recognized until there is considerable nephron loss. CKD is often underdiagnosed and undertreated because patients are often asymptomatic. It has been estimated that about 70% of people with CKD are unaware that they have the disease.

Prognosis and course of CKD are highly variable depending on the etiology, patient's condition and age, and adequacy of health care follow-up. Some individuals live normal, active lives with compensated renal failure, whereas others may rapidly progress to ESRD (stage 5).

Clinical Manifestations

As renal function progressively deteriorates, every body system becomes affected. Manifestations are a result of retained substances including urea, creatinine, phenols, hormones, water, electrolytes, and many other substances. *Uremia* is a syndrome in which kidney function declines to the point that symptoms develop in multiple body systems. It often occurs when the glomerular filtration rate (GFR) is ≤10 mL/min (see Fig. 47-2 in Lewis et al., *Medical-Surgical Nursing,* ed. 8, p. 1172). Manifestations of uremia vary among patients according to the etiology of kidney disease, comorbid conditions, age, and the degree of adherence to the prescribed medical regimen.

- *Urinary system.* Because most people continue to have good urine output, it is often difficult to convince patients they have kidney disease. With progression of CKD, patients will have difficulty with fluid retention and require diuretic therapy. Once on dialysis and after a period of time on dialysis, it is not uncommon for patients to develop anuria.
- *Metabolic disturbances.* As GFR decreases, BUN and serum creatinine levels increase. Serum creatinine and creatinine clearance determinations (calculated glomerular filtration rate) are considered more accurate indicators of kidney function. As BUN increases, nausea, vomiting, lethargy, fatigue, impaired thought processes, and headaches become common. Efforts are made to initiate renal replacement therapy prior to a patient becoming severely symptomatic.
- *Electrolyte and acid base imbalances.* Hyperkalemia results from decreased renal excretion, breakdown of cellular protein, metabolic acidosis, and dietary intake; sodium (Na^+) may also be retained, resulting in water retention, edema, hypertension, and heart failure.
- *Altered carbohydrate metabolism and elevated triglycerides.* Moderate hyperglycemia and hyperinsulinemia occur. Insulin and glucose metabolism may improve after initiation of dialysis. Hyperinsulinemia stimulates hepatic production of triglycerides. Almost all patients with uremia develop dyslipidemia, with elevated very-low-density lipoproteins (VLDLs), normal or decreased low-density lipoproteins (LDLs), and decreased high-density lipoproteins (HDLs).
- *Hematologic system.* Anemia results from a lack of erythropoietin, bleeding tendencies occur because of a defect in platelet function, and cellular and humoral immune responses are suppressed (increased susceptibility to infection results).
- *Cardiovascular system.* The most common cause of death in patients with CKD is cardiovascular disease. Vascular calcification and arterial stiffness are major contributors to cardiovascular disease in CKD. Hypertension is highly prevalent in patients with CKD because hypertension is both a cause and a consequence of CKD. Hypertension is aggravated by sodium retention and increased extracellular fluid volume.

K

Additional systemic signs include pulmonary edema, diarrhea, peripheral neuropathy, osteomalacia, pruritus, hypothyroidism, infertility, and personality and behavior changes.

Diagnostic Studies

- Dipstick evaluation of urine is used to detect protein or microalbuminuria.
- Urinalysis detects protein, red blood cells (RBCs), white blood cells (WBCs), casts, and glucose.
- Urine culture may identify microorganisms in the urine.
- BUN and serum creatinine are elevated.
- GFR, obtained from 24-hour urine creatinine clearance measures, is decreased.
- Reversible renal disease is identified by renal scan, computed tomography (CT) scan, renal ultrasound, and renal biopsy.
- Hematocrit (Hct) and hemoglobin (Hb) levels are decreased.

Collaborative Care

The focus in CKD is on prevention and early identification to deter the progression of kidney disease. Adverse outcomes of CKD can often be prevented or delayed through early detection and treatment. It is important that patients with CKD receive appropriate follow-up and referral to a nephrologist early in the course of the disease. Therapy consists primarily of drug and nutritional therapy and supportive care.

- Acute hyperkalemia may require treatment with intravenous (IV) glucose and insulin to move potassium into the cells, or IV 10% calcium gluconate. Sodium polystyrene sulfonate (Kayexalate), a cation-exchange resin, is used to lower potassium levels in stage 4 CKD. Dialysis may be required to decrease potassium if dysrhythmias are present.
- Control and treatment of hypertension is discussed in Hypertension p. 332. It is recommended that the target BP be <130/80 mm Hg for patients with CKD and 125/75 for patients with significant proteinuria. Treatment of hypertension includes weight loss (if obese), therapeutic lifestyle changes (i.e., exercise, avoidance of alcohol, smoking cessation), diet recommendations, and administration of antihypertensive drugs. Drugs most commonly used include diuretics, ß-adrenergic blockers, calcium channel blockers, angiotensin-converting enzyme (ACE) inhibitors, and angiotensin receptor blockers (ARBs).
- Phosphate binders such as calcium carbonate (e.g., Tums) and calcium acetate (e.g., PhosLo) are used to bind phosphate in the GI tract, which is then excreted in the stool.

Phosphate binders that do not contain calcium include sevelamer (Renagel) and lanthanum (Fosrenol).
- Exogenous erythropoietin (epoetin alfa [Epogen, Procrit]) is available to treat the anemia of CKD.

Many drugs are partially or totally excreted by the kidneys. Delayed and decreased elimination lead to an accumulation of drugs and the potential for drug toxicity. Drugs of particular concern include digoxin, diabetic agents (metformin, glyburide), antibiotics (e.g., vancomycin, gentamicin), and opioid medication.

Nutritional Therapy
The current diet is designed to be as normal as possible to maintain good nutrition. All patients with CKD should be referred to a dietitian for nutritional education and guidance. For CKD stages 1 to 4, many clinicians just encourage a diet with normal protein intake. However, teach patients to avoid high protein diets and supplements as they may overstress the diseased kidneys.

In addition to protein, nutritional therapy also includes the restriction of water, sodium, potassium, and phosphate (see Table 47 10 for specific recommended restrictions in Lewis et al., *Medical-Surgical Nursing*, ed 8, p. 1178).

Nursing Management
Goals
The patient with chronic kidney disease will demonstrate the knowledge and ability to comply with the therapeutic regimen, participate in decision making for the plan of care and future treatment modality, demonstrate effective coping strategies, and continue with activities of daily living (ADLs) within physiologic limitations.

See NCP 47-1 for the patient with chronic kidney disease, Lewis et al., *Medical-Surgical Nursing*, ed. 7, pp. 1180 to 1181.

Nursing Diagnoses
- Excess fluid volume
- Imbalanced nutrition: less than body requirements
- Grieving
- Risk for infection

Nursing Interventions
You should obtain a complete history of any existing kidney disease or family history of kidney disease because some kidney disorders have a hereditary basis including polycystic kidney disease. If a patient has a personal or family history of renal disease, hypertension, or DM, regular checkups, including serum creatinine, BUN, and urinalysis are essential.

K

- Individuals at risk can take measures to prevent or delay the progression of CKD by maintaining glycemic control if diabetic, controlling blood pressure (BP), and obtaining early and definitive treatment of urinary tract infections.
- When potentially nephrotoxic drugs are prescribed, monitor the patient's renal function with serum creatinine and BUN.
- Advise the patient to report any changes in urine appearance (color, odor), frequency, or volume to the health care provider.
- While the patient with CKD is being maintained on conservative therapy, the decision regarding future therapies should be made. This should be done before complications such as mental status changes, bleeding, progressive neuropathies, and fluid overload occur.
- The patient and family need a clear explanation of what is involved in dialysis and transplantation. The patient should be informed that if dialysis is chosen, the option of transplantation still remains, and if a transplanted organ fails, the patient can return to dialysis.

Even though transplantation offers the best therapeutic management for patients with kidney failure, the critical shortage of donor organs has limited this treatment option.

It is important to respect the patient's choice to not receive treatment. Many times, patients will initiate the conversation about palliative care themselves. Discussion needs to focus on moving from the curative approach to promotion of comfort care and consideration for hospice care. Listen to the patient and caregiver, allowing them to do most of the talking and pay special attention to their hopes and fears.

▼ **Patient and Caregiver Teaching**

Teach the patient and family about the diet, drugs, and follow-up medical care (Table 59).

- Teach the patient to take daily BPs, and be able to identify the signs and symptoms of fluid overload, hyperkalemia, and other electrolyte imbalances.
- A dietitian should meet with the patient and caregiver on a regular basis for nutritional planning. A diet history and a consideration of cultural variations will facilitate diet planning and adherence.
- The patient needs to understand the drugs, dosages, and common side effects. It may be helpful to make a list of medications and the times of administration that can be posted in the home. Instruct the patient to avoid certain over-the-counter drugs, such as nonsteroidal antiinflammatory drugs (NSAIDs) and magnesium-based laxatives and antacids.

Table 59	Patient and Caregiver Teaching Guide: Chronic Kidney Disease

You should include the following information in the teaching plan:

1. Necessary dietary (protein, sodium, potassium, phosphate) and fluid restrictions.
2. Difficulties in modifying diet and fluid intake.
3. Signs and symptoms of electrolyte imbalance, especially high potassium.
4. Alternative ways of reducing thirst, such as sucking on ice cubes, lemon, or hard candy.
5. Rationales for prescribed drugs and common side effects. Examples:
   - Phosphate binders (including calcium supplements used as phosphate barriers) should be taken with meals.
   - Calcium supplements prescribed to treat hypocalcemia directly should be taken on an empty stomach (but not at the same time as iron supplements).
   - Iron supplements should be taken between meals.
6. The importance of reporting any of the following:
   - Weight gain greater than 4 lb (2 kg)
   - Increasing BP
   - Shortness of breath
   - Edema
   - Increasing fatigue or weakness
   - Confusion or lethargy
7. Need for support and encouragement. Share concerns about lifestyle changes, living with a chronic illness, and decisions about type of dialysis or transplantation.

BP, Blood pressure.

KIDNEY INJURY, ACUTE

Description

K

Acute kidney injury (AKI), previously known as acute kidney failure, is the term used to encompass the entire range of the syndrome including a very slight deterioration in kidney function to severe impairment.

AKI is characterized by a rapid loss of kidney function demonstrated by a rise in serum creatinine and/or a reduction in urine output. Severity can range from a small increase in serum creatinine or reduction in urine output to the development of azotemia (an accumulation of nitrogenous waste products [urea nitrogen, creatinine] in the blood).

Although AKI is potentially reversible, it has a high mortality rate. AKI usually affects people with other life-threatening conditions. Most commonly AKI follows severe, prolonged hypotension or hypovolemia or exposure to a nephrotoxic agent.

Pathophysiology

AKI is categorized according to three pathophysiologic states of azotemia: prerenal, intrarenal (or intrinsic), and postrenal causes.

- *Prerenal* AKI is caused by factors external to the kidneys that reduce renal blood flow and lead to decreased glomerular perfusion and filtration. In prerenal oliguria there is no damage to the kidney tissue (parenchyma). The oliguria is caused by a decrease in circulating blood volume (e.g., severe dehydration, decreased cardiac output, burns) and is usually reversible. Prerenal disease can lead to intrarenal disease (acute tubular necrosis) if renal ischemia is prolonged.

- *Intrarenal* causes include conditions that cause direct damage to the kidney tissue (parenchyma), resulting in impaired nephron function. Primary renal diseases such as systemic lupus erythematosus and acute pyelonephritis may also cause AKI. Intrarenal AKI is usually caused by prolonged ischemia, nephrotoxins (e.g., antibiotics), myoglobin released from necrotic muscle cells, or hemoglobin released from hemolyzed red blood cells (RBCs). *Acute tubular necrosis* (ATN) is the most common cause of intrarenal AKI, and is primarily the result of ischemia, nephrotoxins, or sepsis.

- *Postrenal* causes involve mechanical obstruction of urinary outflow. As the flow of urine is obstructed, urine refluxes into the renal pelvis, impairing kidney function. The most common causes are prostate cancer, benign prostatic hyperplasia (BPH), urinary tract calculi, trauma, and extrarenal tumors. Unilateral obstruction rarely results in azotemia and if bilateral obstruction is relieved within 48 hours of onset, it is likely that complete recovery of GFR can be achieved; after 12 weeks recovery is unlikely.

Clinical Manifestations

Clinically, acute renal failure may progress through phases: oliguric, diuretic, and recovery. In some situations the patient does not recover from AKI, and CKD results (see Kidney Disease, Chronic, p. 381).

Table 60	RIFLE Classification Used for Staging Acute Kidney Injury	
Stage	**GFR Criteria**	**Urine Output Criteria**
Risk	Serum creatinine increased x 1.5 or GFR decreased by 25%	Urine output <0.5 mL/kg/hr for 6 hr
Injury	Serum creatinine increased x 2 or GFR decreased by 50%	Urine output <0.5 mL/kg/hr for 12 hr
Failure	Serum creatinine increased x 3 or GFR decreased by 75% or Serum creatinine >4 mg/dL with acute rise ≥0.5 mg/dL	Urine output <0.3 mL/kg/hr for 24 hr (oliguria) or anuria for 12 hr
Loss	Persistent acute kidney failure, complete loss of kidney function >4 wk	
End-stage kidney disease	Complete loss of kidney function >3 months	

The RIFLE classification describes the stages of AKI (Table 60). Risk (R) is the first stage of AKI, followed by injury (I) which is the second stage, then increasing in severity to the final or third stage of failure (F). The two outcome variables are loss (L) and end-stage kidney disease (E).

Oliguric Phase

The most common initial manifestation of AKI is oliguria, a reduction in urine output to <400 mL/day. Non-oliguria AKI indicates a urine output >400 mL/day. Oliguria usually occurs within 1 to 7 days of injury to the kidneys. If the cause is ischemia, oliguria will often occur within 24 hours. In contrast, when nephrotoxic drugs are involved, onset may be delayed for up to a week. Oliguric phase lasts on average about 10 to 14 days but can last for months. The longer this phase lasts, the poorer the prognosis for recovery of complete renal function.

K

About 50% of the patients will not be oliguric, making the initial diagnosis more difficult. Urine output generally correlates poorly with a patient's GFR.

- A urinary analysis may show casts, RBCs, white blood cells (WBCs), a specific gravity fixed at around 1.010, and urine osmolality around 300 mOsm/kg (300 mmol/kg). This is the same specific gravity and osmolality as plasma.
- Fluid retention occurs as urinary output decreases; neck veins become distended with a bounding pulse, and edema and hypertension may develop. Fluid overload can lead to heart failure (HF), pulmonary edema, and pericardial and pleural effusions.
- Metabolic acidosis results when the kidneys cannot synthesize ammonia, which is needed for excretion of hydrogen (H^+). The patient may develop Kussmaul (rapid, deep) respirations to increase the excretion of carbon dioxide (CO_2).
- Serum sodium and potassium levels are altered. Damaged tubules cannot conserve sodium; urinary excretion of sodium may increase, resulting in decreased serum sodium. Serum potassium levels In AKI the serum potassium levels increase because the normal ability of the kidneys to excrete potassium is impaired. Cardiac muscle is very intolerant of acute increases in potassium; treatment is essential whenever hyperkalemia develops. The BUN and serum creatinine levels are elevated in kidney failure.
- Leukocytosis is often present. The most common cause of death in AKI is infection. Leukopenia and thrombocytopenia suggest thrombotic thrombocytopenia purpura or systemic lupus erythematosus as possible etiologies for AKI.
- Neurologic changes can occur as nitrogenous waste products accumulate in the brain and other nervous tissue. Symptoms can be as mild as fatigue and difficulty concentrating and can escalate to seizures, stupor, and coma.

Diuretic Phase

The diuretic phase begins with a gradual increase in urine output of 1 to 3 L/day but may reach 3 to 5 L/day or more. The kidneys have recovered their ability to excrete wastes but not to concentrate urine.

- The diuretic phase may last 1 to 3 weeks, with the patient's acid-base, electrolyte, and waste product values beginning to normalize. Because of large losses of fluid and electrolytes, monitor the patient for hypovolemia, hypotension, hyponatremia, and hypokalemia.

Recovery Phase

The recovery phase begins when the GFR increases, allowing the BUN and serum creatinine levels to plateau and then decrease. Although major improvements occur in the first 1 to 2 weeks of this phase, renal function may take up to 12 months to stabilize.

- The outcome of AKI is influenced by the patient's overall health, the severity of renal failure, and the number and type of complications. Some patients do not recover and progress to end-stage kidney disease. Of those who recover, the majority achieve clinically normal kidney function with no complications (e.g., hypertension).

Diagnostic Studies

- History is essential for determining the etiology.
- Urine output and serum creatinine help in diagnosis.
- Urine osmolality, sodium content, and specific gravity help in differentiating the cause. Urinalysis is also done to assess sediment, casts, hematuria, pyuria, and crystals.
- Renal scan and ultrasound are done to assess renal blood flow and integrity of the collecting system.
- Computed tomography (CT) scan can identify masses and vascular abnormalities.

Collaborative Care

Because AKI is potentially reversible, the primary goals of treatment are to eliminate the cause, manage the signs and symptoms, and prevent complications while the kidneys recover. The first step is to determine if there is adequate intravascular volume and CO to ensure adequate perfusion of the kidneys. Diuretic therapy is often administered but not in high doses. If AKI is already established, forcing fluids and diuretics is not effective and may, in fact, be harmful. Conservative therapy may be all that is necessary until renal function improves.

- Fluid intake must be closely monitored during the oliguric phase.
- Hyperkalemia is one of the most serious complications because it can cause cardiac dysrhythmias. Both insulin and sodium bicarbonate temporarily shift potassium into the cells, but it eventually shifts back out. Calcium gluconate raises the threshold at which dysrhythmias occur. Only sodium polystyrene sulfonate (Kayexalate) and dialysis actually remove potassium from the body.

Controversy exists about the timing of renal replacement therapy. Common indications for renal replacement therapy in AKI include (1) volume overload, resulting in compromised cardiac and/or pulmonary status; (2) elevated serum potassium level; (3) metabolic acidosis (serum bicarbonate level <15 mEq/L [15 mmol/L]); (4) BUN level >120 mg/dL (43 mmol/L); (5) significant change in mental status; and (6) pericarditis, pericardial effusion, or cardiac tamponade.

- If renal replacement therapy is required, there is no consensus regarding the best approach. Peritoneal dialysis is considered a viable option for renal replacement, although it is infrequently used. Intermittent hemodialysis (HD) (e.g., at intervals of 4 hours either daily, every other day, or 3 to 4 times per week) and continuous renal replacement therapy (CRRT) have both been used effectively. CRRT is provided continuously over approximately 24 hours duration through cannulation of an artery and vein or cannulation of two veins.

Nutritional Therapy

The challenge of nutritional management is to provide adequate calories to prevent catabolism despite the restrictions required to prevent electrolyte and fluid disorders and azotemia. Adequate energy should be primarily from carbohydrate and fat sources to prevent ketosis from endogenous fat breakdown and gluconeogenesis from muscle protein breakdown.

- To maintain adequate caloric intake, 30 to 35 kcal/kg and 0.8 to 1.0 gram protein/kg is recommended to prevent the further breakdown of body protein for energy purposes. Essential amino acid supplements can be given for amino acid and caloric supplementation.
- Potassium (K^+) and sodium (Na^+) are regulated in accordance with plasma levels. Na^+ is restricted as needed to prevent edema, hypertension, and heart failure.
- Fat emulsion infusions can also be given as a nutritional supplement and provide a good source of nonprotein calories.

If a patient cannot maintain adequate oral intake, enteral nutrition is the preferred route for nutritional support (see Enteral Nutrition, p. 731). When the GI tract is not functional, parenteral nutrition is necessary for the provision of adequate nutrition (see Parenteral Nutrition, p. 752).

Nursing Management

Goals

The patient with AKI will completely recover without any loss of kidney function, maintain normal fluid and electrolyte balance, have decreased anxiety, and adhere to and understand the need for careful follow-up care.

Nursing Diagnoses/Collaborative Problems
- Excess fluid volume
- Risk for infection
- Imbalanced nutrition: less than body requirements
- Fatigue
- Anxiety
- Potential complication: dysrhythmias

Nursing Interventions

Prevention of AKI is essential because of the high mortality rate and is primarily directed toward (1) identifying and monitoring high-risk populations, (2) controlling exposure to industrial chemicals and nephrotoxic drugs, and (3) preventing prolonged episodes of hypotension and hypovolemia. In the hospital the factors that increase the risk for developing AKI are advanced age, massive trauma, extensive burns, cardiac failure, obstetric complications, or preexisting chronic kidney disease.

- Carefully monitor patients for intake and output, as well as for fluid and electrolyte balance. Assess and record extrarenal losses of fluid from vomiting, diarrhea, and hemorrhage.
- Promptly replace significant fluid losses to prevent ischemic tubular damage associated with trauma, burns, and extensive surgery. Intake and output records and the patient's weight provide valuable indicators of fluid volume status.
- Contrast-associated nephropathy occurs when contrast media for diagnostic studies causes nephrotoxic injury. If contrast media must be administered to a high-risk patient, then the patient needs to have optimal hydration and a low dose of the contrast.
- The individual who is taking drugs that are potentially nephrotoxic must have their renal function monitored. Angiotensin-converting enzyme (ACE) inhibitors can also decrease perfusion pressure and cause hyperkalemia. If other measures such as diet modification, diuretics, and sodium bicarbonate cannot control hyperkalemia, the ACE inhibitor may need to be reduced or reconsidered.

During acute intervention you have an important role in managing fluid and electrolyte balance during the oliguric and diuretic phases. Observing and recording accurate intake and output are essential.

- You must be knowledgeable about common signs and symptoms of hypervolemia (in the oliguric phase) or hypovolemia (in the diuretic phase), K^+ and Na^+ disturbances, and other electrolyte imbalances that may occur in AKI.

- Because infection is the leading cause of death in AKI, meticulous aseptic technique is critical. If antibiotics are used to treat infection, the type, frequency, and dosage must be carefully considered because the kidneys are the primary route of excretion for many antibiotics.
- Perform measures to prevent pressure ulcers because the patient usually develops edema, as well as a loss of muscle tone. Mouth care is important to prevent stomatitis.

▼ **Patient and Caregiver Teaching**
- Once kidney function has returned, follow-up care and regular evaluation of renal function should be emphasized.
- Teach the patient the signs and symptoms of recurrent renal disease. Emphasize measures to prevent recurrence of AKI.
- The long-term convalescence of 3 to 12 months may cause psychosocial and financial hardships for both the patient and the family. Make appropriate referrals for counseling as appropriate.

LACTASE DEFICIENCY

Description
Lactase deficiency is a condition in which the lactase enzyme that breaks down lactose into two simple sugars (glucose and galactose) is deficient or absent.

Primary lactase insufficiency is most commonly caused by genetic factors. Certain ethnic or racial groups, especially those with Asian or African ancestry, develop low lactase levels at about age 5. Less common causes include low lactase levels because of premature birth and congenital lactase deficiency, a rare genetic disorder. Lactose malabsorption can also occur when conditions leading to bacterial overgrowth promote lactose fermentation in the small bowel, and when intestinal mucosal damage interferes with absorption (e.g., inflammatory bowel disease, celiac disease).

Clinical Manifestations
Symptoms of lactose intolerance include bloating, flatulence, crampy abdominal pain, and diarrhea. They may occur within one-half hour to several hours after drinking a glass of milk or ingesting a milk product. Undigested lactose creates an osmotic action, pulling fluid into the small intestines, resulting in diarrhea.

Diagnostic Studies
Many lactose-intolerant persons are aware of their milk intolerance and avoid milk and milk products. Lactose intolerance is diagnosed

by a lactose tolerance test, a lactose hydrogen breath test, or genetic testing.

Nursing and Collaborative Management

Treatment consists of eliminating lactose from the diet by avoiding milk and milk products and/or replacing lactase with commercially available preparations. Teach the patient the importance of adherence to the diet.

- A lactose-free diet is given initially and may be gradually advanced to a low-lactose diet.
- Many lactose-intolerant persons may not exhibit symptoms if lactose is taken in small amounts.
- Because avoiding milk and milk products can lead to calcium deficiency, supplements may be necessary to prevent osteoporosis.
- Lactase enzyme (Lactaid) is available as an over-the-counter product. It is mixed with milk and breaks down lactose before the milk is ingested.

LEIOMYOMAS

Leiomyomas (fibroids) are benign smooth muscle tumors within the uterus. They are the most common benign tumors of the female genital tract. By 30 years of age, 10% of white women and 30% of African American women will have uterine leiomyomas.

The cause of leiomyomas is unknown. They appear to depend on ovarian hormones because they grow slowly during the woman's reproductive years and undergo atrophy after menopause.

The majority of women with leiomyomas do not have any symptoms. Of the women who develop symptoms, the most common include abnormal uterine bleeding, pain, and symptoms associated with pelvic pressure. Pain is associated with an infection or twisting of the pedicle from which the tumor is growing.

Pressure on surrounding organs may result in rectal, bladder, and lower abdominal discomfort. Large tumors may cause a general enlargement of the lower abdomen.

Diagnosis is based on the characteristic pelvic findings of an enlarged uterus distorted by nodular masses.

Treatment depends on the symptoms, age of the patient, her desire to bear children, and the location and size of the tumor or tumors. If the symptoms are minimal, the provider may elect to monitor the patient closely for a time.

- Persistent heavy menstrual bleeding causing anemia and large or rapidly growing tumors are indications for surgery.

When so indicated, leiomyomas are removed by hysterectomy or myomectomy. A myomectomy is performed for women who wish to have children. In this case, only the fibroids are removed to preserve the uterus. Small fibroids may be removed using a hysteroscope and laser resection instruments.

- Uterine artery embolization is an alternative treatment for uterine fibroids. In the procedure, embolic material (small plastic or gelatin beads) is injected into the uterine artery and carried to the fibroid branches.
- Cryosurgery and magnetic resonance imaging (MRI)-guided focused ultrasound may also be used to destroy tumors.

LEUKEMIA

Description
Leukemia is a general term used to describe a group of malignant disorders affecting the blood and blood-forming tissues of the bone marrow, lymph system, and spleen. It results in an accumulation of dysfunctional cells because of a loss of regulation in cell division. Although leukemia is often thought of as a disease of children, the number of adults affected is 10 times that of children.

Regardless of the specific type, there is generally no single causative agent in the development of leukemia. Most leukemias result from a combination of factors including genetic and environmental influences.

Classification
Leukemia can be classified as acute versus chronic and by the type of white blood cell (WBC) involved, whether it is of myelogenous origin or of lymphocytic origin. By combining the acute and chronic categories with the cell type involved, four major types of leukemia can be identified. Table 61 summarizes the relative incidence and features of the four types of leukemia.

Acute myelogenous leukemia (AML) represents only one fourth of all leukemias, but it makes up approximately 85% of the acute leukemias in adults. Its onset is often abrupt and dramatic. A patient may have serious infections and abnormal bleeding from the onset of the disease.

Acute lymphocytic leukemia (ALL) is the most common type of leukemia in children and accounts for 15% of acute leukemias in adults. The 5-year survival rate ranges from 17% to 60% for adults. In ALL, immature lymphocytes proliferate in the bone marrow;

Table 61 Types of Leukemia

Type	Age of Onset	Clinical Manifestations	Diagnostic Findings
Acute myelogenous leukemia (AML)	Increase in incidence with advancing age, peak incidence between 60-70 yr of age	Fatigue and weakness, headache, mouth sores; anemia, bleeding, fever, infection, sternal tenderness, gingival hyperplasia, minimal hepatosplenomegaly, and lymphadenopathy	Low RBC count, Hb, Hct; low platelet count; low to high WBC count with myeloblasts; high LDH, greatly hypercellular bone marrow with myeloblasts
Acute lymphocytic leukemia (ALL)	Before 14 yr of age, peak incidence between 2-9 yr of age and in older adults	Fever, pallor; bleeding; anorexia, fatigue and weakness; bone, joint, and abdominal pain; generalized lymphadenopathy; infections; weight loss; hepatosplenomegaly; headache; mouth sores; neurologic manifestations, including CMS involvement, increased intracranial pressure (nausea, vomiting, lethargy, cranial nerve dysfunction) secondary to meningeal infiltration	Low RBC count, Hb, Hct; low platelet count; low, normal, or high WBC count; high LDH; transverse lines of rarefaction at ends of metaphysis of long bones on x-ray; hypercellular bone marrow with lymphoblasts; lymphoblasts also possible in cerebrospinal fluid; presence of Philadelphia chromosome (20%-25% of patients)

Continued

L

Table 61   Types of Leukemia—cont'd

Type	Age of Onset	Clinical Manifestations	Diagnostic Findings
Chronic myelogenous leukemia (CML)	25-60 yr of age, peak incidence around 45 yr of age	No symptoms early in disease, fatigue and weakness, fever, sternal tenderness, weight loss, joint pain, bone pain, massive splenomegaly, increase in sweating	Low RBC count, Hb, Hct; high platelet count early, lower count later; increase in polymorphonuclear neutrophils, normal number of lymphocytes, and normal or low number of monocytes in WBC differential; low leukocyte alkaline phosphatase; presence of Philadelphia chromosome in 90% of patients
Chronic lymphocytic leukemia (CLL)	50-70 yr of age, rare below 30 yr of age, predominance in men	No symptoms frequently, detection of disease often during examination for unrelated condition, chronic fatigue, anorexia, splenomegaly and lymphadenopathy; may progress to fever, night sweats, weight loss, fatigue, and frequent infections	Mild anemia and thrombocytopenia with disease progression; total WBC count >100,000/µL; increase in peripheral lymphocytes; increase in presence of lymphocytes in bone marrow; hypogammaglobulinemia; may have autoimmune hemolytic anemia (4%-11%), idiopathic thrombocytopenia purpura (2%-4%)

CNS, Central nervous system; *Hb*, hemoglobin; *Hct*, hematocrit; *LDH*, lactic dehydrogenase; *RBC*, red blood cell; *WBC*, white blood cell.

most are of B-cell origin. Fever is present in the majority of patients at time of diagnosis. Signs and symptoms may appear abruptly with bleeding or fever, or they may be insidious with progressive weakness, fatigue, and bleeding tendencies.

Chronic myelogenous leukemia (CML) is caused by excessive development of mature neoplastic granulocytes in the bone marrow. These cells contain a distinctive cytogenetic abnormality, the Philadelphia chromosome. CML usually has a chronic stable phase that lasts for several years, followed by the development of an acute aggressive phase (blastic phase) that is often refractory to therapy.

Chronic lymphocytic leukemia (CLL) is the most common leukemia in adults and is characterized by the production and accumulation of functionally inactive but long-lived, small, mature-appearing lymphocytes. The lymphocyte involved is usually the B cell. Lymph node enlargement (lymphadenopathy) throughout the body is present, and there is an increased incidence of infection because of T-cell deficiencies or hypogammaglobulinemia. Because CLL is usually a disease of older adults, treatment decisions must be made by considering disease progression and treatment of side effects. Many individuals in the early stages of CLL require no treatment. Others may be followed closely and receive treatment only when the disease progresses; approximately 30% will require immediate intervention at time of diagnosis.

Clinical Manifestations

Manifestations of leukemia vary (see Table 61). Essentially they relate to problems caused by bone marrow failure and the formation of leukemic infiltrates. The patient is predisposed to anemia, thrombocytopenia, and decreased function of WBCs.

- WBC infiltration into the patient's organs leads to problems such as splenomegaly, hepatomegaly, lymphadenopathy, bone pain, meningeal irritation, and oral lesions.

Diagnostic Studies

- Peripheral blood evaluation and bone marrow examination are the primary methods of diagnosing and classifying the subtypes of leukemia.
- Morphologic, histochemical, immunologic, and cytogenetic methods are all used to identify cell subtypes and the stage of development of leukemic cell populations.
- Studies such as lumbar puncture and computed tomography (CT) scan can determine the presence of leukemic cells outside the blood and bone marrow.

- The malignant cells in most patients with leukemia have chromosomal abnormalities and specific cytogenetic abnormalities are associated with distinct subsets of the disease.

Collaborative Care

Collaborative care first focuses on the initial goal of attaining remission.

- In some cases, such as nonsymptomatic patients with CLL, watchful waiting with active supportive care may be appropriate.
- Because cytotoxic chemotherapy is the mainstay of treatment for some patients, you must understand the principles of cancer chemotherapy, including cellular kinetics, the use of multiple drugs rather than single agents, and the cell cycle (see Chemotherapy, p. 717).
- Corticosteroids and radiation therapy may have a role in therapy for the patient with leukemia. Total body radiation may be used to prepare a patient for bone marrow transplantation, or radiation may be restricted to certain areas (fields), such as the liver, spleen, or other organs affected by infiltrates.
- In ALL, prophylactic intrathecal methotrexate is given to decrease central nervous system (CNS) involvement, which is common in this type of leukemia. When CNS leukemia does occur, cranial radiation may be given. The use of biologic therapy may be indicated for specific leukemias (see Lewis et al., *Medical-Surgical Nursing,* ed. 8, pp. 696 to 698).

Chemotherapeutic agents used to treat leukemia vary. Combination chemotherapy is the mainstay of treatment for leukemia. The three purposes for using multiple drugs are to (1) decrease drug resistance, (2) minimize drug toxicity to the patient by using multiple drugs with varying toxicities, and (3) interrupt cell growth at multiple points in the cell cycle.

Hematopoietic stem cell transplantation (HSCT) is another type of therapy used for patients with different forms of leukemia. The goal of HSCT is to totally eliminate leukemia cells from the body using combinations of chemotherapy with or without total body radiation. This treatment also eradicates the patient's hematopoietic stem cells, which are then replaced with those of a human leukocyte antigen (HLA)-matched sibling, a volunteer donor (allogeneic), or an identical twin (syngeneic) or with the patient's own (autologous) stem cells that were removed (harvested) before the intensive therapy. (See content on HSCT in Lewis et al., *Medical-Surgical Nursing,* ed. 8, p. 697.)

The primary complications of patients with allogeneic HSCT are graft-versus-host disease (GVHD), relapse of leukemia (especially ALL), and infection (especially interstitial pneumonia). Because HSCT has serious associated risks, the patient must weigh the significant risks of treatment-related death or treatment failure (relapse) with the hope of cure.

Nursing Management

Goals

The patient with leukemia will understand and cooperate with the treatment plan, experience minimal side effects and complications associated with both the disease and its treatment, and feel hopeful and supported during the periods of treatment, relapse, or remission.

See NCPs 31-1, pp. 664 to 665; 31-2, p. 683; and 31-3, p. 693, Lewis et al., *Medical-Surgical Nursing,* ed. 8.

Nursing Diagnoses

Nursing diagnoses related to leukemia include those appropriate for anemia (see Anemia, p. 29), thrombocytopenia (see Thrombocytopenic Purpura, p. 642), and neutropenia (see content on neutropenia in Lewis et al., *Medical-Surgical Nursing,* ed. 8, pp. 690 to 692).

Nursing Interventions

The nursing role during acute phases of leukemia is extremely challenging because the patient has many physical and psychosocial needs. As with other forms of cancer, the diagnosis of leukemia can evoke great fear and be equated with death.

- Help the patient realize that although the future may be uncertain, one can have a meaningful quality of life while in remission or with disease control.
- Families need help in adjusting to the stress of the abrupt onset of serious illness (e.g., dependence, withdrawal, changes in role responsibilities, alterations in body image) and the losses imposed by the sick role. The diagnosis of leukemia often brings with it the need to make difficult decisions at a time of profound stress for the patient and family.

You are an important advocate in helping the patient and family understand the complexities of treatment decisions and manage the side effects and toxicities. A patient may require isolation or may need to temporarily relocate to an appropriate treatment center. These situations can lead patients to feel deserted and isolated at a time when support is most needed.

- From a physical care perspective, you are challenged to make assessments and plan care to help the patient deal with the severe side effects of chemotherapy. The life-threatening problems of bone marrow suppression (anemia, thrombocytopenia, neutropenia) require aggressive nursing interventions.

- You must be knowledgeable about all drugs being administered. In addition, you must know how to assess laboratory data reflecting the effects of the drugs. Patient survival and comfort during aggressive chemotherapy are significantly affected by the quality of nursing care.

▼ **Patient and Caregiver Teaching**

Teach the patient, caregiver, and family the importance of their continued diligence in disease management and the need for follow-up care.

- Assistance may be needed to reestablish various relationships that are a part of the patient's life.
- Involving the patient in survivor networks, support groups, or services, such as CanSurmount and Make Today Count, may help the patient adapt to living with a life-threatening illness. Exploring community resources (e.g., American Cancer Society, Leukemia Society) may reduce the financial burden and feelings of dependence. Spiritual support should also be offered.

LIVER CANCER

Description

Primary liver cancer is the fourth most common cancer in the world, with the majority of cases occurring in males. Hepatocellular carcinoma is the most common primary liver cancer. About 80% of people with primary liver cancer have cirrhosis of the liver. Hepatitis C infection is responsible for 50% to 60% of all liver cancers, whereas hepatitis B is responsible for about 20%.

Metastatic carcinoma of the liver is more common than primary carcinoma. The liver is a common site of metastatic cancer growth because of its high rate of blood flow and extensive capillary network. Primary liver tumors commonly metastasize to the lung.

- The prognosis for patients with liver cancer is poor. The cancer grows rapidly, and death may occur within 4 to 7 months as a result of hepatic encephalopathy or massive blood loss from gastrointestinal (GI) bleeding.

Clinical Manifestations

It is difficult to diagnose and differentiate liver cancer from cirrhosis in its early stages because of similar clinical manifestations (e.g., hepatomegaly, splenomegaly, jaundice, weight loss, peripheral edema, ascites, portal hypertension).

- Other common manifestations include dull abdominal pain in the epigastric or right upper quadrant region, anorexia, nausea and vomiting, and increased abdominal girth.

Diagnostic Studies
- Liver scan, ultrasound, computed tomography (CT), magnetic resonance imaging (MRI), magnetic resonance angiography, hepatic angiography, endoscopic retrograde cholangiopancreatography (ERCP), and a liver biopsy assist in diagnosis.
- Serum α-fetoprotein (AFP) may be positive in hepatocellular carcinoma.

Nursing and Collaborative Management
Treatment depends on the size and number of tumors, presence of metastasis, and age and overall health of the patient. Management is similar to that for cirrhosis (see Cirrhosis, p. 138). Surgical excision (partial hepatectomy) is performed when there is no evidence of portal hypertension, normal liver function, and no evidence of invasion of hepatic blood vessels. Only about 15% of patients have surgically resectable disease, but surgical interventions offer the best chance for cure. Liver transplantation is performed when the tumor is localized with underlying liver dysfunction. Other treatment options are radiofrequency ablation, cryosurgery, alcohol injection, and chemotherapy.

Nursing interventions focus on keeping the patient as comfortable as possible. Because the patient with liver cancer manifests the same problems as the patient with advanced liver disease, the nursing interventions discussed for cirrhosis of the liver apply (see Cirrhosis, p. 138).

LOW BACK PAIN, ACUTE

Description
Low back pain is common and probably affects 80% of adults in the United States at least once during their lifetime. Risk factors associated with low back pain include cigarette smoking, stress, poor posture, lack of muscle tone, and excess weight. Jobs that require repetitive heavy lifting, vibration (e.g., jackhammer operator), and prolonged periods of sitting are also associated with low back pain.

Pathophysiology
Low back pain is a common problem because the lumbar region (1) bears most of the weight of the body, (2) is the most flexible

L

region of the spinal column, (3) has nerve roots that are vulnerable to injury or disease, and (4) has an inherently poor biomechanical structure.

Low back pain is most often caused by a musculoskeletal problem.

- The causes of low back pain of musculoskeletal origin include acute lumbosacral strain, instability of lumbosacral bony mechanism, osteoarthritis of the lumbosacral vertebrae, degenerative disk disease, and herniation of the intervertebral disk.

Acute low back pain lasts 4 weeks or less. It is usually associated with some type of activity that causes undue stress (often hyperflexion) on tissues of the lower back. Often symptoms do not appear at the time of injury but develop later because of a gradual increase in pressure on the nerve by an intervertebral disk.

Few definitive diagnostic abnormalities are present with paravertebral muscle strain. The straight-leg raise test is positive for disk herniation when radicular pain occurs. Magnetic resonance imaging (MRI) and computed tomography (CT) scans are generally not done unless trauma or systemic disease (e.g., cancer, spinal infection) is suspected.

Collaborative Care

If the acute muscle spasms and accompanying pain are not severe and debilitating, the patient may be treated on an outpatient basis with a combination of the following: analgesics such as nonsteroidal antiinflammatory drugs (NSAIDs), muscle relaxants, massage and back manipulation, and alternating use of heat and cold compresses. Severe pain may require a brief course of opioid analgesics.

A brief period of rest (1 to 2 days) of rest at home may be necessary for some persons, whereas most persons do better with a continuation of regular activities.

- All patients during this time should avoid activities that aggravate the pain, including lifting, bending, twisting, and prolonged sitting. Most cases improve within 2 weeks.

Nursing Management
Goals

The patient with low back pain will have satisfactory pain relief, avoid constipation secondary to medication and immobility, learn back-sparing practices, and return to previous level of activity within prescribed restrictions.

Nursing Diagnoses
Acute management
- Acute pain
- Impaired physical mobility

Chronic management
- Chronic pain
- Ineffective coping
- Ineffective self-health management

Nursing Interventions

Primary nursing responsibilities in acute low back pain are to assist the patient to maintain activity limitations, promote comfort, and educate the patient about the health problem and appropriate exercises.

- Muscle-strengthening and stretching exercises may be part of the management plan. Although the actual exercises are often taught by the physical therapist, it is your responsibility to ensure that the patient understands the type and frequency of exercise prescribed, as well as the rationale for the program.

▼ **Patient and Caregiver Teaching**

Assess the patient's use of body mechanics and offer instruction regarding activities that could produce back strain (Table 62).

- Advise patients to maintain an appropriate weight. Excess body weight places extra stress on the lower back and weakens abdominal muscles that support the lower back.
- The position assumed while sleeping is also important in preventing low back pain. Tell patients to avoid sleeping in a prone position because it produces excessive lumbar lordosis, placing excessive stress on the lower back. A firm mattress is recommended. The patient should sleep in either a supine or side-lying position, with the knees and hips flexed to prevent unnecessary pressure on support muscles, ligamentous structures, and lumbosacral joints.
- Teach patients the necessity of stopping smoking. Nicotine has been shown to decrease circulation to the vertebral disks and has a causal link to some types of low back pain.

LOW BACK PAIN, CHRONIC

L

Description

Chronic low back pain lasts more than 3 months or is a repeated incapacitating episode. Causes of chronic low back pain include degenerative disk disease, lack of physical exercise, prior injury, obesity, structural and postural abnormalities, and systemic disease.

Table 62	Patient and Caregiver Teaching Guide: Low Back Problems

You should include the following instructions when teaching the patient how to manage low back problems:

Do Not
- Lean forward without bending knees.
- Lift anything above level of elbows.
- Stand in one position for prolonged time.
- Sleep on abdomen or on back or side with legs out straight.
- Exercise without consulting health care provider if having severe pain.
- Exceed prescribed amount and type of exercises without consulting health care provider.

Do
- Prevent lower back from straining forward by placing a foot on a step or stool during prolonged standing.
- Sleep in a side-lying position with knees and hips bent.
- Sleep on back with a lift under knees and legs or on back with 10-inch-high pillow under knees to flex hips and knees.
- Exercise 15 min in the morning and evening regularly; begin exercises with 2- or 3-min warm-up period by moving arms and legs, alternate relaxing and tightening muscles; exercise slowly with smooth movements.
- Carry light items close to body.
- Maintain appropriate body weight.
- Use local heat and cold application.
- Use a lumbar roll or pillow for sitting.

Osteoarthritis (OA) of the lumbar spine may cause chronic pain in the lumbar area in patients over age 50 years or in the thoracic or lumbar area of younger patients with OA.

Spinal stenosis is a narrowing of the vertebral canal or nerve root canals caused by the movement of bone into the space, and when it occurs in the lumbar area, it is a common cause of chronic or recurrent low back pain. When it occurs in the lumbar area of the spine, it is a common cause of chronic or recurrent low back pain. Compression of the nerve roots can result with subsequent disk herniation.

- The pain associated with lumbar spinal stenosis often starts in the low back and then radiates to the buttock and leg. It worsens with walking and standing without walking.

Treatment regimens are much the same as for acute low back pain: a reduction in the pain associated with daily activities, a formal back pain program, and ongoing medical care. Cold, damp weather aggravates the back pain but can be relieved with rest and local heat application.

- Relief of pain and stiffness using mild analgesics, such as nonsteroidal antiinflammatory drugs (NSAIDs), is integral to the daily comfort of the patient with chronic low back pain.
- Weight reduction, sufficient rest periods, local heat/cold application, and exercise and activity throughout the day help keep the muscles and joints mobilized.
- Antidepressants may help with pain relief and sleep problems.
- Surgery may be indicated in patients with severe chronic low back pain who do not respond to conservative care and/ or have continued neurologic deficits. (See Surgical Therapy, Intervertebral Lumbar Disk Damage, p. 371.)

LUNG CANCER

Description

Lung cancer is the leading cause of cancer-related deaths in the United States and accounts for 28% of all cancer deaths. Although incidence and mortality rates for men have dropped in the past decade, a similar trend has not occurred in women.

- Smoking is the greatest risk factor for lung cancer. Smoking is responsible for approximately 80% to 90% of all lung cancers. Tobacco smoke contains 60 carcinogens in addition to substances that interfere with normal cell development. Tobacco smoke causes a change in the bronchial epithelium, which usually returns to normal when smoking is discontinued.

Assessment of lung cancer risk is now divided into three categories: (1) smokers, people who are currently smoking; (2) nonsmokers, people who formerly smoked; and (3) never smokers. The risk of developing lung cancer is directly related to total exposure to tobacco smoke, measured by total number of cigarettes smoked in a lifetime, age of smoking onset, depth of inhalation, tar and nicotine content, and the use of unfiltered cigarettes. Sidestream smoke (smoke from burning cigarettes, cigars) contains the same carcinogens found in mainstream smoke (smoke inhaled and exhaled from the smoker).

- Another risk factor is inhaled carcinogens. These include asbestos, radon, nickel, iron and iron oxides, uranium,

L

polycyclic aromatic hydrocarbons, chromates, arsenic, and
air pollution.

- Female smokers have a higher risk of developing lung
  cancers as compared with male smokers. Those in the risk
  group of never smokers who are diagnosed with adenocarcinoma are 2.5 times more likely to be female.

Pathophysiology

The pathogenesis of lung cancer is not well understood. Most lung
cancers originate from the epithelium of the bronchus (broncho-
genic). They grow slowly, and it takes 8 to 10 years for a tumor to
reach 1 cm, which is the smallest lesion detectable on x-ray. Lung
cancers occur primarily in the segmental bronchi or beyond and
have a preference for the upper lobes of the lungs.

Pathologic changes in the bronchial system show nonspecific
inflammatory changes with hypersecretion of mucus, desquama-
tion of cells, reactive hyperplasia of basal cells, and metaplasia of
normal respiratory epithelium to stratified squamous cells. Primary
lung cancers are often categorized into two broad types: *non–small
cell lung cancer* (NSCLC) (80%) and *small cell lung cancer*
(SCLC) (20%). Lung cancer metastasizes primarily by direct
extension and by way of the blood and lymph system. Common
sites for metastasis are the liver, brain, bones, lymph nodes, and
adrenal glands.

Clinical Manifestations

Manifestations are usually nonspecific, appear late in the disease
process, and depend on the type of primary lung cancer, its location, and metastatic spread.

- Persistent pneumonitis as a result of obstructed bronchi may
  be one of the earliest manifestations, causing fever, chills,
  and cough.
- A significant symptom often reported first is a persistent
  cough that produces sputum. Hemoptysis is not a common
  early symptom.
- Chest pain may be localized or unilateral and range from
  mild to severe.
- Dyspnea and wheezes may be present with bronchial
  obstruction.

Later manifestations include nonspecific symptoms such as
anorexia, fatigue, weight loss, and nausea and vomiting. Hoarseness may be present as a result of involvement of the recurrent
laryngeal nerve. Unilateral paralysis of the diaphragm, dysphagia,
and superior vena cava obstruction may occur because of intrathoracic spread of malignancy. There may be palpable lymph nodes

in the neck or axilla. Mediastinal involvement may lead to pericardial effusion, cardiac tamponade, and dysrhythmias.

Paraneoplastic syndrome is a consequence of the presence of *cancer* in the body, but is not caused by the local presence of cancer cells or direct invasion, obstruction, or metastasis of the cancer. The paraneoplastic effects are mediated by *humoral* factors *(hormones, cytokines)* excreted by tumor cells or by an *immune response* against the *tumor*. Sometimes the symptoms of paraneoplastic syndrome manifest even before the diagnosis of a *malignancy*.

- Examples of paraneoplastic syndrome include hypercalcemia, SIADH secretion, anemia, leukocytosis, hypercoagulable disorders, and neurologic syndromes. SCLCs are most often associated with the paraneoplastic syndrome. These conditions may stabilize with treatment of the underlying neoplasm.

Diagnostic Studies

- Chest x-ray is used for diagnosis, evidence of metastasis, and presence of pleural effusion.
- Computed tomography (CT) scanning is the single most effective noninvasive technique for evaluating lung cancer; scans of brain and bones evaluate metastatic disease.
- Magnetic resonance imaging (MRI) may be used in combination with or instead of CT scans.
- Positron emission tomography (PET) scan measures metabolic activity which increases in malignant tissue.
- Additional diagnostic studies include sputum specimens, biopsy, bronchoscopy, pulmonary angiography, lung scans, and mediastinoscopy.

Staging of non-small cell lung cancer (NSCLC) is performed according to the TNM staging system (see TNM Classification System, p. 799).

Collaborative Care

Surgical resection is the treatment of choice in NSCLC stages I and II without mediastinal involvement because the disease is potentially curable with resection. The 5-year survival in stage I and II disease ranges from 30% to 60%. For other NSCLC stages, patients may require surgery in conjunction with radiation therapy and/or chemotherapy. Fifty percent of all NSCLC lung cancers are not resectable at the time of diagnosis. Surgical procedures that may be performed include pneumonectomy (removal of one entire lung), lobectomy (removal of one or more lung lobes), or segmental or wedge resection procedures.

Radiation therapy may be used as primary therapy in the individual who is unable to tolerate surgical resection because of comorbidities.

- Radiation also relieves symptoms of dyspnea and hemoptysis from bronchial obstruction tumors and treats superior vena cava syndrome.
- Radiation can be used to treat the pain of metastatic bone lesions or cerebral metastasis, to reduce tumor mass preoperatively, or as an adjuvant measure postoperatively.

A newer type of radiation therapy is stereotactic radiotherapy (SRT) that uses high doses of radiation delivered very accurately to the tumor. SRT provides an option to elderly patients, patients with severe lung or heart disease, and other patients with poor health who are not good candidates for surgery.

Chemotherapy is the primary treatment for SCLC. It may be used for nonresectable tumors or as an adjuvant therapy to surgery in NSCLC. A variety of chemotherapy drugs and multidrug regimens (i.e., protocols) have been used. Chemotherapy has improved survival in patients with advanced NSCLC and is now considered standard treatment (see Chemotherapy, p. 717).

One type of targeted therapy approved for patients with NSCLC is erlotinib (Tarceva), which blocks the growth-stimulatory signals in the cancer cells. Another type of targeted therapy inhibits angiogenesis and thus prevents the growth of cancer cells (e.g., bevacizumab [Avastin]).

Nursing Management
Goals
The patient with lung cancer will have effective breathing patterns, adequate airway clearance, adequate oxygenation of tissues, minimal to no pain, and a realistic attitude toward treatment and prognosis.

Nursing Diagnoses
- Ineffective airway clearance
- Anxiety
- Acute pain
- Imbalanced nutrition: less than body requirements
- Ineffective health maintenance
- Ineffective breathing pattern

Nursing Interventions
Care of the patient with lung cancer will initially involve support and reassurance during the diagnostic evaluation. Individualized care will depend on the plan for treatment.

- Assessment and intervention in symptom management is pivotal as well as teaching the patient to recognize signs and symptoms that may indicate progression or recurrence of disease.

- You have a major role in providing patient comfort, teaching methods to reduce pain, monitoring for side effects of prescribed medications, fostering appropriate coping strategies for the patient and caregiver, assessing smoking cessation readiness, and helping access resources to deal with the illness.
- For many individuals who have lung cancer, little can be done to significantly prolong their lives. Radiation therapy and chemotherapy can be used to provide palliative relief from distressing symptoms. Constant pain may become a major problem. See p. 717 for care of the patient with cancer undergoing chemotherapy.
- Nursing care should include referral to social work for evaluation of needs as the patient and family move toward end of life. The patient and family may need information about disability, financial planning, and community resources for end-of-life care such as hospice.

▼ **Patient and Caregiver Teaching**

- The best way to halt the epidemic of lung cancer is for people to stop smoking. Important nursing activities to assist in the progress toward this goal include promoting smoking cessation programs and actively supporting education and policy changes related to smoking.
- There is a wealth of material available to the smoker who is interested in smoking cessation. The Centers for Disease Control (CDC) provides an index of tools on their website *(www.cdc.gov/tobacco/quit_smoking/cessation/index.htm)*. Also see Chapter 12 in Lewis et al., *Medical-Surgical Nursing,* ed. 8.
- Patient teaching needs to include signs and symptoms to report, such as hemoptysis, dysphagia, chest pain, and hoarseness. The patient and family should be encouraged to provide a smoke free environment. This may include smoking cessation for multiple family members. If the treatment plan includes the use of home oxygen, part of the teaching plan must include the safe use of oxygen.
- Discharge instructions for the patient who has had a surgical resection with intent to cure should include manifestations of metastasis. The patient and family should be told to contact the physician if symptoms such as hemoptysis, dysphagia, chest pain, and hoarseness develop.

LYME DISEASE

Description

Lyme disease is a spirochetal infection caused by *Borrelia burgdorferi* and is transmitted by the bite of an infected deer tick. The tick typically feeds on mice, dogs, cats, cows, horses, deer, and humans. Wild animals do not exhibit the illness, but clinical Lyme disease does occur in domestic animals. Person-to-person transmission does not occur.

The peak season for human infection is during the summer months. Most cases occur in three U.S. endemic areas: (1) along the northeastern coast from Maryland to Massachusetts, (2) in Wisconsin and Minnesota, and (3) along the northwestern coast of northern California and Oregon. Reinfection is not uncommon.

Clinical Manifestations

The most characteristic sign is erythema migrans (EM), a skin lesion that occurs at the site of the tick bite within 2 to 30 days after exposure. This lesion begins as a red macule or papule that slowly expands to form a large round lesion with a bright red border and central clearing. The EM lesion is often accompanied by other acute symptoms, such as fever, headache, fatigue, stiff neck, swollen lymph nodes, and migratory joint and muscle pain. Symptoms usually occur in a week but may be delayed for up to 30 days.

- If not treated, the spirochete can disseminate within several weeks or months to the heart, joints, and CNS. Carditis may occur with chronic arthritic pain and swelling in the large joints. Nervous system problems may include severe headaches, temporary facial paralysis (e.g., Bell's palsy), or poor motor coordination.

Diagnostic Studies

Diagnosis is based on the clinical manifestations and history of exposure in an endemic area.

- Complete blood count (CBC) and erythrocyte sedimentation rate (ESR) results are usually normal.
- A two-step laboratory testing process is recommended to confirm diagnosis. The first step is the enzyme-linked immunoassay (ELISA), a test that will have positive results for most persons with Lyme disease. If the ELISA is positive or not conclusive, a Western blot test should be done which will confirm the infection.

- Cerebrospinal fluid should be examined in individuals with neurologic involvement.

Nursing and Collaborative Management

Active lesions can be treated with antibiotic therapy. Oral doxycycline (Vibramycin), cefuroxime (Ceftin), and amoxicillin are often effective in early-stage infection and in prevention of later stages of the disease. Doxycycline has also been shown to be effective in preventing Lyme disease when given within 3 days after the bite of a deer tick. Long-standing infection may require extended intravenous (IV) antibiotic therapy. IV ceftriaxone (Rocephin) is used for cardiac or neurologic abnormalities.

- Patient and caregiver teaching for the prevention of Lyme disease in endemic areas is outlined in Table 65-11, Lewis et al., *Medical-Surgical Nursing*, ed. 8, p. 1662.

MACULAR DEGENERATION

Description

Age-related macular degeneration (AMD) is a degeneration of the retina involving the macula that results in varying degrees of central vision loss. It is the most common cause of irreversible central vision loss in persons over 60 years old. AMD is divided into two classic forms, dry (atrophic), which is more common, and wet (exudative), which is more severe. Wet AMD accounts for 90% of the cases of AMD-related blindness.

Pathophysiology

AMD is related to retinal aging. Family history is a major risk factor, and a gene responsible for some cases of AMD has been identified. In addition, long-term exposure to ultraviolet light, hyperopia, cigarette smoking, and light-colored eyes may be additional risk factors. Nutritional factors such as vitamins C, E, beta-carotene, and zinc may play a role in the progression of AMD.

- In dry AMD, people notice that reading and other close-vision tasks become more difficult. This form starts with the abnormal accumulation of yellowish colored extracellular deposits called *drusen* in the retinal pigment epithelium. Atrophy and degeneration of macular cells then result, leading to a slowly progressive and painless vision loss.
- Wet AMD is characterized by the growth of new blood vessels from their normal location in the choroids to an abnormal location in the retinal epithelium. As the new

M

blood vessels leak, scar tissue gradually forms. Acute vision loss may occur in some cases from bleeding.

Clinical Manifestations

The patient may experience blurred and darkened vision, the presence of scotomas (blind spots in the visual fields), or metamorphopsia (distortion of vision).

Diagnostic Studies

- Visual acuity measurement
- Ophthalmoscopic examination to look for drusen and other changes in the fundus
- Amsler grid test to define the involved area and provide a baseline for future comparison
- Fundus photography and IV fluorescein angiography helps further define the extent and type of AMD

Nursing and Collaborative Management

Vision often does not improve for most people with AMD. Limited treatment options for patients with wet AMD include several medications (i.e., ranibizumab [Lucentis], bevacizumab [Avastin], and pegaptanib [Macugen]) injected directly into the vitreous cavity. These drugs are selective inhibitors of endothelial growth factor and help to slow vision loss.

- Photodynamic therapy is used in wet AMD to destroy abnormal blood vessels without permanent damage to the retinal pigment epithelium and photoreceptor cells. Criteria for its use are very specific.
- Patients at risk for AMD (in consultation with their health care provider) should consider supplements of vitamins and minerals.
- Many patients with low-vision assistive devices can continue reading and retain a license to drive during the daytime and at lowered speeds.

The permanent loss of central vision associated with AMD has significant psychosocial implications for nursing care. Nursing management of the patient with uncorrectable visual impairment is discussed in Lewis and others, *Medical-Surgical Nursing,* ed. 8, pp. 406 to 407 and is appropriate for the patient with AMD. It is especially important when caring for patients to avoid giving them the impression that "nothing can be done" about their problem. Although it is true that therapy will not recover lost vision, much can be done to augment the remaining vision.

MALABSORPTION SYNDROME

Malabsorption results from impaired absorption of fats, carbohydrates, proteins, minerals, and vitamins. The stomach, small intestine, liver, and pancreas regulate normal digestion and absorption. Digestive enzymes ordinarily break down nutrients so that absorption can take place. If there is an interruption in this process at any point, malabsorption may occur.

- Lactose intolerance is the most common malabsorption disorder, followed by inflammatory bowel disease, celiac disease, tropical sprue, and cystic fibrosis.

The most common clinical manifestation of malabsorption is steatorrhea (bulky, foul-smelling, yellow-gray, greasy stools with puttylike consistency). Steatorrhea does not occur with lactose intolerance.

Diagnostic studies include qualitative examination of stool for fat (Sudan stain), a 72-hour stool collection for quantitative measurement of fecal fat, serologic testing for celiac disease, and fecal elastase testing to determine if there is pancreatic insufficiency. A pancreatic secretin test may be performed to rule out pancreatic insufficiency.

Other diagnostic studies include:
- CT scan
- Endoscopy to obtain a small bowel biopsy specimen for diagnosis.
- Tests for carbohydrate malabsorption include the D-Xylose test and the lactose tolerance test.
- Small bowel barium enema is used to identify abnormal mucosal patterns.
- Capsule endoscopy can be used to assess the small intestine for absorption problems.
- Laboratory studies to evaluate nutritional status (complete blood count [CBC], prothrombin, serum vitamin A and carotene levels, serum electrolytes, calcium, and cholesterol) are frequently ordered.

See the specific disorders of Celiac Disease, p. 111; Cystic Fibrosis, p. 163; Inflammatory Bowel Disease, p. 359; Lactase Deficiency, p. 394.

M

MALIGNANT MELANOMA

Description

Malignant melanoma is a tumor arising in cells producing melanin; these are usually the melanocytes of the skin. Melanoma has the ability to metastasize to any organ, including the brain and heart. This is the deadliest form of skin cancer.

The exact cause of melanoma is unknown. Risk factors include long-term ultraviolet (UV) exposure or overexposure to artificial light, such as a tanning booth. Persons with fair skin and eyes and those with a prior diagnosis of melanoma or having a first-degree relative diagnosed with melanoma have an increased risk. Immunosuppression and dysplastic nevi also increase a person's risk.

Clinical Manifestations

About 25% of melanomas occur in existing nevi or moles; about 20% occur in dysplastic nevi. Melanoma frequently occurs on the lower legs in women and on the trunk, head, and neck in men. Because most melanoma cells continue to produce melanin, melanoma tumors are often brown or black. Individuals should consult their health care provider immediately if their moles or lesions show any of the clinical signs (ABCDEs) of melanoma (see Fig. 24-4, Lewis et al., *Medical-Surgical Nursing,* ed. 8, p. 453). The ABCDEs of melanoma include **A**symmetry, **B**order irregularity, **C**olor varied from one area of the lesion to another, **D**iameter >6 mm, and **E** evolving; changing appearance. Any sudden or progressive increase in the size, color, or shape of a mole should be checked. When melanoma begins in the skin it is called *cutaneous melanoma.* Melanoma can also occur in the eyes, meninges, lymph nodes, digestive tract, and anywhere else in the body where melanocytes are found.

Collaborative Care

Pigmented lesions highly suspicious for melanoma should not be shave-biopsied, shave-excised, or electrocauterized. All suspicious lesions should be biopsied using an excisional biopsy technique. The most important prognostic factor is tumor thickness at the time of diagnosis.

- Two methods are used to determine tumor thickness: the *Breslow measurement* which indicates tumor depth in millimeters and the *Clark level* which indicates the depth of invasion of the tumor. The higher the number, the deeper the melanoma.

Treatment depends on the site of the original tumor, stage of the cancer, and patient's age and general health. Initial treatment of malignant melanoma is surgical incision. Melanoma that has spread to the lymph nodes or nearby sites usually requires additional therapy, such as chemotherapy, biologic therapy (e.g., α-interferon, interleukin-2), and/or radiation therapy. Examples of chemotherapy agents include dacarbazine (DTIC), temozolomide (TMZ), procarbazine (Matulane), carmustine (BCNU), and lomustine (CCNU). Topical immune therapy and gene and vaccine therapies are currently being examined as additional treatment options.

Cutaneous melanoma is nearly 100% curable by excision if diagnosed early when the malignant cells are restricted to the epidermis. The most important prognostic factor is tumor thickness at the time of presentation. If spread to regional lymph nodes occurs, the patient has a 45% 5-year survival. If metastasis occurs, treatment is largely palliative.

▼ **Patient and Caregiver Teaching**

Emphasize the importance of protection from the damaging effects of the sun, such as wearing a large-brimmed hat, sunglasses, and a long-sleeved shirt of a lightly woven fabric.

■ Inform patients that the rays of the sun are most dangerous between 10 AM and 2 PM standard time and 11 AM and 3 PM daylight savings time. Recommend patients use a sunscreen with a minimum SPF of 15 on a daily basis.

■ Teach patients to self-examine their skin at least monthly to detect new or persistent skin lesions.

MALNUTRITION

Description

Malnutrition is an excess, deficit, or imbalance of the essential components of a balanced diet. Malnutrition is also described as undernutrition or overnutrition. *Undernutrition* describes a state of poor nourishment as a result of inadequate diet or diseases that interfere with normal appetite and assimilation of ingested foods. *Overnutrition* refers to the ingestion of more food than is required for body needs, as in obesity.

■ The incidence of malnutrition in hospitalized patients is about 30%. The prevalence of malnutrition in older long-term care residents ranges from 37% to 62%.

Pathophysiology

Protein-calorie malnutrition (PCM) is the most common form of undernutrition and can result from primary (nutritional needs not

M

being met) or secondary (alteration or defect in ingestion, digestion, absorption, or metabolism) factors. Secondary malnutrition
may occur as a result of gastrointestinal (GI) obstruction, surgical
procedures, cancer, malabsorption syndromes, drugs, or infectious
diseases.

- In the initial process of starvation, the body's selective use
  of carbohydrates (glycogen) rather than fat and protein to
  meet metabolic needs will deplete glycogen stores within 18
  hours.
- When carbohydrate stores are depleted, skeletal protein
  begins to be converted to glucose for energy, resulting in a
  negative nitrogen balance. However, within 5 to 9 days,
  body fat is mobilized to supply needed energy.
- In prolonged starvation up to 97% of calories are provided
  by fat, and protein is conserved. Depletion of fat stores
  depends on the amount available, but fat stores are generally
  used up in 4 to 6 weeks. Once fat stores are used, body
  proteins, including those in internal organs and plasma, can
  no longer be spared and rapidly decrease because they are
  the only remaining body source of available energy.
- When the diet is extremely deficient in calories and
  essential proteins, the sodium-potassium exchange pump
  fails, leaving sodium inside the cell (along with water
  causing cell expansion), and potassium levels in extracellular fluid rise.
- The liver is the body organ that loses the most mass during
  protein deprivation. It gradually becomes infiltrated with fat
  secondary to decreased synthesis of lipoproteins. Immediate
  restoration to a diet of protein and other necessary constituents must be instituted or death rapidly ensues.

Clinical Manifestations

Malnutrition signs range from mild to emaciation and death. The
most obvious clinical signs on physical examination are apparent
in the skin (dry and scaly skin, brittle nails, rashes, hair loss),
mouth (crusting and ulceration, changes in tongue), muscles
(decreased mass and weakness), and CNS (mental changes such as
confusion, irritability).

- The person is susceptible to infection. Both humoral
  and cell-mediated immunity are deficient in PCM. There is
  a decrease in leukocytes in the peripheral blood. Phagocytosis is altered as a result of the lack of energy necessary to
  drive the process. Many malnourished persons are also
  anemic.

Diagnostic Studies

- Serum albumin, prealbumin, and transferrin levels are decreased.
- Serum potassium (K^+) is often elevated.
- Red blood cell (RBC) count and hemoglobin (Hb) levels indicate the presence and degree of anemia.
- White blood cell (WBC) count and total lymphocyte count are decreased.
- Liver enzyme studies may be elevated.
- Anthropometric measurements help evaluate response to therapy.

Collaborative Care

Early management of uncomplicated PCM is usually achieved without hospitalization by means of a diet high in calories and protein and by close supervision. In severe PCM the patient may be hospitalized for correction of fluid and electrolyte imbalances and for infections secondary to a compromised immune system. Enteral feedings, both oral and tube, can be used to supplement the diet. In cases of severe PCM, parenteral nutrition (PN) may be initiated (see Enteral Nutrition, p. 731, and Parenteral Nutrition, p. 752).

Nursing Management

Goals

The patient with malnutrition will achieve weight gain, consume a specified number of calories per day (with a diet individualized for the patient), and have no adverse consequences related to malnutrition or nutrition therapies.

Nursing Diagnoses

- Imbalanced nutrition: less than body requirements
- Self-care deficit (feeding)
- Constipation or diarrhea
- Deficient fluid volume
- Risk for impaired skin integrity
- Activity intolerance

Nursing Interventions

Assess the patient's nutritional status, as well as focus on the other physical problems of the patient. Identify patients who are at risk, why they are at risk, and how to intervene appropriately.

- Daily weight can give an ongoing record of body weight gain or loss. The body weight, in conjunction with accurate recording of food and fluid intake, provides a picture of the patient's fluid and nutritional state.
- You and the dietitian can assist the patient and caregiver in the selection of high-calorie and high-protein foods.

M

- Provide between-meal supplements for the undernourished patient. If the patient is unable to consume enough nutrition with a high-calorie, high-protein diet, oral liquid nutrition supplements can be added.
- Encourage the family to bring the patient's favorite food while the patient is hospitalized.
- Some patients may benefit from appetite stimulants, such as megestrol acetate (Megace) or dronabinol (Marinol), to improve nutritional intake.

▼ **Patient and Caregiver Teaching**
- Teach the patient and caregiver the importance of good nutrition and the rationale for recording the daily weight, intake, and output.
- Assess the patient's ability to comply with the dietary instructions in light of past eating habits, religious and ethnic preferences, age, income, other resources, and state of health.
- Consider with the patient the availability and acceptability of community resources that provide meals. In discharge planning, ensure proper follow-up such as visits by the home health nurse.

MÉNIÈRE'S DISEASE

Description
Ménière's disease is an inner ear disease characterized by episodic vertigo, tinnitus, aural fullness, and fluctuating sensorineural hearing loss. Symptoms are incapacitating as a result of sudden, severe attacks of vertigo with nausea and vomiting. Symptoms usually begin between ages 30 and 60 years.

Pathophysiology
The cause of the disease is unknown, but it results in an excessive accumulation of endolymph in the membranous labyrinth. The volume of endolymph increases until the membranous labyrinth ruptures, mixing high-potassium endolymph with low-potassium perilymph.

Clinical Manifestations
- Attacks may occur without warning or be preceded by an aura consisting of a sense of fullness in the ear, increasing tinnitus, and muffled hearing.
- The patient may report a whirling sensation and experience the feeling of being pulled to the ground ("drop attack").

- Autonomic symptoms include pallor, sweating, nausea, and vomiting.
- The duration of the attacks may be hours or days, and attacks may occur several times per year. The clinical course is highly variable.
- Low-pitched tinnitus may be present continuously in the affected ear or may be intensified during an attack.
- Hearing loss fluctuates, decreasing with each vertigo attack and eventually leading to permanent hearing loss.

Diagnostic Studies

- Audiogram results demonstrate mild, low-frequency hearing loss.
- Vestibular tests
- Glycerol test supports the diagnosis if hearing improvement occurs.

Nursing and Collaborative Management

During an acute attack, antihistamines, anticholinergics, and benzodiazepines can be used to decrease the abnormal sensation and lessen symptoms such as nausea and vomiting. Acute vertigo is treated symptomatically with bed rest, sedation, and antiemetics or antivertigo drugs for motion sickness. Diazepam (Valium), meclizine (Antivert), and fentanyl with droperidol (Innovar) may be used to reduce the vertigo. Most patients respond to the prescribed medications but must learn to live with the unpredictability of the attacks and the loss of hearing.

- During an acute attack a patient needs reassurance that the condition is not life threatening.
- Focus on providing only essential care, because movement aggravates vertigo.
- Side rails should be up and the bed in low position if the patient is in bed. Avoid the use of lights and TV, which exacerbate symptoms. Have an emesis basin available because vomiting is common. Assist with ambulation because unsteadiness remains after an attack.

Management between attacks may include calcium channel blockers, diuretics, antihistamines, and a low-sodium diet.

With frequent incapacitating attacks and reduced quality of life, surgical therapy is indicated. Surgical options include endolymphatic shunt, vestibular nerve resection, and labyrinth ablation. Careful management can decrease the possibility of progressive sensorineural loss in many patients.

M

MENINGITIS

Description

Meningitis is an acute inflammation of the meningeal tissues surrounding the brain and spinal cord. Meningitis specifically refers to infection of the arachnoid mater and cerebrospinal fluid (CSF). Bacterial meningitis is considered a medical emergency; if it is left untreated, the mortality rate approaches 100%. See Table 37, p. 210, for a comparison of meningitis and encephalitis.

Pathophysiology

Meningitis usually occurs in the fall, winter, or early spring and is often secondary to viral respiratory disease. *Streptococcus pneumoniae* and *Neisseria meningitidis* are the leading causes of bacterial meningitis. Organisms usually gain entry to the central nervous system (CNS) through the upper respiratory tract or bloodstream, but they may enter by direct extension from penetrating wounds of the skull or through fractured sinuses in basal skull fractures.

The inflammatory response to the infection tends to increase CSF production with a moderate increase in intracranial pressure (ICP). The purulent secretion produced by bacteria quickly spreads to other areas of the brain through the CSF.

- All patients with meningitis must be observed closely for manifestations of increased ICP, which is thought to be a result of swelling around the dura and increased CSF volume. (See Increased Intracranial Pressure, p. 352).

Clinical Manifestations

Fever, severe headache, nausea, vomiting, and nuchal rigidity (resistance to flexion of the neck) are essential signs.

- Photophobia, a decreased level of consciousness (LOC), and signs of increased ICP may also be present.
- If the infecting organism is a meningococcus, a skin rash is common and petechiae may be seen.
- Seizures occur in one third of all cases of meningitis.
- Coma is associated with a poor prognosis and occurs in 5% to 10% of patients with bacterial meningitis.

Complications

In bacterial meningitis, cranial nerve dysfunction, which usually disappears within a few weeks, often occurs with cranial nerves III, IV, VI, VII, or VIII.

- Cranial nerve irritation can have serious sequelae; the optic nerve (CN II) is compressed by increased ICP. Papilledema is often present, and blindness may occur.
- When the oculomotor (CN III), trochlear (CN IV), and abducens (CN VI) nerves are irritated, ocular movements are affected. Ptosis, unequal pupils, and diplopia are common.
- Irritation of the trigeminal nerve (CN V) is evidenced by sensory losses and loss of the corneal reflex, with irritation of the facial nerve (CN VII) resulting in facial paresis. Irritation of the vestibulocochlear nerve (CN VIII) causes tinnitus, vertigo, and deafness.
- Hemiparesis, dysphasia, and hemianopsia may also occur, with these signs resolving over time.
- Acute cerebral edema may occur with bacterial meningitis, causing seizures, optic nerve palsy, bradycardia, hypertensive coma, and death.
- Headaches may occur for months after the diagnosis of meningitis until the irritation and inflammation have completely resolved.
- A noncommunicating hydrocephalus may occur if the exudate causes adhesions that prevent the normal flow of the CSF from the ventricles. CSF reabsorption by the arachnoid villi may also be obstructed by the exudate. Surgical implantation of a shunt is the only treatment.
- A complication of meningococcal meningitis is the Waterhouse-Friderichsen syndrome. The syndrome is manifested by petechiae, disseminated intravascular coagulation (DIC), and adrenal hemorrhage.

Diagnostic Studies

Diagnosis is usually verified by doing a lumbar puncture with analysis of the CSF.

- CSF protein levels are usually elevated and higher in bacterial than in viral meningitis. CSF glucose concentration is commonly decreased in bacterial meningitis but may be normal in viral meningitis. CSF is purulent and turbid in bacterial meningitis; it may be the same or clear in viral meningitis.
- CSF, sputum, and nasopharyngeal secretions are used to identify the causative organism.
- Skull x-rays may detect infected sinuses.
- Computed tomography (CT) scans may reveal increased ICP or hydrocephalus.

M

Collaborative Care

A rapid diagnosis based on a history and physical examination is crucial because the patient is usually in a critical state when health care is sought. When meningitis is suspected, antibiotic therapy is instituted after the collection of specimens for cultures, even before the diagnosis is confirmed. Penicillin, ampicillin, vancomycin, and a third-generation cephalosporin (e.g., ceftriaxone [Rocephin] or cefotaxime [Claforan]) are common drugs of choice to treat bacterial meningitis. Dexamethasone may be prescribed before or with the first dose of antibiotics to decrease mortality rate and reduce the incidence of hearing loss in patients with bacterial meningitis.

Nursing Management

Goals

The patient with meningitis will have a return to maximal neurologic functioning, resolution of infection, and control of pain and discomfort.

See NCP 57-2 for the patient with bacterial meningitis, Lewis et al., *Medical-Surgical Nursing,* ed. 8, p. 1454.

Nursing Diagnoses/Collaborative Problems

- Ineffective intracranial adaptive capacity
- Risk for ineffective cerebral tissue perfusion
- Disturbed sensory perception
- Acute pain
- Hyperthermia
- Potential complication: seizure activity

Nursing Interventions

Prevention of respiratory infections through vaccination programs for pneumococcal pneumonia and influenza is very important. A vaccine is available for protection against *Neisseria meningitidis* and is recommended for children and adolescents ages 11 or 18 years. In addition, early and vigorous treatment of respiratory and ear infections is important. Persons who have close contact with anyone who has meningitis should be given prophylactic antibiotics.

The patient with meningitis is acutely ill. The fever is high, and head pain is severe. Irritation of the cerebral cortex may result in seizures with changes in mental status and LOC dependent on the level of ICP.

- Assessment of vital signs, neurologic evaluation, fluid intake and output, and evaluation of lung fields and skin should be performed at regular intervals based on the patient's condition.

- Head and neck pain secondary to movement requires attention. Codeine provides some pain relief without undue sedation for most patients. A darkened room and cool cloth over the eyes relieve the discomfort of photophobia. For the delirious patient, additional low lighting may be necessary to decrease hallucinations.
- All patients suffer some degree of mental distortion and hypersensitivity and may be frightened and misinterpret the environment. Make every attempt to minimize environmental stimuli and the resulting exaggerated perception.

If seizures occur, take protective measures. Antiseizure medications are administered as ordered. Problems associated with increased ICP need to be managed (see Increased Intracranial Pressure, p. 352). Avoid restraints if possible. The presence of a familiar person at the bedside may have a calming effect.

Fever must be vigorously managed because it increases cerebral edema and the frequency of seizures. Aspirin or acetaminophen may be used to reduce fever. If the fever is resistant to aspirin or acetaminophen, more vigorous means are necessary, such as an automatic cooling blanket. If a cooling blanket is not available, tepid sponge baths with water may be effective. Because high fever greatly increases the metabolic rate, the patient should be assessed for dehydration and adequacy of intake. Supplemental feedings to maintain adequate nutritional intake by means of tube or oral feedings may be necessary.

- Meningitis generally requires respiratory isolation until the cultures are negative. Meningococcal meningitis is highly contagious, whereas other causes of meningitis may pose a minimal to no infection risk with patient contact.
- After the acute period has passed, stress the importance of good nutrition with an emphasis on a high-protein, high-caloric diet in small, frequent feedings.
- Muscle rigidity may persist in the neck and backs of the legs. Progressive range-of-motion (ROM) exercises and warm baths are useful. Have the patient gradually increase activity as tolerated, but encourage adequate rest and sleep.
- Residual effects can result in sequelae such as dementia, seizures, deafness, hemiplegia, and hydrocephalus. Assess vision, hearing, cognitive skills, and motor and sensory abilities after recovery with appropriate referrals as indicated.
- Throughout the acute and convalescent periods, be aware of the anxiety and stress experienced by individuals close to the patient.

M

METABOLIC SYNDROME

Description

Metabolic syndrome, also known as *syndrome X, insulin resistance syndrome,* and *dysmetabolic syndrome,* is a collection of risk factors that increase an individual's chance of developing cardiovascular disease and diabetes mellitus. It is estimated that about 25% of Americans have metabolic syndrome.

Pathophysiology

The main underlying risk factor for metabolic syndrome is insulin resistance. In insulin resistance the body's cells have a diminished ability to respond to the action of insulin. To compensate, the pancreas secretes more insulin, thus resulting in hyperinsulinemia (Fig. 10). Most people with metabolic syndrome are overweight or obese. African Americans, Hispanics, American Indians, and Asians are at an increased risk for metabolic syndrome.

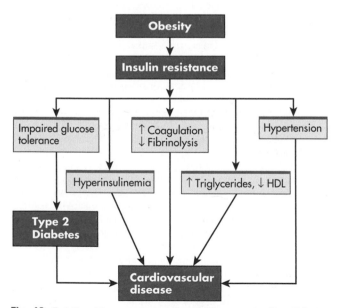

Fig. 10. Relationship among insulin resistance, obesity, diabetes mellitus, and cardiovascular disease.

- Patients diagnosed with metabolic syndrome typically have diabetes and cannot maintain a proper level of glucose, have hypertension, and secrete a large amount of insulin, or who have survived a heart attack and have hyperinsulinemia.

Clinical Manifestations

Signs of metabolic syndrome include impaired fasting blood glucose, hypertension, abnormal cholesterol levels, and obesity. Patients with this syndrome are at a higher risk of developing heart disease, stroke, diabetes, renal disease, and polycystic ovary syndrome.

Nursing and Collaborative Management

Lifestyle modifications are the first-line interventions to reduce the risk factors for metabolic syndrome. Management or reversal of metabolic syndrome can be achieved by reducing the major risk factors of cardiovascular disease: reducing LDL cholesterol, smoking cessation, lowering BP, and reducing glucose levels. For long-term risk reduction, weight should be decreased, physical activity increased, and healthy dietary habits established.

Nurses should assist patients by providing information on healthy diets, exercise, and positive lifestyle changes. Although there is no specific medication for metabolic syndrome, cholesterol lowering medication and antihypertensives can be used. Metformin (Glucophage) has also been used to prevent diabetes by lowering glucose levels and enhancing the cells' sensitivity to insulin.

MULTIPLE MYELOMA

Description

Multiple myeloma, or plasma cell myeloma, is a condition in which neoplastic plasma cells infiltrate the bone marrow and destroy bone. The disease is twice as common in men as in women and usually develops after age 40 years. Although it was previously not considered curable, many patients are living 7 or more years because of the variety of treatments that can be provided throughout the course of the disease.

Pathophysiology

The cause of multiple myeloma is unknown. Exposure to radiation, organic chemicals (e.g., benzene), herbicides, and insecticides may play a role. Genetic factors and viral infection may also influence the risk of developing multiple myeloma.

M

The disease process involves the excessive production of plasma cells that infiltrate the bone marrow and produce abnormal and excessive amounts of immunoglobulins (usually IgG [most common], IgA, IgD, and IgE). The abnormal immunoglobulin is known as myeloma protein.

Production of excessive and abnormal amounts of interleukins (IL-4, IL-5, IL-6) also contributes to the pathologic process of bone destruction. The body's normal immune response is compromised by the reduction of normal plasma cells. In some patients, excessive production and secretion of free light-chain proteins (called *Bence Jones* proteins) from the myeloma cell is also seen and can be detected in the urine.

- Ultimately the end-organ effects of myeloma are seen in the bones and kidneys and possibly the spleen, lymph nodes, and liver.

Clinical Manifestations

Multiple myeloma develops slowly and insidiously.

- The patient often does not manifest symptoms until the disease is advanced, at which time skeletal pain is the major symptom. Pain in the pelvis, spine, and ribs is common.
- Diffuse osteoporosis develops as the myeloma protein destroys more bone. Osteolytic lesions are seen in the skull, vertebrae, and ribs. Vertebral destruction can lead to vertebral collapse with compression of the spinal cord.
- Loss of bone integrity can lead to the development of pathologic fractures. Bony degeneration causes calcium loss from bones, resulting in hypercalcemia. Hypercalcemia may cause renal, gastrointestinal (GI), or neurologic changes, such as polyuria, anorexia, confusion, and ultimately seizures, coma, and cardiac problems.
- High protein levels caused by the myeloma protein can result in renal failure from renal tubular obstruction and interstitial nephritis.
- The patient may display symptoms of anemia, thrombocytopenia, and granulocytopenia, all of which are related to the replacement of normal bone marrow with plasma cells.

Diagnostic Studies

- Pancytopenia, hyperuricemia, hypercalcemia, and elevated creatinine may be found.
- Monoclonal (M) antibody protein is found in blood and urine.
- Bence Jones protein is often found in urine.
- Bone marrow analysis shows significantly increased numbers of plasma cells.

- X-rays show distinct areas of bone erosions, generalized thinning of the bones, and/or fractures, especially in the vertebrae, ribs, pelvis, and bones of the thigh and upper arms.
- The simplest measure of prognosis in multiple myeloma is based on blood levels of two markers: β_2-microglobulin and albumin. In general, higher levels of these two markers are associated with a poorer prognosis.

Collaborative Care

The therapeutic approach involves managing both the disease and its symptoms. Multiple myeloma is seldom cured, but treatment can relieve symptoms, produce remission, and prolong life. Current treatment options include "watchful waiting" (for early multiple myeloma), chemotherapy, biologic therapy, and hematopoietic stem cell transplantation (HSCT).

Ambulation and adequate hydration are used to treat hypercalcemia, dehydration, and potential renal damage. Weight bearing helps the bones reabsorb some calcium, and fluids dilute calcium and prevent protein precipitates from causing renal tubular obstruction.

Control of pain and prevention of pathologic fractures are other goals of collaborative care. Analgesics, orthopedic supports, and localized radiation help reduce skeletal pain.

Chemotherapy with corticosteroids is usually the first treatment recommended and is used to reduce the number of plasma cells (see Chemotherapy, p. 717). High-dose chemotherapy followed by autologous HSCT has evolved as the standard of care in eligible patients. α-Interferon has been used after chemotherapy. Radiation therapy is another important component of treatment, primarily because of its effect on localized lesions.

Surgical procedures, such as vertebroplasty, may be done to support degenerative vertebrae. Bisphosphonates, such as pamidronate (Aredia), zoledronic acid (Zometa), and etidronate (Didronel), inhibit bone breakdown and are used for skeletal pain and hypercalcemia.

- Drugs may be used to treat the complications of multiple myeloma. For example, allopurinol (Zyloprim) may be given to reduce hyperuricemia, and intravenous (IV) furosemide (Lasix) promotes renal excretion of calcium.

Nursing Management

Maintaining adequate hydration is a primary nursing consideration to minimize problems from hypercalcemia. Fluids are administered to attain a urinary output of 1.5 to 2 L/day. Because of the myeloma

M

proteins, the patient is at additional risk of renal dysfunction. You need to monitor electrolytes and fluid balance.

Because of the potential for pathologic fractures, you must be careful when moving and ambulating the patient. A slight twist or strain in the wrong area (e.g., weak area in patient's bones) may be sufficient to cause a fracture.

Pain management requires innovative and knowledgeable nursing interventions. Analgesics, such as nonsteroidal anti-inflammatory drugs (NSAIDs), acetaminophen, or acetaminophen with codeine, may be more effective than opioids alone in diminishing bone pain. Braces, especially for the spine, may also help control pain.

- Assessment and prompt treatment of infection are important. Hematologic function is impaired as a result of the disease and effects of treatment. Nursing care presented in NCP 31-1, pp. 664 to 665; NCP 31-2, p. 683; and NCP 31-3, p. 693, Lewis et al., *Medical-Surgical Nursing,* ed. 8 applies to the patient with multiple myeloma.
- The patient's psychosocial needs require sensitive, skilled management. As with leukemia (see Leukemia, p. 396), it is important to help the patient and significant others adapt to changes fostered by chronic illness and adjust to the losses related to the disease process.
- The way in which patients and caregivers deal with confronting death may be affected by the manner in which they have learned to accept and live with the chronic nature of the disease.

MULTIPLE SCLEROSIS

Description

Multiple sclerosis (MS) is a chronic, progressive, degenerative disorder of the central nervous system (CNS) characterized by demyelination of the nerve fibers of the brain and spinal cord. MS is considered a disease of young to middle-age adults, with the onset usually being between 20 and 50 years of age. Women are affected more often than men.

- Incidence of MS is highest in temperate climates (between 45 and 65 degrees of latitude), such as those found in Europe, Canada, and the northern United States, as compared with tropical regions.

Pathophysiology

The cause of MS is unknown, although research findings suggest MS is related to infectious (viral), immunologic, and genetic factors and perpetuated as a result of intrinsic factors (e.g., faulty immunoregulation). Susceptibility to MS appears to have an inherited tendency; first-, second-, and third-degree relatives of patients with MS are at a slightly increased risk. Possible precipitating factors include infection, physical injury, emotional stress, excessive fatigue, and pregnancy.

MS is characterized by chronic inflammation, demyelination, and gliosis (scarring) in the CNS. The primary neuropathologic condition is an autoimmune disease caused by autoreactive T cells (lymphocytes). A virus in genetically susceptible individuals may initially trigger this process. The activated T cells migrate to the CNS. This is likely the initial event in the development of MS. Subsequent antigen–antibody reaction within the CNS results in an inflammatory response and leads to axon demyelination.

- The disease process consists of loss of myelin, disappearance of oligodendrocytes, and proliferation of astrocytes.
- Early in the disease the damaged myelin can regenerate, the symptoms will disappear, and the patient experiences a remission.
- In addition to myelin disruption, the axon also becomes involved. Myelin is replaced by glial scar tissue, which forms hard, sclerotic plaques in multiple regions of the CNS. Without myelin, nerve impulses slow down.
- With destruction of nerve axons, impulses are totally blocked, resulting in permanent loss of function. In many chronic lesions, demyelination continues with progressive loss of nerve function.

Clinical Manifestations

Because the onset is often insidious and gradual, with vague symptoms that occur intermittently over months or years, the disease may not be diagnosed until long after the onset of the first symptom.

- Because the disease process has a spotty distribution in the CNS, signs and symptoms vary over time. The disease is characterized by chronic progressive deterioration in some persons and remissions and exacerbations in others. Clinical manifestations vary according to areas of the CNS involved. A classification scheme of MS by clinical course has been developed (Table 63).
- Common signs and symptoms include motor, sensory, cerebellar, and emotional problems.

M

Table 63	Clinical Courses of Multiple Sclerosis
Category	**Characteristics**
Relapsing-remitting	Clearly defined relapses with full recovery or sequelae and residual deficit on recovery.
	Approximately 85% of people are initially diagnosed with this type of MS.
Primary-progressive	Slowly worsening neurologic function from the beginning with no distinct relapses or remissions.
	About 10% of people are diagnosed with this type of MS.
Secondary-progressive	A relapsing-remitting initial course, followed by progression with or without occasional relapses, minor remissions, and plateaus.
	New treatments may be slowing this progression.
	About 50% of people with relapsing remitting MS develop this type within 10 years.
Progressive-relapsing	Progressive disease from onset, with clear acute relapses, with or without full recovery; periods between relapses are characterized by continuing progression.
	Only 5% of people experience this type of MS.

- Motor symptoms include weakness or paralysis of the limbs, trunk, or head; diplopia; and spasticity of muscles.
- Sensory symptoms include numbness and tingling, patchy blindness (scotomas), blurred vision, vertigo, tinnitus, decreased hearing, and chronic neuropathic pain.
- Cerebellar signs include nystagmus, ataxia, dysarthria, and dysphagia.
- Bowel and bladder function can be affected if the sclerotic plaque is located in the areas of the CNS that control elimination. Problems usually include constipation and a spastic (uninhibited) bladder.

- Sexual dysfunction occurs in many persons. Physiologic erectile dysfunction may result from spinal cord involvement in men. Women may experience decreased libido, difficulty with orgasmic response, painful intercourse, and decreased vaginal lubrication.
- Persons may experience anger, depression, or euphoria. Signs and symptoms are aggravated or triggered by physical and emotional trauma, fatigue, and infection.

The average life expectancy after the onset of symptoms is more than 25 years. Death usually occurs because of the infectious complications (e.g., pneumonia) of immobility or because of unrelated disease.

Diagnostic Studies

Because there is no definitive diagnostic test for MS, the diagnosis is based primarily on the history, clinical manifestations, and presence of multiple sclerotic plaques identified by magnetic resonance imaging (MRI). Laboratory tests are adjuncts to the clinical examination.

- Cerebrospinal fluid (CSF) analysis may show an increase in immunoglobulin G (IgG) or a high number of lymphocytes and monocytes.
- Evoked potential response testing results are often delayed as a result of decreased nerve conduction from the eye and ear to the brain.
- MRI may be helpful because sclerotic plaques as small as 3 to 4 mm in diameter can be detected. Characteristic white-matter lesions scattered through the brain or spinal cord may also be evident.

Collaborative Care

Because there is currently no cure for MS, collaborative care is aimed at treating the disease process and providing symptomatic relief. The disease process is treated with drugs, and the symptoms are controlled with a variety of medications and other therapy.

Drug Therapy

- Adrenocorticotropic hormone (ACTH), methylprednisolone (Medrol), and prednisone are helpful in treating acute exacerbations.
- Immunomodulator drugs help modify disease progression and prevent relapses. These drugs include interferon β-1b (Betaseron), interferon β-1a (Avonex, Rebif), glatiramer acetate (Copaxone), and natalizumab (Tysabri),

M

■ Immunosuppressive drugs, such as azathioprine (Imuran), methotrexate, mitoxantrone (Novantrone), and cyclophosphamide (Cytoxan), have been shown to produce some beneficial effects in patients with MS.

Many other drugs are used to treat the symptoms of MS. Antispasmodics are used for spasticity. Amantadine (Symmetrel), CNS stimulants (pemoline [Cylert], methylphenidate [Ritalin], and modafinil [Provigil]) are used for fatigue. Anticholinergics are used to treat bladder symptoms. Donepezil (Aricept), an acetylcholinesterase inhibitor, is used to treat cognitive impairment. Tricyclic antidepressants and antiseizure medications are used for chronic pain. Table 59-15, Lewis et al., *Medical-Surgical Nursing,* ed. 8, p. 1503 lists drugs used for symptomatic treatment of MS.

Other Therapy

Surgery (e.g., neurectomy, rhizotomy, cordotomy), dorsal-column electrical stimulation or intrathecal baclofen (Lioresal) delivered by pump may be required if spasticity is not controlled with antispasmodics.

Tremors that become unmanageable with medication are sometimes treated by thalamotomy or deep brain stimulation.

Neurologic dysfunction sometimes improves with physical therapy and speech therapy.

Nutritional Therapy

A nutritious, well-balanced diet is essential. Although there is no standard prescribed diet, a high-protein diet with supplementary vitamins is often advocated. A diet high in roughage may help relieve constipation.

Nursing Management

Goals

The patient with MS will maximize neuromuscular function, maintain independence in activities of daily living for as long as possible, manage disabling fatigue, optimize psychosocial well-being, adjust to the illness, and reduce factors that precipitate exacerbations.

See NCP 59-3 for the patient with multiple sclerosis, Lewis et al., *Medical-Surgical Nursing,* ed. 8, pp. 1505 to 1506.

Nursing Diagnoses

■ Impaired physical mobility
■ Impaired urinary elimination
■ Sexual dysfunction
■ Interrupted family processes
■ Ineffective self-health management

Nursing Interventions

The patient with MS should be aware of triggers that may cause exacerbations or worsening of the disease. Exacerbations of MS are triggered by infection (especially upper respiratory infections), trauma, childbirth, stress, fatigue, and climatic changes. Assist the patient to identify particular triggers and develop ways to avoid them or minimize their effects.

- During the diagnostic phase the patient needs reassurance that even though there is a tentative diagnosis of MS, certain diagnostic studies must be made to rule out other neurologic disorders. The patient with recently diagnosed MS may need assistance with the grieving process.
- During an acute exacerbation the patient may be immobile and confined to bed. The focus of nursing intervention at this phase is to prevent the hazards of immobility, such as respiratory and urinary tract infections and pressure ulcers.

▼ **Patient and Caregiver Teaching**

- Focus teaching on building a general resistance to illness. This includes avoiding fatigue, extremes of heat and cold, and exposure to infection.
- It is important to teach the patient to achieve a good balance of exercise and rest, eat nutritious and well-balanced meals, and avoid the hazards of immobility (contractures and pressure sores).
- Patients should know their treatment regimens, the side effects of drugs, and drug interactions with over-the-counter medications.
- Some patients may need to be taught self-catheterization to control bladder problems.
- Increasing dietary fiber may help some patients achieve regularity in bowel habits.
- Inform patients about the National Multiple Sclerosis Society, which offers a variety of services to meet the needs of MS patients and their families.

MYASTHENIA GRAVIS

Description

Myasthenia gravis (MG) is an autoimmune disease of the neuro-muscular junction characterized by fluctuating weakness of certain skeletal muscle groups. Women are affected more often than men. The peak age at onset in women is during the childbearing years.

M

Pathophysiology

MG is caused by an autoimmune process in which antibodies are produced that attack acetylcholine (ACh) receptors. A reduction in the number of ACh receptor sites at the neuromuscular junction prevents ACh molecules from attaching to the receptors and stimulating muscle contraction. Anti-ACh receptor antibodies are detectable in the serum of most patients with MG. Thymic tumors are found in about 15% of all patients with MG, and abnormal thymus tissue is found in most others.

Clinical Manifestations

The primary feature is fluctuating weakness of skeletal muscle. Strength is usually restored after a period of rest. The muscles most often involved are those used for moving the eyes and eyelids, chewing, swallowing, speaking, and breathing. The muscles are generally the strongest in the morning and become exhausted with continued activity. By the end of the day, muscle weakness is prominent.

- In 90% of cases, the eyelid muscles or extraocular muscles are involved. Facial mobility and expression can be impaired. There may be difficulty in chewing and swallowing food. Speech is affected, and the voice often fades during long conversations.
- No other signs of neural disorder accompany MG; there is no sensory loss, reflexes are normal, and muscle atrophy is rare.
- The course of the disease is highly variable. Some patients may have short-term remissions, others may stabilize, and still others may have severe progressive involvement. Restricted ocular myasthenia, usually seen only in men, has a good prognosis.
- Exacerbations of MG can be precipitated by emotional stress, pregnancy, menses, secondary illness, trauma, temperature extremes, and hypokalemia. Ingestion of drugs, including β-adrenergic blockers and psychotropic drugs, can aggravate MG.

The major complications of MG result from muscle weakness in areas that affect swallowing and breathing. An acute exacerbation of MG that results in aspiration, respiratory infection, and respiratory insufficiency is known as a *myasthenic crisis*.

Diagnostic Studies

The diagnosis of MG can be made on the basis of history and physical examination.

- Electromyogram (EMG) may show a decremental response to repeated stimulation of the hand muscles, indicative of muscle fatigue.

- The Tensilon test reveals improved muscle contractility after an intravenous (IV) injection of the anticholinesterase agent edrophonium chloride (Tensilon chloride).

Collaborative Care

Drug Therapy

Drug therapy for MG includes anticholinesterase drugs, alternate-day corticosteroids, and immunosuppressants.

- Acetylcholinesterase is the enzyme responsible for the breakdown of ACh in the synaptic cleft. Acetylcholinesterase inhibitors prolong the action of ACh and facilitate transmission of impulses at the neuromuscular junction. Pyridostigmine (Mestinon) is the most successful drug in this group.
- Because of the autoimmune nature of MG, corticosteroids (specifically prednisone) are used to suppress the immune response. Cytotoxic drugs such as azathioprine (Imuran) and cyclophosphamide (Cytoxan) may also be used for immunosuppression.
- Corticosteroids (prednisone) are used to suppress the immune response. Drugs such as azathioprine (Imuran), mycophenolate (CellCept), and cyclosporine (Sandimmune) may also be used for immunosuppression.

Other Therapies

Because the presence of the thymus gland in the patient with MG appears to enhance the production of AChR antibodies, removal of the thymus gland results in improvement in a majority of patients.

- Plasmapheresis can yield a short-term improvement in symptoms, and is indicated for patients in crisis or in preparation for surgery when corticosteroids must be avoided.
- Intravenous (IV) immunoglobulin G has been used with some success and is recommended as a second-line treatment for MG.

Nursing Management

Goals

The patient with MG will have a return of normal muscle endurance, manage fatigue, avoid complications, and maintain a quality of life appropriate to disease course.

Nursing Diagnoses

- Ineffective breathing pattern
- Ineffective airway clearance
- Impaired verbal communication
- Imbalanced nutrition: less than body requirements
- Disturbed sensory perception
- Activity intolerance
- Disturbed body image

M

Nursing Interventions

The patient with MG who is admitted to the hospital usually has a respiratory tract infection or is in acute myasthenic crisis. Nursing care is aimed at maintaining adequate ventilation, continuing drug therapy, and watching for side effects of therapy. You need to be able to distinguish cholinergic from myasthenic crisis because the causes and treatment of the two differ greatly (Table 64).

- As with other chronic illnesses, care focuses on the neurologic deficits and their impact on daily living.
- A balanced diet that can be chewed and swallowed easily should be prescribed. Semisolid foods may be easier to eat than solids or liquids. Scheduling doses of medication so that peak action is reached at mealtime may make eating less difficult.
- Arrange diversional activities that require little physical effort and match the interests of the patient.

▼ **Patient and Caregiver Teaching**

Teaching should focus on the importance of following the medical regimen, potential adverse reactions to specific drugs, planning

Table 64	Comparison of Myasthenic Crisis and Cholinergic Crisis

Myasthenic Crisis	Cholinergic Crisis
Causes	
Exacerbation of myasthenia following precipitating factors or failure to take drug as prescribed or drug dose too low	Overdose of anticholinesterase drugs, resulting in increased ACh at the receptor sites, remission (spontaneous or after thymectomy)
Differential Diagnosis	
Improved strength after IV administration of anticholinesterase drugs; increased weakness of skeletal muscles manifesting as ptosis, bulbar signs (e.g., difficulty in swallowing, difficulty in articulating words), or dyspnea	Weakness within 1 hr after ingestion of anticholinesterase; increased weakness of skeletal muscles manifesting as ptosis, bulbar signs, dyspnea; effects on smooth muscle include pupillary miosis, salivation, diarrhea, nausea or vomiting, abdominal cramps, increased bronchial secretions, sweating, or lacrimation

ACh, Acetylcholine; *IV*, intravenous.

activities of daily living to avoid fatigue, availability of community resources, and complications of the disease and therapy (crisis conditions) and what to do about them.

- Contact with the Myasthenia Gravis Society or an MG support group may be helpful and should be explored.

MYOCARDIAL INFARCTION

Myocardial infarction is a serious manifestation of coronary artery disease and is part of the spectrum referred to as acute coronary syndrome. See Acute Coronary Syndrome, p. 5 for the discussion of this disorder.

MYOCARDITIS

Description

Myocarditis is a focal or diffuse inflammation of the myocardium that has been associated with viruses, bacteria, fungi, radiation therapy, pharmacologic and chemical factors, and autoimmune disorders. Coxsackie A and B viruses are the most common etiologic agents. Myocarditis is frequently associated with acute pericarditis, particularly when it is caused by coxsackievirus B strains.

Pathophysiology

When the myocardium becomes infected, the causative agent invades the myocytes and causes cellular damage and necrosis. The immune response is activated, cytokines and oxygen-free radicals are released, and an autoimmune response occurs, resulting in further destruction of myocytes. Myocarditis results in cardiac dysfunction and possibly dilated cardiomyopathy (see Cardiomyopathy, p. 102).

Clinical Manifestations

Clinical features of myocarditis are variable, ranging from a benign course without overt manifestations to severe heart involvement or sudden cardiac death. Fever, fatigue, malaise, myalgias, pharyngitis, dyspnea, lymphadenopathy, and nausea and vomiting are early systemic manifestations of the viral illness.

- Early cardiac manifestations appear 7 to 10 days after viral infection and include pericardial chest pain with a pericardial friction rub and effusion.

M

- Late cardiac signs relate to the development of heart failure and may include S_3, crackles, jugular venous distention, syncope, peripheral edema, and angina.

Diagnostic Studies

- Electrocardiogram (ECG) changes are often nonspecific and reflect associated pericardial involvement, including diffuse ST segment abnormalities. Dysrhythmias and conduction disturbances may be present.
- Laboratory findings are often inconclusive, with mild to moderate leukocytosis and atypical lymphocytes, increased erythrocyte sedimentation rate (ESR) and C-reactive protein (CRP) levels, elevated levels of myocardial markers such as troponin, and elevated viral titers. (Virus is generally only present in tissue and fluid samples during the initial 8 to 10 days of illness.)
- Histologic confirmation is possible through endomyocardial biopsy. A biopsy done during the initial 6 weeks of acute illness is most diagnostic because this is the period in which lymphocytic infiltration and myocyte damage indicative of myocarditis are present.
- Other studies include the use of echocardiography, nuclear scans, and magnetic resonance imaging (MRI) to evaluate cardiac function.

Collaborative Care

The treatment for myocarditis consists of managing associated cardiac symptoms.

- Digoxin improves myocardial contractility and reduces ventricular rate but is used cautiously in patients with myocarditis because of the increased sensitivity of the heart to the adverse effects of this drug (e.g., dysrhythmias, potential toxicity).
- Angiotensin-converting enzyme (ACE) inhibitors and β-blockers are used if the heart is enlarged or to treat heart failure.
- Diuretics reduce fluid volume and decrease preload. If hypertension is not present, nitroprusside (Nitropress), inamrinone (Inocor), and milrinone (Primacor) may be used to reduce afterload and improve cardiac output by decreasing systemic vascular resistance.

Immunosuppression therapy with agents such as prednisone, azathioprine (Imuran), and cyclosporine may reduce myocardial inflammation and prevent irreversible myocardial damage. Evidence of the success of this therapy is inconclusive, and the use of these agents for the treatment of myocarditis remains controversial.

Nursing Management

Your interventions should focus on assessing for the signs and symptoms of heart failure and instituting measures to decrease cardiac workload (e.g., use of semi-Fowler's position, spaced activity and rest periods, provisions for a quiet environment). Medications that increase the heart's contractility and decrease the preload, afterload, or both require careful monitoring.

The patient may be anxious about the diagnosis of myocarditis, recovery from myocarditis, and therapy. Assess the level of anxiety, institute measures to decrease anxiety, and keep the patient and caregivers informed about the therapeutic plan.

The patient who receives immunosuppressive therapy has additional problems of alterations in immune response with the potential for infection. Monitor for complications and provide the patient with a clean, safe environment by following proper infection control standards.

NAUSEA AND VOMITING

Description

Nausea and vomiting are the most common manifestations of gastrointestinal (GI) diseases. Although each symptom can occur independently, they are closely related and usually treated as one problem. They occur in a wide variety of conditions unrelated to GI disease, including pregnancy, infection, central nervous system (CNS) disorders (e.g., meningitis), cardiovascular problems (e.g., myocardial infarction [MI], heart failure [HF]), metabolic disorders (e.g., diabetes mellitus), side effects of drugs (e.g., chemotherapy, digitalis), and psychologic factors (e.g., stress, fear).

Nausea is a feeling of discomfort in the epigastrium with a conscious desire to vomit. Anorexia usually accompanies nausea and is brought on by unpleasant stimulation involving any of the five senses. Generally, nausea occurs before vomiting. It is related to slowing of gastric motility and emptying.

Vomiting is the forceful ejection of partially digested food and secretions *(emesis)* from the upper GI tract. It is a complex act that results in the forceful ejection of partially digested food and secretions from the upper GI tract.

Pathophysiology

A vomiting center in the brainstem coordinates the multiple components involved in vomiting. Neural impulses reach the vomiting center by way of afferent pathways through branches of the autonomic nervous system. Receptors for these afferent fibers are located in the GI tract, kidneys, heart, and uterus. When stimulated, these receptors relay information to the vomiting center, which initiates the vomiting reflex. The simultaneous closure of the glottis, deep inspiration with contraction of the diaphragm in the inspiratory position, closure of the pylorus, relaxation of the stomach and lower esophageal sphincter, and contraction of the abdominal muscles with increasing intraabdominal pressure force stomach contents up and out of the mouth.

In addition, the chemoreceptor trigger zone (CTZ) located in the brain responds to chemical stimuli of drugs and toxins. Once stimulated (e.g., motion sickness), the CTZ transmits impulses to the vomiting center.

Clinical Manifestations

Signs of severe or prolonged nausea and vomiting include rapid dehydration with loss of essential electrolytes (e.g., potassium [K^+], hydrogen [H^+]). As vomiting persists, there may be severe electrolyte imbalances, loss of extracellular fluid (ECF) volume, decreased plasma volume, and eventual circulatory failure. Metabolic alkalosis may result from loss of gastric hydrochloric acid. Less frequently metabolic acidosis can occur when the contents of the small intestine are vomited. Weight loss may occur in a short time when vomiting is severe.

- The threat of pulmonary aspiration is a concern when vomiting occurs in elderly or unconscious patients or those with other conditions that impair the gag reflex.

Collaborative Care

The goals of management are to determine and treat the underlying cause of nausea and vomiting and provide symptomatic relief. Determining the cause is often difficult because nausea and vomiting are manifestations of many conditions.

Many different drugs are used to treat nausea and vomiting, but they are used with caution until the cause of the vomiting is determined. Drugs may include anticholinergics (e.g., scopolamine), antihistamines (e.g., promethazine [Phenergan]), phenothiazines (e.g., prochlorperazine [Compazine]), and butyrophenones (e.g., droperidol [Inapsine]). Other drugs with antiemetic effects include benzamides (metoclopramide [Reglan]) and 5-HT (serotonin) receptor antagonists (e.g., ondansetron [Zofran]). A comprehensive list of drugs used for nausea and vomiting is included in Table 42-1, Lewis et al., *Medical-Surgical Nursing,* ed. 8, p. 965.

Alternative therapies such as acupressure or acupuncture have been shown to be effective in reducing postoperative nausea and vomiting, and herbs such as ginger and peppermint oil may be used by patients.

The patient with severe vomiting requires intravenous (IV) fluid therapy with electrolyte replacement until able to tolerate oral intake. In some cases a nasogastric (NG) tube and suction are used to decompress the stomach. Once symptoms have subsided, oral nourishment beginning with clear liquids is started. Water is the initial fluid of choice for rehydration. As the condition improves, a diet high in carbohydrates and low in fatty foods is preferred.

Nursing Management
Goals
The patient with nausea and vomiting will experience minimal or no nausea and vomiting, have normal electrolyte levels and hydration status, and return to a normal pattern of fluid balance and nutrient intake.

See NCP 42-1 for the patient with nausea and vomiting, Lewis et al., *Medical-Surgical Nursing,* ed. 8, p. 967.

Nursing Diagnoses
- Nausea
- Deficient fluid volume
- Imbalanced nutrition: less than body requirements

Nursing Interventions
Until a diagnosis is confirmed, the patient is kept on nothing by mouth (NPO) status and given IV fluids. An NG tube connected to suction may be necessary for persistent vomiting. Secure the NG tube to prevent its movement in the nose and back of the throat because this can stimulate nausea and vomiting.

- The environment should be quiet, free of noxious odors, and well ventilated.
- Use of relaxation techniques and diversional tactics may help prevent or relieve nausea and vomiting.
- Cleansing the face and hands with a cool washcloth and providing mouth care between episodes increase the person's comfort level. When symptoms occur, all foods and medications should be stopped until the acute phase is past.

With prolonged vomiting, interventions include recording intake and output with vital signs, assessment for dehydration, positioning to prevent aspiration, and observation for changes in comfort and mentation.

▼ Patient and Caregiver Teaching
- Provide explanations for diagnostic tests and procedures.
- Instruct the patient and caregiver on how to deal successfully with the unpleasant sensations of nausea, methods of preventing

nausea and vomiting, and strategies to maintain fluid and nutritional intake.

- When food is identified as the precipitating cause of nausea and vomiting, help the patient identify the specific food and when it was eaten, prior history with that food, and whether anyone else in the family is sick.

NEPHROTIC SYNDROME

Description

Nephrotic syndrome results when the glomerulus of the kidney is excessively permeable to plasma protein, causing proteinuria and leading to low plasma albumin and tissue edema. Common causes include primary glomerular disease (e.g., focal glomerulonephritis), infections (e.g., hepatitis, streptococcal), neoplasms (e.g., Hodgkin's lymphoma), allergens (e.g., bee sting), drugs (e.g., nonsteroidal antiinflammatory agents [NSAIDs]), and multisystem diseases (e.g., diabetes mellitus [DM]).

Pathophysiology and Clinical Manifestations

The increased glomerular membrane permeability found in nephrotic syndrome is responsible for massive excretion of protein in the urine. This results in decreased serum protein and subsequent edema formation, including ascites and anasarca.

- Diminished plasma oncotic pressure from the decrease in serum proteins stimulates hepatic lipoprotein synthesis, which results in hyperlipidemia. Fat bodies (fatty casts) commonly appear in the urine.
- Immune responses, both humoral and cellular, are altered in nephrotic syndrome. As a result, infection is a major cause of morbidity and mortality.
- Calcium and skeletal abnormalities may occur, including hypocalcemia, blunted calcemic response to parathyroid hormone, hyperparathyroidism, and osteomalacia.
- With nephrotic proteinuria, loss of clotting factors can result in a relative hypercoagulable state. Hypercoagulability with thromboembolism is potentially the most serious complication of nephrotic syndrome. The renal vein is the most commonly involved site for thrombus formation. Pulmonary emboli occur in about 40% of nephrotic patients with thrombosis.

Characteristic manifestations include peripheral edema, massive proteinuria, hyperlipidemia, and hypoalbuminemia. Characteristic blood chemistries include decreased serum albumin, decreased total serum protein, and elevated serum cholesterol.

Collaborative Care

The goals of treatment are to relieve edema and cure or control the primary disease. Management of edema includes the cautious use of angiotensin-converting enzyme (ACE) inhibitors, NSAIDs, low-sodium intake (2 to 3 g/day), and a low to moderate protein diet (0.5 to 0.6 g/kg/day).

- Dietary salt restrictions are essential to managing edema. In some patients, thiazide or loop diuretics may be needed.
- If protein loss exceeds 10 g/24 hr, additional dietary protein may be needed.
- Treatment of hyperlipidemia is often unsuccessful. However, treatment with lipid-lowering agents, such as colestipol (Colestid) and lovastatin (Mevacor), may result in moderate decreases in serum cholesterol levels.
- Corticosteroids and cyclophosphamide (Cytoxan) may be used for the treatment of severe cases. Prednisone has been effective in some persons with early-stage nephrosis, membranous glomerulonephritis, proliferative glomerulonephritis, and lupus nephritis.
- Management of DM and treatment of edema are the only measures used for nephrotic syndrome related to DM.

Nursing Management

The major focus of care is related to edema. It is important to assess edema by weighing the patient daily, accurately recording intake and output, and measuring abdominal girth or extremity size. Comparing this information daily provides you with a tool for assessing the effectiveness of treatment. Clean the edematous skin carefully. Avoid trauma and the effectiveness of diuretic therapy must be monitored.

The patient has the potential to become malnourished from the excessive loss of protein in the urine. Maintaining a low to moderate protein diet that is also low in sodium is not always easy. The patient is usually anorexic; serving small, frequent meals in a pleasant setting may encourage better dietary intake.

- Because the patient is susceptible to infection, measures should be taken to avoid exposure to persons with known infections.
- Support for the patient, in terms of coping with an altered body image, is essential because there is often embarrassment and shame associated with the edematous appearance.

NON-HODGKIN'S LYMPHOMAS

Description

Non-Hodgkin's lymphomas (NHLs) are a heterogeneous group of malignant neoplasms of primarily B- or T-cell origin that affect all ages. B-cell lymphomas constitute about 90% of all NHLs. They are classified according to different cellular and lymph node characteristics. A variety of clinical presentations and courses are recognized, from indolent (slowly developing) to rapidly progressive disease. NHL is the most commonly occurring hematologic cancer and the fifth leading cause of cancer death.

Pathophysiology

The cause of NHLs is usually unknown, but an increased incidence is associated with advanced age, use of immunosuppressive medications, and having received chemotherapy or radiation therapy. Epstein-Barr virus is associated with Burkitt's lymphoma, Hodgkin's lymphoma, and immunoblastic lymphoma. Although there is no hallmark feature in NHL, all NHLs involve lymphocytes arrested in various stages of development.

Clinical Manifestations

NHLs can originate outside the lymph nodes, and the method of spread can be unpredictable. The majority of patients have widely disseminated disease at the time of diagnosis. The primary clinical manifestation is painless lymph node enlargement *(adenopathy)*. Because the disease is usually disseminated when diagnosed, other symptoms are present depending on where the disease has spread (e.g., hepatomegaly with liver involvement, neurologic symptoms with central nervous system disease). NHL can also present nonspecifically with airway obstruction, renal failure, pericardial tamponade, and gastrointestinal complaints.

- Patients with high-grade (very aggressive) lymphomas may have lymphadenopathy and constitutional ("B") symptoms, such as fever, night sweats, and weight loss. The peripheral blood is usually normal, but some lymphomas may occur in a "leukemic" phase.

Diagnostic Studies

Diagnostic studies for NHL resemble those used for Hodgkin's lymphoma. Lymph node biopsy establishes the cell type and pattern. Staging, as described for Hodgkin's lymphoma, is used to guide therapy. The prognosis for NHL is generally not as good as that for Hodgkin's lymphoma.

Nursing and Collaborative Management

Treatment for NHL involves chemotherapy and sometimes radiation therapy (see Chemotherapy, p. 717). Ironically, aggressive lymphomas are more responsive to treatment and more likely to be cured. Indolent lymphomas have a naturally long course but are more difficult to treat effectively.

- Hematopoietic stem cell transplants in NHL may have benefit in certain subtypes with aggressive or refractory lymphoma
- Rituximab (Rituxan), a genetically engineered monoclonal antibody against the CD20 antigen on the surface of normal and malignant B lymphocytes is used to treat NHL.
- Numerous chemotherapy combinations have been used to try to overcome the resistant nature of this disease (see Table 31-30 p. 702, Lewis et al., *Medical-Surgical Nursing*, ed. 8). Rituximab with chemotherapy, such as cyclophosphamide (Cytoxan) with or without prednisone or the CHOP regimen (cyclophosphamide, doxorubicin [Adriamycin], vincristine [Oncovin], prednisone, and rituximab) may be used.
- Complete remissions are uncommon, but the majority of patients respond with improvement in symptoms.
- Other therapies for some types of NHL include the monoclonal antibodies ibritumomab tiuxetan (Zevalin) and tositumomab (Bexxar).

Nursing care for patients with NHL is similar to those with Hodgkin's lymphoma, but NHL is often more extensive and involves specific organs.

- Care is based on managing problems related to the disease (pain, spinal cord compression, tumor lysis syndrome), pancytopenia, and other effects of therapy.
- Because most of these patients receive therapy that is potentially myelosuppressive, nursing care presented in NCPs 31-1, pp. 664 to 665; 31-2, p. 683; and 31-3, p. 693, Lewis et al., *Medical-Surgical Nursing*, ed. 8, applies.
- Psychosocial considerations are very important. Helping the patient and family understand the disease, treatment, and expected and potential untoward side effects is paramount in enlisting their help in the patient's well-being and safety.

OBESITY

Description

Obesity is an abnormal increase in the proportion of fat cells. Obesity has reached epidemic proportions in the United States with the highest prevalence occurring between the ages of 40 to 59 for both men and women. The morbidly obese (>100 pounds overweight) appear to be the fastest growing group. Between the years 2000 and 2005 those considered to be morbidly obese increased by more than 50%. The precentage of Americans greater than age of 20 who are either overweight or obese is 66%.

Classifications of Body Weight and Obesity

The majority of obese persons have primary obesity, which is excess calorie intake for the body's metabolic demands. Others have secondary obesity, which can result from various congenital anomalies, chromosomal anomalies, metabolic problems, or CNS lesions and disorders.

- The degree to which a patient is classified as underweight, healthy (normal) weight, overweight, or obese is assessed by using a body mass index (BMI) chart.
- Waist circumference is another way to assess and classify weight (Table 65).
- The waist-to-hip ratio can also be used to assess the health risks associated with obesity. Health risks increase if the waist circumference is >40 inches in men and >35 inches in women.
- Individuals with fat located primarily in the abdominal area (*apple-shaped body*) are at a greater risk for obesity-related complications than those whose fat is primarily located in the upper legs (*pear-shaped body*).

Pathophysiology

The cause of obesity involves significant genetic/biologic susceptibility factors that are highly influenced by environmental and psychosocial factors.

- Strong evidence of a genetic predisposition to obesity is suggested in studies of twins, adoptees, and families.
- Increased circulating plasma levels of leptin, insulin, ghrelin, and decreased levels of peptide YY interacting at the level of the hypothalamus may be important factors contributing to obesity.
- Adipocytes (fat cells) themselves secrete a number of hormones and cytokines known as adipokines that are altered by visceral fat accumulation.
- Environmental factors include greater access to prepackaged and fast foods, larger portion sizes, lack of physical activity and sedentary recreation, and high-calorie foods that may be more accessible to those of low socioeconomic status.
- The association of food with comfort, reward, pleasure, and fun is a powerful incentive for overeating,

Table 65 Hormones and Peptides in Obesity

Hormone/Peptide	Where Produced	Normal Function	Alteration in Obesity
Leptin	Adipocytes	Suppresses appetite and hunger Regulates eating behavior	Obesity is associated with high levels; leptin resistance develops, thus obese people may lose the effect of appetite suppression
Insulin	Pancreas	Decreases appetite	Frequently have high circulating levels
Ghrelin	Stomach (primarily)	Stimulates appetite ↑ After food deprivation ↓ In response to the presence of food in the stomach	Normal postprandial decline does not occur, which can lead to increased appetite and overeating
Peptide YY	Descending colon and rectum	Inhibits appetite by slowing GI motility and gastric emptying	Circulating levels are decreased; decreased release after eating
Cholecystokinin	Duodenum, Jejunum	Inhibits gastric emptying and sends satiety signals to hypothalamus	Unknown role

GI, Gastrointestinal.

There is a 20% to 40% increase in mortality for both men and women who are overweight in midlife. Many problems occur in obese people at higher rates than people of normal weight including cardiovascular disease, respiratory problems, cancer, diabetes mellitus, and musculoskeletal, gastrointestinal, and liver problems.

Diagnostic Studies

- History and physical examination to reveal extent and duration of obesity.
- Laboratory tests of liver function, fasting glucose level, triglyceride level, and low- and high-density lipoprotein cholesterol levels to assist in evaluating the cause and effects of obesity.
- Classifications of body weight and obesity defined by BMI, standardized height-weight charts, anthropometric measurements, or hip/waist ratio.

Collaborative Care

When no organic cause can be found for obesity, it should be considered a chronic, complex illness. A supervised plan of care should focus on:

- Successful weight loss, requiring a short-term energy deficit
- Successful weight control, requiring long-term behavioral changes

A multipronged approach should be taken with attention to dietary intake, physical activity, behavioral modification, and perhaps drug therapy. Restricting food intake is an essential component for any weight loss or maintenance program. A good weight loss plan should contain foods from the basic food groups (see Table 40-1 Nutritional Therapy in Lewis et al., *Medical-Surgical Nursing,* ed. 8, p. 922). Weight reduction diets found in popular media that advocate the elimination of any one category of foods should be discouraged. A well-balanced, low-calorie diet is essential to weight loss and weight control.

- The loss of 1 to 2 pounds per week is a realistic and healthy goal to set with the patient.
- During normal plateau periods, when no weight is lost for several days to several weeks, patients need encouragement and support to prevent giving up on the weight loss plan.

Daily exercise of at least 30 to 60 minutes per day is an essential part of a weight control program. Walking, swimming, and cycling are good forms of exercise.

- The patient should be encouraged to wear a pedometer to document the recommended goal of 10,000 steps per day.
- Psychologic benefits of exercise include enhanced self-confidence, reduced tension and stress, better quality sleep and

rest, and increased stamina and energy, which are all factors that improve the patient's overall health.

- Behavior therapy to deemphasize the diet and change eating behaviors uses the basic techniques of self-monitoring, stimulus control, and rewards. Persons who have undergone behavior therapy are more successful in maintaining their losses over an extended time than those who do not participate in such training.
- The person who is on a weight control program may be encouraged to join a support or self-help group if the support of others having the same experiences is helpful.

Drug Therapy

Medications have been used in the treatment of obesity as adjuncts to diet, exercise, and behavioral modification. Drugs approved for weight loss can be classified into two categories: those that decrease food intake by reducing appetite or increasing satiety (sense of feeling full after eating) and those that decrease nutrient absorption. Drugs that increase energy expenditure (e.g., ephedrine) are not approved by the Food and Drug Administration for weight loss in the United States.

- Mixed noradrenergic-serotonergic agents are used in weight management. Sibutramine (Meridia) inhibits both serotonin and norepinephrine uptake, thus increasing their levels in the CNS.
- Nutrient absorption-blocking drugs such as orlistat (Xenical) work by blocking fat breakdown and absorption in the intestine.

Drugs will not cure obesity without substantial changes in food intake and increased physical activity. Weight gain occurs when short-term drug therapy is stopped. As with any drug treatment, teach patients about administration and side effects. Discourage the purchase of over-the-counter diet aids.

Surgical Therapy

Bariatric surgery is a surgical procedure that is used to treat obesity. Criteria for bariatric surgery include having a BMI ≥ 40 kg/m^2 or a BMI ≥ 35 kg/m^2 with one or more severe obesity-related medical complications (e.g., hypertension, type 2 diabetes mellitus, heart failure, sleep apnea).

- Bariatric surgeries are categorized as restrictive, malabsorptive, or a combination of restrictive and malabsorptive. In restrictive procedures the stomach is reduced in size (less food eaten), and in malabsorptive procedures the length of the small intestine is decreased (less food absorbed).
- Gastric restrictive surgeries include vertical-banded gastroplasty, adjustable gastric banding, and vertical sleeve gastrectomy; gastric malabsorptive surgeries include biliopancreatic

diversion and biliopancreatic diversion with duodenal switch; a combination procedure is a Roux-en-Y gastric bypass. These surgeries are discussed further on pp. 955 to 957 in Lewis et al., *Medical-Surgical Nursing,* ed. 8.

Cosmetic surgeries may be used to reduce fatty tissue and skinfolds. These procedures include a *lipectomy* (adipectomy) to remove unsightly adipose folds and *liposuction* for cosmetic purposes.

Nursing Management

Goals

The overall goals are that the patient with obesity will modify eating patterns, participate in a regular physical activity program, achieve weight loss to a specified level, maintain weight loss at a specified level, and minimize or prevent health problems related to obesity.

Nursing Diagnoses

- Imbalanced nutrition: more than body requirements
- Impaired skin integrity
- Ineffective breathing pattern
- Chronic low self-esteem
- Health-seeking behaviors

Nursing Interventions

Working closely with other members of the health care team, assist in the planning for and management of the obese patient. You are in a pivotal position to help overweight and obese people deal with negative experiences and educate other health care professionals to prevent bias against overweight patients. It is essential that you have a nonjudgmental approach in helping patients manage their problems related to obesity.

Before selecting a weight loss strategy with the patient, assess motivation because it is essential for a favorable outcome.

Preoperative care for gastric surgery includes planning for special needs of an obese patient, such as the availability of an oversized blood pressure (BP) cuff, oversized bed and chair; and a reinforced trapeze bar. Consideration should be given to questions such as how the patient will be weighed, transported through the hospital, and turned.

Instruct the patient in the proper coughing technique, deep breathing, use of an incentive spirometer, and methods of turning and positioning to prevent pulmonary complications after surgery.

Postoperative care and teaching emphasize facilitating patient respiratory efforts (elevating the head of the bed, turning, coughing, deep breathing), monitoring the abdominal wound for healing, early ambulation, and monitoring nasogastric (NG) tube patency. Extra nurses and other personnel may be necessary to turn and ambulate the patient.

- The patient has considerable abdominal pain after surgery, and pain medications should be given as frequently as necessary during the immediate postoperative period.

- Anticipate and recognize several potential psychologic problems after surgery. Some patients express guilt feelings concerning the fact that the only way they could lose weight was by surgical means rather than by the "sheer willpower" of reduced dietary intake. Be ready to provide support so that the patient does not dwell on negative feelings.

- Discharge teaching includes the importance of strict adherence to a diet high in protein and low in carbohydrates, fat, and roughage, with six small feedings daily, and prompt recognition of complications such as anemia, diarrhea, vitamin deficiencies, and psychiatric problems.

- Reinforce physical activity programs and cognitive training such as self-help support groups or professional counseling to facilitate the patient's adjustment to a new body image and social reintegration.

ORAL CANCER

Description
There are two types of oral cancer: oral cavity cancer, which starts in the mouth, and oropharyngeal cancer, which develops in the part of the throat just behind the mouth (called the oropharynx). Head and neck squamous cell carcinoma (HNSCC) is a term for cancers of the oral cavity, pharynx, and larynx and accounts for 90% of malignant oral tumors. Carcinoma of the lip has the most favorable prognosis of any oral tumor because these cancers are usually diagnosed earlier.

- The 5-year survival rate for all stages of cancer of the oral cavity and pharynx is 59%.

Pathophysiology
Although the definitive cause of oral cancer is unknown, there are a number of predisposing factors, including a diet low in fruits and vegetables, prolonged exposure to sunlight, tobacco use (cigar, cigarette, pipe, snuff), excessive alcohol intake, and chronic irritation, such as from a jagged tooth or poor dental care. Human papillomavirus (HPV) contributes to 30% to 40% of oral cancer cases.

Clinical Manifestations

Common manifestations include:

- *Leukoplakia,* called "smoker's patch," is a whitish precancerous lesion on the mucosa of the mouth or tongue that results from chronic irritation, especially from smoking. The patch becomes keratinized (hard and leathery) and is sometimes described as hyperkeratosis.

- *Erythroplakia,* which is a red velvety patch on the mouth or tongue, is also a precancerous lesion. More than 50% of cases of erythroplakia progress to squamous cell carcinoma.

Later symptoms of oral cancer are pain, dysphagia (difficulty swallowing), and difficulty in moving the jaw (e.g., chewing and speaking).

Cancer of the lip usually appears as an indurated, painless lip ulcer. The first sign of tongue cancer is an ulcer or area of thickening. Soreness or pain of the tongue may occur, especially on eating hot or highly seasoned foods. Later symptoms of tongue cancer include increased salivation, slurred speech, dysphagia, toothache, and earache.

Diagnostic Studies

- Biopsy of suspected lesion with cytologic examination
- Oral exfoliative cytology and toluidine blue test to screen for oral cancer
- Once cancer is diagnosed, computed tomography (CT), magnetic resonance imaging (MRI), and positron emission tomography (PET) are used in staging.

Collaborative Care

Management usually consists of surgery, radiation, chemotherapy, or a combination of these. Surgery remains the most effective treatment. Many of the operations are radical procedures involving extensive resections. Some examples are hemiglossectomy (removal of one half of the tongue), glossectomy (removal of the entire tongue), and radial neck dissection (wide excision of the lymph nodes and their lymphatic channels). A tracheostomy (see Tracheostomy, p. 754) is commonly done with radical neck dissection.

Chemotherapy and radiation are used together when the lesions are more advanced or involve several structures of the oral cavity. Chemotherapy may also be used when surgery and radiation fail or as the initial therapy for smaller tumors (see Chemotherapy, p. 717).

Palliative treatment may be indicated when the prognosis is poor, the cancer is inoperable, or the patient decides against surgery. If it becomes difficult for the patient to swallow, a gastrostomy may be performed to provide adequate nutritional intake and frequent suctioning will be necessary when swallowing becomes difficult.

Nursing Management

Goals

The patient with carcinoma of the oral cavity will have a patent airway, be able to communicate, have adequate nutritional intake to promote wound healing, and have relief of pain and discomfort.

Nursing Diagnoses

- Imbalanced nutrition: less than body requirements
- Chronic pain
- Anxiety
- Ineffective coping
- Ineffective health maintenance

Nursing Interventions

You have a significant role in early detection and treatment of oral cancer. Identify patients at risk (users of tobacco products, alcoholism, poor dental care, pipe smokers) and provide information regarding predisposing factors. Refer any individual with an ulcerative lesion that does not heal within 2 to 3 weeks to a health care provider.

Preoperative care for the patient who is having radical neck dissection involves consideration of the patient's physical and psychosocial needs with a special emphasis on oral hygiene. Assess alcohol intake and implement measures early to assess and treat withdrawal if it is a problem (see Chapter 12, Lewis et al., *Medical-Surgical Nursing*, ed. 8). Explanations and emotional support are of special significance and should include postoperative measures relating to communication and feeding.

Postoperative care for a radical neck dissection focuses on the maintenance of a patent airway, including tracheostomy care and observing for signs of respiratory distress (see NCP 27-1 and NCP 27-2 for the patient with a tracheostomy and the patient with a radical neck surgery, Lewis et al., *Medical-Surgical Nursing*, ed. 8, pp. 532 to 534 and 539 to 540). See Head and Neck Cancer, p. 275, for further discussion and teaching.

OSTEOARTHRITIS

Description

Osteoarthritis (OA), the most common form of joint (articular) disease in North America, is a slowly progressive noninflammatory disorder of the diarthrodial (synovial) joints. Currently 21 million Americans are affected by OA, with the numbers expected to greatly increase as the population ages. Osteoarthritis involves the formation of new joint tissue in response to cartilage destruction.

OA is not considered to be a normal part of the aging process, but aging is one risk factor for disease development. Cartilage destruction can actually begin between the ages of 20 and 30 years, and the majority of adults are affected by age 40. Few patients experience symptoms until after age 50 or 60 years, but more than half of those older than 65 years of age have x-ray evidence of the disease in at least one joint. Women are more often affected than men, and they may have more severe OA. The increased incidence in aging women is believed to result from estrogen reduction at menopause.

- Genetic factors appear to play a significant role in the occurrence of OA. Modifiable risk factors include obesity, which contributes to hip and knee OA. Regular moderate exercise decreases the likelihood of disease development and progression. Anterior cruciate ligament injury, which is associated with quick stops and pivoting as in football and soccer, has been linked to an increased risk of knee OA. Occupations that require frequent kneeling and stooping are also linked to a higher risk of knee OA.

Pathophysiology

OA results from cartilage damage that triggers a metabolic response at the level of the chondrocytes. Progression of OA causes cartilage to gradually become softer, less elastic, and less able to resist wear with heavy use. Continued changes in the cartilage collagen lead to fissuring and erosion of the articular surfaces. Incongruity in joint surfaces creates an uneven distribution of stress across the joint and contributes to a reduction in motion.

Although inflammation is not characteristic of OA, a secondary synovitis may result when phagocytic cells try to rid the joint of small pieces of cartilage torn from the joint surface. These inflammatory changes contribute to the early pain and stiffness of OA. Contact between exposed bony joint surfaces after cartilage has completely deteriorated can occur in later stages of OA.

Clinical Manifestations

Systemic manifestations such as fatigue or fever are not present in OA. This is an important differentiation between OA and inflammatory joint disorders, such as rheumatoid arthritis (Table 66).

Joints. Manifestations of OA range from mild discomfort to significant disability. Joint pain is the predominant symptom of OA. Pain generally worsens with joint use. In the early stages of OA, joint pain is relieved by rest. In advanced disease, however, the patient may complain of pain with rest or experience sleep disruptions resulting from increasing joint discomfort. The pain of OA may be referred to the groin, buttock, or medial side of the thigh or knee. Sitting down becomes difficult, as does rising from a chair when the hips are lower than the knees. As OA develops in intervertebral (apophyseal) joints of the spine, localized pain and stiffness are common.

Unlike pain, which is typically provoked by activity, joint stiffness occurs after periods of rest or static position. Early-morning stiffness is common but generally resolves within 30 minutes, a factor distinguishing OA from inflammatory arthritic disorders.

- Overactivity can temporarily increase stiffness. *Crepitation,* a grating sensation caused by loose particles of cartilage in the joint cavity, can also contribute to stiffness.
- OA usually affects joints asymmetrically. The most commonly involved joints are shown in Fig. 65-2, Lewis et al., *Medical-Surgical Nursing,* ed. 8, p. 1644.

Deformity. Deformity or instability associated with OA is specific to the involved joint. For example, *Heberden's nodes* occur on the distal interphalangeal joints as an indication of osteophyte formation and loss of joint space. *Bouchard's nodes* on the proximal interphalangeal joints indicate similar disease involvement. Heberden's and Bouchard's nodes are often red, swollen, and tender. These bony enlargements do not usually cause significant loss of function.

Knee OA often leads to joint malalignment as a result of cartilage loss in the medial compartment. The patient has a characteristic bow-legged appearance and may develop an altered gait. In advanced hip OA, one of the patient's legs may become shorter because of loss of joint space.

Diagnostic Studies

- A bone scan, computed tomography (CT) scan, or magnetic resonance imaging (MRI) may be useful to diagnose OA. X-rays also confirm disease and monitor the progression of joint damage.
- No laboratory abnormalities or biomarkers are specific diagnostic indicators. The erythrocyte sedimentation rate (ESR) is

| Table 66 | Comparison of Rheumatoid Arthritis and Osteoarthritis |

Parameter	Rheumatoid Arthritis	Osteoarthritis
Age at onset	Young to middle age	Usually >age 40
Gender	Female/male ratio is 2:1 or 3:1; less marked gender difference after age 60	Before age 50, more men than women; after age 50, more women than men
Weight	Lost or maintained weight	Often overweight
Disease	Systemic disease with exacerbations and remissions	Localized disease with variable, progressive course
Affected joints	Small joints first (PIPs, MCPs, MTPs), wrists, elbows, shoulders, knees; usually bilateral, symmetric	Weight-bearing joints of knees and hips, small joints (MCPs, DIPs, PIPs), cervical and lumbar spine; often asymmetric
Pain characteristics	Stiffness lasts 1 hr all day and may decrease with use, pain is variable, may disrupt sleep	Stiffness occurs on arising but usually subsides after 30 min, pain gradually worsens with joint use and disease progression, relieved with rest
Effusions	Common	Uncommon
Nodules	Present, especially on extensor surfaces	Heberden's (DIPs) and Bouchard's (PIPs) nodes
Synovial fluid	WBC count >2000/μL with mostly neutrophils	WBC count <2000/μL (mild leukocytosis)
X-rays	Joint space narrowing and erosion with bony overgrowths, subluxation with advanced disease; osteoporosis related to corticosteroid use	Joint space narrowing, osteophytes, subchondral cysts, sclerosis
Laboratory findings	RF positive in 80% of patients	RF negative
	Elevated ESR, CRP indicative of active inflammation	Transient elevation in ESR related to synovitis

CRP, C-reactive protein; DIP, distal interphalangeal; ESR, erythrocyte sedimentation rate; MCP, metacarpophalangeal; MTP, metatarsophalangeal; PIP, proximal interphalangeal; RF, rheumatoid factor; WBC, white blood cell.

normal except in instances of acute synovitis, when minimal elevations may be noted.

- Synovial fluid analysis allows differentiation between OA and other forms of inflammatory arthritis. In OA, fluid remains clear yellow with few or no signs of inflammation.

Collaborative Care

Therapy focuses on managing pain and inflammation, preventing disability, and maintaining and improving joint function. Nondrug interventions are the foundation of management. Drug therapy serves as an adjunct to nondrug treatments. Symptoms are often managed conservatively for many years, but the patient's loss of joint function, unrelieved pain, and diminished ability to independently perform self-care may require surgery. Arthroscopic surgery to repair cartilage or ligament tears or remove bone bits or cartilage may be effective in OA.

Rest and Joint Protection

The affected joint should be rested during any periods of acute inflammation and maintained in a functional position with splints or braces if necessary. Immobilization should not exceed 1 week because joint stiffness increases with inactivity. The patient may need to modify usual activities or use an assistive device to decrease stress on affected joints.

Heat and Cold Applications

Applications of heat and cold may help reduce complaints of pain and stiffness. Heat therapy is helpful for stiffness, including hot packs, whirlpool, ultrasound, and paraffin wax baths.

Nutritional Therapy and Exercise

If the patient is overweight, a weight reduction program is a critical part of the treatment plan. You should help the patient evaluate the current diet to make appropriate changes. Aerobic conditioning, range of motion exercises, and specific programs for strengthening the quadriceps have been beneficial for many patients with knee OA.

Complementary and Alternative Therapies

Complementary and alternative therapies for symptom management of arthritis have become increasingly popular with patients who have failed to find relief through traditional medical care. Therapies include yoga, acupuncture, massage, guided imagery, and therapeutic touch. Nutritional supplements such as glucosamine and chondroitin may be helpful in some patients for relieving moderate to severe arthritis and improving joint mobility.

Drug Therapy

Drug therapy is based on the severity of the patient's symptoms (see Table 65-3, Lewis et al., *Medical-Surgical Nursing,* ed. 8, pp. 1645 to 1647). The patient with mild to moderate joint pain may receive relief from acetaminophen (Tylenol). The patient may receive up to 1000 mg every 6 hours, with a daily dose not to exceed 4 g. A topical agent such as capsaicin cream (Zostrix) may also be beneficial. It blocks pain by locally interfering with substance P, which is responsible for pain impulse transmission. Other topical over-the-counter products that contain salicylates, camphor, eucalyptus oil, and menthol may also provide temporary pain relief.

For the patient who cannot obtain adequate pain management with acetaminophen, or for the patient with moderate to severe OA pain, a nonsteroidal antiinflammatory drug (NSAID) may provide greater relief. NSAID therapy is typically initiated in low-dose, over-the-counter strengths (e.g., ibuprofen [Motrin], 200 mg up to 4 times per day), with the dose increased as the patient's symptoms indicate. If the patient is at risk for or experiences gastrointestinal (GI) side effects with NSAID use, supplemental treatment with a protective agent such as misoprostol (Cytotec) may be indicated. As an alternative to traditional NSAIDs, treatment with the COX-2 inhibitor celecoxib (Celebrex) may be considered in selected patients.

- Intraarticular injections of corticosteroids may be appropriate for the older patient with local inflammation and effusion. Systemic use of corticosteroids is not indicated and may actually accelerate the disease process.
- Another treatment for mild to moderate knee OA is intraarticular injections of hyaluronic acid (HA). HA is found in normal joint fluid and articular cartilage. Synthetic and naturally occurring HA derivatives (Orthovisc, Synvisc, Supartz, Euflexxa, Hyalgan) are administered in three weekly injections directly into the joint space.
- Medications thought to slow the progression of OA or support joint healing are known as disease-modifying osteoarthritis drugs (DMOADs). A number of drugs are under investigation (e.g., doxycycline [Vibramycin]) with mixed results as to whether they are effective and safe.

Nursing Management
Goals
The patient with OA will maintain or improve joint function through a balance of rest and activity, use joint protection measures to improve activity tolerance, achieve independence in self-care and maintain optimal role function, and use drug and nondrug pain management techniques to manage pain satisfactorily.

Nursing Diagnoses
- Acute and chronic pain
- Insomnia
- Impaired physical mobility
- Self-care deficits
- Imbalanced nutrition: more than body requirements
- Chronic low self-esteem

Nursing Interventions
Community education should focus on decreasing modifiable risk factors for OA through weight loss and the reduction of occupational and recreational hazards. Athletic instruction and physical fitness programs should include safety measures that protect and reduce trauma to the joint structures.

The patient with OA is usually treated on an outpatient basis, often by an interdisciplinary team of health care providers that includes a rheumatologist, a nurse, an occupational therapist, and a physical therapist.

- Drugs are administered for the treatment of pain and inflammation. Nondrug pain management strategies may include massage, the application of heat (thermal packs) or cold (ice packs), relaxation, and guided imagery.
- Splints may be prescribed to rest and stabilize painful or inflamed joints. Once an acute flare has subsided, a physical therapist can provide valuable assistance in planning an exercise program.
- Urge the patient to continue all prescribed therapies at home and also be open to the discussion of new approaches to symptom management.
- Home and work environment modification is essential for patient safety, accessibility, and self-care. Measures include removing scatter rugs, providing rails at the stairs and bathtub, using night-lights, and wearing well-fitting supportive shoes. Assistive devices such as canes, walkers, elevated toilet seats, and grab bars reduce joint load and promote safety.
- Sexual counseling may help the patient and significant other to enjoy physical closeness by introducing the idea of alternate positions and timing for intercourse.

▼ **Patient and Caregiver Teaching**
Patient and caregiver teaching related to OA is an important nursing responsibility in any care setting and is the foundation of successful disease management.

- Provide information about the nature and treatment of the disease, pain management, correct posture and body mechanics, and correct use of assistive devices such as a cane or walker, principles of joint protection and energy conservation, and a therapeutic exercise program.

- You need to assist the patient in developing long-term strategies to manage OA.
- Individualize home management goals to meet the patient's needs. Include the caregiver, family, and significant others in goal setting and teaching.
- Support and understanding of the disease process can be gained through community resources such as the Arthritis Foundation's Self-Help Course (www.arthritis.org).

OSTEOMALACIA

Osteomalacia in the United States is an uncommon condition of adult bone associated with vitamin D deficiency, resulting in bone decalcification and softening. This disease is the same as rickets in children except that the epiphyseal growth plates are closed in the adult.

- Vitamin D is required for absorption of calcium from the intestine. Insufficient vitamin D intake can interfere with the normal bone mineralization, causing failure or insufficient calcification of bone, which results in bone softening.
- Etiologic factors include lack of exposure to ultraviolet rays (which is needed for vitamin D synthesis), GI malabsorption, extensive burns, chronic diarrhea, pregnancy, kidney disease, and drugs such as phenytoin (Dilantin).

The most common clinical features are localized bone pain, difficulty rising from a chair, and difficulty walking. Other manifestations include low back and bone pain, progressive muscular weakness especially in the pelvic girdle, weight loss, and progressive deformities of the spine (kyphosis) or extremities. Fractures are common and demonstrate delayed healing.

Laboratory findings include decreased serum calcium or phosphorus levels, decreased serum 25-hydroxyvitamin D, and elevated serum alkaline phosphatase. X-rays may demonstrate the effects of generalized bone demineralization, especially a loss of calcium in the bones of the pelvis, and the presence of associated bone deformity.

- *Looser's transformation zones* (ribbons of decalcification in bone found on x-ray) are diagnostic of osteomalacia. Significant osteomalacia may exist without demonstrable x-ray changes.

Collaborative care is directed toward the correction of the vitamin D deficiency. Vitamin D_3 (cholecalciferol) and vitamin D_2 (ergocalciferol) can be supplemented, and the patient often shows a dramatic response. Calcium or phosphorus supplements may also be prescribed. Dietary ingestion of eggs, meat, oily fish, and milk and breakfast cereals fortified with calcium and vitamin D is encouraged. Exposure to sunlight (and ultraviolet rays) is also valuable, along with weight-bearing exercise.

OSTEOMYELITIS

Description
Osteomyelitis is a severe infection of the bone, bone marrow, and surrounding soft tissue. The most common infecting microorganism is *Staphylococcus aureus*. A variety of microorganisms can cause osteomyelitis, and aerobic gram-negative bacteria alone or mixed with gram-positive organisms are often found (Table 67).

- Use of antibiotics in conjunction with surgical treatment has significantly reduced the mortality rate and complications associated with osteomyelitis.

Pathophysiology
Infecting microorganisms can invade by indirect or direct entry. The *indirect entry (hematogenous)* of microorganisms in

Table 67	Causative Organisms in Osteomyelitis
Organism	**Possible Predisposing Problem**
Staphylococcus aureus	Pressure ulcer, penetrating wound, open fracture, orthopedic surgery, vascular insufficiency disorders (e.g., diabetes, atherosclerosis)
Staphylococcus epidermidis	Indwelling prosthetic devices (e.g., joint replacements, fracture fixation devices)
Streptococcus viridans	Abscessed tooth, gingival disease
Escherichia coli	Urinary tract infection
Mycobacterium tuberculosis	Tuberculosis
Neisseria gonorrhoeae	Gonorrhea
Pseudomonas	Puncture wounds, IV drug use
Salmonella	Sickle cell disease
Fungi, mycobacteria	Immunocompromised host

osteomyelitis most frequently affects growing bone in boys younger than 12 years old and is associated with their higher incidence of blunt trauma. Adults with vascular insufficiency disorders (e.g., diabetes mellitus) and genitourinary and respiratory infections are at higher risk for a primary infection to spread by way of the blood to the bone. The pelvis, tibia, and vertebrae, which are vascular-rich sites of bone, are the most common sites of infection.

Direct-entry osteomyelitis can occur at any age when there is an open wound (e.g., penetrating wounds, fractures) and microorganisms gain entry to the body. Osteomyelitis may also occur in the presence of a foreign body, such as an implant or an orthopedic prosthetic device (e.g., plate, total joint prosthesis).

After gaining entrance to the bone by way of the blood, the microorganisms then lodge in an area of bone in which circulation slows, usually the metaphysis.

- The microorganisms grow, resulting in increased pressure because of the nonexpanding nature of most bone. This leads to ischemia and vascular compromise of the periosteum.
- Eventually the infection passes through the bone cortex and marrow cavity, ultimately resulting in cortical devasculariza-tion and necrosis. Once ischemia occurs, the bone dies.

The area of devitalized bone eventually separates from surround-ing living bone, forming *sequestra.* Once formed, a sequestrum continues to be an infected island of bone, surrounded by pus and difficult to reach by blood-borne antibiotics or white blood cells (WBCs). Sequestrum may enlarge and serve as a site for microorganisms that spread to other sites, including the lungs and brain. If necrotic sequestrum is not resolved naturally or surgically, it may develop a sinus tract, resulting in a chronic, purulent cutane-ous drainage.

Chronic osteomyelitis is either a continuous, persistent problem (result of inadequate acute treatment) or a process of exacerbations and remission. Granulation tissue turns to scar tissue, and this avascular tissue provides an ideal site for continued microorganism growth and is impenetrable to antibiotics.

Clinical Manifestations

Acute osteomyelitis refers to the initial infection or an infection of less than 1 month in duration.

- Systemic manifestations include fever, night sweats, restless-ness, nausea, and malaise.
- Local manifestations include constant bone pain that is unre-lieved by rest and worsens with activity; swelling, tenderness, and warmth at the infection site; and restricted movement of the affected part.

- Later signs include drainage from the sinus tracts to the skin and/or fracture site.
- *Chronic osteomyelitis* refers to a bone infection that persists for longer than 1 month or an infection that has failed to respond to the initial course of antibiotic therapy.
- Systemic signs may be diminished, with local signs of infection more common, including constant bone pain and swelling, tenderness, and warmth at the infection site.

Diagnostic Studies

- Bone or soft tissue biopsy is the definitive way to determine the causative microorganism.
- Blood and/or wound cultures are frequently positive for microorganisms.
- Elevated WBC and erythrocyte sedimentation rate (ESR) may be found.
- Radiologic signs suggestive of osteomyelitis usually do not appear until 10 days to weeks after the appearance of clinical symptoms, by which time the disease will have progressed.
- Radionuclide bone scans (gallium and indium) are helpful in diagnosis and usually positive in the area of infection.
- Magnetic resonance imaging (MRI) and computed tomography (CT) scans may be used to help identify the extent of the infection including soft tissue involvement.

Collaborative Care

Vigorous and prolonged intravenous (IV) antibiotic therapy is the treatment of choice if bone ischemia has not occurred. If antibiotic therapy is delayed, surgical debridement and decompression are often necessary.

Patients are often discharged to home care with IV antibiotics delivered through a central venous catheter or peripherally inserted central catheter (PICC). IV antibiotic therapy may initially be started in the hospital and continued in the home for 4 to 6 weeks or as long as 3 to 6 months. A variety of antibiotics may be prescribed depending on the microorganism. These drugs include penicillin, nafcillin (Nafcil), neomycin, vancomycin, and cephalexin (Keflex).

- In adults with chronic osteomyelitis, oral therapy with a fluoroquinolone (ciprofloxacin [Cipro]) for 6 to 8 weeks may be prescribed instead of IV antibiotics.
- Oral antibiotic therapy may also be given after IV therapy is complete to ensure resolution of the infection.
- Patient response to drug therapy is monitored through bone scans and ESR tests.

- Surgical treatment for chronic osteomyelitis includes removal of the poorly vascularized tissue and dead bone and extended use of antibiotics. Antibiotic-impregnated polymethylmethacrylate bead chains may also be implanted during surgery.
- Intermittent or constant irrigation of the affected bone with antibiotics may also be initiated.
- Hyperbaric oxygen therapy using 100% oxygen may be administered as an adjunct therapy in refractory cases of chronic osteomyelitis.

Orthopedic prosthetic devices may need to be removed. Muscle flaps or skin grafting provide wound coverage over the dead space (cavity) in the bone. Bone grafts may help to restore blood flow. Amputation of the extremity may be indicated to preserve life or improve quality of life (see Amputation, p. 697).

- Rare complications of osteomyelitis include septicemia, septic arthritis, pathologic fractures, squamous cell carcinoma, and amyloidosis.

Nursing Management
Goals
The patient with osteomyelitis will have satisfactory pain and fever control, not experience any complications associated with osteomyelitis, cooperate with the treatment plan, and maintain a positive outlook on the disease outcome.

A nursing care plan for the patient with osteomyelitis is available on the Evolve website at http://evolve.elsevier.com/Lewis/medsurg.

Nursing Diagnoses
- Acute pain
- Impaired physical mobility
- Ineffective self-health management

Nursing Interventions
Control of infections already in the body (e.g., urinary and respiratory tract) is important in preventing osteomyelitis. Adults who are immunocompromised, have orthopedic devices, and/or have vascular insufficiencies such as diabetes mellitus are especially susceptible.

- Instruct these patients and their families regarding manifestations of osteomyelitis and to immediately report symptoms of bone pain, fever, swelling, and restricted limb movement to the health care provider.

Some immobilization of the affected limb (e.g., splint, traction) is usually indicated to decrease pain. Carefully handle the involved limb to avoid excessive manipulation, which increases pain and may cause a pathologic fracture.

- Assess the patient's pain. Minor to severe pain may be experienced with muscle spasms. Nonsteroidal antiinflammatory drugs (NSAIDs), opioid analgesics, and muscle relaxants may be prescribed.
- Dressings are used to absorb the exudate from draining wounds and to debride devitalized tissue from the wound site when removed. When the dressing is changed, sterile technique is essential.

The patient is frequently on bed rest in the early stages of acute infection. Good body alignment and frequent position changes prevent complications associated with immobility and promote comfort.

- Instruct the patient to avoid any activities such as exercise or heat application that increase circulation and serve as stimuli to the spread of infection.
- Peak and trough blood levels of most antibiotics must be carefully monitored throughout the course of therapy to avoid adverse drug effects.

▼ **Patient and Caregiver Teaching**

- Teach the patient potential adverse and toxic reactions associated with prolonged and high-dose antibiotic therapy. These reactions include hearing deficit, fluid retention, and neurotoxicity, which can occur with the aminoglycosides. Jaundice, colitis, and photosensitivity have been noted with extended use of cephalosporins.
- Long-term antibiotic therapy can result in an overgrowth of *Candida albicans* and *Clostridium difficile* in the genitourinary and oral cavities. Instruct the patient to report any whitish yellow, curdlike lesions to the health care provider.
- If at home, instruct the patient and family on the management of the venous access device. Also teach how to administer the antibiotic when scheduled and the need for follow-up laboratory testing.
- The patient and caregiver are often frightened and discouraged because of the serious nature of the disease, uncertainty of the outcome, and the lengthy cost and course of treatment. Continued psychologic and emotional support is an integral part of nursing management.

OSTEOPOROSIS

Description

Osteoporosis, or porous bone (fragile bone disease), is a chronic, progressive metabolic bone disease characterized by low bone mass and structural deterioration of bone tissue, leading to increased bone fragility. At least 10 million persons in the United States (80% of them women) have osteoporosis, and with the projected increase in life expectancy, this number is expected to grow. One in two women and one in eight men over the age of 50 will sustain an osteoporosis-related fracture during their lifetime.

Osteoporosis is more common in women than in men for several reasons: (1) women tend to have lower calcium intake than men throughout their lives (men between 15 and 50 years old consume twice as much calcium as women); (2) women have less bone mass because of their generally smaller frame; (3) pregnancy and breast-feeding can deplete a woman's skeletal system; (4) bone resorption begins at an earlier age in women and is accelerated at menopause; and (5) longevity increases the likelihood of osteoporosis.

Risk factors for osteoporosis are female gender, increasing age, white or Asian race, oophorectomy, family history, small stature, anorexia, early menopause, sedentary lifestyle, and insufficient dietary calcium. Increased risk is also associated with cigarette smoking and alcoholism. Decreased risk is associated with regular weight-bearing exercise and fluoride and vitamin D ingestion.

- Women >65 years old should be routinely screened for osteoporosis. Screening should begin by age 60 for women at increased risk of osteoporotic fractures.

Pathophysiology

Peak bone mass (maximum bone tissue) is mainly achieved before age 20 years. It is determined by a combination of four major factors: heredity, nutrition, exercise, and hormone function. Heredity may be responsible for up to 70% of peak bone mass.

- Bone loss from midlife (age 35 to 40 years) onward is inevitable, but the rate of loss varies. At menopause, women experience rapid bone loss when the decline in estrogen production is the sharpest. This rate of loss then slows and eventually matches the rate of bone lost by men 65 to 70 years old.

Bone is continually being deposited by osteoblasts and resorbed by osteoclasts, a process called *remodeling.* Normally the rates of bone deposition and resorption are equal to each other so that the total bone mass remains constant. In osteoporosis, bone resorption exceeds bone deposition.

- Although resorption affects the entire skeletal system, osteoporosis occurs most commonly in the bones of the spine, hips, and wrists. Over time, wedging and fractures of the vertebrae produce a gradual loss of height and a humped back known as *dowager's hump* or *kyphosis.*
- The usual first signs of osteoporosis are back pain or spontaneous fractures. The loss of bone substance causes the bone to become mechanically weakened and prone to either spontaneous fractures or fractures from minimal trauma.
- Specific diseases associated with osteoporosis include inflammatory bowel disease, intestinal malabsorption, kidney disease, rheumatoid arthritis, hyperthyroidism, chronic alcoholism, cirrhosis of the liver, and diabetes mellitus (DM).
- Many drugs can interfere with bone metabolism, including corticosteroids, antiseizure drugs (phenytoin [Dilantin]), heparin, aluminum-containing antacids, certain cancer treatments, and excessive thyroid hormones.

Clinical Manifestations

Osteoporosis is often called the "silent disease" because bone loss occurs without symptoms. People may not know they have osteoporosis until their bones become so weak that a sudden strain, bump, or fall causes a hip, wrist, or vertebral fracture.

- Collapsed vertebrae may initially be manifested as back pain, loss of height, or spinal deformities, such as kyphosis or severely stooped posture.

Diagnostic Studies

Osteoporosis often goes unnoticed because it cannot be detected by conventional x-ray until more than 25% to 40% of the calcium in the bone is lost.

- Serum calcium, phosphorus, and alkaline phosphatase levels remain normal, although alkaline phosphatase may be elevated after a fracture.

Bone mineral density (BMD) measurements are used to measure bone density. Types of BMD include quantitative ultrasound (QUS) and dual-energy x-ray absorptiometry (DEXA).

- QUS measures bone density with sound waves in the heel, kneecap, or shin.
- One of the most common BMD studies is DEXA, which measures bone density in the spine, hips, and forearm (the most common sites of fractures resulting from osteoporosis). DEXA studies are also useful to evaluate changes in bone density over time and to assess the effectiveness of treatment.

- DEXA results are frequently reported as T-scores: The T-score is the number of standard deviations below the average for normal bone density. A T-score of ≥−1 indicates normal bone density. Osteoporosis is defined as a BMD of ≤−2.5 (at least 2.5 standard deviations) below the mean BMD of young adults.

Osteopenia is defined as bone loss that is more than normal (a T-score between −1 and −2.5), but not yet at the level for a diagnosis of osteoporosis. More than 14 million women over age 50 have osteopenia. Bone biopsy can be used to differentiate the diagnosis of osteoporosis from osteomalacia.

Nursing and Collaborative Management

Care of the patient with osteoporosis focuses on proper nutrition, calcium and vitamin D supplementation, exercise, prevention of fractures, and medications. Treatment is recommended for postmenopausal women treatment who have (1) a T-score of ≤−2.5, (2) a T-score between −1 and −2.5 with additional risk factors, or (3) prior history of a hip or vertebral fracture.

Prevention and treatment of osteoporosis focus on adequate calcium intake (1000 mg/day in premenopausal women and postmenopausal women taking estrogen and 1500 mg/day in postmenopausal women who are not receiving supplemental estrogen).

- If dietary intake of calcium is inadequate, supplemental calcium may be recommended. The amount of elemental calcium varies in different calcium preparations (see Table 64-15, Lewis et al., *Medical-Surgical Nursing,* ed. 8, p. 1636). Calcium supplementation inhibits age-related bone loss.
- Moderate amounts of exercise are important to build up and maintain bone mass. The best exercises are those that are weight bearing and force an individual to work against gravity, such as walking, hiking, weight training, stair climbing, tennis, and dancing. Walking is preferred to high-impact aerobics or running, both of which may put too much stress on the bones of patients with osteoporosis.
- Instruct patients to quit smoking and limit alcohol intake to decrease the likelihood of losing bone mass.

Vertebroplasty and kyphoplasty are minimally invasive procedures that may be used to treat osteoporotic vertebral fractures. In vertebroplasty, bone cement is injected into the collapsed vertebra to stabilize it, but it does not correct the deformity. In kyphoplasty, an air bladder is inserted into the collapsed vertebra and inflated to regain vertebral body height and then bone cement is injected.

Drug Therapy

Estrogen replacement therapy after menopause is no longer given as primary treatment to prevent osteoporosis because of the associated increased risk of heart disease and breast and uterine cancer. If estrogen is being used to treat menopausal symptoms, it will also protect the woman against bone loss and fractures of the hip and vertebrae. It is believed that estrogen inhibits osteoclast activity, leading to decreased bone resorption.

Calcitonin is secreted by the thyroid gland and inhibits osteoclastic bone resorption by directly interacting with active osteoclasts. It is available in intramuscular (IM), subcutaneous, and intranasal forms. When calcitonin is used, calcium supplementation is necessary to prevent secondary hyperparathyroidism.

- Bisphosphonates inhibit osteoclast-mediated bone resorption, thereby increasing BMD and total bone mass. This group of drugs includes etidronate (Didronel), alendronate (Fosamax), pamidronate (Aredia), risedronate (Actonel), clodronate (Bonefos), tiludronate (Skelid), and ibandronate (Boniva). Alendronate is available as a weekly oral tablet, and ibandronate and risedronate are available as once-per-month oral tablet. Zoledronic acid (Reclast) has been approved for a once-yearly intravenous infusion and been shown to prevent osteoporosis for two years after a single infusion.
- Another type of drug used in treating osteoporosis is selective estrogen receptor modulators, such as raloxifene (Evista). These drugs mimic the effect of estrogen on bone by reducing bone resorption without stimulating the tissues of the breast or uterus.
- Teriparatide (Forteo) is a portion of human parathyroid hormone that is used for the treatment of osteoporosis by increasing the action of osteoblasts. It is the first drug for osteoporosis that stimulates new bone formation rather than just preventing further bone loss. This drug is expensive, and long-term use (>2 years) may slightly increase the risk for osteosarcoma.

Medical management of patients receiving corticosteroids includes prescribing the lowest possible dose of the drug. In addition, an adequate intake of calcium and vitamin D is needed including supplementation when osteoporosis drugs are prescribed. If osteopenia is evident on bone densitometry, treatment with bisphosphonate agents, such as alendronate (Fosamax), should be considered.

OVARIAN CANCER

Description

Ovarian cancer is a malignant tumor of the ovaries. Because most patients with ovarian cancer have advanced disease at diagnosis, it causes more deaths than any other cancer of the female reproductive system. White women of North American or European descent are at greater risk for ovarian cancer than are African American women. Currently only 20% of ovarian cancers are diagnosed at an early stage.

The cause of ovarian cancer is unknown, but multiple factors increase the risk for women to develop this type of cancer (Table 68). Protective factors that decrease the risk of ovarian cancer reduce the number of ovulatory cycles, and thus reduce exposure to estrogen.

Pathophysiology

About 90% of ovarian cancers are epithelial carcinomas. Germ cell tumors account for another 10%. Histologic grading is an important prognostic determinant.

Ovarian cancer can metastasize directly by shedding malignant cells that frequently implant on the uterus, bladder, bowel, and omentum. Metastasis can also occur by lymphatic spread.

Clinical Manifestations

Symptoms are vague in the early stages. An accumulation of fluid initially causes abdominal enlargement. Nonspecific symptoms

Table 68	Risk Factors for Ovarian Cancer	
Increased Risk		**Decreased Risk**
■ Family or personal history of ovarian, breast, or colon cancer		■ Oral contraceptive use (>5 yr)
■ Personal history of hereditary nonpolyposis colorectal cancer		■ Breast-feeding
■ Hormone replacement therapy		■ Multiple pregnancies
■ Mutant BRCA gene		■ Early age at first birth
■ Early menarche and late menopause		
■ Increasing age		
■ Nulliparity		
■ High-fat diet		

warranting further evaluation if they occur on an almost daily basis for at least 3 weeks include: pelvic or abdominal pain, bloating, urinary urgency or frequency, and difficulty in eating or feeling full quickly. Women who have one or more of these symptoms, especially if they are new, persistent, or worsening are advised to see their health care provider.

- Vaginal bleeding rarely occurs and pain is not an early symptom. Later signs are increased abdominal girth, unexplained weight loss or gain, and menstrual irregularities.

Diagnostic Studies

- No screening test exists for ovarian cancer. Yearly bimanual pelvic examinations should be performed to identify the presence of an ovarian mass. Abdominal or vaginal ultrasound can be used to detect ovarian masses.
- For women with a high risk of ovarian cancer, a combination of serum CA-125 (a tumor marker) and ultrasound is recommended in addition to a yearly pelvic examination. CA-125 is positive in 80% of women with epithelial ovarian cancer and is used to monitor the disease course.

Collaborative Care

Women identified as being at high risk based on family and health history may require counseling regarding options such as prophylactic oophorectomy and oral contraceptives. Although oophorectomy will significantly reduce the risk of ovarian cancer, it will not completely eliminate the possibility of the disease.

The usual treatment for stage I disease (limited to the ovaries) is a total abdominal hysterectomy and bilateral salpingo-oophorectomy with the removal of as much of the tumor as possible (i.e., tumor debulking). The addition of chemotherapy or the instillation of intraperitoneal radioisotopes is usually done for stage I disease that is poorly differentiated (see Chemotherapy, p 117).

The patient with stage II disease (limited to the true pelvis) may receive external abdominal and pelvic radiation, intraperitoneal radiation, or systemic combined chemotherapy after tumor-reducing surgery. After the completion of systemic chemotherapy in patients who are clinically free of symptoms, a "second-look" surgical procedure is often performed to determine whether there is any evidence of disease. This option does not necessarily improve the outcome. If no disease is found, the patient is monitored for recurrent disease.

Chemotherapy (e.g., cisplatin [Platinol], carboplatin [Paraplatin]) is used for the treatment of stage III (limited to the abdominal cavity) and stage IV (distant metastases) diseases. Altretamine

(Hexalen) is used for the palliative treatment of persistent, recurrent ovarian cancer. Paclitaxel (Taxol) and topotecan (Hycamtin) are used to treat metastatic ovarian cancer. Surgical debulking is often done in conjunction with chemotherapy for advanced disease. Intraperitoneal chemotherapy may be used for patients who have minimum residual disease after surgery for advanced disease. Gemcitabine (Gemzar) in combination with carboplatin is used to treat recurrent ovarian cancer.

- Palliative radiation and chemotherapy may be used to shrink the size of metastatic tumors to relieve pressure and pain.

Nursing Management: Cancers of the Female Reproductive Tract
See Cervical Cancer, p. 113.

PAGET'S DISEASE

Description
Paget's disease (osteitis deformans) is a chronic skeletal bone disorder in which there is excessive bone resorption followed by replacement of normal marrow by vascular, fibrous connective tissue and new bone that is larger, more disorganized, and weaker. Up to 40% of all patients with Paget's disease have a relative with the disorder. Compared with women, men are affected 2:1. The etiology of Paget's disease is unknown, although a viral etiology has been proposed. Regions of the skeleton commonly affected are the pelvis, long bones, spine, ribs, sternum, and cranium.

Clinical Manifestations
In milder forms of Paget's disease, patients may remain free of symptoms, and the disease may be discovered incidentally on x-ray or serum chemistry.

- Initial manifestations are usually an insidious development of skeletal pain (which may progress to severe intractable pain), fatigue, and progressive development of a waddling gait.
- Headaches, dementia, visual deficits, and loss of hearing can result with an enlarged, thickened skull.
- Pathologic fracture is the most common complication and may be the first indication of the disease. Other complications include osteosarcoma, osteoclastoma (giant cell) tumors, or fibrosarcoma.

Diagnostic Studies

- There are markedly elevated serum alkaline phosphatase (ALP) levels (indicating high bone turnover) in advanced forms of the disease.
- X-rays may reveal that the normal contour of the affected bone is curved and the bone cortex is thickened, especially in weight-bearing bones and the cranium.
- Bone scans using a radiolabeled bisphosphate demonstrate bone lesions.

Nursing and Collaborative Management

Management is usually limited to symptomatic and supportive care and correction of secondary deformities by either surgical intervention or braces. Bone resorption, relief of acute symptoms, and lowering of the serum ALP levels may be significantly influenced by the administration of calcitonin, which inhibits osteoclastic activity. Response to calcitonin therapy is not permanent and often stops when therapy is discontinued.

- Bisphosphonate drugs such as etidronate (Didronel), alendronate (Fosamax), risedronate (Actonel), and ibandronate (Boniva) are also used to retard bone resorption.
- Calcium and vitamin D are often given to decrease hypocalcemia, a common side effect of bisphosphonates.
- Pain is usually managed by nonsteroidal antiinflammatory drugs (NSAIDs).
- Orthopedic surgery for fractures, hip and knee replacements, and knee realignment may be necessary.

A firm mattress should be used to provide back support and relieve pain. The patient may be required to wear a corset or light brace to relieve back pain and provide support when in the upright position. The patient should be proficient in the correct application of such devices and know how to regularly examine areas of the skin for friction damage.

- Discourage activities such as lifting and twisting. Good body mechanics are essential. Physical therapy may increase muscle strength.
- A properly balanced nutritional program, especially as it pertains to vitamin D, calcium, and protein, is important for bone formation.
- Prevention measures such as patient education, the use of an assistive device, and environmental changes should be actively pursued to prevent falls and subsequent fractures.

PANCREATIC CANCER

Description

Pancreatic cancer is the fourth leading cause of death from cancer in the United States, with the peak incidence occurring between 65 and 80 years. Most pancreatic tumors are adenocarcinomas occurring in the head of the pancreas. As the tumor grows, the common bile duct becomes obstructed and obstructive jaundice develops.

The majority of cancers have metastasized at the time of diagnosis, and the prognosis is poor. Most patients die within 5 to 12 months of the initial diagnosis, and the 5-year survival rate is less than 5%.

Pathophysiology

The cause of pancreatic cancer is unknown. Risk factors are diabetes mellitus; chronic pancreatitis; family history of pancreatic cancer; cigarette smoking; high-fat diet; and exposure to chemicals such as benzidine. Pancreatic cancer develops twice as frequently in smokers as in nonsmokers.

Clinical Manifestations

Manifestations include abdominal pain (dull or aching), anorexia, rapid and progressive weight loss, nausea, and jaundice.

- Pain is common and related to the tumor location. Extreme, unrelenting pain is related to the extension of the cancer into the retroperitoneal tissues and nerve plexuses. The pain is frequently located in the upper abdomen or left hypochondrium and radiates to the back. It is commonly related to eating, and it also occurs at night. Weight loss is because of poor digestion and absorption caused by lack of pancreatic digestive enzymes.

Diagnostic Studies

- Ultrasound and computed tomography (CT) scan are the most commonly used imaging techniques.
- Magnetic resonance imaging (MRI) and MR cholangiopancreatography (MRCP) may be used for diagnosing and staging pancreatic cancer.
- Endoscopic retrograde cholangiography (ERCP) allows for visualization and collection of secretions and tissues from the pancreatic duct and biliary system.
- Tumor markers such as CA19-9 are used for establishing the diagnosis and monitoring treatment response.

Collaborative Care

Surgery provides the most effective treatment, but only 15% to 20% of patients have resectable tumors. The classic surgery is a *radical pancreaticoduodenectomy* or *Whipple's procedure.* This procedure is a resection of the proximal pancreas (proximal pancreatectomy), the adjoining duodenum (duodenectomy), the distal portion of the stomach (partial gastrectomy), and the distal segment of the common bile duct. An anastomosis of the pancreatic duct, common bile duct, and stomach to the jejunum is done.

- Radiation therapy alters survival rates little, but is effective for pain relief. External radiation is usually used, but implantation of internal radiation seeds into the tumor has also been used.
- The role of chemotherapy in pancreatic cancer is limited. Chemotherapy usually consists of fluorouracil (5-FU) and gemcitabine (Gemzar) either alone or in combination with agents such as capecitabine (Xeloda) or erlotinib (Tarceva).

Nursing Management

Because the patient with pancreatic cancer has many of the same problems as the patient with pancreatitis, nursing care includes the same measures (see section on Acute Pancreatitis below).

- Provide symptomatic and supportive nursing care, including medications and comfort measures to relieve pain.
- Psychologic support is essential, especially during times of anxiety or depression.
- Adequate nutrition is an important part of the nursing care plan. Frequent and supplemental feedings may be necessary. Measures to stimulate the appetite as much as possible and overcome anorexia, nausea, and vomiting should be included.
- A significant component of nursing care is helping the patient and caregiver through the grieving process.

PANCREATITIS, ACUTE

Description

Acute pancreatitis is an acute inflammatory process of the pancreas, with the degree of inflammation varying from mild edema to severe hemorrhagic necrosis. Some patients recover completely; others have recurring attacks, and chronic pancreatitis develops in others. Acute pancreatitis can be life threatening.

- It is most common in middle-aged men and women, with the rate of pancreatitis three times higher in African Americans than whites.

Pathophysiology

Many factors can cause injury to the pancreas. The primary etiologic factors are biliary tract disease (more common in women) and alcoholism (more common in men). In the United States the most common cause is gallbladder disease. Less common causes of acute pancreatitis include trauma (postsurgical, abdominal), viral infections (mumps, HIV), penetrating duodenal ulcers, cysts, abscesses, cystic fibrosis, certain drugs (corticosteroids, sulfonamides, nonsteroidal antiinflammatory drugs [NSAIDs]), and metabolic disorders (hyperparathyroidism, renal failure). In some cases the cause is not known (idiopathic).

- The most common pathogenic mechanism is believed to be autodigestion of the pancreas. The etiologic factors cause injury to pancreatic cells or activation of the pancreatic enzymes in the pancreas rather than in the intestine.

The pathophysiologic involvement of acute pancreatitis is classified as either *mild pancreatitis* (also known as edematous or interstitial) or *severe pancreatitis* (also called *necrotizing pancreatitis*). Patients with severe pancreatitis are at high risk for developing pancreatic necrosis, organ failure, and septic complications.

Clinical Manifestations

Abdominal pain is the predominant symptom. The pain is usually located in the left upper quadrant but may be in the midepigastrium. It commonly radiates to the back because of the retroperitoneal location of the pancreas.

- The pain has a sudden onset and is described as severe, deep, piercing, and continuous or steady. It is aggravated by eating and frequently has its onset when the patient is recumbent; it is not relieved by vomiting. The pain may be accompanied by flushing, cyanosis, and dyspnea.

Other manifestations include nausea and vomiting, low-grade fever, leukocytosis, hypotension, tachycardia, and jaundice. Abdominal tenderness with muscle guarding is common. Bowel sounds may be decreased or absent. Ileus may occur and causes marked abdominal distention. The lungs are frequently involved, with crackles present.

- Intravascular damage from circulating trypsin may cause areas of cyanosis or greenish to yellow-brown discoloration of the abdominal wall. Other areas of ecchymoses are the flanks (*Grey Turner's spots* or *sign*, a bluish flank discoloration) and the periumbilical area (*Cullen's sign,* a bluish periumbilical discoloration).

- Shock may occur because of hemorrhage into the pancreas, toxemia from the activated pancreatic enzymes, or hypovolemia as a result of massive fluid shifts into the retroperitoneal space.

Complications

Local complications of acute pancreatitis are pseudocyst and abscess.

- A pancreatic *pseudocyst* is a cavity continuous with or surrounding the outside of the pancreas. Manifestations are abdominal pain, palpable epigastric mass, nausea, vomiting, and anorexia. The serum amylase level remains elevated. These cysts usually resolve spontaneously within a few weeks, but may perforate, causing peritonitis, or rupture into the stomach or duodenum. Treatment consists of an internal drainage procedure with an anastomosis between the pancreatic duct and the jejunum.
- A *pancreatic abscess* is a large fluid-containing cavity within the pancreas. It results from extensive necrosis in the pancreas. It may become infected or perforate into adjacent organs. Manifestations include upper abdominal pain, abdominal mass, high fever, and leukocytosis. Pancreatic abscesses require prompt surgical drainage to prevent sepsis.

Systemic complications of acute pancreatitis include pleural effusion, atelectasis, pneumonia, hypotension, and hypocalcemia leading to tetany.

Diagnostic Studies

- Elevations of serum amylase and lipase are primary diagnostic findings.
- Liver enzymes, triglycerides, glucose, and bilirubin are also elevated with a decrease in calcium.
- Abdominal ultrasound, x-ray, or contrast-enhanced computed tomography (CT scan) can identify pancreatic problems, including pseudocysts and abscesses.
- Other diagnostic tests are endoscopic retrograde cholangiopancreatography (ERCP), endoscopic ultrasound (EUS), magnetic resonance cholangiopancreatography (MRCP), and angiography.

Collaborative Care

Objectives of management for acute pancreatitis include relief of pain, prevention or alleviation of shock, reduction of pancreatic secretions, control of fluid and electrolyte imbalance, prevention or treatment of infections, and removal of the precipitating cause, if possible.

- A primary consideration is the relief and control of pain. Morphine may be used and may be combined with an antispasmodic.
- If shock is present, blood volume replacements and expanders such as dextran or albumin may be given.

It is important to reduce or suppress pancreatic enzymes to decrease stimulation of the pancreas and allow it to rest. The patient is allowed to take nothing by mouth (NPO). Nasogastric (NG) suction may be used to reduce vomiting and gastric distention and prevent gastric digestive juices from entering the duodenum. Drugs that neutralize or suppress formation of hydrochloric (HCl) acid in the stomach, such as antacids, histamine H_2-receptor antagonists, and proton pump inhibitors, also help suppress pancreatic activity.

- Inflamed and necrotic pancreatic tissue is a good medium source for bacterial growth. Antibiotic therapy should be instituted early if an infection occurs.
- When food is allowed, small, frequent feedings are given. The diet is usually high in carbohydrate content because it is the least stimulating to the exocrine portion of the pancreas.

When the acute pancreatitis is related to gallstones, an urgent ERCP plus endoscopic sphincterotomy may be performed. This may be followed by laparoscopic cholecystectomy to reduce the potential for recurrence. Surgical intervention may be indicated when the diagnosis is uncertain and in patients who do not respond to conservative therapy. Patients with severe acute pancreatitis may require drainage of necrotic fluid collections. This can be done surgically, under CT guidance, or endoscopically. Percutaneous drainage of a pseudocyst can be performed, and a drainage tube is left in place.

Several different drugs may be used in the treatment of both acute and chronic pancreatitis (see Table 44-20, Lewis et al., *Medical-Surgical Nursing,* ed. 8, p. 1091).

Nursing Management
Goals
The patient with acute pancreatitis will have relief of pain, normal fluid and electrolyte balance, minimal to no complications, and no recurrent attacks.

See nursing care plan for the patient with acute pancreatitis at http://evolve.elsevier.com/Lewis/medsurg.

Nursing Diagnoses
- Acute pain
- Deficient fluid volume

- Imbalanced nutrition: less than body requirements
- Ineffective self-health management

Nursing Interventions

Encourage early diagnosis and treatment of biliary tract disease, such as cholelithiasis. Encourage the patient to eliminate alcohol intake, especially if there have been any previous episodes of pancreatitis.

During the acute phase, a major focus of your care is the relief of pain. Pain and restlessness can increase the metabolic rate and subsequent stimulation of pancreatic enzymes. Assess and document the duration of pain relief. Measures such as comfortable positioning, frequent changes in position, and relief of nausea and vomiting assist in reducing the restlessness that usually accompanies the pain.

- Assuming positions that flex the trunk and draw the knees up to the abdomen may decrease pain. A side-lying position with the head elevated 45 degrees decreases tension on the abdomen and may help ease the pain.
- For the patient who is on NPO status or has an NG tube, provide frequent oral and nasal care to relieve dryness of the mouth and nose.
- Observation for fever and other manifestations of infection is important. Respiratory infections are common because the retroperitoneal fluid raises the diaphragm, which causes the patient to take shallow, guarded abdominal breaths. Prevention of respiratory infections includes turning, coughing, deep breathing, and assuming a semi-Fowler's position.

Most patients need follow-up home care. The patient may have lost physical reserve and muscle strength. Physical therapy may be needed. Continued care to prevent infection and detect any complications is important.

▼ **Patient and Caregiver Teaching**

- Counseling regarding abstinence from alcohol is important to prevent the patient from experiencing future attacks of acute pancreatitis and development of chronic pancreatitis. Because cigarettes can stimulate the pancreas, smoking should be avoided.
- Dietary teaching should include the restriction of fats because they stimulate the secretion of cholecystokinin, which then stimulates the pancreas. Carbohydrates are less stimulating to the pancreas, so they should be encouraged. Instruct the patient to avoid crash dieting and binge eating because these can precipitate attacks.
- Instruct the patient and caregiver regarding the recognition and reporting of symptoms of infection, diabetes mellitus, or

steatorrhea (foul-smelling, frothy stools). These changes indicate possible destruction of pancreatic tissue.

- Teach the patient and caregiver about the prescribed regimen, including the importance of taking the required medications and following the recommended diet.

PANCREATITIS, CHRONIC

Description
Chronic pancreatitis is a continuous, prolonged, inflammatory, and fibrosing process of the pancreas. The pancreas becomes progressively destroyed as it is replaced with fibrotic tissue. Strictures and calcifications may also occur in the pancreas. Chronic pancreatitis may follow acute pancreatitis, but it may also occur in the absence of any history of an acute condition.

Pathophysiology
The most common cause of obstructive pancreatitis is inflammation of the sphincter of Oddi associated with cholelithiasis (gallstones). Cancer of the ampulla of Vater, duodenum, or pancreas can also cause chronic pancreatitis.

In nonobstructive pancreatitis there is inflammation and sclerosis, mainly in the head of the pancreas and around the pancreatic duct. This type of chronic pancreatitis is the most common form. In the United States, chronic pancreatitis is found almost exclusively in individuals who abuse alcohol.

Clinical Manifestations
As with acute pancreatitis, a major manifestation of chronic pancreatitis is abdominal pain. The patient may have episodes of acute pain, but it usually is chronic (recurrent attacks at intervals of months or years). The attacks may become more and more frequent until they are almost constant, or they may diminish as the pancreatic fibrosis develops. The pain is located in the same areas as in acute pancreatitis but is usually described as a heavy, gnawing feeling or sometimes as burning and cramplike. The pain is not relieved with food or antacids.

- Other manifestations include symptoms of pancreatic insufficiency, including malabsorption with weight loss, constipation, mild jaundice with dark urine, steatorrhea, and diabetes mellitus. The steatorrhea may become severe with voluminous, foul, fatty stools. Urine and stool may be frothy. Some abdominal tenderness may be found.

- Complications of chronic pancreatitis may include pseudocyst formation, bile duct or duodenal obstruction, pancreatic ascites or pleural effusion, and pancreatic cancer.

Diagnostic Studies

Confirming the diagnosis of chronic pancreatitis can be challenging and is based on the patient's signs and symptoms, lab studies, and imaging.

- Serum amylase and lipase levels may be elevated slightly or not at all.
- Serum bilirubin and alkaline phosphatase levels may be elevated.
- Mild leukocytosis and elevated sedimentation rate may be found.
- Endoscopic retrograde cholangiopancreatography (ERCP) is used to visualize changes in the pancreatic and biliary ductal system.
- Imaging studies such as computed tomography (CT), magnetic resonance imaging (MRI), MR cholangiopancreatography (MRCP), transabdominal ultrasound, and endoscopic ultrasound may be useful.

Nursing and Collaborative Management

When the patient with chronic pancreatitis is experiencing an acute attack, the therapy is similar to that for acute pancreatitis. At other times the focus is on the prevention of further attacks, relief of pain, and control of pancreatic exocrine and endocrine insufficiency. Sometimes large, frequent doses of analgesics are needed to relieve the pain.

- Diet, pancreatic enzyme replacement (e.g., Viokase, Cotazym), and control of the diabetes are measures used to control the pancreatic insufficiency. The diet is bland, low in fat, and high in carbohydrates. Alcohol must be totally eliminated.
- Treatment of chronic pancreatitis sometimes requires surgery. When biliary disease is present or obstruction or pseudocyst develops, surgery may be indicated to divert bile flow or relieve ductal obstruction.

▼ Patient and Caregiver Teaching

- Instruct the patient to take measures to prevent further attacks. Dietary control, along with consistency of other treatment measures such as taking pancreatic enzymes, is essential. Observe the patient's stools for steatorrhea to help determine the effectiveness of the enzymes. Instruct the patient and caregiver to observe the stools.

- Alcohol must be avoided, and the patient may need assistance with this problem. If the patient has developed a dependence on alcohol, a referral to other agencies or resources may be necessary.
- If diabetes has developed, the patient needs instruction regarding testing of blood glucose levels and drugs (see Diabetes Mellitus, p. 168).

PARKINSON'S DISEASE

Description

Parkinson's disease (PD) is a chronic, progressive neurodegenerative disorder characterized by slowness in the initiation and execution of movement *(bradykinesia),* increased muscle tone *(rigidity),* tremor at rest, and gait disturbance. PD is the most common form of *parkinsonism* (a syndrome characterized by similar symptoms).

The prevalence of PD is about 160 per 100,000 people. The diagnosis increases with age, with the peak onset in the 70s. Many autosomal dominant and recessive genes have been linked to familial PD. PD is more common in men by a ratio of $3:2$.

Pathophysiology

It is thought that PD is the result of a complex interplay between environmental factors and the genetic makeup of the individual. There are many forms of parkinsonism other than PD. Encephalitis lethargica, or type A encephalitis, has been clearly associated with the onset of parkinsonism. Parkinson-like symptoms have also occurred after intoxication with a variety of chemicals, including carbon monoxide, manganese (among copper miners), and an analog of meperidine (MPTP). Drug-induced parkinsonism can follow reserpine (Serpasil), methyldopa (Aldomet), lithium, haloperidol (Haldol), and phenothiazine (Thorazine) therapy. It is also seen following the use of amphetamine and methamphetamine.

- The pathology of PD involves the degeneration of the dopamine-producing neurons in the substantia nigra of the midbrain, which in turn disrupts the normal balance between dopamine (DA) and acetylcholine (ACh) in the basal ganglia.
- Dopamine is a neurotransmitter essential for normal functioning of the extrapyramidal motor system, including control of posture, support, and voluntary motion. Symptoms do not occur until 80% of neurons in the substantia nigra are lost.

Clinical Manifestations

Onset of PD is gradual and insidious, with a prolonged progression and course. Classic manifestations include tremor, rigidity, and bradykinesia, which are often called the triad of PD. In the beginning stages, only a mild tremor, slight limp, or decreased arm swing may be evident. Later the patient may have a shuffling, propulsive gait with arms flexed and loss of postural reflexes. In some patients there may be a slight change in speech patterns.

- *Tremor,* often the first sign, may initially be minimal, so that the patient is the only one who notices it. This tremor is more prominent at rest and is aggravated by emotional stress or increased concentration. The hand tremor is described as "pill rolling" because the thumb and forefinger appear to move in a rotary fashion as if rolling a pill, coin, or other small object. Tremor can involve the diaphragm, tongue, lips, and jaw.

- *Rigidity* is increased resistance to passive motion when the limbs are moved through their range of motion. Parkinsonian rigidity is typified by a jerky quality, as if there were intermittent catches in the movement of a cogwheel, when the joint is moved. This is called *cogwheel rigidity.*

- *Bradykinesia* (slow and retarded movement) is particularly evident in the loss of automatic movements, which is secondary to the physical and chemical alteration of the basal ganglia. In the unaffected person, automatic movements are involuntary and occur subconsciously; these include the blinking of the eyelids, swinging of the arms while walking, swallowing of saliva, self-expression with facial and hand movements, and minor movement of postural adjustment. The patient with PD does not execute these movements. This lack of spontaneous activity accounts for the "old man" image with stooped posture, masked facies ("deadpan" expression), drooling of saliva, and shuffling gait. There is difficulty in initiating movement.

- Nonmotor symptoms include depression, anxiety, apathy, fatigue, pain, impotence, and short-term memory impairment.

- As the disease progresses, complications such as *dyskinesia, akinesia,* dementia, and neuropsychiatric problems occur. Dementia occurs in up to 40% of patients with PD.

- Swallowing may become very difficult *(dysphagia),* leading to malnutrition or aspiration.

- General debilitation may lead to pneumonia, urinary tract infections, and skin breakdown.

- Orthostatic hypotension may occur and, along with the loss of postural reflexes, may result in falls or other injury.

Sleep disorders are common, potentially severe, often under-recognized, and ineffectively treated. It is important for you to include an assessment of problems relating to sleep in these patients.

Diagnostic Studies

Because there is no specific diagnostic test for PD, the diagnosis is based solely on the history and clinical features.

- A definitive diagnosis can be made only when there are at least two of the three characteristic signs of the classic triad: tremor, rigidity, and bradykinesia.
- The ultimate confirmation is a positive response to antiparkinsonian medication.

Collaborative Care

Because there is no cure, management is aimed at relieving symptoms.

Drug Therapy

Drug therapy for PD is aimed at correcting the imbalance of central nervous system (CNS) neurotransmitters. Antiparkinsonian drugs either enhance the release or supply of DA (dopaminergic) or antagonize or block the effects of acetylcholine (ACh) in the striatum. Levodopa with carbidopa (Sinemet) is often the first drug to be used. Levodopa is a precursor of dopamine and can cross the blood-brain barrier. It is converted to dopamine in the basal ganglia.

Some health care providers believe that, after a few years of therapy, the effectiveness of Sinemet wears off. Therefore they prefer to initiate therapy with a DA receptor agonist instead. These drugs include bromocriptine (Parlodel), pergolide (Permax), ropinirole (Requip), and pramipexole (Mirapex). These drugs directly stimulate DA receptors. When more moderate to severe symptoms are present, levodopa with carbidopa (Sinemet) is added to the drug regimen.

- Anticholinergic drugs are also used to manage PD. These drugs act by decreasing ACh activity. Antihistamines with anticholinergic properties or a β-adrenergic blocker (e.g., propranolol [Inderal]) are used to manage tremors. The antiviral agent amantadine (Symmetrel) is also an effective antiparkinsonian drug.
- Select monoamine oxidase (MAO) inhibitors (e.g., selegiline [Eldepryl]) may be used in combination with Sinemet, and catechol-O-methyltransferase (COMT) inhibitors (e.g., entacapone [Comtan], tolcapone [Tasmar]) may be used as adjuncts to levodopa. Rasagiline (Azilect), a MAO-B inhibitor, is used

as an initial drug therapy in early PD and as an addition to levodopa in patients with more advanced disease.

Table 69 summarizes drugs commonly used in Parkinson's disease, the symptoms they relieve, and their common side effects.

Surgical Therapy

Surgical therapy is usually used to relieve symptoms in patients with PD who are unresponsive to drug therapy or who have developed severe motor complications. Procedures fall into three categories: ablation (destruction), deep brain stimulation (DBS), and transplantation. Ablation therapy involves stereotactic ablation of areas in the thalamus, globus pallidus, and subthalamic nucleus. Ablative procedures have been largely replaced by DBS, which involves placing an electrode in the thalamus, globus pallidus, or subthalamic nucleus that delivers a specific current to the targeted brain location. Ablative and DBS procedures work by reducing the increased neuronal activity produced by DA depletion.

Transplantation of fetal neural tissue into the basal ganglia is designed to provide DA-producing cells in the brain, but this form of therapy is still in experimental stages.

Nutritional Therapy

Diet is of major importance because malnutrition and constipation can be serious consequences of inadequate nutrition. Patients who have dysphagia and bradykinesia need appetizing foods that are easily chewed and swallowed. The diet should contain adequate roughage and fruit to avoid constipation. Ample time should be planned for eating to avoid frustration and encourage independence.

Nursing Management

Goals

The patient with PD will maximize neurologic function, maintain independence in activities of daily living for as long as possible, and optimize psychosocial well-being.

See NCP 59-4 for the patient with PD, Lewis et al., *Medical-Surgical Nursing*, ed. 8, pp. 1511 to 1512.

Nursing Diagnoses

- Impaired physical mobility
- Impaired verbal communication
- Imbalanced nutrition: less than body requirements
- Deficient diversional activity

Nursing Interventions

Promotion of physical exercise and a well-balanced diet are major concerns for nursing care. Exercise can limit the consequences of decreased mobility such as muscle atrophy, contractures, and constipation. Overall muscle tone as well as specific exercises to

Table 69 Drug Therapy: Parkinson's Disease

Drug	Mechanism of Action	Symptoms Relieved
Dopaminergics		
Dopamine Precursors		
levodopa (L-dopa)	Converted to dopamine in basal ganglia	Bradykinesia, tremor, rigidity
levodopa-carbidopa (Sinemet, Parcopa [orally dissolving tablet])		
Dopamine Receptor Agonists		
bromocriptine mesylate (Parlodel)	Stimulate dopamine receptors	
pramipexole (Mirapex)		
ropinirole (Requip, Requip XL)		
rotigotine (Neupro) (skin patch)		
Dopamine Agonists		
amantadine (Symmetrel)	Blocks reuptake of dopamine into presynaptic neurons	
apomorphine (Apokyn)	Stimulates postsynaptic dopamine receptors	

Anticholinergics	Block cholinergic receptors, thus helping to	Tremor
trihexyphenidyl (Artane)	balance cholinergic and dopaminergic activity	
benztropine (Cogentin)		
biperiden (Akineton)		
Antihistamine	Has anticholinergic effect	Tremor, rigidity
diphenhydramine (Benadryl)		
Monoamine Oxidase Inhibitors	Block breakdown of dopamine	Bradykinesia, rigidity, tremor
selegiline (Eldepryl, Carbex)		
rasagiline (Azilect)		
Catechol-O-Methyl Transferase (COMT) Inhibitors	Block COMT and slow the breakdown of levodopa,	
entacapone (Comtan)	thus prolonging the action of levodopa	
tolcapone (Tasmar)		

strengthen the muscles involved with speaking and swallowing should be included.

Because PD is a chronic degenerative disorder with no acute exacerbations, you should focus on teaching and nursing care directed toward the maintenance of good health, encouragement of independence, and avoidance of complications such as contractures.

▼ **Patient and Caregiver Teaching**

- For patients who are at risk for falling and tend to "freeze" while walking, have them think consciously about stepping over imaginary lines on the floor, drop rice kernels and step over them, rock from side to side, lift the toes when stepping, take one step backward and two steps forward.
- Getting out of a chair can be facilitated by using an upright chair with arms and placing the back legs on small (2-inch) blocks.
- Rugs and excess furniture should be removed to avoid stumbling.
- Clothing can be simplified by the use of slip-on shoes and Velcro hook-and-loop fasteners or zippers on clothing instead of buttons and hooks.
- An elevated toilet seat can facilitate getting on and off the toilet.
- As the disease progresses, the impact on the psychologic well-being of the patient and family also increases. You can assist the patient and family caregivers through listening, providing education, encouraging social interactions, and referral to the American Parkinson Disease Association (www. apdaparkinson.org).

PELVIC INFLAMMATORY DISEASE

Description
Pelvic inflammatory disease (PID) is an infectious condition of the pelvic cavity that may involve the fallopian tubes (salpingitis), ovaries (oophoritis), and pelvic peritoneum (peritonitis). PID may be "silent" with no symptoms, whereas other women may be in acute distress. PID is a major cause of infertility.

Chronic pelvic pain is noncyclical pain greater than 6 months in duration, involving the pelvis, lower back, buttocks, and abdomen. Up to one third of women have chronic pelvic pain after PID.

Pathophysiology
PID is often the result of untreated cervicitis. The organism infecting the cervix ascends higher into the uterus, fallopian tubes,

ovaries, and peritoneal cavity. The most frequent causative organisms are *Chlamydia trachomatis* and *Neisseria gonorrhoeae*. These organisms, as well as mycoplasma, streptococci, and anaerobes, may gain entrance during sexual intercourse or after pregnancy termination, pelvic surgery, or childbirth.

Factors associated with chronic pelvic pain include interstitial cystitis, lower genital tract inflammation, irritable bowel syndrome, untreated uterine fibroids, endometriosis, and dysmenorrhea.

Clinical Manifestations

The woman with PID usually goes to a health care provider because of lower abdominal pain.

- The pain starts gradually and then becomes constant. The intensity may vary from mild to severe; movement such as walking and intercourse increase the pain.
- Spotting after intercourse and purulent vaginal discharge are common.
- Fever and chills may also be present.
- Women with less acute symptoms notice increased cramping pain with menses, irregular bleeding, and some pain with intercourse. Women who have mild symptoms may go untreated either because they did not seek care or the health care provider misdiagnosed their complaints.

Complications

Immediate complications of PID include septic shock and *Fitz-Hugh-Curtis syndrome,* a perihepatitis that can occur when PID spreads through the peritoneum to the liver. The patient has symptoms of right upper quadrant pain, but liver function tests are normal. Tubo-ovarian abscesses may "leak" or rupture, resulting in pelvic or generalized peritonitis.

- Long-term complications include ectopic pregnancy, infertility, and chronic pelvic pain. PID can cause adhesions and strictures to develop in the fallopian tubes.

Diagnostic Studies

Diagnosis is based on data obtained during the bimanual portion of the pelvic examination. Women with PID have lower abdominal tenderness, bilateral adnexal tenderness, and positive cervical motion tenderness.

- Diagnostic criteria also include fever and abnormal vaginal or cervical discharge.
- Cultures for gonorrhea and chlamydia are also obtained from the endocervix.

- A pregnancy test should be done to rule out ectopic pregnancy.
- When pain or obesity compromises the pelvic examination and a tubo-ovarian abscess may be present, a vaginal ultrasound is indicated.

Collaborative Care

Treatment of PID is usually on an outpatient basis. The patient is given a combination of antibiotics such as cefoxitin (Mefoxin) and doxycycline (Vibramycin) to provide broad coverage against the causative organisms. The patient must have no intercourse for 3 weeks. Her partner(s) must be examined and treated. Physical rest and oral fluids are also important. Reevaluation in 48 to 72 hours, even if symptoms are improving is essential.

If outpatient treatment is not successful or the patient is acutely ill or in severe pain, hospital admission is indicated. Maximum doses of parenteral antibiotics are then given with analgesics to relieve pain and intravenous (IV) fluids to prevent dehydration. Application of heat to the lower abdomen or sitz baths may be used to improve circulation and decrease pain. Bed rest in semi-Fowler's position promotes pelvic cavity drainage and may prevent the development of abscesses.

Indications for surgery include the presence of abscesses that fail to resolve with IV antibiotics. The abscesses may be drained by laparotomy or laparoscopy. Childbearing function in young women is preserved whenever possible.

Treatment for chronic pelvic pain should focus on the underlying disorder. If the source of the pain is unknown, treatment is directed at managing the symptoms.

Nursing Management

Prevention, early recognition, and prompt treatment of vaginal and cervical infections can help prevent PID and its serious complications. Provide information regarding factors that place a woman at increased risk for PID. Urge women to seek medical attention for any unusual vaginal discharge or possible infection of their reproductive organs.

During hospitalization for PID, you have an important role in implementing drug therapy, monitoring the patient's health status, and providing symptom relief and patient education. Explain the need for limited activity (bed rest in a semi-Fowler's position) and increased fluid intake should increase patient cooperation.

- The patient may have guilt feelings about PID, especially if it was associated with a sexually transmitted disease. She may also be concerned about the complications associated with PID, such as adhesions and strictures of the fallopian tubes, infertility, and the increased incidence of ectopic pregnancy. Discuss with the patient her feelings and concerns to assist her to cope effectively with them.

PEPTIC ULCER DISEASE

Description

Peptic ulcer disease is an erosion of the gastrointestinal (GI) mucosa resulting from the digestive action of hydrochloric (HCl) acid and pepsin. Any portion of the GI tract that comes into contact with gastric secretions is susceptible to ulcer development, including the lower esophagus, stomach, duodenum, and at the margin of a gastrojejunal anastomosis site after surgical procedures.

Peptic ulcers can be classified as acute or chronic, depending on the degree and duration of mucosal involvement, and gastric or duodenal, according to the location.

- An *acute ulcer* is associated with superficial erosion and minimal inflammation. It is of short duration and resolves quickly when the cause is identified and removed.
- A *chronic ulcer* is of long duration, eroding through the muscular wall with the formation of fibrous tissue. It is continuously present for many months or intermittently throughout the person's lifetime. Chronic ulcers are more common than acute erosions.
- *Gastric* and *duodenal* ulcers, although defined as peptic ulcers, are distinctly different in etiology and incidence (Table 70). Generally, the treatment of all ulcer types is similar.

Pathophysiology

Peptic ulcers develop only in the presence of an acid environment. The back-diffusion of HCl into the gastric mucosa results in cellular destruction and inflammation. Histamine is released from the damaged mucosa, resulting in vasodilation and increased capillary permeability and further secretion of acid and pepsin. The critical pathologic process in gastric ulcer formation may not be the amount of acid that is secreted, but the amount that is able to penetrate the mucosal barrier. A variety of factors are known to destroy the mucosal barrier (see Gastritis, p. 242).

In addition to chronic gastritis, *H. pylori* are associated with peptic ulcer development. In the stomach the bacterium colonizes the gastric epithelial cells within the mucosal layer. In one patient, *H. pylori* may lead to intestinal metaplasia in the stomach resulting in chronic atrophic gastritis, whereas in other patients *H. pylori*

Table 70 Comparison of Gastric and Duodenal Ulcers

	Gastric Ulcers	Duodenal Ulcers
Lesion	Superficial; smooth margins; round, oval, or cone shaped	Penetrating (associated with deformity of duodenal bulb from healing of recurrent ulcers)
Location of lesion	Predominantly antrum, also in body and fundus of stomach	First 1-2 cm of duodenum
Gastric secretion	Normal to decreased	Increased
Incidence	Greater in women	Greater in men, but increasing in women, especially postmenopausal
	Peak age 50-60 yr	Peak age 35-45 yr
	More common in persons of lower socioeconomic status	Associated with psychologic stress
	Increased with smoking, drug use (aspirin, NSAID), and alcohol use	Increased with smoking, drug use, and alcohol use
	Increased with incompetent pyloric sphincter and bile reflux	Associated with other diseases (e.g., chronic obstructive pulmonary disease, pancreatic disease, hyperparathyroidism, Zollinger-Ellison syndrome, chronic renal failure)

Clinical manifestations	Burning or gaseous pressure in high left epigastrium and back and upper abdomen Pain 1-2 hr after meals; if penetrating ulcer, aggravation of discomfort with food Occasional nausea and vomiting, weight loss	Burning, cramping, pressure-like pain across midepigastrium and upper abdomen; back pain with posterior ulcers Pain 2-4 hr after meals and midmorning, midafternoon, middle of night; periodic and episodic Pain relief with antacids and food; occasional nausea and vomiting
Recurrence rate	High	High
Complications	Hemorrhage, perforation, gastric outlet obstruction, intractability	Hemorrhage, perforation, obstruction

NSAID, Nonsteroidal antiinflammatory drug.

may alter gastric secretion and produce tissue damage leading to peptic ulcer disease. Response to *H. pylori* is likely influenced by many factors, including genetics, environment, and diet.

Clinical Manifestations

Pain associated with gastric ulcer is located high in the epigastrium and occurs about 1 to 2 hours after meals. The pain is described as burning or gaseous. If the ulcer has eroded through the gastric mucosa, food tends to aggravate rather than alleviate the pain.

Duodenal ulcer symptoms occur when gastric acid comes in contact with the ulcer, generally 2 to 5 hours after a meal. The pain is described as "burning" or "cramplike." It is most often located in the midepigastric region beneath the xiphoid process. Duodenal ulcers can also produce back pain. A characteristic of duodenal ulcer is its tendency to occur continuously for a few weeks or months and then disappear for a time, only to recur some months later.

- Not all patients with gastric or duodenal ulcers will experience pain or discomfort. Silent peptic ulcers are more likely to occur in older adults and those taking NSAIDs. The presence or absence of symptoms is not directly related to the size of the ulcer or the degree of healing.

Complications

Major complications of peptic ulcers are hemorrhage, perforation, and gastric outlet obstruction. All are considered emergency situations and may require surgical interventions.

Hemorrhage is the most common complication. It develops from the erosion of granulation tissue at the base of the ulcer during healing or from the erosion of an ulcer through a major blood vessel. Duodenal ulcers account for a greater percentage of upper GI bleeding than gastric ulcers.

Perforation, the most lethal complication, occurs when the ulcer penetrates the serosal surface with spillage of either gastric or duodenal contents into the peritoneal cavity. Contents may contain air, saliva, food particles, HCl acid, pepsin, bacteria, bile, and pancreatic fluid and enzymes. Bacterial peritonitis may occur within 6 to 12 hours.

- Manifestations of perforation are sudden with a dramatic onset and include severe upper abdominal pain that quickly spreads throughout the abdomen. Respirations become shallow and rapid, and bowel sounds are usually absent.

Gastric outlet obstruction may occur with acute or chronic peptic ulcer disease. The patient with gastric outlet obstruction generally has a long history of ulcer pain. Symptoms include upper abdomen discomfort and swelling that worsens toward the end of the day, vomiting (often projectile), and constipation.

Diagnostic Studies

- Endoscopy is used to determine the characteristics and nature of the ulcer, obtain a tissue biopsy, obtain specimens to test for *H. pylori,* and assess the degree of ulcer healing after treatment.
- Biopsy of the antral mucosa and testing for urease (rapid urease testing) confirms a diagnosis of *H. pylori* infection. Noninvasive tests include a urea breath test, which checks for active infection by *H. pylori.*
- Complete blood count (CBC), urinalysis, liver enzyme studies, serum amylase determination, and stool examination may be performed for further diagnostic information.

Collaborative Care

Conservative Therapy

The regimen consists of adequate rest, dietary manifestations, drug therapy, elimination of smoking, and long-term follow-up care. Drugs are a vital part of therapy, and strict adherence to the prescribed regimen of drugs is important because peptic ulcer recurrence is high without treatment.

Drug therapy includes the use of histamine H_2-receptor antagonists (e.g., cimetidine [Tagamet], famotidine [Pepcid]), proton pump inhibitors (e.g., omeprazole [Prilosec]), antisecretory agents (e.g., misoprostol [Cytotec]), cytoprotective agents (e.g., sucralfate [Carafate]), antacids, and anticholinergics. Aspirin and NSAIDs should be discontinued or the doses reduced. The patient is given antibiotics to eradicate *H. pylori* infection. See Drug Therapy Tables 42-20 to 42-22, Lewis et al., *Medical-Surgical Nursing,* ed. 8, p. 991.

Healing of a peptic ulcer requires many weeks of therapy. Pain disappears after 3 to 6 days, but ulcer healing is much slower. Complete healing may take 3 to 9 weeks, depending on the ulcer size, treatment regimen, and patient adherence.

An acute exacerbation is frequently accompanied by bleeding, increased pain and discomfort, and nausea and vomiting.

- In hemorrhage, management is similar to that described for upper GI bleeding. The first-line management of upper GI bleeding is endoscopy and endotherapy. The goal of endoscopy is to coagulate or thrombose the bleeding vessel. Emergency assessment and management of the patients with a massive hemorrhage is described in Lewis et al., *Medical-Surgical Nursing,* ed. 8, pp. 981 to 982.

- In perforation, the focus of therapy is to stop the spillage of gastric contents by NG tube or surgery. Blood volume is replaced with lactated Ringer's and albumin solutions, and packed red blood cells (RBCs) may be necessary. Broad-spectrum antibiotic therapy is started immediately to treat bacterial peritonitis. Pain medication is also given.
- In gastric outlet obstruction the aim of therapy is to decompress the stomach by way of an NG tube.

Nutritional Therapy

There are no recommended dietary modifications for peptic ulcer disease. Patients are taught to eat and drink foods and fluids that do not cause any distressing symptoms. Caffeine-containing beverages and foods can increase symptom distress in some patients. Teach the patient to eliminate alcohol because it can delay healing. Foods that commonly cause gastric irritation include hot, spicy foods and pepper, carbonated beverages, and broth (meat extract).

Surgical Therapy

With the use of antisecretory and antibiotic agents, surgery for PUD is uncommon. Surgery is performed on those patients who have complications that are unresponsive to medical management and when there is a concern about gastric cancer.

Surgical procedures include partial gastrectomy, vagotomy, or pyloroplasty. Partial gastrectomy with removal of the distal two thirds of the stomach and anastomosis of the gastric stump to the duodenum is called a *gastroduodenostomy* or *Billroth I* operation; removal of the distal two thirds of the stomach with anastomosis of the gastric stump to the jejunum is called a *gastrojejunostomy* or *Billroth II* operation. *Vagotomy* is done to decrease gastric acid secretion, and involves severing the vagus nerve. *Pyloroplasty* is the surgical enlargement of the pyloric sphincter to facilitate the passage of contents from the stomach.

Postoperative complications from surgery are dumping syndrome, postprandial hypoglycemia, and bile reflux gastritis.

- *Dumping syndrome* occurs when surgery drastically reduces the reservoir capacity of the stomach and causes loss of control over the amount of gastric chyme entering the small intestine. The large bolus of hypertonic fluid entering the intestine causes a fluid shift into the bowel, creating a decrease in plasma volume along with distention of the bowel lumen and rapid intestinal transit. The patient usually describes feelings of generalized weakness, sweating, palpitations, and dizziness caused by the decrease in plasma volume. The patient also complains of abdominal cramps, borborygmi, and the urge to defecate as a result of fluid being drawn into the bowel lumen. The onset of symptoms occurs at the end of a meal or within 15 to 30 minutes of eating, and symptoms usually last about 1 hour after meals.

- *Postprandial hypoglycemia* is considered a variant of dumping syndrome, because it is the result of uncontrolled gastric empty- ing of a bolus of fluid high in carbohydrates, resulting in hyper- glycemia and the release of excessive amounts of insulin into the circulation. Symptoms are similar to a hypoglycemic reac- tion, including sweating, weakness, mental confusion, palpita- tions, and tachycardia.

- Gastric surgery that involves the pylorus can result in reflux of bile into the stomach. The major symptom of *reflux alkaline gastritis* is continual epigastric distress that increases after meals. Vomiting relieves distress but only temporarily. The administration of cholestyramine (Questran) to bind with the bile salts, either before or with meals, has been helpful.

Because of surgical changes, the stomach's reservoir is dimin- ished and meal size must be reduced accordingly. Dry foods with a low-carbohydrate content and moderate protein and fat content are better tolerated initially. Fluids should be taken between meals but not with the meal, and the patient should plan rest periods of at least 30 minutes after each meal.

Nursing Management
Goals
The overall goals are that the patient with peptic ulcer disease will adhere to the prescribed therapeutic regimen, experience a reduc- tion or absence of discomfort, exhibit no signs of GI complications, have complete healing of the peptic ulcer, and make appropriate lifestyle changes to prevent recurrence.

See NCP 42-2 for the patient with peptic ulcer disease, Lewis et al., *Medical-Surgical Nursing,* ed. 8, pp. 993 to 994.

Nursing Diagnoses/Collaborative Problems
- Acute pain
- Ineffective self-health management
- Nausea
- Potential complication: perforation of GI mucosa
- Potential complication: hemorrhage

Nursing Interventions
During an acute phase the patient may be NPO for a few days, have an NG tube inserted and connected to intermittent suction, and have IV fluid replacement. Convey the rationale for this therapy to the patient and caregiver. The volume of fluid lost, signs and symptoms of the patient, and laboratory test results determine the type and amount of IV fluids administered. When the stomach is kept empty of gastric secretions, the ulcer pain diminishes and

ulcer healing begins. Take vital signs initially and at least hourly to detect and treat shock. The patient's immediate environment should be quiet and restful.

If the patient has surgery, postoperative care is similar to post-operative care after abdominal laparotomy (see Abdominal Pain, Acute, p. 3). Additional considerations for a patient with a partial gastrectomy include:

- Gastric aspirate from the NG tube must be carefully observed for color, amount, and odor during the immediate postoperative period.
- It is essential that the NG suction is working and that the tube remains patent so that accumulated gastric secretions do not put a strain on the anastomosis.
- Observe the patient for signs of decreased peristalsis and lower abdominal discomfort that may indicate impending intestinal obstruction.
- Keep the patient comfortable and free of pain by the administration of prescribed medications and frequent changes in position.
- Observe the dressing for signs of bleeding or odor and drainage indicative of an infection.
- Encourage early ambulation.
- Rest, adequate nutrition, adherence to prescribed drug therapy, and avoidance of known irritants and stressors are keys to recovery.

▼ **Patient and Caregiver Teaching**
General instructions should cover aspects of the disease process, drugs, possible changes in lifestyle, and regular follow-up care (Table 71).

- Stress the need for long-term follow-up care. Because success-ful treatment is frequently followed by a recurrence of ulcer disease, the patient should be encouraged to seek immediate intervention if symptoms return.

PERICARDITIS, ACUTE

Description
Pericarditis is a condition caused by inflammation of the pericar-dium. The pericardium provides lubrication to decrease friction during systolic and diastolic heart movements and assists in pre-venting excessive dilation of the heart during diastole.

| Table 71 | Patient and Caregiver Teaching Guide: Peptic Ulcer Disease |

When teaching the patient and caregiver about management of peptic ulcer disease, you should:

1. Explain dietary modifications, including avoidance of foods that cause epigastric distress. This may include black pepper, spicy foods, and acidic foods.
2. Explain the rationale for avoiding cigarettes. In addition to promoting ulcer development, smoking will delay ulcer healing.
3. Encourage the reduction or elimination of alcohol intake.
4. Explain the rationale for avoiding OTC drugs unless approved by the patient's health care provider. Many preparations contain ingredients, such as aspirin, that should not be taken unless approved by the health care provider. Check with the health care provider regarding the use of nonsteroidal antiinflammatory drugs.
5. Explain the rationale for not interchanging brands of antacids, H_2-receptor blockers, and proton pump inhibitors that can be purchased OTC without checking with the health care provider. This can lead to harmful side effects.
6. Emphasize the need to take all medications as prescribed. This includes both antisecretory and antibiotic drugs. Failure to take medications as prescribed can result in relapse.
7. Explain the importance of reporting any of the following:
   - Increased nausea and/or vomiting
   - Increase in epigastric pain
   - Bloody emesis or tarry stools
8. Explain the relationship between symptoms and stress. Stress management strategies are encouraged.
9. Encourage patient and caregiver to share concerns about lifestyle changes and living with a chronic illness.

OTC, Over-the-counter.

Pathophysiology

Acute pericarditis is most often idiopathic with a variety of suspected viral causes. The coxsackievirus B group is the most commonly identified virus. Other causes include uremia, bacterial infection, acute myocardial infarction (MI), tuberculosis, neoplasm, and trauma.

Pericarditis in the patient with an acute MI may be described as two distinct syndromes. *Acute pericarditis* may occur within the initial 48- to 72-hour period after an MI. The second is

Dressler's syndrome (late pericarditis), which appears 4 to 6 weeks after an MI.

An inflammatory response is the characteristic pathologic finding in acute pericarditis. There is an influx of neutrophils, increased pericardial vascularity, and eventual fibrin deposition on the pericardium.

Clinical Manifestations

In acute pericarditis, clinical manifestations include progressive, frequently severe chest pain that is sharp and pleuritic in nature. The pain is generally worse with deep inspiration and when lying supine. It is relieved by sitting up and leaning forward. The pain may radiate to the neck, arms, or left shoulder, mimicking angina, but pericardial pain has the distinction of referral to the trapezius muscle. The pain is relieved by sitting up and leaning forward.

- Dyspnea that accompanies acute pericarditis is related to the patient's need to breathe in rapid, shallow breaths to avoid chest pain and may be aggravated by fever and anxiety.
- The hallmark finding is the *pericardial friction rub*. The rub is a scratching, grating, high-pitched sound believed to arise from friction between the roughened pericardial and epicardial surfaces. It is best heard with the stethoscope diaphragm firmly placed at the lower left sternal border of the chest. The pericardial friction rub does not radiate widely or vary in timing from the heartbeat. It can require frequent auscultation to identify because it may be intermittent and short-lived. Timing the pericardial friction rub with the pulse (and not respirations) helps to distinguish it from pleural friction rub.

Complications

Complications that may result from acute pericarditis are pericardial effusion and cardiac tamponade.

Pericardial effusion is an accumulation of excess fluid in the pericardium. Large effusions may compress nearby structures. Pulmonary tissue compression can cause cough, dyspnea, and tachypnea. Phrenic nerve compression can induce hiccups, and compression of the recurrent laryngeal nerve may result in hoarseness. Heart sounds are generally distant and muffled. Blood pressure (BP) is usually maintained.

Cardiac tamponade develops as the pericardial effusion increases in volume, compressing the heart. The patient may report chest pain and is often confused, anxious, and restless. Heart sounds become muffled, pulse pressure is narrowed, and the patient develops tachypnea, tachycardia, and decreased cardiac output. Neck veins are usually markedly distended because of jugular venous pressure elevation, and a pulsus paradoxus is present. *Pulsus paradoxus* is a decrease in systolic BP with inspiration that is exaggerated in cardiac tamponade. (See Table 37-8, Lewis et al., *Medical-Surgical Nursing,* ed. 8, p. 847 for measurement technique.)

Diagnostic Studies

- Electrocardiogram (ECG) is useful in diagnosis, with abnormalities (e.g., diffuse ST segment elevations) noted in approximately 90% of the cases.
- Echocardiography is used to determine the presence of pericardial effusion or cardiac tamponade.
- Tissue Doppler imaging and color M-mode of early left-ventricular flow help assess diastolic function.
- Laboratory findings include leukocytosis and elevation of erythrocyte sedimentation rate (ESR) and C-reactive protein (CRP).
- Computed tomography (CT) scan and magnetic resonance imaging (MRI) provide for visualization of the pericardium and pericardial space.

Collaborative Care

Management is directed toward identification and treatment of the underlying problem. Antibiotics should be used to treat bacterial pericarditis, and nonsteroidal antiinflammatory drugs (NSAIDs) (e.g., salicylates [aspirin], ibuprofen [Motrin]) control the pain and inflammation of acute pericarditis. Corticosteroids are generally reserved for patients with pericarditis secondary to systemic lupus erythematosus, patients already taking corticosteroids for a rheumatologic or other immune system condition, or those who do not respond to NSAIDs. When necessary, prednisone is given in a tapering dosage schedule.

- Pericardiocentesis is usually performed for pericardial effusion with acute cardiac tamponade, purulent pericarditis, or a high suspicion of a neoplasm. Hemodynamic support for the patient undergoing pericardiocentesis may include the administration of volume expanders and inotropic agents (e.g., dopamine [Intropin]) and the discontinuation of any anticoagulants.

Nursing Management

Management of the patient's pain and anxiety is your primary nursing consideration. Assess the amount, quality, and location of the pain to distinguish the pain of myocardial ischemia (angina) from the pain of pericarditis. Pericarditic pain is usually located in the precordium or left trapezius ridge and has a sharp, pleuritic quality that increases with inspiration. Relief from this pain is often obtained by sitting or leaning forward and is worsened when lying supine.

- Pain relief measures include maintaining the patient on bed rest with the head of the bed elevated to 45 degrees and providing an overhead padded table for support.
- Antiinflammatory medications help to alleviate the patient's pain. Because of the potential for gastrointestinal (GI) bleeding, administer these drugs with food and instruct the patient to avoid alcohol.
- Monitor for the signs and symptoms of tamponade and prepare for possible pericardiocentesis.
- Anxiety-reducing measures for the patient include providing simple, complete explanations of all procedures performed. These explanations are particularly important for the patient whose diagnosis is being established and for the patient who has previously experienced angina or an acute MI.

PERIPHERAL ARTERY DISEASE (LOWER EXTREMITIES)

Description
Peripheral artery disease (PAD) involves thickening of artery walls, which results in a progressive narrowing of the arteries of the upper and lower extremities. PAD is strongly related to other types of cardiovascular disease (CVD) and their risk factors.

Pathophysiology
The leading cause of PAD is *atherosclerosis*, a gradual thickening of the intima and media of arteries, which leads to progressive narrowing of the vessel lumen. These pathologic changes consist of migration and replication of smooth muscle cells, deposition of connective tissue, lymphocyte and macrophage infiltration, and accumulation of lipids. Significant risk factors for PAD are hyperlipidemia, uncontrolled hypertension, and diabetes mellitus, with the highest risk being tobacco use.

Clinical Manifestations
Severity of the manifestations depends on the site, extent of obstruction, and extent and amount of collateral circulation.

- The classic symptom is *intermittent claudication,* which is ischemic muscle ache or pain that is precipitated by exercise and relieved by resting.

- Paresthesia, manifested as numbness or tingling in the toes or feet, may result from nerve tissue ischemia. Gradually diminishing perfusion to neurons produces loss of both pressure and deep pain sensation.
- Pallor of the foot is noted in response to leg elevation. *Reactive hyperemia* (redness) develops when the limb is allowed to hang in a dependent position *(dependent rubor)*. The skin becomes shiny and taut, and there is hair loss on the lower legs. Diminished or absent pedal, popliteal, or femoral pulses are present.
- As the disease process advances and involves multiple arterial segments, continuous pain develops at rest. Rest pain most often occurs in the forefoot or toes and is aggravated by limb elevation.

The most serious complications are nonhealing arterial ulcers and gangrene, which may result in lower extremity amputation. If PAD has been present for an extended period, collateral circulation may prevent gangrene of the extremity.

Diagnostic Studies

- Doppler ultrasound and duplex imaging assess blood flow.
- Segmental blood pressure (BP) readings of the thigh, below the knee, and at ankle level with the patient supine.
- Angiography or magnetic resonance angiography (MRA) delineates location and extent of PAD.

Collaborative Care

The first treatment goal is to aggressively modify cardiovascular risk factors in all patients with PAD regardless of the severity of symptoms because of the high risk for myocardial infarction (MI), ischemic stroke, and cardiovascular-related death. Smoking cessation is essential. Aggressive lipid management is essential. Treatment with a lipid-lowering agents such as a statin (e.g., simvastatin [Zocor]) lowers cholesterol levels and also reduces CVD morbidity and mortality. Hypertension and diabetes mellitus also need to be properly controlled.

Antiplatelet agents such as aspirin, ticlopidine (Ticlid), and clopidogrel (Plavix) are critically important for reducing the risks of CVD events and death in PAD patients.

- Guidelines for oral antiplatelet therapy recommend aspirin (81 to 325 mg/day) or clopidogrel (Plavix).
- The use of angiotensin-converting enzyme (ACE) inhibitors (e.g., ramipril [Altace]) decreases morbidity and mortality.
- Two drugs available to treat intermittent claudication are pentoxifylline (Trental) and cilostazol (Pletal). Pentoxifylline increases erythrocyte flexibility and reduces blood viscosity,

whereas cilostazol is a phosphodiesterase inhibitor that inhibits platelet aggregation and increases vasodilation.

The primary nondrug treatment for claudication is a formal exercise-training program. Walking is the most effective exercise. Teach the patient to walk to the point of discomfort, stop and rest, and then resume walking until the discomfort recurs. Walking should be done for 30 to 40 minutes per day, three to five times per week.

- Teach PAD patients to adjust their overall caloric intake so that ideal body weight can be achieved and maintained, dietary cholesterol should be <200 mg/day, and sodium intake should be no more than 2 g/day.

- Patients taking antiplatelet agents, nonsteroidal antiinflammatory agents, or anticoagulants should consult with their health care provider before using any dietary or herbal supplements because of potential interactions and bleeding risks.

Conservative management goals of the patient with *critical limb ischemia* resulting from PAD include protecting the extremity from trauma, decreasing ischemic pain, preventing and controlling infection, and maximizing perfusion. Carefully inspect, cleanse, and lubricate both feet to prevent cracking of the skin and infection. Optimal therapy is revascularization via surgery or endovascular procedure.

Interventional radiology catheter-based procedures are alternatives to open surgical approaches for treatment of lower extremity PAD. Determining which intervention to use depends on stenosis location along with lesion type and severity. Most patients ambulate the day of the procedure and return to normal activity within 24 to 48 hours.

- *Percutaneous transluminal balloon angioplasty* uses a catheter that contains a cylindrical balloon at the tip. The end of the catheter is advanced to the stenotic area of the artery. When in position, the balloon is inflated, compressing the confining atherosclerotic intimal lining while also stretching the underlying media.

- *Stents,* expandable metallic devices, are positioned within the artery immediately after the balloon angioplasty is performed. The stent acts as a scaffold to keep the artery open and is used as a treatment for peripheral artery dissection.

- *Atherectomy* removes the obstructing plaque. A directional atherectomy device uses a high-speed cutting disc built into the catheter end that cuts long strips of the atheroma. Laser atherectomy uses ultraviolet energy to break the molecular bonds of the atheroma to reduce the stenosis.

Various surgical approaches can be used to improve arterial blood flow beyond a stenotic or occluded artery. The most common is a peripheral arterial bypass operation with autogenous vein or synthetic graft material to bypass or carry blood around the lesion.

- Other surgical options include *endarterectomy* (opening the artery and removing the obstructing plaque) and *patch graft angioplasty* (opening the artery, removing plaque, and sewing a patch to the opening to widen the lumen).
- Amputation is the least desirable surgical option, but may be required if gangrene is extensive, infection is present in the bone (osteomyelitis), or all major arteries in the limb are occluded.

Nursing Management

Goals

The patient with lower extremity PAD will have adequate tissue perfusion, relief of pain, increased exercise tolerance, and intact, healthy skin on extremities.

See NCP 38-1 for the patient with peripheral arterial disease of the lower extremities, Lewis et al., *Medical-Surgical Nursing,* ed. 8, pp. 878 to 879.

Nursing Diagnoses

- Ineffective peripheral tissue perfusion
- Risk for impaired skin integrity
- Activity intolerance
- Ineffective self-health management

Nursing Interventions

After surgical or radiologic intervention, the operative extremity should be checked every 15 minutes initially and then hourly for color, temperature, capillary refill, presence of peripheral pulses, and movement and sensation. Loss of palpable pulses necessitates immediate intervention.

After transfer from the recovery area, continue to monitor perfusion to the extremities and assess for potential complications such as bleeding, hematoma, thrombosis, embolization, and compartment syndrome. A dramatic increase in pain, loss of previously palpable pulses, extremity pallor or cyanosis, decreasing ankle-brachial indexes (ABI), numbness or tingling, or a cold extremity suggest occlusion of the graft or stent. Report these findings to the physician immediately.

- Knee-flexed positions should be avoided except for exercise. Sitting for long periods is discouraged because leg dependency may cause pain and edema, resulting in discomfort and stress to suture lines and increased risk of venous thrombosis. If edema develops, a reclining position is preferred, with the edematous leg elevated above heart level. Walking even short distances is desirable.

▼ **Patient and Caregiver Teaching**
- Strongly encourage the patient to stop smoking, if appropriate. Encourage physical activity and explain that it improves a number of CVD risk factors, including hypertension, hyperlipidemia, obesity, and glucose levels.
- Teach foot care to all patients with PAD. Meticulous foot care is especially important in the diabetic patient with PAD. Also teach patients to check skin temperature, capillary refill, and palpate pulses. Emphasize that they must report any changes in these findings or the development of any ulceration or inflammation to their health care provider. Encourage patients to wear clean, all-cotton or all-wool socks, and comfortable shoes with rounded (not pointed) toes and soft insoles.

PERITONITIS

Description
Peritonitis results from a localized or generalized inflammatory process of the peritoneum. Primary peritonitis occurs when blood-borne organisms enter the peritoneal cavity. Secondary peritonitis is much more common and occurs when abdominal organs perforate or rupture and release their contents (bile, enzymes, bacteria) into the peritoneal cavity. Common causes are listed in Table 72.

Pathophysiology
Intestinal contents and bacteria irritate the normally sterile peritoneum and produce an initial chemical peritonitis that is followed a few hours later by a bacterial peritonitis. Patients who use peritoneal dialysis are also at high risk. The resulting inflammatory response leads to massive fluid shifts (peritoneal edema) and adhesions as the body attempts to wall off the infection.

Clinical Manifestations
- Abdominal pain is the most common symptom.
- A universal sign is tenderness over the involved area. Rebound tenderness, muscular rigidity, and spasm are other major signs of peritoneum irritation.
- Abdominal distention or ascites, fever, tachycardia, tachypnea, nausea, vomiting, and altered bowel habits may also be present.

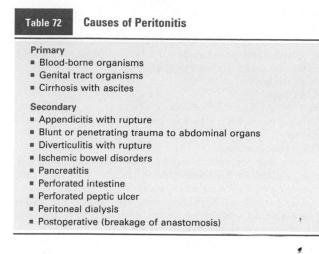

Table 72   Causes of Peritonitis

Primary
- Blood-borne organisms
- Genital tract organisms
- Cirrhosis with ascites

Secondary
- Appendicitis with rupture
- Blunt or penetrating trauma to abdominal organs
- Diverticulitis with rupture
- Ischemic bowel disorders
- Pancreatitis
- Perforated intestine
- Perforated peptic ulcer
- Peritoneal dialysis
- Postoperative (breakage of anastomosis)

P

Complications include hypovolemic shock, sepsis, intraabdominal abscess formation, paralytic ileus, and acute respiratory distress syndrome. If treatment is delayed, death may occur.

Diagnostic Studies
- Complete blood count (CBC) will determine hemoconcentration and leukocytosis.
- Peritoneal fluid aspiration and analysis can detect blood, bile, pus, bacteria, fungi, and amylase content.
- Abdominal x-ray may show dilated loops of bowel consistent with paralytic ileus, free air if there is a perforation, or air and fluid levels if an obstruction is present.
- Computed tomography (CT) scan or ultrasound may be useful in identifying ascites or abscesses.
- Peritoneoscopy may be helpful in patients without ascites.

Collaborative Care
Surgery is usually indicated to locate the cause, drain purulent fluid, and repair the damage. Patients with milder cases of peritonitis or those who are poor surgical risks may be managed nonsurgically. Treatment consists of antibiotics, nasogastric (NG) suction, analgesics, and intravenous (IV) fluid administration. Patients who require surgery need preoperative preparation.

Nursing Management
Goals
The patient with peritonitis will have resolution of inflammation, relief of abdominal pain, freedom from complications (especially hypovolemic shock), and normal nutritional status.
Nursing Diagnoses
- Acute pain
- Risk for deficient fluid volume
- Imbalanced nutrition: less than body requirements
- Anxiety
Nursing Interventions
The patient with peritonitis is extremely ill and needs skilled supportive care. An IV line is inserted to replace fluids lost to the peritoneal cavity and as an access for antibiotic therapy. Monitor the patient for pain and response to analgesic therapy. The patient may be positioned with knees flexed to increase comfort. Sedatives may be given to allay anxiety.
- Accurate monitoring of fluid intake and output and electrolyte status is necessary to determine replacement therapy. Monitor vital signs frequently.
- Antiemetics may be administered to decrease nausea and vomiting and prevent further fluid and electrolyte losses. The patient is on nothing by mouth (NPO) status and may have an NG tube in place to decrease gastric distention.
- If the patient has an open-incision surgical procedure, drains are inserted to remove purulent drainage and excessive fluid. Postoperative care of the patient is similar to the care of the patient with an exploratory laparotomy (see Abdominal Pain, Acute, p. 3).

PNEUMONIA

Description
Pneumonia is an acute inflammation of the lung parenchyma caused by a microorganism. Despite new antimicrobial agents to treat pneumonia, it is still common, with significant morbidity and mortality rates. Pneumonia can be caused by bacteria, viruses, *Mycoplasma,* fungi, parasites, and chemicals.

A clinically effective way to classify pneumonia is to classify it as *community-acquired pneumonia* (CAP) or *hospital-acquired pneumonia* (HAP). Classifying pneumonia is important because of the differences in the likely causative organisms (Table 73) and the selection of appropriate treatment.

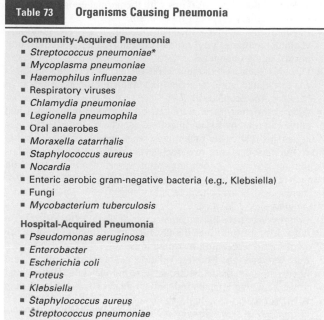

Table 73   **Organisms Causing Pneumonia**

Community-Acquired Pneumonia
- *Streptococcus pneumoniae**
- *Mycoplasma pneumoniae*
- *Haemophilus influenzae*
- Respiratory viruses
- *Chlamydia pneumoniae*
- *Legionella pneumophila*
- Oral anaerobes
- *Moraxella catarrhalis*
- *Staphylococcus aureus*
- *Nocardia*
- Enteric aerobic gram-negative bacteria (e.g., Klebsiella)
- Fungi
- *Mycobacterium tuberculosis*

Hospital-Acquired Pneumonia
- *Pseudomonas aeruginosa*
- *Enterobacter*
- *Escherichia coli*
- *Proteus*
- *Klebsiella*
- *Staphylococcus aureus*
- *Streptococcus pneumoniae*
- Oral anaerobes

*Most common cause of community-acquired pneumonia (CAP).

- *CAP* is a lower respiratory tract infection of the lung paren-chyma with onset in the community or during the first 2 days of hospitalization.
- *HAP* is pneumonia occurring 48 hours or longer after hospital admission and not incubating at the time of hospitalization. Two types of HAP are ventilator-associated pneumonia (VAP) and health care–associated pneumonia (HCAP).

Pathophysiology

Normally the airway distal to the larynx is sterile because of protec-tive defense mechanisms. Pneumonia is more likely to result when defense mechanisms become incompetent or are overwhelmed by infectious agents.

Factors predisposing a patient to pneumonia include:
- Decreased consciousness depresses the cough and epiglottal reflexes.

- Tracheal intubation interferes with the normal cough reflex and the mucociliary escalator mechanism.
- Impaired mucociliary mechanism caused by air pollution, cigarette smoking, viral upper respiratory tract infections, and normal aging changes
- Diseases such as leukemia, alcoholism, and diabetes mellitus are associated with an increased frequency of gram-negative bacilli in the oropharynx.
- Altered oropharyngeal flora can occur after a patient has had antibiotic therapy for an infection elsewhere in the body.

Organisms that cause pneumonia reach the lungs by aspiration from the nasopharynx or oropharynx, inhalation of microbes present in the air, or hematogenous spread from an infection elsewhere in the body.

There are four characteristic stages of *pneumococcal pneumonia:*

1. *Congestion.* After the organisms reach the alveoli, there is an outpouring of fluid into the alveoli. Organisms multiply in the serous fluid, spreading the infection.
2. *Red hepatization.* Massive dilation of capillaries; alveoli are filled with organisms, neutrophils, red blood cells (RBCs), and fibrin. The lung appears red and granular, or liverlike, which is why the process is called hepatization.
3. *Gray hepatization.* Blood flow decreases, and leukocytes and fibrin consolidate in the affected part of the lung.
4. *Resolution.* Complete resolution and healing occur if there are no complications.

Clinical Manifestations and Complications

Usually the onset of symptoms is sudden including fever, chills, cough productive of purulent sputum, and pleuritic chest pain (in some cases). In the elderly or debilitated patient, confusion or stupor (possibly related to hypoxia) may be the only finding.

- On physical examination signs of pulmonary consolidation, such as dullness to percussion, increased fremitus, bronchial breath sounds, and crackles, may be found.
- The typical pneumonia syndrome is related to infections with *Streptococcus pneumonia* and *Haemophilus influenzae.*

Pneumonia may also present atypically with a more gradual onset, dry cough, and extrapulmonary manifestations such as fever, headache, myalgias, fatigue, sore throat, nausea, vomiting, and diarrhea. On physical examination crackles are often heard. This symptom pattern is associated with *Mycoplasma pneumoniae, Legionella pneumophila,* and *Chlamydia pneumoniae.*

Initial manifestations of viral pneumonia are highly variable. Symptoms may include chills; fever; dry, nonproductive cough; and extrapulmonary symptoms. Primary viral pneumonia can be caused by influenza virus infection. Viral pneumonia may also be a complication of systemic viral diseases such as measles, varicella-zoster, and herpes simplex.

Complications include pleurisy (inflammation of the pleura), pleural effusion, atelectasis (collapsed, airless alveoli), bacteremia, lung abscess, pericarditis, arthritis, meningitis, and endocarditis.

Diagnostic Studies

- History, physical examination, and chest x-ray often provide enough information for making management decisions without further testing.
- Chest x-ray often shows a pattern characteristic of the infecting organism.
- Sputum culture and sensitivity test may be done.
- Blood cultures may be done.
- Gram stain of sputum and blood cultures is used to identify causative organism.
- Arterial blood gases (ABGs) to assess for hypoxemia, hypercapnia, and acidosis.
- White blood count (WBC) count often reveals leukocytosis.

Collaborative Care

Pneumococcal vaccine is used to prevent *Streptococcus pneumoniae* (pneumococcus) pneumonia. Initial Pneumomax vaccine is indicated for patients (1) with chronic illnesses such as lung and heart disease and diabetes mellitus, (2) with lowered resistance to infection such as leukemia and kidney failure, (3) at least 65 years old, (4) who smoke cigarettes or have asthma, or (5) in a long-term care facilities. Revaccination should occur at >5 years for patients aged 65 years and older and also for patients with lowered resistance to infection.

Currently there is no definitive treatment for viral pneumonia. Care is generally supportive. Prompt treatment with appropriate antibiotics almost always cures bacterial and *Mycoplasma* pneumonia. In uncomplicated cases, the patient responds to drug therapy within 48 to 72 hours. Table 28-6 in Lewis et al., *Medical-Surgical Nursing,* ed. 8, p. 550, outlines drugs for bacterial CAP. Indications of improvement include decreased temperature, improved breathing, and reduced chest pain.

- Supportive measures may be used, including oxygen therapy, analgesics to relieve chest pain, and antipyretics such as aspirin or acetaminophen. Individualize rest and activity to the patient's tolerance.

- Hydration is important. If the patient has heart failure, fluid intake is carefully monitored. If the patient cannot maintain adequate oral intake, intravenous (IV) administration of fluids and electrolytes becomes necessary.
- It is important to provide nutritional intake to meet the needs of the patient. Small, frequent meals are easier for some patients to tolerate.

Nursing Management

Goals

The patient with pneumonia will have clear breath sounds, normal breathing patterns, no signs of hypoxia, normal chest x-ray, and no complications related to pneumonia.

See NCP 28-1 for the patient with pneumonia, Lewis et al., *Medical-Surgical Nursing,* ed. 8, pp. 552 to 553.

Nursing Diagnoses

- Impaired gas exchange
- Ineffective breathing pattern
- Acute pain

Nursing Interventions

Interventions focus on preventing the occurrence of pneumonia. If possible, exposure to upper respiratory infections (URIs) should be avoided. If a URI occurs, it should be treated promptly with supportive measures (e.g., rest, fluids). If symptoms persist for more than 7 days, the person should seek medical care. The individual at increased risk for pneumonia should be encouraged to obtain both influenza and pneumococcal vaccines.

In the hospital, your role involves identifying the patient at risk and taking measures to prevent the development of pneumonia.

- Place the patient with altered consciousness in positions (e.g., side-lying, upright) that will prevent or minimize aspiration. Turn and reposition the patient at least every 2 hours to facilitate adequate lung expansion and discourage the pooling of secretions.
- The patient who has a feeding tube requires attention to prevent aspiration.
- In the intensive care unit, strict adherence to "Ventilator Bundle" interventions has been shown to significantly reduce VAP. These interventions are: elevation of the head of the bed 30 to 45 degrees, daily "sedation vacations," assessment of readiness to extubate, and peptic ulcer disease and venous thromboembolism prophylaxis.

- The patient who has difficulty swallowing (e.g., a stroke patient) needs assistance in eating, drinking, and taking medication to prevent aspiration. In the patient who has had local anesthesia to the throat, assess for a gag reflex before giving food or fluids.
- Patients with impaired mobility from any cause need assistance with turning and moving as well as encouragement to deep breathe at frequent intervals.
- Practice strict medical asepsis and adherence to infection control guidelines to reduce the incidence of hospital-acquired infections.

▼ **Patient and Caregiver Teaching**
- Teach the patient about the importance of taking every dose of the prescribed antibiotic, any drug–drug and food–drug interactions for the prescribed antibiotic, and the need for adequate rest to maintain progress toward recovery.
- Teaching should also include information about available influenza and pneumococcal vaccines.

PNEUMOTHORAX

Description
A pneumothorax is a complete or partial collapse of a lung as a result of an accumulation of air in the pleural space. This condition should be suspected after any blunt trauma to the chest wall. A pneumothorax may be closed or open.

Pathophysiology
Closed pneumothorax has no associated external wound; the most common form is spontaneous pneumothorax, which is caused by the rupture of small blebs on the visceral pleural space. Blebs, the result of airway inflammation, are most commonly because of smoking. The risk increases with the amount of smoking. Males who are heavy smokers (>22 cigarettes/day) are more likely to have a spontaneous pneumothorax than nonsmokers. Other risk factors include male gender, family history, and previous spontaneous pneumothorax.

- Injury to the lung from broken ribs can also cause pneumothorax, as well as laceration or puncture of the lung during subclavian catheter insertion. If excessive pressure is used during manual or mechanical ventilation, alveoli or bronchioles can rupture.
- The esophagus may also be involved in pneumothorax. The esophagus may tear during forceful vomiting or emergency

intubation with a gastric tube. Air from the esophagus will enter the mediastinum and pleural space.

Open pneumothorax occurs when air enters the pleural space through an opening in the chest wall. Examples include stab or gunshot wounds and surgical thoracotomy. A penetrating chest wound is often referred to as a sucking chest wound.

Tension pneumothorax results when a rapid accumulation of air in the pleural space causes high intrapleural pressures that create tension on the heart and great vessels. It may result from an open or closed pneumothorax. In an open chest wound, a flap may act as a one-way valve; thus air can enter on inspiration but cannot escape. Intrathoracic pressure increases, the lung collapses, and the mediastinum shifts toward the unaffected side, which is subsequently compressed. As pressure increases, cardiac output (CO) decreases because venous return is decreased.

- Tension pneumothorax can occur with mechanical ventilation or resuscitative efforts or if chest tubes are clamped or become blocked after insertion for a pneumothorax. Unclamping the tube or relieving the obstruction will remedy the situation.

Hemothorax is an accumulation of blood in the pleural space from an intercostal blood vessel, the internal mammary artery, the lung, the heart, or the great vessels. It is frequently found in association with open pneumothorax and is then called a *hemopneumothorax*.

Clinical Manifestations

If the pneumothorax is small, only mild tachycardia and dyspnea may be present. If it is a large pneumothorax, shallow, rapid respirations, dyspnea, air hunger, and oxygen desaturation may occur.

- Chest pain and a cough with or without hemoptysis may also be present.
- On auscultation there are no breath sounds over the affected area.
- Chest x-ray shows the presence of air or fluid in the pleural space and reduction in lung volume.

Tension pneumothorax is a medical emergency, with both the respiratory and cardiovascular systems affected. If the tension in the pleural space is not relieved, the patient is likely to die from inadequate cardiac output or severe hypoxemia. Emergency management is to insert a large-bore needle into the anterior chest wall at the fourth or fifth intercostal space to release the trapped air. A chest tube is then inserted and connected to water-seal drainage.

Collaborative Care

If the patient is stable and the amount of air or fluid accumulated in the intrapleural space is minimal, no treatment may be needed because the pneumothorax resolves spontaneously, or the pleural space can be aspirated with a large-bore needle (thoracentesis).

The most common treatment for a pneumothorax and hemothorax is to insert a chest tube and connect it to water-seal drainage (see Chest Tubes and Pleural Drainage, p. 724). Repeated spontaneous pneumothoraces may need to be treated surgically by a partial pleurectomy, stapling, or pleurodesis to promote the adherence of pleurae to one another.

P

POLYCYSTIC KIDNEY DISEASE

Polycystic kidney disease (PKD) is the most common life-threatening genetic disease in the world. It is characterized by large, thin-walled cysts that fill the cortex and the medulla and destroy surrounding tissue by compression. The cysts range in size from several millimeters to several centimeters in diameter, involve both kidneys, and are filled with fluid, including blood or pus.

The *childhood form* of PKD is a rare autosomal recessive disorder that is often rapidly progressive. The *adult form* of PKD is an autosomal dominant disorder that is latent for many years and usually manifests between 30 and 40 years old.

Symptoms appear when the cysts begin to enlarge. Often the first manifestations are hypertension, hematuria (from rupture of cysts), or a feeling of heaviness in the back, side, or abdomen. On physical examination, palpable bilateral enlarged kidneys are often found.

- Sometimes the first manifestations are a urinary tract infection (UTI) and/or urinary calculi.
- Chronic pain is one of the most common problems, and in some people it can be constant and quite severe.
- Usually the disease progresses to end-stage renal failure (ESRD) occurring by age 60 in 50% of patients.
- Polycystic kidney disease can also affect the liver (liver cysts), heart (abnormal heart valves), blood vessels (aneurysms), and intestines (diverticulosis). The most serious complication is a cerebral aneurysm, which can rupture.

Diagnosis is based on clinical manifestations, family history, intravenous pyelogram (IVP), ultrasound (best screening measure), or computed tomography (CT) scan.

There is no specific treatment for PKD. A major aim of treatment is to prevent infections of the urinary tract or to treat them with appropriate antibiotics if they occur. Nephrectomy may be necessary if pain, bleeding, or infection becomes a chronic, serious problem. When the patient begins to experience progressive renal failure, interventions are determined by the remaining renal function. Dialysis and kidney transplant may be needed to treat ESRD.

Nursing measures are those used for management of end-stage renal disease (see Kidney Disease, Chronic, p. 381). They include diet modification, fluid restriction, medications (e.g., antihypertensives), assisting the patient to accept the chronic disease process, assisting the patient and family to deal with financial concerns, and other issues related to the hereditary nature of the disease.

- The patient who has adult PKD often has children by the time the disease is diagnosed. The patient will need appropriate counseling regarding plans for having more children. In addition, genetic counseling resources should be provided for the children.

POLYCYTHEMIA

Description

Polycythemia is the production and presence of increased number of red blood cells (RBCs). The increase in RBCs can be so great that blood circulation is impaired as a result of the increased blood viscosity (hyperviscosity) and volume (hypervolemia).

Pathophysiology

The two types of polycythemia are *primary polycythemia (polycythemia vera)* and *secondary polycythemia* (Fig. 11). Their etiologies and pathogeneses differ, although their complications and clinical manifestations are similar.

Polycythemia vera is considered a chronic myeloproliferative disorder arising from a chromosomal mutation in a single pluripotent stem cell. Therefore not only are RBCs involved, but also white blood cells and platelets, leading to increased production of each of these blood cells. The disease develops insidiously and follows a chronic, vacillating course. The median age at diagnosis is 60 years old. Patients have enhanced blood viscosity and blood volume and congestion of organs and tissues with blood. Splenomegaly and hepatomegaly are common.

Secondary polycythemia can be either *hypoxia driven* or *hypoxia independent*. In hypoxia-driven polycythemia, hypoxia stimulates erythropoietin (EPO) production in the kidney, which in turn stimulates RBC production. The hypoxia may be because of high altitude, pulmonary and cardiovascular disease, defective O_2 transport,

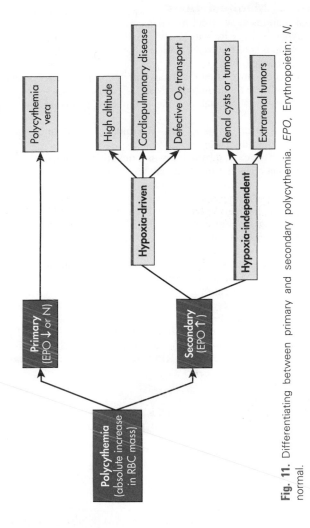

Fig. 11. Differentiating between primary and secondary polycythemia. *EPO*, Erythropoietin; *N*, normal.

or tissue hypoxia. In hypoxia-independent polycythemia, EPO is produced by a malignant or benign tumor tissue.

Clinical Manifestations

Initial manifestations from hypertension caused by hypervolemia and hyperviscosity include:

- Complaints of headache, vertigo, dizziness, tinnitus, and visual disturbances

The major cause of morbidity and mortality from polycythemia vera is related to thrombosis. Manifestations caused by blood vessel distention, circulatory stasis, thrombosis, and tissue hypoxia include:

- Angina, heart failure (HF), intermittent claudication, and venous thrombosis

Hemorrhage caused by either vessel rupture from overdistention or inadequate platelet function may result in:

- Petechiae, ecchymoses, epistaxis, or gastrointestinal (GI) bleeding

Other clinical manifestations include:

- Generalized pruritus that may be a striking symptom and is related to histamine release from an increased number of basophils
- Hepatomegaly and splenomegaly that contribute to patient complaints of satiety and fullness
- Pain from peptic ulcer caused by increased gastric secretions
- Paresthesia and erythromelalgia (painful burning and redness of the hands and feet)
- Plethora (ruddy complexion) may be present
- Hyperuricemia resulting from the increase in RBC destruction that accompanies excessive RBC production; may cause a form of gout

Diagnostic Studies

- Elevated hemoglobin (Hb) and RBC count with microcytosis
- Low to normal EPO level (polycythemia vera); high EPO level (secondary polycythemia)
- Elevated white blood cell (WBC) count with basophilia
- Elevated platelets (thrombocytosis) and platelet dysfunction
- Elevated leukocyte alkaline phosphatase, uric acid, and cobalamin levels
- Elevated histamine levels
- Bone marrow examination showing hypercellularity of RBCs, WBCs, and platelets
- Splenomegaly found in 90% of patients with primary polycythemia

Collaborative Care

Treatment is directed toward reducing blood volume and viscosity and bone marrow activity. Phlebotomy is the mainstay of treatment. At the time of diagnosis 300 to 500 mL of blood may be removed every other day until the hematocrit (Hct) level is reduced to normal. The aim of phlebotomy is to reduce and keep the Hct to less than 45% to 48%. An individual managed with repeated phlebotomies eventually becomes iron deficient, although this effect is rarely symptomatic. Iron supplementation should be avoided.

- Hydration therapy is used to reduce the blood's viscosity.
- Myelosuppressive agents such as busulfan (Myleran), hydroxyurea (Hydrea), melphalan (Alkeran), and imatinib mesylate (Gleevec) are used.
- Low-dose aspirin is used as primary prophylaxis for vascular events. Interferon alpha (IFN-α) is used in women of childbearing age or those with intractable pruritus.
- Anagrelide (Agrylin) may be used to reduce the platelet count and inhibit platelet aggregation.
- Allopurinol (Zyloprim) may reduce the number of acute gouty attacks.

Nursing Management

Primary polycythemia vera is not preventable. However, because secondary polycythemia is generated by any source of hypoxia, maintaining adequate oxygenation may prevent problems. Therefore controlling chronic pulmonary disease, stopping smoking, and avoiding high altitudes may be important.

When acute exacerbations of polycythemia vera develop, assist with or perform phlebotomies, depending on the institution's policies.

- Evaluate fluid intake and output during hydration therapy to avoid fluid overload (which further complicates circulatory congestion) and underhydration (which can cause even greater blood viscosity).
- If myelosuppressive agents are used, administer the drugs as ordered, observe the patient, and teach the patient about medication side effects.
- An assessment of the patient's nutritional status in collaboration with the dietitian may be necessary to offset the inadequate food intake that can result from GI symptoms of fullness, pain, and dyspepsia.
- Activities and/or medications must be instituted to decrease thrombus formation. Active or passive leg exercises and ambulation when possible should be initiated.

- Because of its chronic nature, polycythemia vera requires ongoing evaluation. Phlebotomy may need to be done every 2 to 3 months. Evaluate the patient for the development of complications.

PRESSURE ULCER

Description
A pressure ulcer is localized injury to the skin and/or underlying tissue (usually over a bony prominence) as a result of pressure or pressure in combination with shear and/or friction. The most common site for pressure ulcers is the sacrum, with heels being second. Factors influencing development of pressure ulcers include amount of pressure (intensity), length of time pressure is exerted on the skin (duration), and ability of the patient's tissue to tolerate externally applied pressure. Besides pressure, shearing force (pressure exerted on skin when it adheres to the bed and skin layers slide in the direction of body movement), friction (two surfaces rubbing against each other), and excessive moisture contribute to pressure ulcer formation.
- Factors that put a patient at risk for the development of pressure ulcers include immobility, advanced age, obesity, impaired circulation, incontinence, diabetes mellitus, neurologic disorders, contractures, anemia, and prolonged surgery.

Clinical Manifestations
Pressure ulcers are graded or staged according to their deepest level of tissue damage or "wounding." Table 74 describes the pressure ulcer stages.
- A pressure ulcer may be unstageable. The actual depth of tissue loss is obscured by slough (yellow, tan, gray, green, or brown) and/or eschar (tan, brown, or black) in the wound bed. If the pressure ulcer becomes infected, signs of systemic infection, such as leukocytosis and fever, may occur.

Collaborative Care
Care of a patient with a pressure ulcer requires local wound care as well as support measures such as adequate nutrition, pain management, and pressure relief. The current trend is to keep a pressure ulcer slightly moist, rather than dry, to enhance reepithelialization. Both conservative and surgical strategies are used in the treatment of pressure ulcers, depending on the ulcer's stage and condition.

| Table 74 | Staging of Pressure Ulcers |

Definition/Description	Further Description

Suspected Deep Tissue Injury

| Purple or maroon localized area of discolored intact skin or blood-filled blister caused by damage of underlying soft tissue from pressure and/or shear. The area may be preceded by tissue that is painful, firm, mushy, boggy, warmer, or cooler as compared with adjacent tissue. | Deep tissue injury may be difficult to detect in individuals with dark skin tones. Evolution may include a thin blister over a dark wound bed. May further evolve and become covered by thin eschar. Evolution may be rapid, exposing additional layers of tissue even with optimal treatment. |

Stage I

| Intact skin with nonblanchable redness of a localized area usually over a bony prominence. Darkly pigmented skin may not have visible blanching; its color may differ from the surrounding area. | Area may be painful, firm, soft, warmer, or cooler as compared with adjacent tissue. Stage I may be difficult to detect in individuals with dark skin tones. May indicate "at risk" persons. |

Stage II

| Partial thickness loss of dermis presenting as a shallow open ulcer with a red pink wound bed, without slough. May also present as an intact or open/ruptured serum-filled blister. | Presents as a shiny or dry shallow ulcer without slough or bruising (indicates suspected deep tissue injury). This stage should not be used to describe skin tears, tape burns, perineal dermatitis, maceration, or excoriation. |

Continued

| Table 74 | Staging of Pressure Ulcers—cont'd |

Definition/Description	Further Description
Stage III Full thickness tissue loss. Subcutaneous fat may be visible but bone, tendon, or muscle are not exposed. Slough may be present but does not obscure the depth of tissue loss. May include undermining and tunneling.	Depth of a stage III pressure ulcer varies by anatomic location. The bridge of the nose, ear, occiput, and malleolus do not have subcutaneous tissue, and stage III ulcers can be shallow. In contrast, areas of significant adiposity can develop extremely deep stage III pressure ulcers. Bone/tendon is not visible or directly palpable.
Stage IV Full thickness tissue loss with exposed bone, tendon, or muscle. Slough or eschar may be present on some parts of the wound bed. Often include undermining and tunneling.	Depth of a stage IV pressure ulcer varies by anatomic location. The bridge of the nose, ear, occiput, and malleolus do not have subcutaneous tissue and these ulcers can be shallow. Stage IV ulcers can extend into muscle and/or supporting structures (e.g., fascia, tendon or joint capsule) making osteomyelitis possible. Exposed bone/tendon is visible or directly palpable.
Unstageable Ulcer Full thickness tissue loss in which the base of the ulcer is covered by slough (yellow, tan, gray, green, or brown) and/or eschar (tan, brown, or black) in the wound bed.	Until enough slough and/or eschar is removed to expose the base of the wound, the true depth, and therefore stage, cannot be determined. Stable (dry, adherent, intact without erythema or fluctuance) eschar on the heels serves as "the body's natural (biologic) cover" and should not be removed.

Source: National Pressure Ulcer Advisory Board at www.npuap.org.

Nursing Management

Goals
The patient with a pressure ulcer will have no deterioration of the ulcer stage, reduce or eliminate the factors that lead to pressure ulcers, not develop an infection in the pressure ulcer, have healing of pressure ulcers, and have no recurrence.

Nursing Diagnosis
* Impaired skin integrity

Nursing Interventions
Patients should be assessed for pressure ulcer risk initially on admission and at periodic intervals (see Table 13-12, Lewis et al., *Medical-Surgical Nursing*, ed. 8, p. 199).

- Devices such as alternating pressure mattresses, foam mattresses with adequate stiffness and thickness, wheelchair cushions, padded commode seats, foam boots, and lift sheets are useful in reducing pressure and shearing force. However, they are not adequate substitutes for frequent repositioning.

  Once a person has been identified as being at risk for pressure ulcer development, prevention strategies should be implemented. (Table 75 and NCP 13-1, Lewis et al., *Medical-Surgical Nursing*, ed. 8, p. 202, list guidelines for preventing pressure ulcers.)

  Once a pressure ulcer has developed, initiate interventions based on the ulcer's characteristics (e.g., size, stage, location, presence of infection, or pain) and the patient's general status, to document the size of the ulcer.

  Local ulcer care may involve debridement, wound cleaning, relief of pressure, and the application of a dressing.

- A pressure ulcer that has necrotic tissue or eschar (except for dry, stable necrotic heels, must have the tissue removed by surgical, mechanical, enzymatic, or autolytic debridement methods. Once the pressure ulcer has been successfully debrided and has a clean granulating base, the goal is to provide an appropriate wound environment that supports moist wound healing and prevents disruption of newly formed granulation tissue.

- Reconstruction of the pressure ulcer site by operative repair, including skin grafting, skin flaps, musculocutaneous flaps, or free flaps, may be necessary.

- Pressure ulcers should be cleaned with noncytotoxic solutions that do not kill or damage cells, especially fibroblasts.

- After the pressure ulcer has been cleansed, it needs to be covered with an appropriate dressing. (Dressings are discussed in Table 13-10, Lewis et al., *Medical-Surgical Nursing*, ed. 8, p. 197.)

Table 75	Patient and Caregiver Teaching Guide: Pressure Ulcer

When teaching the patient and/or caregiver to prevent and care for pressure ulcers, you should:

1. Identify and explain risk factors and etiology of pressure ulcers to the patient and caregiver.
2. Assess all at-risk patients at time of first hospital and/or home visit or whenever the patient's condition changes. Thereafter assess at regular intervals based on care setting (every 24 hours for acute care or every visit for home care).
3. Teach the caregiver techniques for incontinence. If incontinence occurs, cleanse skin at time of soiling and use pads or briefs that are absorbent.
4. Demonstrate correct positioning to decrease risk of skin breakdown. Instruct caregiver to reposition a bed-bound patient at least every 2 hours, a chair-bound patient every hour. NEVER position the patient directly on the pressure ulcer.
5. Assess resources (i.e., adequacy of caregiver's availability and skill, finances, and equipment) of patients requiring pressure ulcer care at home. When selecting ulcer care dressing, consider cost and amount of caregiver time.
6. Teach patient and/or caregiver to place clean dressings over sterile dressings using "no touch" technique when changing dressings. Instruct caregiver on disposal of contaminated dressings.
7. Teach patient and caregiver to inspect skin daily. Assess and document pressure ulcer status at least weekly.
8. Teach patient and caregiver the importance of good nutrition to enhance ulcer healing.
9. Evaluate program effectiveness.

- Maintenance of adequate nutrition is an important nursing responsibility for the patient with a pressure ulcer. Often the patient is debilitated and has a poor appetite secondary to inactivity.
- Oral feedings must be adequate in calories, protein, fluids, vitamins, and minerals to meet the patient's nutritional requirements.
- Enteral feedings can be used to supplement oral feedings. If necessary, parenteral nutrition may be used.

▼ Patient and Caregiver Teaching

Because recurrence of pressure ulcers is common, it is extremely important to educate both the patient and the caregiver in prevention techniques (see Table 75).

- Teach the caregiver about the etiology of pressure ulcers, prevention techniques, early signs, nutritional support, and care techniques for pressure ulcers.
- Because the patient with a pressure ulcer often requires extensive care for other health problems, it is important that you support the caregiver.

PROSTATE CANCER

Description

Prostate cancer is the most common form of cancer in men, with one in five men developing prostate cancer at some point in their lives. It is the second leading cause of cancer death in men after lung cancer. Most cases occur in men older than age 65 years, but many cases occur in younger men, who sometimes have a more aggressive type of cancer.

- African American men have a higher incidence of prostate cancer than any other male group worldwide.
- A history of benign prostatic hyperplasia (BPH) is not a risk factor for prostate cancer.

Pathophysiology

Prostate cancer is an androgen-dependent adenocarcinoma. The tumor usually is slow growing. Tumor spread is by three routes: direct extension, lymphatics, and bloodstream. Spread by direct extension involves the seminal vesicles, urethral mucosa, bladder wall, and external sphincter. Later spread occurs through the lymphatic system to the regional lymph nodes. Venous spread from the prostate involves the pelvic bones, head of the femur, lower lumbar spine, liver, and lungs.

Clinical Manifestations

Prostate cancer is often asymptomatic in the early stages. Eventually the patient may have symptoms similar to those of BPH, including dysuria, hesitancy, dribbling, frequency, urgency, hematuria, nocturia, and retention.

- Pain in the lumbosacral area that radiates down to the hips or legs, when coupled with urinary symptoms, may indicate metastasis. As the cancer spreads to the bones, pain can become severe, especially in the back and legs, because of spinal cord compression and bone destruction.

Diagnostic Studies

- In a digital rectal examination (DRE) of the prostate gland, it may feel hard, nodular, and asymmetric.
- Elevated levels of prostate specific antigen (PSA) are indicative of prostatic pathologic conditions, but not necessarily prostate cancer.
- Elevated prostatic acid phosphatase (PAP) levels are specific for prostate cancer.
- Biopsy using transrectal ultrasound can confirm the diagnosis.
- Computed tomography (CT) scan, bone scan, or magnetic resonance imaging (MRI) can assess cancer spread.
- Elevated serum alkaline phosphatase may indicate bone metastasis.

Collaborative Care

The management of prostate cancer depends on the stage and overall health of the patient. Prostate cancer is staged on the basis of tumor growth and spread (Whitmore-Jewett stages A to D) and graded on tumor histology (Gleason score). The 5-year survival rate with an initial diagnosis at stage A is 100%.

At all stages, there is more than one possible treatment option. The decision of which treatment course to pursue is a joint decision between the patient and the health care provider. Various treatment options are summarized in Table 55-6, Lewis et al., *Medical-Surgical Nursing,* ed. 8, p. 1388.

- A conservative approach to slow-growing tumors is "watchful waiting" that involves follow-up with frequent PSA testing and DREs to monitor the progress of the disease. Significant changes in PSA, DRE, or symptoms warrant a reevaluation of treatment options.

Surgical therapy for patients with a stage A or B tumor involves a radical prostatectomy as the treatment of choice for long-term survival. With radical prostatectomy, the entire prostate gland, seminal vesicles, and part of the bladder neck (ampulla) are removed. A retroperitoneal lymph node dissection is also usually done. The two most common approaches for radical prostatectomy are retropubic (low abdominal incision) and perineal (incision between the scrotum and anus).

- Surgery is usually not considered an option for stage D cancer, except to relieve obstruction, because metastasis has already occurred.
- The two major complications following a radical prostatectomy are erectile dysfunction and urinary incontinence.

A nerve-sparing technique is sometimes used to prevent erectile dysfunction caused by radical prostatectomy. This surgery is the preferred choice for most men undergoing prostatectomy in the early stage of disease with cancer confined to the prostate gland. The degree of success varies.

Cryotherapy in another surgical technique that destroys cancer cells by freezing. The treatment takes about 2 hours, with the patient under general or spinal anesthesia.

Radiation therapy is a common option for prostate cancer. Radiation therapy may be offered as the only treatment, or it may be offered in combination with surgery or hormonal therapy. Salvage radiation therapy given for cancer recurrence after a radical prostatectomy has shown promise in improving survival in some men.

- External beam radiation is the most widely used method. Brachytherapy using radioactive seed implants placed in the prostate gland is best suited for patients with stage A or B prostate cancer.

Chemotherapy is generally reserved for late-stage disease and has not been shown to improve survival. The goal of chemotherapy is palliation.

Prostate cancer growth is largely dependent on the presence of androgens. Therefore androgen deprivation is a primary therapeutic approach. Hormone therapy also known as *androgen deprivation therapy* focuses on reducing the levels of circulating androgens to reduce tumor growth.

- Luteinizing hormone-releasing hormone (LHRH) agonists (e.g., leuprolide [Lupron, Eligard, Viadur], goserelin [Zoladex], triptorelin [Trelstar]) produce a chemical castration similar to the effects of an orchiectomy.
- Androgen receptor blockers (e.g., flutamide [Eulexin], nilutamide [Nilandron], bicalutamide [Casodex]) compete with circulating androgens at the receptor sites and can be used in combination with goserelin or leuprolide.
- Combining an androgen receptor blocker with an LH-RH agonist is an often used treatment, which results in combined androgen blockade.
- Estrogen has been used as a form of androgen deprivation therapy but is declining in popularity because of development of more effective hormone therapies.

A bilateral orchiectomy is the surgical removal of the testes that may be done alone or in combination with prostatectomy. For advanced stages of prostate cancer (stage D) an orchiectomy is one treatment option for cancer control. Although this procedure is less costly when compared with chemical hormone manipulation using LH-RH agonists, it is also permanent.

Nursing Management

Goals

The patient with prostate cancer will be an active participant in the treatment plan, have satisfactory pain control, follow the therapeutic plan, understand the effect of the therapeutic plan on sexual function, and find a satisfactory way to manage the impact on bladder or bowel function.

Nursing Diagnoses

- Decisional conflict
- Acute pain
- Urinary retention
- Impaired urinary elimination
- Constipation or diarrhea
- Sexual dysfunction
- Anxiety

Nursing Interventions

One of your most important roles is to encourage patients (in consultation with their health care provider) to have an annual prostate screening (PSA and DRE) starting at the age of 50 years or younger if risk factors are present.

- Provide psychologic support for the patient and the family to help them cope with the cancer diagnosis and decisions regarding treatment choices.
- Care during the preoperative and postoperative phases of radical prostatectomy is similar to surgical procedures for Benign Prostatic Hyperplasia (see p. 69).
- Nursing interventions for the patient undergoing chemotherapy are discussed on p. 717.
- Pain control is the primary nursing intervention for the terminally ill patient.
- In advanced prostate cancer, hospice care is often appropriate and beneficial to the patient and family. (Hospice care is discussed in Chapter 11, Lewis et al., *Medical-Surgical Nursing,* ed. 8.)

▼ Patient and Caregiver Teaching

If the patient is discharged with an indwelling catheter in place, teach appropriate catheter care.

- Instruct the patient to clean the urethral meatus with soap and water once each day; maintain a high fluid intake; keep the collecting bag lower than the bladder at all times; keep the catheter securely anchored to the inner thigh or abdomen; and report any signs of bladder infection, such as bladder spasms, fever, or hematuria.
- If urinary incontinence is a problem, the patient should be encouraged to practice pelvic floor muscle exercises

(Kegel) at every urination and throughout the day. Continuous practice during the 4- to 6-week healing process improves the success rate.

PULMONARY EMBOLISM

Description

Pulmonary embolism (PE) is blockage of pulmonary arteries by a thrombus, fat, or air embolus or tumor tissue. PE is associated with a mortality rate of up to 30% in patients who are not treated. Risk factors for PE are immobility, surgery within the last 3 months (especially pelvic and lower extremity surgery), stroke, paralysis, history of deep vein thrombosis (DVT), malignancy, obesity in women, heavy cigarette smoking, and hypertension.

Pathophysiology

Most PEs arise from DVT in the deep leg veins. Venous thromboembolism (VTE) is the preferred terminology to describe the spectrum of pathology from DVT to pulmonary embolism (PE).

Lethal pulmonary emboli most commonly originate in the femoral or iliac veins. *Emboli* are mobile clots that generally do not stop moving until they lodge at a narrowed part of the circulatory system. The lower lobes of the lung are most frequently affected because they have a higher blood flow than other lobes.

- Thrombi in the deep veins can dislodge spontaneously. However, it is more common for mechanical forces (e.g., sudden standing) and changes in the rate of blood flow (e.g., those that occur with the Valsalva maneuver) to dislodge the thrombus. The majority of patients with PE because of DVT have no leg symptoms at the time of diagnosis.

Clinical Manifestations

Manifestations of PE are varied and nonspecific, making diagnosis difficult. The classic triad—dyspnea, chest pain, and hemoptysis—occurs in only about 20% of patients. Symptoms may begin slowly or suddenly. A mild to moderate hypoxemia with a low $PaCO_2$ is a common finding.

- Other signs are cough, chest pain, crackles, fever, accentuation of the pulmonic heart sound, and a sudden change in mental status resulting from hypoxemia.

Massive emboli may produce abrupt hypotension, shock, pallor, severe dyspnea, and hypoxemia. An electrocardiogram (ECG) and chest x-ray may indicate right ventricular hypertrophy secondary to pulmonary hypertension. The mortality rate of those with massive PE and shock is approximately 33%.

Medium-sized emboli often cause pleuritic chest pain accompanied by dyspnea, slight fever, and a productive cough with blood-streaked sputum. A physical examination may indicate tachycardia and a pleural friction rub.

Small emboli frequently go undetected or produce vague, transient symptoms. The exception to this is the patient with underlying cardiopulmonary disease, in whom even small or medium-sized emboli may result in severe cardiopulmonary compromise.

Complications

Pulmonary infarction (death of lung tissue) is most likely when (1) the occlusion is of a large or medium-sized pulmonary vessel (>2 mm in diameter), (2) insufficient collateral blood flows from the bronchial circulation, or (3) preexisting lung disease is present. Infarction results in alveolar necrosis and hemorrhage. Concomitant pleural effusion is frequent.

Pulmonary hypertension results from hypoxemia or involvement of more than 50% of the area of the normal pulmonary bed. As a single event, an embolus does not cause pulmonary hypertension unless it is massive. Recurrent emboli may result in chronic pulmonary hypertension. Pulmonary hypertension eventually results in dilation and hypertrophy of the right ventricle. Depending on the degree of pulmonary hypertension and its rate of development, outcomes can vary, with some patients dying within months of the diagnosis and others living for decades (see Pulmonary Hypertension, p. 534).

Diagnostic Studies

- Spiral (or helical) computed tomography (CT) scan is the most frequently used test for PE. If the patient is unable to tolerate the contrast media used in a spiral CT, then a ventilation perfusion (V/Q) scan is done.
- D-dimer testing assists in screening for an embolism.
- Pulmonary angiography is a definitive test for emboli.
- Venous ultrasound can detect DVT as a source of PE.
- Arterial blood gases (ABGs) are abnormal with pulmonary occlusion but are not diagnostic of PE.

Collaborative Care

Objectives of treatment are to (1) prevent further growth or multiplication of thrombi in the lower extremities, (2) prevent embolization from the upper or lower extremities to the pulmonary vascular system, and (3) provide cardiopulmonary support if indicated.

Supportive therapy for the patient's cardiopulmonary status varies according to the severity of the pulmonary embolism.

- Administration of oxygen (O_2) by mask or cannula may be adequate for some patients. O_2 is given in a concentration determined by ABG analysis. In some situations, endotracheal intubation and mechanical ventilation may be needed to maintain adequate oxygenation.
- Respiratory measures such as turning, coughing, and deep breathing are important to prevent or treat atelectasis.
- If shock is present, vasopressor agents may be necessary to support systemic circulation. If heart failure is present, diuretics are used.

Pain resulting from pleural irritation or reduced coronary blood flow is treated with opioids, usually morphine. Properly managed anticoagulant therapy is effective for many patients. Although unfractionated heparin has been traditionally used, low molecular-weight heparin (e.g., enoxaparin [Lovenox]) is becoming more common. Warfarin (Coumadin) should be initiated within the first 24 hours and is typically administered for 3 to 6 months. Some health care providers are using factor Xa inhibitors and direct thrombin inhibitors in treating PE.

- Fibrinolytic agents, such as tissue plasminogen activator (tPA [Activase]) or alteplase (Activase), may be used to dissolve the PE as well as the thrombus source.

If the degree of pulmonary arterial obstruction is severe (usually >50%) and the patient does not respond to conservative therapy, an immediate embolectomy may be indicated. This is a rarely performed procedure that has a 50% mortality rate.

- To prevent further pulmonary embolization, an inferior vena cava (IVC) filter may be surgically placed in the vena cava to prevent migration of large clots from the lower extremities into the pulmonary system. It can be used for patients with absolute contraindications to anticoagulant therapy or for patients at high risk for PE (see Venous Thrombosis, p. 687).

Nursing Management

Nursing measures aimed at prevention of pulmonary embolism are similar to those for prevention of deep vein thrombosis (see Venous Thrombosis, p. 687).

The prognosis of a patient with pulmonary emboli is good if therapy is promptly instituted. Keep the patient in bed in a semi-Fowler's position to facilitate breathing. Maintain an intravenous (IV) line for medications and fluid therapy. Administer O_2 therapy as ordered. Carefully monitor vital signs, electrocardiogram (ECG), blood gases, and lung sounds to assess the patient's status.

- The patient is usually anxious because of pain, an inability to breathe, and a fear of death. Carefully explain the situation and provides emotional support and reassurance to help relieve the patient's anxiety.
- In addition to thromboembolic problems, the patient may have an underlying chronic illness requiring long-term treatment. To provide supportive therapy, you must understand and differentiate between the various problems caused by the underlying disease and those related to thromboembolic disease.

▼ **Patient and Caregiver Teaching**
- Long-term management is similar to that for the patient with venous thrombosis (see p. 687).
- Patient teaching regarding long-term anticoagulant therapy is critical. Anticoagulant therapy continues for at least 3 to 6 months; patients with recurrent emboli are treated indefinitely. INR (international normalized ratio) levels are drawn at intervals and warfarin dosage is adjusted.
- Discharge planning is aimed at limiting the progression of the condition and preventing complications and recurrence. Reinforce the need for the patient to return to the health care provider for regular follow-up examinations.

PULMONARY HYPERTENSION

Description
Pulmonary hypertension is elevated pulmonary pressures resulting from an increase in pulmonary vascular resistance to blood flow. Pulmonary hypertension can occur as a primary disease *(primary pulmonary hypertension [PPH])* or as a secondary complication of a respiratory, cardiac, autoimmune, or hepatic disorder *(secondary pulmonary hypertension)*.

Primary Pulmonary Hypertension
PPH is a rare and potentially fatal disease whose cause is unknown. It is characterized by mean pulmonary arterial pressure above 25 mm Hg at rest (normal 12 to 16 mm Hg) or above 30 mm Hg with exercise in the absence of a demonstrable cause. PPH affects more women than men, and it may have a genetic component because the incidence is higher in families. The mean age is 36 years.

Pathophysiology

- Normally the pulmonary circulation is characterized by low resistance and low pressure. In pulmonary hypertension the pulmonary pressures are elevated.
- An essential mechanism involved in PPH is a deficient release of vasodilator mediators from the pulmonary epithelium with a resultant cascade of injury.
- Vasoconstriction, remodeling of the walls of the pulmonary vessels, and thrombosis in situ are the three elements that combine to increase vascular resistance.

Clinical Manifestations

Classic symptoms are dyspnea on exertion and fatigue. Exertional chest pain, dizziness, and exertional syncope are other symptoms. Eventually, as the disease progresses, dyspnea occurs at rest. Pulmonary hypertension increases the workload of the right ventricle and causes right ventricular hypertrophy (a condition called *cor pulmonale*) (see Cor Pulmonale, p. 154) and eventually heart failure (see Heart Failure, p. 285).

PPH is a diagnosis of exclusion, and evaluation includes electrocardiogram (ECG), chest x-ray, echocardiogram, and spiral computed tomography (CT). Cardiac catheterization measures pulmonary artery pressures and cardiac output.

Collaborative Care

Although there is no cure for PPH, treatment can relieve symptoms, increase quality of life, and prolong life.

- Diuretic therapy relieves dyspnea and peripheral edema and may be useful in reducing right ventricular volume overload.
- Anticoagulation therapy prevents thrombus formation.
- Hypoxia is a potent pulmonary vasoconstrictor, and use of low-flow oxygen provides symptomatic relief.
- Some patients can be effectively managed with calcium channel blocker therapy.

In the past decade, new drugs have been approved for the treatment of PPH. All of them promote vasodilation of the pulmonary blood vessels, reduce right ventricular overload, and reverse remodeling. One class of drugs is the prostacyclin analogs (e.g., epoprostenol [Flolan], treprostinil [Remodulin], iloprost [Ventavis]).

Epoprostenol administration requires an indwelling central line catheter and continuous infusion pump. If the central line is disrupted, stopped, or dislodged for any reason, clinical deterioration can occur within minutes. With careful teaching and training of the patient and family, epoprostenol has been successful in improving quality of life of patients with PPH.

A second class of drugs used to treat PPH is endothelin receptor blockers that work by blocking the hormone endothelin, which causes blood vessels to constrict. Two oral drugs in this class are bosentan (Tracleer) and ambrisentan (Letairis). Monthly liver function tests are needed because of risk of hepatotoxicity.

The third class of drugs are phosphodiesterase inhibitors (e.g., sildenafil [Revatio]). It prolongs the vasodilatory effect of nitric oxide and is effective in decreasing pulmonary vascular resistance.

Surgical interventions for pulmonary hypertension include atrial septostomy (AS), pulmonary thromboendarterectomy (PTE), and lung transplantation. Lung transplantation is recommended for those patients who do not respond to drug therapy and progress to severe right-sided heart failure. Recurrence of the disease has not been reported in individuals who have undergone transplantation.

- A patient education and support site for pulmonary hypertension is located at www.phassociation.org.

Secondary Pulmonary Hypertension

Secondary pulmonary hypertension (SPH) occurs when a primary disease causes a chronic increase in pulmonary artery pressures. The disease pathology may result in anatomic or vascular changes causing pulmonary hypertension.

Anatomic changes causing increased vascular resistance include loss of capillaries as a result of alveolar wall damage (e.g., chronic obstructive pulmonary disease [COPD]), stiffening pulmonary vasculature (e.g., pulmonary fibrosis connective tissue disorders), and obstruction of blood flow (chronic emboli).

Vasomotor increases in pulmonary vascular resistance are found in conditions characterized by alveolar hypoxia. Hypoxia causes localized vasoconstriction and shunting of blood away from poorly ventilated alveoli.

- It is possible to have a combination of anatomic restriction and vasomotor constriction. This is found in the patient with long-standing chronic bronchitis who has chronic hypoxia in addition to loss of lung tissue.

Symptoms can reflect the underlying disease, but some are directly attributable to SPH, including dyspnea, fatigue, lethargy, and chest pain.

- Treatment of SPH consists mainly of treating the underlying primary disorder. When irreversible pulmonary vascular damage has occurred, therapies used for PPH are initiated.

PYELONEPHRITIS

Description

Pyelonephritis is an inflammation of the renal parenchyma and the collecting system (including the renal pelvis). *Urosepsis* is a systemic infection arising from a urologic source. Its prompt diagnosis and effective treatment are critical because it can lead to septic shock, the outcome of unresolved bacteremia involving a gram-negative organism (see Shock, p. 572).

Pathophysiology

Pyelonephritis usually begins with colonization and infection of the lower urinary tract via the ascending urethral route. Bacteria normally found in the intestinal tract, such as *Escherichia coli,* frequently cause pyelonephritis.

A preexisting factor is often present, such as *vesicoureteral reflux* (retrograde or backward movement of urine from lower to upper urinary tract) or dysfunction of lower urinary tract function, such as obstruction from benign prostatic hyperplasia or a urinary stone. In residents of long-term care facilities, urinary tract catheterization and the use of indwelling catheters are common causes of pyelonephritis and urosepsis.

Acute pyelonephritis commonly starts in the renal medulla and spreads to the adjacent cortex. Recurring episodes of pyelonephritis, especially in the presence of obstructive abnormalities, can lead to scarred, poorly functioning kidneys and a condition called *chronic pyelonephritis.*

Chronic pyelonephritis may also occur in the absence of an existing infection, recent infection, or history of urinary tract infections (UTIs). It often progresses to end-stage renal disease when both kidneys are involved, even if the underlying infection or problem is successfully eradicated (see Kidney Disease, Chronic, p. 381).

Clinical Manifestations

Acute pyelonephritis manifestations vary from mild fatigue to the sudden onset of chills, fever, vomiting, malaise, flank pain, and costovertebral tenderness on the affected side. Dysuria, urinary urgency, and frequency that are characteristic of bladder infections may also be present.

Acute manifestations generally subside within a few days even without specific therapy, although bacteriuria or pyuria usually persists.

Diagnostic Studies

- Urinalysis shows pyuria, bacteriuria, hematuria, and white blood cell (WBC) casts.
- Complete blood cell (CBC) count with WBC differential to identify leukocytosis.
- Intravenous pyelogram (IVP) and computed tomography (CT) are not recommended in early stages to prevent spread of infection.
- Ultrasound is used to identify anatomic abnormalities, hydronephrosis, renal abscesses, or stones.

Chronic pyelonephritis is diagnosed by radiologic and histologic testing rather than clinical features. Pathologic analysis reveals loss of functioning nephrons, infiltration of the parenchyma with inflammatory cells, and fibrosis.

Collaborative Care

Patients with severe infections or complicating factors such as nausea and vomiting with dehydration require hospital admission. Parenteral antibiotics are often given initially in the hospital to rapidly establish high serum and urinary drug levels.

The patient with mild symptoms may be treated as an outpatient with antibiotics for 14 to 21 days. Symptoms and signs typically improve or resolve within 48 to 72 hours after starting therapy. Relapses may be treated with a 6-week course of antibiotics. Antibiotic prophylaxis may also be used for recurrent infections.

Nursing Management

Goals

The patient with pyelonephritis will have normal renal function, normal body temperature, no complications, relief of pain, and no recurrence of symptoms.

See NCP 46-1 for the patient with a UTI, Lewis et al., *Medical-Surgical Nursing,* ed. 8, p. 1126.

Nursing Diagnoses/Collaborative Problem

- Impaired urinary elimination
- Readiness for enhanced self-health management
- Potential complication: urosepsis

Nursing Interventions

It is important that the patient receive early treatment for cystitis to prevent ascending infections. Because the patient with structural abnormalities of the urinary tract is at increased risk for infection, stress the need for regular medical care.

- Instruct the patient regarding the need to continue medications as prescribed and the need for follow-up urine cultures to ensure proper management and identification of recurrence of infection or relapse.

- In addition to antibiotic therapy, encourage the patient to drink at least eight glasses of fluid every day, even after the infection has been treated.
- Rest is often indicated to increase patient comfort.
- The patient with frequent relapses or reinfections may be treated with long-term, low-dose antibiotics. Understanding the rationale for therapy is important to enhance patient compliance.

RAYNAUD'S PHENOMENON

Description

R

Raynaud's phenomenon is an episodic vasospastic disorder of the small cutaneous arteries, most frequently involving the fingers and toes. It occurs primarily in young women; the exact etiology is unknown. It may occur secondary to an exaggerated response to sympathetic nervous system stimulation. Other contributing factors include occupationally related trauma and pressure to fingertips, as noted in typists, pianists, and those who use hand-held vibrating equipment. Exposure to heavy metals (e.g., lead) may also be a contributing etiologic factor. Exposure to cold, emotional upsets, tobacco use, and caffeine usually precipitate symptoms.

- *Primary Raynaud's phenomenon,* the more common form of the disease, is associated with significantly lower physical and mental health-related quality of life.
- When symptoms occur in association with autoimmune diseases (e.g., rheumatoid arthritis, systemic lupus erythematosus [SLE]), it is called *secondary Raynaud's phenomenon.*

Clinical Manifestations

- The disorder is characterized by vasospasm-induced color changes (white, red, and blue) of the fingers, toes, ears, and nose. Decreased perfusion results in pallor (white). The digits then appear cyanotic (bluish purple). These changes are subsequently followed by rubor (red) caused by the hyperemic response that occurs when perfusion is restored.
- The patient usually describes cold and numbness in the vasoconstrictive phase, with throbbing and aching pain, tingling, and swelling in the hyperemic phase. An episode usually lasts only minutes, but in severe cases it may persist for several hours.

- Complications include punctate (small hole) lesions of the fingertips and superficial gangrenous ulcers in advanced stages.

Diagnosis is based on persistent symptoms for at least 2 years.

Nursing and Collaborative Management

When a patient's episodes are severe and other therapies are ineffective, drug therapy is considered. Calcium channel blockers (e.g., diltiazem [Cardizem]) are the first-line drug therapy. Calcium channel blockers relax smooth muscles of the arterioles by blocking the influx of calcium into the cells, thus reducing vasospastic attacks.

Sympathectomy is considered only in advanced cases. Patients with Raynaud's phenomenon should receive routine follow-up to monitor for development of connective tissue or autoimmune diseases because Raynaud's phenomenon may be an early sign of scleroderma.

▼ **Patient and Caregiver Teaching**

Teaching should be directed toward prevention of recurrent episodes.

- Loose, warm clothing should be worn for protection from cold, including gloves when the refrigerator-freezer is used or cold objects are being handled.
- Temperature extremes should be avoided. Immersing hands in warm water often decreases the spasm.
- Patients should stop using all tobacco products and avoid caffeine and other drugs with vasoconstrictive effects (e.g., pseudoephedrine).
- Biofeedback, relaxation training, and stress management are effective for some patients whose symptoms are exacerbated by stress.

REACTIVE ARTHRITIS

Reactive arthritis *(Reiter's syndrome)* is associated with a symptom complex that includes urethritis or cervicitis, conjunctivitis, and mucocutaneous lesions. It occurs more commonly in young men as compared with young women. Although the exact etiology is unknown, reactive arthritis appears to occur after a genitourinary or gastrointestinal tract infection. *Chlamydia trachomatis* is most often implicated in sexually transmitted reactive arthritis. Men and women appear to have equal risk for developing dysenteric reactive arthritis, which typically occurs within days or weeks after infection with *Shigella, Salmonella, Campylobacter,* or

Yersinia. Individuals with inherited HLA-B27 are at increased risk of developing reactive arthritis after sexual contact or exposure to certain enteric pathogens, supporting the likelihood of a genetic predisposition.

- Urethritis develops within 1 to 2 weeks after sexual contact or dysentery. Low-grade fever, conjunctivitis, and arthritis may occur over the next several weeks.
- This arthritis tends to be asymmetric, frequently involving large joints of the lower extremities and toes. Lower back pain may occur with severe disease.
- Mucocutaneous lesions commonly occur as small, painless, superficial ulcerations on the tongue, oral mucosa, and glans penis. Soft tissue manifestations commonly include enthesopathies such as Achilles tendinitis or plantar fasciitis.
- Few laboratory abnormalities occur, although the erythrocyte sedimentation rate (ESR) may be elevated.

Prognosis is favorable, with most patients recovering after 2 to 16 weeks. Because reactive arthritis is often associated with *Chlamydia trachomatis* infection, treatment of patients and their sexual partners with doxycycline (Vibramycin) is widely recommended.

Joints may heal completely, and many patients have complete remission with full joint function. Up to 50% may develop chronic or recurring disease, which can result in major disability. Treatment of chronic reactive arthritis is symptomatic.

REFRACTIVE ERRORS

Refractive errors are the most common visual problem. This defect in vision prevents light rays from converging into a single focus on the retina. Defects result from corneal curvature irregularities, lens-focusing power, or eye length.

Types of refractive errors include the following:

- *Myopia* (nearsightedness), the most common refractive error, is caused by light rays focusing in front of the retina, resulting in an inability to accommodate for objects at a distance.
- *Hyperopia* (farsightedness) is caused by light rays focusing behind the retina and requires the person to use accommodation to focus the light rays on the retina for near and far objects.
- *Presbyopia* is a loss of accommodation resulting from age, with the crystalline lens becoming larger, firmer, and less elastic. This condition generally appears about the age of 45 years and results in an inability to accommodate for near objects.

- *Astigmatism* is caused by an irregular corneal curvature so that incoming light rays are bent unequally and light rays do not come to a single point of focus on the retina.
- The major symptom of refractive errors is blurred vision. Additional complaints may include ocular discomfort, eye strain, or headaches.
- Management of refractive errors is correction, which may include eyeglasses, contact lenses, refractive surgery, or surgical implantation of an artificial lens to improve the focus of light rays on the retina.

RESPIRATORY FAILURE, ACUTE

Description

The major function of the respiratory system is gas exchange, which involves the transfer of oxygen (O_2) and carbon dioxide (CO_2) between inhaled tidal volumes and circulating blood volume within the pulmonary capillary bed. Respiratory failure results when one or both of these gas-exchanging functions are inadequate. *Respiratory failure* is not a disease but a symptom of an underlying pathology affecting lung tissue function, O_2 delivery, cardiac output (CO), or the baseline metabolic state. It is a condition that occurs because of one or more diseases involving the lungs or other body systems (Table 76). Respiratory failure is classified as hypoxemic or hypercapnic.

- *Hypoxemic respiratory failure* is also referred to as oxygenation failure because the primary problem is inadequate O_2 transfer between the alveoli and the pulmonary capillary bed. Although no universal definition exists, hypoxemic respiratory failure is commonly defined as a partial pressure of oxygen in arterial blood (PaO_2) of 60 mm Hg or less when the patient is receiving an inspired O_2 concentration of $\geq 60\%$.
- *Hypercapnic respiratory failure* is also referred to as ventilatory failure because the primary problem is insufficient CO_2 removal. Hypercapnic respiratory failure is commonly defined as a partial pressure of carbon dioxide in arterial blood ($PaCO_2$) >45 mm Hg in combination with acidemia (pH <7.35).

Many patients experience both hypoxemic and hypercapnic respiratory failure.

Pathophysiology

Hypoxemic respiratory failure. Four physiologic mechanisms may cause hypoxemia and subsequent hypoxemic respiratory

Table 76	Common Causes of Hypoxemic and Hypercapnic Respiratory Failure

Hypoxemic Respiratory Failure*	Hypercapnic Respiratory Failure*
Respiratory System ■ Acute respiratory distress syndrome ■ Pneumonia ■ Toxic inhalation (e.g., smoke inhalation) ■ Hepatopulmonary syndrome (e.g., low-resistance flow state, V/Q mismatch) ■ Massive pulmonary embolism (e.g., thrombus emboli, fat emboli) ■ Pulmonary artery laceration and hemorrhage ■ Inflammatory state and related alveolar injury **Cardiac System** ■ Anatomic shunt (e.g., ventricular septal defect) ■ Cardiogenic pulmonary edema ■ Shock (decreasing blood flow through pulmonary vasculature) ■ High cardiac output states: Diffusion limitation	**Respiratory System** ■ Asthma ■ COPD ■ Cystic fibrosis **Central Nervous System** ■ Brainstem injury/infarction ■ Sedative and opioid overdose ■ Spinal cord injury ■ Severe head injury **Chest Wall** ■ Thoracic trauma (e.g., flail chest) ■ Kyphoscoliosis ■ Pain ■ Morbid obesity **Neuromuscular System** ■ Myasthenia gravis ■ Critical illness polyneuropathy ■ Acute myopathy ■ Toxin exposure/ingestion (e.g., tree tobacco, acetylcholinesterase inhibitors, carbamate, or organophosphate poisoning) ■ Amyotrophic lateral sclerosis ■ Phrenic nerve injury ■ Guillain-Barré syndrome ■ Poliomyelitis ■ Muscular dystrophy ■ Multiple sclerosis

COPD, Chronic obstructive pulmonary disease.
*This list is not all inclusive.

R

failure: (1) mismatch between ventilation (V) and perfusion (Q) commonly referred to as V/Q mismatch, (2) shunt, (3) diffusion limitation, and (4) hypoventilation. The most common causes are V/Q mismatch and shunt.

■ Many diseases and conditions alter *V/Q mismatch*. The most common are those in which increased secretions are present in the airways (e.g., chronic obstructive pulmonary disease [COPD]) or alveoli (e.g., pneumonia) or when bronchospasm is present (e.g., asthma). V/Q mismatch may also result when alveoli collapse (atelectasis) or as a result of pain.

- *Shunt* occurs when blood exits the heart without having participated in gas exchange. A shunt can be viewed as an extreme V/Q mismatch. There are two types of shunt: anatomic and intrapulmonary. O_2 therapy alone may be ineffective in increasing the PaO_2 if hypoxemia is caused by shunt.

- *Diffusion limitation* occurs when a process that thickens or destroys the membrane compromises the gas exchange across the alveolar-capillary membrane. Diffusion limitation may worsen by conditions that affect the pulmonary vascular bed, such as severe emphysema or recurrent pulmonary emboli. Some diseases cause the alveolar-capillary membrane to become thicker (fibrotic), which slows gas transport. These diseases include pulmonary fibrosis, interstitial lung disease, and acute respiratory distress syndrome (ARDS). The classic sign of diffusion limitation is hypoxemia that is present during exercise but not at rest.

- *Alveolar hypoventilation* is a generalized decrease in ventilation that results in an increase in the $PaCO_2$ and a consequent decrease in PaO_2. Alveolar hypoventilation may be the result of restrictive lung disease, central nervous system (CNS) disease, chest wall dysfunction, or neuromuscular disease.

- Frequently, hypoxemic respiratory failure is caused by a combination of V/Q mismatch, shunting, diffusion limitation, and hypoventilation.

Hypercapnic respiratory failure. Hypercapnic respiratory failure results from an imbalance between ventilatory supply and ventilatory demand. Normally, ventilatory supply far exceeds ventilatory demand. However, patients with preexisting lung disease such as severe COPD cannot effectively increase lung ventilation in response to exercise or metabolic demands. Hypercapnic respiratory failure is sometimes called ventilatory failure because the primary problem is the inability of the respiratory system to ventilate out sufficient CO_2 to maintain a normal $PaCO_2$.

- Many diseases can cause a limitation in ventilatory supply (see Table 76). They can be grouped into four categories: (1) abnormalities of the airways and alveoli, (2) abnormalities of the CNS, (3) abnormalities of the chest wall, and (4) neuromuscular conditions.

Clinical Manifestations
Respiratory failure may develop suddenly (in minutes or hours) or gradually (taking several days or longer). A sudden decrease in

PaO_2 or a rapid rise in $PaCO_2$ implies a serious condition that can rapidly become a life-threatening emergency.

Manifestations are related to the extent of the change in PaO_2 and $PaCO_2$, the rapidity of change (acute versus chronic), and the ability to compensate to overcome this change. When the patient's compensatory mechanisms fail, respiratory failure occurs. Because manifestations are variable, it is important to monitor trends in arterial blood gas (ABG) values or use pulse oximetry to evaluate the extent of change.

- Mental status changes such as restlessness, confusion, and combative behavior will occur early, frequently before ABG results indicate changes.
- Tachycardia, tachypnea, and mild hypertension are also early signs. A severe morning headache may suggest that hypercapnia occurred during the night. Rapid shallow breaths suggest that the tidal volume may be inadequate to remove CO_2 from the lungs.
- As the PaO_2 decreases and acidosis increases, the myocardium becomes dysfunctional, resulting in angina and dysrhythmias. Permanent brain damage may occur if the hypoxia is severe and prolonged. Renal function may be impaired, and sodium (Na^+) retention, edema formation, acute tubular necrosis, and uremia may result.
- The patient may have a rapid, shallow breathing pattern or a respiratory rate that is slower than normal. A change from a rapid to a slower rate in a patient in acute respiratory distress suggests extreme fatigue and the possibility of an impending respiratory arrest.
- Respiratory behaviors such as assumption of tripod position, pursed-lip breathing, and two- or three-word dyspnea also indicate respiratory distress.
- There may be a change in the inspiratory (I) to expiratory (E) (I/E) ratio. Normally the I/E ratio is 1 : 2. In patients in respiratory distress, the ratio may increase to 1 : 3 or 1 : 4. This change signifies airflow obstruction.
- You may observe *retraction* (inward movement) of the intercostal spaces or the supraclavicular area and the use of accessory muscles during inspiration or expiration. Use of the accessory muscles signifies moderate distress. Paradoxic breathing indicates severe distress.

Report immediately any change in mental status, such as combative behavior, confusion, or a decreased level of consciousness (LOC), because this change may indicate the onset of rapid deterioration and the need for mechanical ventilation.

Diagnostic Studies

- ABG analysis is used to determine $PaCO_2$, PaO_2, bicarbonate, and pH.
- Chest x-ray helps to identify possible causes of respiratory failure.
- A catheter may be inserted into a peripheral artery for monitoring blood pressure (BP) and obtaining ABGs.
- Pulse oximetry is used for the monitoring of oxygenation status, but in respiratory failure, ABGs are necessary to obtain oxygenation (PaO_2) and ventilation ($PaCO_2$) status, as well as acid-base information.
- Other studies may include complete blood count (CBC), serum electrolytes, urinalysis, and electrocardiogram (ECG).
- Sputum and blood cultures are obtained as necessary to determine sources of possible infection.
- If pulmonary embolus is suspected, a ventilation-perfusion (V/Q) lung scan or CT scan may be done.

In severe respiratory failure requiring endotracheal intubation, end-tidal CO_2 ($ETCO_2$) may be used to assess tube placement within the trachea immediately following intubation. $ETCO_2$ may also be used during ventilator management to assess trends in lung ventilation. A central venous or pulmonary artery (PA) catheter is often used to measure hemodynamic parameters (e.g., central venous pressure, PA pressures, CO, pulmonary artery wedge pressure, central/mixed venous O_2 saturation [$ScvO_2$/SvO_2]).

Nursing and Collaborative Management

Because many different problems can cause respiratory failure, specific care of the patient varies.

Goals

The patient in acute respiratory failure will have normal ABG values or value's within the patient's baseline, normal or breath sounds within the patient's baseline, no dyspnea or breathing patterns within the patient's baseline, and effective cough and ability to clear secretions.

Nursing Diagnoses

- Impaired gas exchange
- Ineffective airway clearance
- Ineffective breathing pattern
- Risk for imbalanced fluid volume

Respiratory Therapy

The major goals of care for acute respiratory failure include maintaining adequate oxygenation and ventilation. Interventions include O_2 therapy, mobilization of secretions, and positive pressure ventilation (PPV).

O_2 therapy. The primary goal of O_2 therapy is to correct hypoxemia (see Oxygen Therapy, p. 743). If hypoxemia is secondary to V/Q mismatch, supplemental O_2 administered at 1 to 3 L/min by nasal cannula or 24% to 32% by simple face mask or Venturi mask should improve the PaO_2 and SaO_2. Hypoxemia secondary to an intrapulmonary shunt is usually not responsive to high O_2 concentrations, and the patient usually requires PPV (see Mechanical Ventilation, p. 736).

- Patients with chronic hypercapnia frequently have CO_2 narcosis and should receive O_2 through a low-flow device, such as a nasal cannula at 1 to 2 L/min or a Venturi mask at 24% to 28%. Closely monitor these patients for changes in mental status, respiratory rate, and ABG results until their PaO_2 level has reached their baseline normal value.

Mobilization of secretions. Retained pulmonary secretions may cause or exacerbate acute respiratory failure by blocking O_2 movement into the alveoli and pulmonary capillary blood and the removal of CO_2. Secretions can be mobilized through effective coughing, adequate hydration and humidification, chest physical therapy, ambulation when possible, and tracheal suctioning.

Effective coughing and positioning. If secretions are obstructing the airway, encourage the patient to cough. The patient with a neuromuscular weakness from disease or exhaustion may not be able to generate sufficient airway pressures to produce an effective cough. *Augmented coughing (quad coughing)* may be helpful. Perform augmented coughing by placing the palm of your hand (or the palms of both hands) on the patient's abdomen below the xiphoid process. As the patient ends a deep inspiration and begins the expiration, move your hands forcefully downward, increasing abdominal pressure and facilitating the cough.

- Positioning the patient by elevating the head of the bed to at least 45 degrees or using a reclining chair bed may help maximize thoracic expansion.
- All patients should be side-lying if there is a possibility that the tongue will obstruct the airway or aspiration may occur. An oral or nasal artificial airway should be kept at the bedside for use if necessary.

Hydration and humidification. Thick and viscous secretions are difficult to expel. Adequate fluid intake (2 to 3 L/day) is necessary to keep secretions thin and easy to remove. If the patient is unable to take sufficient fluids orally, intravenous (IV) hydration will be used. Assess for signs of fluid overload by clinical evaluation (e.g., crackles, dyspnea) and invasive monitoring (e.g., increased central venous pressure) at regular intervals.

Airway suctioning. If the patient is unable to expectorate secretions, nasopharyngeal, oropharyngeal, or nasotracheal suctioning is done. Suctioning through an artificial airway, such as an endotracheal tube, is also performed as needed. At all times, suctioning is done cautiously because it may precipitate hypoxia.

Positive pressure ventilation. If intensive measures fail to improve ventilation and oxygenation, ventilatory assistance may be initiated. (See Mechanical Ventilation, p. 736.)

Drug Therapy

Goals of drug therapy for patients in acute respiratory failure include relief of bronchospasm, reduction of airway inflammation and pulmonary congestion, treatment of pulmonary infection, and reduction of severe anxiety and restlessness.

Relief of bronchospasm. Relief of bronchospasm increases alveolar ventilation. Short-acting bronchodilators, such as metaproterenol (Alupent) and albuterol (Ventolin), reverse bronchospasm, using either a hand-held nebulizer or a metered-dose inhaler with a spacer. These drugs may be given at 15- to 30-minute intervals until you determine that a response is occurring.

Reduction of airway inflammation. Corticosteroids (e.g., methylprednisolone [Solu-Medrol]) may be used in conjunction with bronchodilating agents when bronchospasms and inflammation are present. Inhaled corticosteroids are not used for acute respiratory failure, because they require 4 to 5 days before optimum effects are seen.

Reduction of pulmonary congestion. IV diuretics (e.g., furosemide [Lasix]) and nitroglycerin (e.g., Tridil) are used to decrease the pulmonary congestion caused by heart failure. If atrial fibrillation is also present, calcium channel blockers and β-adrenergic blockers may be used to decrease heart rate and improve cardiac output.

Treatment of pulmonary infections. Pulmonary infections can either cause or exacerbate acute respiratory failure. IV antibiotics are frequently administered to inhibit bacterial growth.

Reduction of severe anxiety and restlessness. Anxiety, restlessness, and agitation result from cerebral hypoxia. In addition, fear caused by the inability to breathe and a sense of loss of control may exacerbate anxiety. Anxiety, pain, and agitation increase O_2 consumption, which may worsen the degree of hypoxemia. Anxiety, pain, and agitation also increase CO_2 production, affect ventilator management, and increase morbidity.

- Sedation and analgesia with drug therapy are used to decrease anxiety, agitation, and pain. You must monitor patients closely receiving any sedative medication for respiratory and cardiovascular depression.

Collaborative Care

Goals and related interventions to maximize O_2 delivery are essential to improving the patient's oxygenation and ventilation status. The primary goal is to treat the underlying cause of the respiratory failure. Other supportive goals include maintaining an adequate CO and hemoglobin concentration.

- Interventions are directed toward reversing the disease process that resulted in the development of acute respiratory failure.
- Decreased cardiac output is treated by administration of IV fluids, medications, or both.
- If hemoglobin concentration is <9 g/dL (<90 g/L), packed red blood cells may be transfused.

Nutritional Therapy

Maintenance of protein and energy stores is especially important because nutritional depletion causes a loss of muscle mass, including the respiratory muscles, and may prolong recovery. During the acute manifestations of respiratory failure, the risk of aspiration typically prevents oral nutritional intake. Therefore enteral (preferred) or parenteral nutrition may be administered until acute manifestations subside.

RESTLESS LEGS SYNDROME

Description

Restless legs syndrome (RLS) is characterized by unpleasant sensory (paresthesias) and motor abnormalities of one or both legs. Prevalence rates vary from 5% to 15%, although the numbers may be higher, because the condition is underdiagnosed.

There are two distinct types of RLS, primary (idiopathic) and secondary. The majority of cases are primary, and many patients with this type of RLS report a positive family history. Secondary RLS can be seen in metabolic abnormalities associated with iron deficiency, renal failure, polyneuropathy associated with diabetes mellitus, rheumatoid arthritis, or pregnancy. Anemia, deficient iron condition, and certain medications can cause or worsen symptoms.

Pathophysiology

Primary RLS is related to abnormal iron metabolism and functional alterations in central dopaminergic neurotransmitter systems. Although primary RLS may be related to nervous system dysfunction, the exact cause remains to be determined. Several theories include (1) an alteration in dopaminergic transmission in the basal ganglia, (2) axonal neuropathy, or (3) a brainstem disinhibition phenomenon resulting in motor and sensory disturbances. Recent research has found a strong association between RLS and cardiovascular disease.

Clinical Manifestations

The severity of RLS sensory symptoms ranges from infrequent minor discomfort (paresthesias including numbness, tingling, "pins and needles") to severe pain. Sensory symptoms often appear first and are manifested as an annoying and uncomfortable (but usually not painful) sensation in the legs.

- The sensation is often compared with the sensation of bugs creeping or crawling on the skin.
- Patients can also experience pain in the upper extremities and trunk that occurs when the patient is sedentary and usually in the evening or at night.
- Pain at night can produce sleep disruptions and is often relieved by physical activity such as walking, stretching, rocking, or kicking.

Motor abnormalities associated with RLS consist of voluntary restlessness and periodic, involuntary movements that usually occur during sleep. Symptoms are aggravated by fatigue. Over time, RLS advances to more frequent and severe episodes.

Diagnostic Studies

RLS is a clinical diagnosis based in large part on the patient's history or the report of the bed partner related to nighttime activities. Diagnostic criteria include (1) an urge to move the legs, usually accompanied by uncomfortable and unpleasant sensations in the legs that begin or worsen during periods of rest or inactivity; (2) the urge to move or unpleasant sensations are partially or totally relieved by movement; and (3) symptoms that are worse in the evening or night.

- Polysomnography studies during sleep may be performed to distinguish the problem from other clinical conditions (e.g., sleep apnea).
- Blood tests, such as a complete blood count, serum ferritin levels, and renal function tests (e.g., serum creatinine) may help to exclude secondary causes of RLS.

Nursing and Collaborative Management

The goal of collaborative management is to reduce patient discomfort and distress and improve sleep quality. When RLS is secondary to uremia or iron deficiency, correction of these conditions will decrease symptoms.

■ Nondrug approaches include establishing regular sleep habits, encouraging exercise, avoiding activities that cause symptoms, and eliminating aggravating factors such as alcohol, caffeine, and certain drugs (neuroleptics, lithium, antihistamines, antidepressants).

If nondrug measures fail to provide symptom relief, drug therapy may be started. The drugs of choice in treating RLS are dopaminergic agents such as carbidopa-levodopa (Sinemet) and dopamine agonists (e.g., pergolide [Permax], bromocriptine [Parlodel], pramipexole [Mirapex]). Ropinirole (Requip), a drug used to treat Parkinson's disease, is used to treat moderate to severe RLS. These agents are effective in managing sensory and motor symptoms.

Other agents that may be used include antiseizure drugs, benzodiazepines, clonidine (Catapres), and propranolol (Inderal). Opioids (e.g., oxycodone) are usually reserved for those patients with severe symptoms who fail to respond to other drug therapies.

RETINAL DETACHMENT

Description
Retinal detachment is a separation of the sensory retina and underlying pigment epithelium with fluid accumulation between the two layers. Risk factors include increasing age, severe myopia, aphakia, diabetic retinopathy, cataract or glaucoma surgery, eye trauma, and family or personal history.

Pathophysiology
The most common cause is a retinal break, which is an interruption in the full thickness of the retinal tissue. Retinal holes are spontaneous atrophic breaks and retinal tears occur when the vitreous shrinks with aging and pulls on the retina.

Once there is a retinal break, liquid vitreous enters between the sensory and retinal pigment epithelium layers, causing detachment. Untreated retinal detachment leads to blindness in the involved eye.

Clinical Manifestations
Symptoms of a detaching retina include photopsia ("light flashes"), floaters, and a "cobweb" or ring in the vision field. Once the retina is detached, a painless loss of peripheral or central vision is described.

Diagnostic Studies
- Visual acuity measurements
- Direct and indirect ophthalmoscopy or slit lamp microscopy
- Ultrasound to help identify a detachment

Collaborative Care
Retinal breaks are evaluated to determine if prophylactic laser photocoagulation or cryopexy is necessary to avoid retinal detachment. Some breaks do not progress to detachment, so the patient may be observed and given precise information about the warning signs of impending detachment and instructions to seek immediate evaluation if these signs occur. The ophthalmologist usually refers the patient with a detachment to a retinal specialist.

Treatment objectives are to seal any retinal breaks and relieve inward traction on the retina. Surgical treatment to seal breaks may include laser photocoagulation and cryopexy. Management of inward retinal traction can involve scleral buckling, pneumatic retinopexy, and vitrectomy.

- Reattachment is successful in 90% of all cases, with visual prognosis dependent on the extent, length, and area of detachment.

Nursing Management
Goals
The patient with a retinal detachment will experience minimal anxiety throughout the event and maintain an acceptable level of comfort postoperatively.

Nursing Diagnoses
- Acute pain
- Anxiety

Nursing Interventions
Retinal detachment is a situation with an urgent need for surgery. The patient needs emotional support, especially during the immediate preoperative period.

- The level of activity restriction following retinal detachment surgeries varies greatly. Verify the prescribed level of activity with each patient's surgeon and help the patient plan for any necessary assistance related to activity restrictions.
- With postoperative pain, administer prescribed pain medications and teach the patient to take medication as necessary when discharged.
- Discharge planning is important. Begin this process as early as possible because the patient may not be hospitalized long.

▼ **Patient and Caregiver Teaching**
- Instruct the patient with an increased risk of retinal detachment about the signs of detachment and to seek immediate evaluation if any of those signs or symptoms occurs.
- Promote the use of proper protective eyewear to help avoid retinal detachments related to trauma.
- After eye surgery for retinal detachment, review the signs of retinal detachment with the patient because the risk of detachment in the other eye is increased.

RHEUMATIC FEVER AND HEART DISEASE

Description
Rheumatic fever is an acute, inflammatory disease of the heart. The resulting damage to the heart from rheumatic fever is called *rheumatic heart disease,* a chronic condition characterized by scarring and deformity of the heart valves.

Pathophysiology
Rheumatic fever occurs as a delayed sequela (usually 2 to 3 weeks) after a group A streptococcal pharyngitis. Manifestations of rheumatic fever (RF) appear to be related to an abnormal immunologic response to group A streptococcal cell membrane antigens. RF affects the heart, joints, central nervous system (CNS), and skin.

About 40% of RF episodes are marked by carditis, and all layers of the heart (endocardium, myocardium, pericardium) are involved.
- Rheumatic endocarditis is found primarily in the valves, with swelling and erosion of the valve leaflets. Vegetations form and create a fibrous thickening of the valve leaflets, fusion of commissures and chordae tendineae, and fibrosis of the papillary muscle. Stenosis and regurgitation may occur in valve leaflets. The mitral and aortic valves are most commonly affected.
- Myocardial involvement is characterized by *Aschoff bodies,* which are nodules formed by a reaction to inflammation with accompanying swelling and fragmentation of collagen fibers.
- Rheumatic pericarditis develops and affects both layers of the pericardium, which becomes thickened and covered with a fibrinous exudate.

The lesions of rheumatic fever are systemic and involve the joints (polyarthritis), skin (subcutaneous [SC] nodules), and CNS (chorea).

Clinical Manifestations

The presence of two major criteria, or one major and two minor criteria, plus evidence of a preceding group A streptococcal infection indicates a high probability of RF.

Major Criteria

- *Carditis* is the most important manifestation of RF and results in three signs: (1) an organic heart murmur or murmurs of mitral or aortic regurgitation, or mitral stenosis; (2) cardiac enlargement and heart failure (HF) occurring secondary to myocarditis; and (3) pericarditis resulting in distant heart sounds, chest pain, a pericardial friction rub, or signs of effusion.

- *Monoarthritis or polyarthritis,* the most common finding in RF, involves swelling, heat, redness, tenderness, and limitation of motion. The larger joints are most frequently affected.

- *Sydenham's chorea* is the major CNS manifestation. It is characterized by involuntary movements, especially of the face and limbs, muscle weakness, and disturbances of speech and gait.

- *Erythema marginatum* lesions are a less common feature. The bright pink, nonpruritic, maplike macular lesions occur mainly on the trunk and proximal extremities and may be exacerbated by heat (e.g., a warm bath).

- *Subcutaneous nodules* are firm, small, hard, painless swellings found most commonly over extensor surfaces of the joints, especially knees, wrists, and elbows.

Minor Criteria

Minor clinical manifestations are frequently present and helpful in recognizing the disease. These include fever, polyarthralgia, and certain laboratory tests (e.g., elevated C-reactive protein, elevated white blood cell count).

Evidence of infection. Evidence of a preceding group A streptococcal infection include a positive rapid antigen test for group A streptococci, an elevated antistreptolysin-O titer, or a positive throat culture.

Diagnostic Studies

- Chest x-ray may show an enlarged heart if HF is present.
- Echocardiogram may show valvular insufficiency and pericardial fluid or thickening.
- Electrocardiogram (ECG) reveals a prolonged PR interval with delayed atrioventricular (AV) conduction.

Collaborative Care

Treatment consists of drug therapy and supportive measures. Antibiotic therapy does not modify the course of the acute disease or the development of carditis, but it does eliminate residual group A streptococci remaining in the tonsils and pharynx and prevents the spread of organisms to close contacts. Salicylates, nonsteroidal antiinflammatory drugs (NSAIDs), and corticosteroids are effective in controlling the fever and joint manifestations. Corticosteroids are also used if severe carditis is present.

Nursing Management
Goals
The patient with RF and rheumatic heart disease will have normal or baseline heart function, resumption of daily activities without joint pain, and verbalization of the ability to manage the disease sequelae.
Nursing Diagnoses
- Activity intolerance
- Decreased cardiac output
- Ineffective self-health management

Nursing Interventions
RF is one of the cardiovascular diseases that is preventable. Prevention involves the early detection and immediate treatment of group A streptococcal pharyngitis. Adequate treatment of streptococcal pharyngitis prevents initial attacks of RF. Your role is to educate the community to seek medical attention for symptoms of streptococcal pharyngitis and emphasize the need for adequate treatment of a streptococcal sore throat.

The primary goals of managing a patient with RF are to control and eradicate the infecting organism; prevent cardiac complications; and relieve joint pain, fever, and other symptoms.
- Administer antibiotics as ordered and teach the patient that oral antibiotics require adherence to the full course of therapy.
- Administer antipyretics, NSAIDs, and corticosteroids and monitor fluid intake.
- Promotion of optimal rest is essential to reduce the cardiac workload and diminish the metabolic needs of the body. After acute symptoms have subsided, the patient without carditis should ambulate.
- If the patient has carditis with HF, strict bed rest restrictions apply. Encourage nonstrenuous activities once recovery has begun.

▼ Patient and Caregiver Teaching
- Teach the patient with a previous history of RF about the disease process, possible sequelae, and the need for continuous prophylactic antibiotics.
- Patient teaching should include good nutrition, hygiene practices, and adequate rest.

- Caution the patient about the possibility of developing valvular heart disease. Teach the patient to seek medical attention if symptoms such as excessive fatigue, dizziness, palpitations, or exertional dyspnea develop.

RHEUMATOID ARTHRITIS

Description

Rheumatoid arthritis (RA) is a chronic, systemic autoimmune disease characterized by inflammation of connective tissue in the diarthrodial (synovial) joints, typically with periods of remission and exacerbation. RA is frequently accompanied by extraarticular manifestations.

RA occurs globally, affecting all ethnic groups. It can occur at any time of life, but the incidence increases with age, peaking between 30 and 50 years old. Women are affected by RA more frequently than men. Smoking significantly increases the risk of RA in both men and women who are genetically predisposed to the disease.

Pathophysiology

The cause of RA is unknown. No infectious agent has been cultured from blood and synovial tissue or fluid with enough reproducibility to suggest an infectious cause. An autoimmune etiology is currently the most widely accepted cause.

1. *Autoimmunity.* The autoimmune theory suggests that changes associated with RA begin when a susceptible host experiences an initial immune response to an antigen. The antigen, which is probably not the same in all patients, triggers the formation of an abnormal immunoglobulin G (IgG). RA is characterized by the presence of autoantibodies against this abnormal IgG. The autoantibodies are known as *rheumatoid factor* (RF), and they combine with IgG to form immune complexes that initially deposit on synovial membranes or superficial articular cartilage in the joints.

   - Immune complex formation leads to the activation of complement, and an inflammatory response results. Neutrophils are attracted to the site of inflammation, where they release proteolytic enzymes that damage articular cartilage and cause the synovial lining to thicken.
   - Other inflammatory cells include T helper ($CD4^+$) cells and proinflammatory cytokines, such as interleukin-1 (IL-1), interleukin-6 (IL-6), and tumor necrosis factor (TNF).
   - Joint changes from chronic inflammation begin when the hypertrophied synovial membrane invades the surrounding

Table 77	Anatomic Stages of Rheumatoid Arthritis

Stage I: Early
No destructive changes on x-ray, possible x-ray evidence of osteoporosis

Stage II: Moderate
X-ray evidence of osteoporosis, with or without slight bone or cartilage destruction; no joint deformities (although possibly limited joint mobility); adjacent muscle atrophy; possible presence of extraarticular soft tissue lesions (e.g., nodules, tenosynovitis)

Stage III: Severe
X-ray evidence of cartilage and bone destruction in addition to osteoporosis; joint deformity, such as subluxation, ulnar deviation, or hyperextension, without fibrous or bony ankylosis; extensive muscle atrophy; possible presence of extraarticular soft tissue lesions (e.g., nodules, tenosynovitis)

Stage IV: Terminal
Fibrous or bony ankylosis, stage III criteria
Data from American College of Rheumatology: Classification criteria for determining progression of rheumatoid arthritis.

Available at www.hopkins-arthritis.org/physician-corner/education/acr/acr.html.

cartilage, ligaments, tendons, and joint capsule. *Pannus* (highly vascular granulation tissue) forms within the joint. It eventually covers and erodes the entire surface of the articular cartilage.
2. *Genetic factors.* Genetic predisposition appears to be important in the development of RA. The strongest evidence for a familial influence is the increased occurrence of a human leukocyte antigen (HLA) known as HLA-DR4 in white RA patients. Other HLA variants have also been identified in patients from other ethnic groups.

The pathogenesis of RA is more clearly understood than its etiology. If unarrested, the disease progresses through four stages, which are identified in Table 77.

Clinical Manifestations

RA typically develops insidiously. Nonspecific manifestations such as fatigue, anorexia, weight loss, and generalized stiffness may precede the onset of arthritic complaints. The stiffness becomes more localized after weeks to months. Some patients report a history of a precipitating stressful event, such as infection, work stress, physical exertion, childbirth, surgery, or emotional upset.

Articular involvement is manifested by pain, stiffness, limitation of motion, and signs of inflammation (heat, swelling, tenderness). Joint symptoms occur symmetrically and frequently affect the small joints of the hands and feet, as well as the larger peripheral joints, including wrists, elbows, shoulders, knees, hips, ankles, and jaw.

- The patient characteristically has joint stiffness after periods of inactivity. (See Table 66, p. 458, for a comparison of the manifestations of RA and osteoarthritis [OA].)
- As RA progresses, inflammation and fibrosis of the joint capsule and supporting structures may lead to deformity and disability. Atrophy of muscles and destruction of tendons around the joint cause one articular surface to slip past the other *(subluxation)*. Typical hand deformities include "ulnar drift," "swan neck," and boutonniere deformities.

Extraarticular manifestations. RA can affect nearly every system in the body. Extraarticular manifestations of RA are depicted in Fig. 65-5, Lewis et al., *Medical-Surgical Nursing,* ed. 8, p. 1652. The three most common manifestations are rheumatoid nodules, Sjögren's syndrome, and Felty syndrome.

Rheumatoid nodules develop in up to 25% of all patients with RA. They appear subcutaneously as firm, nontender, granuloma-type masses and are usually found over the extensor surfaces of joints such as the fingers and elbows. Nodules at the base of the spine and back of the head are common in older adults. Nodules that appear on the sclera or lungs indicate active disease and have a poorer prognosis. They are usually not removed because of the high probability of recurrence.

Sjögren's syndrome is seen in 10% to 15% of patients with RA. Sjögren's syndrome can occur as a disease by itself or in conjunction with other arthritic disorders, such as RA and systemic lupus erythematosus (SLE). Affected patients have diminished lacrimal and salivary gland secretion, leading to complaints of burning, gritty, itchy eyes. They experience decreased tearing and photosensitivity (see Sjögren's Syndrome, p. 589).

Felty syndrome occurs most commonly in patients with severe, nodule-forming RA. It is characterized by inflammatory eye disorders, splenomegaly, lymphadenopathy, pulmonary disease, and blood dyscrasias (anemia, thrombocytopenia, granulocytopenia).

Diagnostic Studies

A diagnosis is often made based on history and physical findings, but some laboratory tests are useful for confirmation and to monitor disease progression.

- Erythrocyte sedimentation rate (ESR) and C-reactive protein are general indicators of active inflammation.
- Positive RF occurs in 80% of patients and rises during active disease.
- Antinuclear antibody (ANA) titers may be noted in some patients.
- Antibodies to cyclic citrulline protein (Anti-CCP) are showing important potential as a marker for early RA detection. CCP antibodies have been found in the patient's blood for up to 10 years before symptoms appear.
- Synovial fluid analysis in early disease often shows a straw-colored fluid with many fibrin flecks. The white blood cell (WBC) count of synovial fluid is elevated (up to 25,000/μL).
- Inflammatory changes in the synovium can be confirmed by tissue biopsy.
- X-ray findings (not specifically diagnostic) may reveal bone demineralization and soft tissue swelling during the early months of RA. Later, narrowing of the joint space, destruction of articular cartilage, erosion, subluxation, and deformity are seen. Malalignment and ankylosis are seen in advanced disease.

Collaborative Care

Management of RA begins with a comprehensive program of drug therapy and education. Teaching regarding drug therapy includes correct administration, reporting of side effects, and frequent medical and laboratory follow-up visits. Physical therapy maintains joint motion and muscle strength. Occupational therapy develops upper-extremity function and encourages joint protection through the use of splints, pacing techniques, and assistive devices.

Drug Therapy

Drugs remain the cornerstone of RA treatment. Instead of maintaining the patient on high doses of aspirin or NSAIDs until x-rays show clear evidence of disease, health care providers now aggressively prescribe disease-modifying antirheumatic drugs (DMARDs) because irreversible joint changes can occur early in the disease process. Drugs have the potential to lessen the permanent effects of RA, such as joint erosion and deformity. Choice of drug is based on disease activity, patient's level of function, and lifestyle considerations, such as the desire to bear children.

- Treatment of early RA often involves methotrexate (Rheumatrex) because it reduces clinical symptoms in days to weeks, is inexpensive, and has a lower toxicity compared with other drugs.

- Sulfasalazine (Azulfidine) and the antimalarial drug hydroxychloroquine (Plaquenil) may be effective DMARDs for mild to moderate disease.
- Leflunomide (Arava) is a synthetic DMARD that blocks immune cell overproduction and has efficacy similar to methotrexate and sulfasalazine.
- Biologic/targeted therapy drugs (e.g., etanercept [Enbrel], infliximab [Remicade], adalimumab [Humira]), are also used to slow disease progression in patients with moderate to severe disease who have not responded to DMARDs or in combination therapy with an established DMARD. Two newer tumor necrosis factor (TNF) inhibitors, golimumab (Simponi) and certolizumab (Cimzia), improve symptoms in patients with moderate-to-severe RA. Both drugs are given in combination with methotrexate.
- Additional drugs used infrequently for treating RA include antibiotics (minocycline [Minocin]), immunosuppressants (azathioprine [Imuran]), penicillamine (Cuprimine), and gold compounds (auranofin [Ridaura], gold sodium thiomalate [Myochrysine]).
- Corticosteroid therapy can be used to aid in symptom control. Intraarticular injections may temporarily relieve the pain and inflammation associated with disease flare-ups.
- Various NSAIDs and salicylates are included in the drug regimen to treat arthritis pain and inflammation. Enteric-coated aspirin is often used in high dosages of four to six per day (10 to 18 tablets). NSAIDs have antiinflammatory, analgesic, and antipyretic properties. Although many NSAIDs inhibit inflammation, they do not appear to alter the course of RA. A newer generation of NSAIDs, COX-2 inhibitors, are effective in RA as well as in OA. The drug celecoxib (Celebrex) is currently the only available COX-2 inhibitor.

Nursing Management
Goals
The patient with RA will have satisfactory pain relief and minimal loss of functional ability of the affected joints, participate in planning and carrying out the therapeutic regimen, maintain a positive self-image, and perform self-care to the maximum amount possible.

See NCP 65-1 for the patient with rheumatoid arthritis, Lewis et al., *Medical-Surgical Nursing,* ed. 8, pp. 1656 to 1657.

Nursing Diagnoses
- Chronic pain
- Impaired physical mobility
- Disturbed body image
- Ineffective self-health management
- Self-care deficit (bathing, feeding dressing, toileting)

Nursing Interventions

Prevention of RA is not possible at this time. However, community education programs should include information on symptom recognition to promote early diagnosis and treatment. The primary goals in the management of RA are reduction of inflammation, management of pain, maintenance of joint function, and prevention or correction of joint deformity.

Interventions begin with a careful physical assessment (joint pain, swelling, range of motion, general health status), psychosocial assessment (family support, sexual satisfaction, emotional stress, financial constraints, vocation and career limitations), and environmental assessment (transportation, home, and work modifications).

- Suppression of inflammation may be effectively achieved through the administration of NSAIDs, DMARDs, and biologic/targeted therapies. Discuss the action and side effects of each drug and the importance of necessary laboratory monitoring. Make the drug regimen as understandable as possible.
- Nondrug management may include the use of therapeutic heat and cold, rest, relaxation techniques, joint protection, biofeedback, transcutaneous electrical nerve stimulation (TENS), and hypnosis.
- Lightweight splints are sometimes used to rest an inflamed joint and prevent deformity from muscle spasms and contractures. Remove the splints at regular intervals to give the skin care and perform range-of-motion (ROM) exercises. Reapply the splints as prescribed.
- Morning care and procedures should be planned around the patient's morning stiffness. Sitting or standing in a warm shower, sitting in a tub with warm towels around the shoulders, or soaking the hands in a basin of warm water may help to relieve joint stiffness and allow the patient to comfortably perform activities of daily living.
- Alternating scheduled rest periods with activity throughout the day helps relieve fatigue and pain. Help the patient identify ways to modify activities to avoid overexertion.
- Good body alignment while resting can be maintained through the use of a firm mattress or bed board. Positions of extension

should be encouraged and positions of flexion avoided. Pillows should never be placed under the knees. A small, flat pillow may be used under the head and shoulders. Splints and casts may be helpful in maintaining proper alignment and promoting rest, especially when joint inflammation is present.

Protecting the joints from stress is important. Nursing interventions include helping the patient identify ways to modify tasks. Sample activities that protect small joints are listed in Table 65-10, Lewis et al., *Medical-Surgical Nursing,* ed. 8, p. 1658.

- Patient independence may be increased by occupational therapy training with assistive devices that help simplify tasks, such as built-up utensils, button hooks, and raised toilet seats. A cane or a walker offers support and relief of pain when walking.
- Heat and cold therapy helps to relieve stiffness, pain, and muscle spasm. Application of ice may be beneficial during periods of disease exacerbation, whereas moist heat appears to offer better relief of chronic stiffness.
- Reinforce participation in an exercise program and ensure that the exercises are being done correctly. Gentle ROM exercises are usually done daily to keep the joints functional.

▼ **Patient and Caregiver Teaching**

Self-management and adherence to an individualized home program can only be accomplished if the patient has a thorough understanding of RA, the nature and course of the disease, and the goals of therapy. In addition, the patient's perception of the disease and value system must be considered.

- Help the patient recognize fears and concerns faced by all people living with a chronic illness. Evaluation of the family support system is important.
  - Financial planning may be necessary. Community resources such as a home care nurse, homemaker services, and vocational rehabilitation may be considered. Self-help groups are beneficial for some patients.

SEIZURE DISORDERS

Description

A seizure is a paroxysmal, uncontrolled electrical discharge of neurons in the brain that interrupts normal function. It is frequently a symptom of underlying illness. Seizures may accompany a variety of disorders, or they may occur spontaneously without any apparent cause.

- In the adult, metabolic disturbances that cause seizures include acidosis, electrolyte imbalances, hypoglycemia, hypoxia, alcohol and barbiturate withdrawal, dehydration, and water intoxication.

- Extracranial disorders that can cause seizures include heart, lung, liver, and kidney disease; systemic lupus erythematosus; diabetes mellitus (DM); hypertension; and septicemia.

Epilepsy is a condition in which a person has spontaneously recurring seizures caused by a chronic underlying condition. National trends show that incidence of epilepsy is decreasing in children and increasing in people >60 years old. Some populations are at higher risk to develop epilepsy, including those with Alzheimer's disease, stroke, and persons with a parent who has epilepsy.

Pathophysiology

The most common causes of seizure during the first 6 months of life are severe birth injury, congenital defects involving the central nervous system (CNS), infections, and inborn errors of metabolism. In individuals between 20 and 30 years old, seizure disorder usually occurs as a result of structural lesions such as trauma, brain tumors, or vascular disease. After the age of 50 years, primary causes of seizure are stroke and metastatic brain tumors. Although many causes of seizure disorders have been identified, three fourths of all cases cannot be attributed to a specific cause and are considered *idiopathic.*

The etiology of recurring seizures (epilepsy) has long been attributed to a group of abnormal neurons *(seizure focus)* that seem to undergo spontaneous firing. This firing spreads by physiologic pathways to involve adjacent or distant areas of the brain. The factor that causes this abnormal firing is not clear. Any stimulus that causes the cell membrane of the neuron to depolarize induces a tendency to spontaneous firing. Often the brain area from which epileptic activity arises is found to have scar tissue *(gliosis).* Scarring is thought to interfere with the normal chemical and structural environment of brain neurons, making them more likely to fire abnormally.

New evidence indicates that *astrocytes,* or cerebral support cells, may play a key role in recurring seizures. Astrocytes release glutamate that triggers synchronous firing of neurons. Drug therapy focused on suppressing astrocyte signaling or decreasing glutamate release might be a mechanism to control seizures.

Clinical Manifestations

The specific clinical manifestations of a seizure are determined by the site of the electrical disturbance. The preferred method of classifying epileptic seizures is the International Classification System (see Table 59-6, Lewis et al., *Medical-Surgical Nursing,* ed. 8, p. 1492). The system is based on the clinical and electroencephalographic (EEG) manifestations of seizures.

In this system, seizures are divided into two major classes, *generalized* and *partial.* Depending on the type, a seizure may progress through several phases: (1) *prodromal phase* with signs or activity that precedes a seizure, (2) *aural phase* with a sensory warning, (3) *ictal phase* with full seizure, and (4) *postictal phase,* which is the period of recovery after the seizure.

Generalized Seizures

Generalized seizures are characterized by bilateral synchronous epileptic discharge in the brain. In most cases the patient loses consciousness for a few seconds to several minutes.

- *Tonic-clonic* (formerly known as grand mal) seizures are the most common generalized seizures. This type of seizure is characterized by a loss of consciousness and falling to the ground if the patient is upright, followed by stiffening of the body (tonic phase) for 10 to 20 seconds and subsequent jerking of the extremities (clonic phase) for another 30 to 40 seconds. Cyanosis, excessive salivation, tongue or cheek biting, and incontinence may accompany the seizure. In the postictal phase the patient usually has muscle soreness, is very tired, and may sleep for several hours. The patient has no memory of the seizure activity.

- *Typical absence* (petit mal) seizures usually occur only in children and rarely continue beyond adolescence. This type of seizure may cease totally as the child ages, or it may evolve into another type of seizure. The typical clinical manifestation is a brief staring spell that lasts only a few seconds. There may be an extremely brief loss of consciousness. When untreated, the seizures may occur up to 100 times each day. Typical absence seizures are often precipitated by hyperventilation and flashing lights.

- *Atypical absence* seizures are another type of generalized seizure characterized by a staring spell. A brief warning, peculiar behavior during the seizure and confusion after the seizure are also common.

- Other types of generalized seizures include myoclonic, atonic, tonic, and clonic seizures.

Partial Seizures

Partial (focal) seizures are caused by focal irritations and begin in a specific region of the cortex, as indicated by the EEG and clinical manifestations. Partial seizures may be confined to one side of the brain and remain partial or focal in nature, or they may spread to involve the entire brain, culminating in a generalized tonic-clonic seizure. Any tonic-clonic seizure preceded by an aura or warning is a partial seizure that generalizes secondarily.

Partial seizures are further divided into simple partial seizures (those with simple motor or sensory phenomena) and complex partial seizures (those with complex symptoms). The terms *focal motor, focal sensory,* and *jacksonian* have been used to describe seizures of the simple partial type. Complex partial seizures include *temporal lobe seizures, temporal lobe absence seizures,* and *psychomotor seizures.*

Complications

Status epilepticus is a state of continuous seizure activity or a condition in which seizures recur in rapid succession without return to consciousness between seizures. It can occur with any type of seizure. Status epilepticus is the most serious complication of epilepsy and is a neurologic emergency.

- During repeated seizures the brain uses more energy than can be supplied. Neurons become exhausted and cease to function. Permanent brain damage may result.
- Tonic-clonic status epilepticus is the most dangerous because it can cause ventilatory insufficiency, hypoxemia, cardiac dysrhythmias, and systemic acidosis, all of which can be fatal.
- Another complication of seizures is severe injury and even death from trauma experienced during a seizure. Patients who lose consciousness during a seizure are at greatest risk.

Perhaps the most common complication of seizure disorder is the effect it has on a patient's lifestyle. Although attitudes have improved in recent years, epilepsy still carries a social stigma that can lead to discrimination in employment and educational opportunities. Transportation may also be difficult because of legal sanctions against driving in most states.

Diagnostic Studies

- Most important in diagnosis are accurate and comprehensive descriptions of the seizures and the patient's health history.
- The EEG is useful only if it shows abnormalities. It is not a definitive test because some patients who do not have seizure disorders have abnormal EEG patterns, whereas many patients with seizure disorders have normal EEGs between seizures.
- Complete blood count (CBC), serum chemistries, studies of liver and kidney function, and urinalysis can rule out metabolic disorders.

- Computed tomography (CT) scan and magnetic resonance imaging (MRI) can rule out a structural lesion.
- Cerebral angiography, single photon emission computed tomography (SPECT), magnetic resonance spectroscopy (MRS), magnetic resonance angiography (MRA), and positron emission tomography (PET) may be used in selected situations.

Collaborative Care

Most seizures do not require professional emergency medical care because they are self-limiting and rarely cause body injury. However, if status epilepticus occurs, significant body harm occurs, or the event is a first-time seizure, medical care should be sought immediately. Table 59-8, Lewis et al., *Medical-Surgical Nursing,* ed. 8, p. 1495, summarizes the emergency care of the patient with a generalized tonic-clonic seizure.

Drug Therapy

Seizure disorders are treated primarily with antiseizure drugs (see Table 59-9, Lewis et al., *Medical-Surgical Nursing,* ed. 8, p. 1496). Medications generally act by stabilizing the nerve cell membranes and preventing the spread of the epileptic discharge.

The primary goal of antiseizure drug therapy is to obtain maximum seizure control with a minimum of toxic side effects. The principle of drug therapy is to begin with a single drug based on patient age and weight with consideration of the type, frequency, and cause of seizure and increase the dosage until the seizures are controlled or toxic side effects occur. If seizure control is not achieved with a single drug, the drug dosage and timing or administration may be changed or a second drug may be added.

- Newer antiseizure drugs include gabapentin (Neurontin), lamotrigine (Lamictal), topiramate (Topamax), tiagabine (Gabitril), levetiracetam (Keppra), and zonisamide (Zonegran). Some of these drugs are broad spectrum and appear to be effective for multiple seizure types.
- Treatment of status epilepticus requires initiation of a rapid-acting antiseizure medication given intravenously. Drugs most commonly used are lorazepam (Ativan) and diazepam (Valium).
- Antiseizure drugs should not be discontinued abruptly because this can precipitate seizures.
- Alternative therapies, such as vagal nerve stimulation and biofeedback, may also be used.

Surgical interventions for patients whose epilepsy cannot be controlled with drug therapy include limbic resection, primarily anterior temporal lobe resection; amygdalohippocampectomy;

neocortical resection, including extratemporal resection and lesionectomies; hemispherectomies; multilobar resections; and corpus collosum sections.

Nursing Management

Goals

The patient with seizures will be free from injury during a seizure, have optimal mental and physical functioning while taking antiseizure medication, and have satisfactory psychosocial functioning.

Nursing Diagnoses

- Ineffective breathing pattern
- Risk for injury
- Ineffective self-health management

Nursing Interventions

The patient with a seizure disorder should practice good general health habits (e.g., maintaining a proper diet, getting adequate rest, exercising). Help the patient to identify events or situations that precipitate the seizures and give suggestions for avoiding them or handling them better.

Nursing care for a hospitalized patient or for a person who has had seizures as a result of metabolic factors should focus on observation and treatment of the seizure, education, and psychosocial intervention.

- When a seizure occurs, you should carefully observe and record all aspects of the event because the diagnosis and subsequent treatment depend on the seizure description. The description should include the exact onset of the seizure (which body part was affected first and how); the course and nature of the seizure activity (loss of consciousness, tongue biting, automatisms, stiffening, jerking, total lack of muscle tone); the body parts involved and their sequence of involvement; and the presence of autonomic signs (dilated pupils, excessive salivation, altered breathing, cyanosis, flushing, diaphoresis, or incontinence).

- Assessment of the postictal period should include a detailed description of the level of consciousness (LOC), vital signs, memory loss, muscle soreness, speech disorders (aphasia, dysarthria), weakness or paralysis, sleep period, and the duration of each sign or symptom.

- During the seizure it is important to maintain a patent airway. This may involve protecting the head, turning the patient to the side, loosening constrictive clothing, or easing the patient to the floor if sitting in a chair. After the seizure the patient may require suctioning and oxygen.

S

- A seizure can be a frightening experience for the patient and for others who may witness it. You should assess the level of their understanding and provide information about how and why the event occurred.

▼ **Patient and Caregiver Teaching**

Prevention of recurring seizures is the major goal in the treatment of epilepsy. Because seizure disorders cannot be cured, drugs must be taken regularly and continually, often for a lifetime. You have an important role in teaching the patient and the caregiver. Guidelines for teaching are shown in Table 78.

- Caution the patient not to adjust medications without professional guidance because this can increase seizure frequency and even cause status epilepticus.
- Ensure that the patient knows the specifics of the medication regimen and what to do if a dose is missed.
- Encourage the patient to report any medication side effects and keep regular appointments with the health care provider.

Table 78	Patient and Caregiver Teaching Guide: Seizure Disorders and Epilepsy

You should include the following information in the teaching plan for the patient with a seizure disorder:

1. Take drugs as prescribed. Report any and all side effects of drugs to the health care provider. When necessary, blood is drawn to ensure that therapeutic levels are maintained.
2. Use nondrug techniques, such as relaxation therapy and biofeedback training, to potentially reduce the number of seizures.
3. Be aware of availability of resources in the community.
4. Wear a medical alert bracelet, necklace, and identification card.
5. Avoid excessive alcohol intake, fatigue, and loss of sleep.
6. Eat regular meals and snacks in between if feeling shaky, faint, or hungry.

Caregivers should receive the following information:

1. For first aid treatment of tonic-clonic seizure, it is not necessary to call an ambulance or send the patient to the hospital after a single seizure unless the seizure is prolonged, another seizure immediately follows, or extensive injury has occurred.
2. During an acute seizure, it is important to protect the patient from injury. This may involve supporting and protecting the head, turning the patient to the side, loosening constrictive clothing, and easing the patient to the floor, if seated.

- Teach the caregiver, family members, and significant others the first-aid treatment of tonic-clonic seizures.
- Provide psychosocial support for the patient by providing education and helping to identify coping mechanisms.

SEXUALLY TRANSMITTED DISEASES

Sexually transmitted diseases (STDs) are infectious diseases transmitted most commonly through sexual contact. Historically, they have been referred to as *venereal diseases*. Common diseases that are transmitted sexually are listed in Table 79.

Diseases that are associated with sexual transmission can also be contracted by other routes, such as through blood, blood products, and autoinoculation. See Gonorrhea, p. 258; Syphilis, p. 621; Herpes, Genital, p. 315; Warts, Genital, p. 693; and Chlamydial Infections, p. 117.

An estimated 65 million people in the United States are currently infected with one or more STDs. In the United States all gonorrhea and syphilis and, in most states, chlamydial infection

S

Table 79	Microorganisms Responsible for Sexually Transmitted Diseases
Microorganisms	**Disease**
Bacteria	
Chlamydia trachomatis	Nongonococcal urethritis (NGU), cervicitis, lymphogranuloma venereum
Neisseria gonorrhoeae	Gonorrhea
Treponema pallidum	Syphilis
Viruses	
Cytomegalovirus (CMV)	Encephalitis, esophagitis, retinitis, pneumonitis in immunocompromised patients
Hepatitis B virus	Hepatitis B
Herpes simplex virus (HSV)	Genital herpes
Human immunodeficiency virus (HIV)	HIV infection, acquired immunodeficiency syndrome (AIDS)
Human papillomavirus (HPV)	Genital warts, cervical cancer
Poxvirus	Molluscum contagiosum

must be reported to the state or local public health authorities. In spite of this requirement, there are many unreported cases of these infections.

Many factors contribute to the increased incidence of STDs. Earlier reproductive maturity and increased longevity has resulted in a longer sexual life span. An increase in the total population has resulted in an increase in the number of susceptible hosts.

- Other factors include greater sexual freedom, lack of barrier methods (e.g., condoms) during sexual activity, and an increased emphasis on sexuality in the media.
- Changes in the methods of contraception are also reflected in the incidence of STDs. The preference for oral contraceptives and intrauterine devices (IUDs) that offer no protection against STDs over barrier contraceptives such as condoms increases the risk of transmission of disease.

Nursing Management: Sexually Transmitted Diseases

Goals

The patient with an STD will demonstrate understanding of the mode of transmission and the risks posed by STDs, complete treatment and return for appropriate follow-up care, notify or assist in notification of sexual contacts about their need for testing and treatment, abstain from intercourse until infection is resolved, and demonstrate knowledge of safe sex practices.

Nursing Diagnoses

- Risk for infection
- Ineffective health maintenance
- Anxiety

Nursing Interventions

The diagnosis of an STD may be met with a variety of emotions, such as shame, guilt, anger, and a desire for vengeance. Try to help the patient verbalize feelings. A referral for professional counseling to explore ramifications of an STD may be indicated.

All patients should return to the treatment center for a repeat culture from infected sites or serologic testing at designated times to determine effectiveness of treatment.

- Inform the patient that cures are not always obtained on first treatment to reinforce the need for a follow-up visit.
- Advise the patient to inform sexual partners of the need for treatment, regardless of whether they are free of symptoms or experiencing symptoms.
- The patient with an STD should have certain hygiene measures emphasized.

- An important measure is frequent hand washing and bathing; this results in destruction of many of the causative organisms of STDs.
- Bathing and cleaning of involved areas can provide local comfort and prevent secondary infection.
- Douching may spread infection and is therefore contraindicated.
- Sexual abstinence is indicated during the communicable phase of the disease. If sexual activity occurs before the patient has completed treatment, the use of condoms may prevent spread of infection and reinfection.

▼ **Patient Teaching**

- Be prepared to discuss safe sex practices with all patients, not only those who are perceived to be at risk. These practices include abstinence, monogamy with an uninfected partner, avoidance of certain high-risk sexual practices, and use of condoms and other barriers to limit contact with potentially infectious body fluids or lesions. A patient teaching guide related to the patient with a STD is presented in Table 53-9, Lewis et al., *Medical-Surgical Nursing*, ed. 8, p. 1340.
- All sexually active women should be screened for cervical cancer. Women with a history of STDs are at greater risk for cervical cancer than those without this history.
- Consider initiating an interview to establish the patient's risk for contracting an STD. Questions to ask include number of partners, type of birth control used, use of condoms, use of intravenous (IV) drugs, and sexual preference. Plan patient teaching based on responses to these questions.
- An inspection of the sexual partner's genitals before coitus is recommended. The presence of discharge, sores, blisters, or rash should be viewed with concern.
- Tell men that some protection is provided if they void immediately after intercourse and wash their genitals and adjacent areas with soap and water.
- Women may also benefit from postcoital voiding and washing. Spermicidal jellies and creams have not been shown to reduce STD risk.
- Proper use of a latex condom provides a highly effective barrier to infection. The condom should be undamaged and correctly in place throughout all phases of sexual activity.
- Sexual contact with persons known or suspected to have human immunodeficiency virus (HIV) infection should be avoided. A sexually active homosexual man can reduce risk by minimizing the number of sexual contacts. Unprotected anal intercourse

should be eliminated, and condoms should be used if sexual contact continues.

- Actively encourage communities to provide better education related to STDs for their citizens. Teenagers, who are known to have a high incidence of infection, should be a prime target for such educational programs.
- Highly effective HPV vaccines which protect against cervical cancer and genital warts should be encouraged before the start of sexual activity.

SHOCK

Description

Shock is a syndrome characterized by decreased tissue perfusion and impaired cellular metabolism. The four main categories of shock are cardiogenic, hypovolemic, distributive, and obstructive.

- Although the cause, initial presentation, and management strategies vary for each type of shock, the physiologic responses of the cells to hypoperfusion are similar.

Cardiogenic Shock

Cardiogenic shock occurs when either systolic or diastolic dysfunction of the pumping action of the heart results in reduced cardiac output (CO). The heart's inability to pump the blood forward is classified as systolic dysfunction. Causes include myocardial infarction (MI), cardiomyopathies, severe systemic or pulmonary hypertension, blunt cardiac injury, bradydysrhythmias, and myocardial depression from metabolic problems. Diastolic dysfunction is an impaired ability of the right or left ventricle to fill during diastole. This results in decreased stroke volume. Causes of diastolic dysfunction include ventricular hypertrophy and cardiomyopathy

- The patient presents with tachycardia, hypotension, and a narrowed pulse pressure. A low CO (<4 L/min) and a low *cardiac index* (<2.5 L/min/m^2) result when systolic dysfunction is present.
- The patient has tachypnea and pulmonary congestion that is evident by the presence of crackles. An increase in the pulmonary artery wedge pressure (PAWP) and pulmonary vascular resistance is also noted.
- Signs of peripheral hypoperfusion (e.g., cyanosis, pallor, diaphoresis, diminished pulses, decreased capillary refill time) are apparent.

- Decreased renal blood flow results in sodium and water retention and decreased urine output. Anxiety, confusion, and agitation may develop since cerebral perfusion is impaired.

Studies helpful in diagnosing cardiogenic shock include laboratory studies (e.g., cardiac enzymes, b-type natriuretic peptide [BNP]), troponin levels), electrocardiogram (ECG), chest x-ray, and echocardiogram.

Hypovolemic Shock

Hypovolemic shock occurs when there is a loss of intravascular fluid volume. The volume loss may be either an absolute or a relative volume loss.

- *Absolute hypovolemia* results when fluid is lost through hemorrhage, gastrointestinal (GI) loss (e.g., vomiting, diarrhea), fistula drainage, diabetes insipidus, or diuresis.
- In *relative hypovolemia*, fluid volume moves out of the vascular space into the extravascular space (e.g., interstitial space). This fluid shift is called *third spacing* that can be seen in sepsis and burns.

In hypovolemic shock, the vascular compartment size remains unchanged while the volume of blood or plasma decreases. A reduction in intravascular volume results in decreased venous return to the heart, decreased preload, decreased stroke volume, and decreased CO. A cascade of events results in decreased tissue perfusion and impaired cellular metabolism, the hallmarks of shock (Fig. 12). A total blood loss of 15% to 30% results in a sympathetic nervous system (SNS)–mediated response that causes an increase in heart rate, cardiac output, and respiratory rate and depth. If hypovolemia is corrected at this time, tissue dysfunction is generally reversible.

- If volume loss is >30%, blood volume must be replaced aggressively with blood or blood products. A loss of >40% of the total blood volume results in irreversible tissue destruction.

Laboratory studies include serial measurements of hemoglobin and hematocrit levels, electrolytes, lactate, blood gases, and central venous oxygenation (ScvO$_2$), and hourly urine outputs.

Distributive Shock (Spinal, Septic, Anaphylactic)

Neurogenic shock is a hemodynamic phenomenon that can occur within 30 minutes after a spinal cord injury at the fifth thoracic (T5) vertebra or above and last up to 6 weeks. The injury results in a massive vasodilation without compensation because of the loss

S

PATHOPHYSIOLOGY MAP

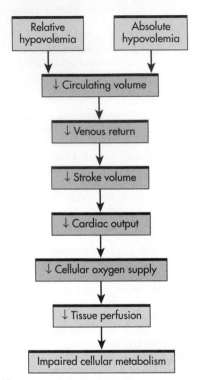

Fig. 12. The pathophysiology of hypovolemic shock.

of SNS vasoconstrictor tone. This leads to a pooling of blood in the blood vessels, tissue hypoperfusion, and ultimately impaired cellular metabolism.

Spinal anesthesia can also block transmission of impulses from the SNS. Depression of the vasomotor center of the medulla from drugs (e.g., opioids, benzodiazepines) may result in decreased vasoconstrictor tone of the peripheral blood vessels, resulting in neurogenic shock.

- Clinical manifestations are hypotension (from massive vaso-dilation) and bradycardia (from unopposed parasympathetic stimulation).

The patient in neurogenic shock may not be able to regulate temperature. The inability to regulate temperature, combined with massive vasodilation, promotes heat loss. Initially, the patient's skin will be warm because of the massive dilation. As the heat disperses, the patient is at risk for hypothermia.

The pathophysiology of neurogenic shock is described in Fig. 67-4, Lewis et al., *Medical-Surgical Nursing,* ed. 8, p. 1722.

Anaphylactic shock is an acute and life-threatening hypersensitivity (allergic) reaction to a sensitizing substance, such as a drug, chemical, vaccine, food, or insect venom. Usually it is an immediate reaction that causes massive vasodilation, release of vasoactive mediators, and an increase in capillary permeability.

- As capillary permeability increases, fluid leaks from the vascular space into the interstitial space. Anaphylactic shock can lead to respiratory distress as a result of laryngeal edema or severe bronchospasm, and circulatory failure as a result of massive vasodilation.
- Patients present with a sudden onset of symptoms, including dizziness, chest pain, incontinence, swelling of the lips and tongue, wheezing, and stridor. Skin changes include flushing, pruritus, urticaria, and angioedema.
- A patient can develop a severe allergic reaction, possibly leading to anaphylactic shock after contact, inhalation, ingestion, or injection with an antigen (allergen) to which the person has previously been sensitized.

Septic shock is the presence of sepsis with hypotension despite fluid resuscitation along with the presence of tissue perfusion abnormalities. The main organisms that cause sepsis are gram-negative and gram-positive bacteria. Parasites, fungi, and viruses can also lead to the development of sepsis and septic shock. The pathophysiology of septic shock is described in Fig. 67-5, Lewis et al., *Medical-Surgical Nursing,* ed. 8, p. 1723.

- When a microorganism enters the body, the normal immune/inflammatory cascade responses are initiated and work together to destroy the antigen. However, in severe sepsis and septic shock the response to an antigen is exaggerated. There is an increase in inflammation and coagulation and a decrease in fibrinolysis. Endotoxins from the microorganism cell wall stimulate the release of cytokines and other proinflammatory mediators. The combined effects of the mediators result in damage to the endothelium, vasodilation, increased capillary permeability, and neutrophil and platelet aggregation and adhesion to the endothelium.
- Clinical manifestations include an initial decreased ejection fraction with the ventricles dilating so as to maintain stroke

volume. The ejection fraction typically improves and the ventricular dilation resolves over 7 to 10 days. Persistence of a high CO and a low SVR beyond 24 hours is an ominous finding and is often associated with an increased development of hypotension and MODS.

■ Respiratory failure is common. The patient initially hyperventilates, resulting in respiratory alkalosis. Once the patient can no longer compensate, respiratory acidosis develops.

■ Other clinical signs include decreased urine output, alteration in neurologic status, and GI dysfunction, such as GI bleeding and paralytic ileus.

Obstructive Shock

Obstructive shock develops when a physical obstruction to blood flow occurs with a decreased CO. This can be caused from a restriction to diastolic filling of the right ventricle because of compression (e.g., cardiac tamponade, tension pneumothorax, pulmonary embolism, superior vena cava syndrome). The pathophysiology of obstructive shock is described in Fig. 67-6, Lewis et al., *Medical-Surgical Nursing,* ed. 8, p. 1724.

■ Patients experience a decreased CO, increased afterload, and variable left ventricular filling pressures depending on the obstruction. Other clinical signs include jugular vein distention and pulsus paradoxus. Rapid assessment and immediate treatment are important to prevent further hemodynamic compromise and possibly cardiac arrest.

Stages of Shock

The shock continuum begins with the initial stage that occurs at a cellular level and is usually not clinically apparent. Metabolism changes at the cellular level from aerobic to anaerobic cause lactic acid buildup. The removal of lactic acid by the liver requires oxygen, which is unavailable because of decreased tissue perfusion.

Shock is categorized into three clinically apparent but overlapping stages: the compensatory stage, the progressive stage, and the irreversible stage.

In the *compensatory stage,* the body activates neural, hormonal, and biochemical mechanisms to overcome the increasing consequences of anaerobic metabolism and maintain homeostasis.

■ One of the classic signs of shock is a fall in blood pressure (BP). The SNS stimulates vasoconstriction and the release of epinephrine and norepinephrine; both are potent vasoconstrictors. Blood flow to the most essential organs, the heart and the brain, is maintained; and blood flow to the kidneys, GI tract, and lungs is shunted or diverted.

- Decreased blood flow to the kidneys activates the renin-angiotensin-aldosterone system, resulting in vasoconstriction and sodium and water reabsorption.
- Shunting blood from the lungs has an important effect on the patient in shock. Areas of the lungs participating in ventilation are not perfused because of decreased blood flow to the lungs. The patient has a compensatory increase in the rate and depth of respirations.
- The myocardium responds to SNS stimulation and the increase in oxygen demand by increasing heart rate and contractility.

If the cause of shock is corrected at this stage, the patient recovers with few or no residual effects. If the perfusion deficit is not corrected and the body is unable to compensate, the patient goes on to the progressive stage of shock.

The *progressive stage* of shock begins as compensatory mechanisms fail. Continued decreased cellular perfusion and resulting altered capillary permeability are the distinguishing features of this stage. The patient may have diffuse and profound edema (anasarca).

- CO begins to fall, with a resultant decrease in BP and peripheral perfusion, including a decrease in coronary artery, cerebral, and peripheral perfusion. Myocardial dysfunction from decreased perfusion results in dysrhythmias, myocardial ischemia, and potentially myocardial infarction.
- The combined effects of pulmonary vasoconstriction and bronchoconstriction are impaired gas exchange, decreased compliance, and worsening ventilation-perfusion mismatch. The patient presents with tachypnea, crackles, and an overall increased work of breathing.
- Renal function is markedly impaired. The patient has a decreased urine output and an elevated blood urea nitrogen (BUN) and serum creatinine. Metabolic acidosis occurs from an inability to excrete acids and reabsorb bicarbonate.
- Decreased tissue perfusion predisposes the patient to ulcers and GI bleeding.
- Loss of the functional ability of the liver leads to a failure to metabolize drugs and waste products such as ammonia and lactate. Jaundice results from an accumulation of bilirubin.

S

- Dysfunction of the hematologic system places the patient at risk for the development of disseminated intravascular coagulation (DIC).

In the final stage of shock, the *irreversible stage,* decreased perfusion from peripheral vasoconstriction and decreased cardiac output exacerbate anaerobic metabolism (see Fig. 67-9, Lewis et al., *Medical-Surgical Nursing,* ed. 8, p. 1729). The loss of intravascular volume worsens hypotension and tachycardia and decreases coronary blood flow. Cerebral blood flow cannot be maintained and cerebral ischemia results.

- The patient demonstrates profound hypotension and hypoxemia. In this final stage, recovery is unlikely. The organs are in failure, and the body's compensatory mechanisms are overwhelmed.

Diagnostic Studies

- Obtaining a thorough medical and surgical history, and a history of recent events (e.g., surgery, chest pain, trauma, medications) provides valuable data.
- Blood studies, which may include complete blood count (CBC), DIC screen, cardiac enzymes, BUN, glucose, electrolytes, arterial blood gases (ABGs), lactate, blood cultures, and liver enzymes.
- Twelve-lead ECG, continuous cardiac monitoring, chest x-ray, continuous pulse oximetry, and hemodynamic monitoring (e.g., arterial pressure, central venous or PA pressure, $ScvO_2/SvO_2$).

See Table 67-3, Lewis et al., *Medical-Surgical Nursing,* ed. 8, p. 1720 for further information. See Table 67-2, Lewis et al., *Medical-Surgical Nursing,* ed. 8, p. 1719 for the hemodynamic effects of shock.

Collaborative Care: General Measures

Critical factors in management are early recognition and treatment. Prompt intervention can alter the shock process and prevent the progressive or irreversible stage. Successful management depends on (1) identification of patients at risk for shock; (2) integration of the patient's history, physical examination, and clinical findings to establish a diagnosis; (3) interventions to control or eliminate the cause of the decreased perfusion; (4) protection of target and distal organs from dysfunction; and (5) provision of multisystem supportive care. Emergency care of the patient in shock is presented in Table 80.

General management strategies begin with ensuring that the patient has a patent airway. Once the airway is established, either

Table 80 Emergency Management: Shock

Etiology*	Assessment Findings	Interventions
Surgical	■ Restlessness	**Initial**
■ Postoperative bleeding	■ Confusion	■ Assess ABCs.
■ Ruptured organ/vessel	■ Anxiety	■ Stabilize cervical spine as appropriate.
■ Gastrointestinal bleeding	■ Feeling of impending doom	■ Administer high-flow oxygen (100%) by non-rebreather
■ Aortic dissection	■ Decreased level of	mask or bag-valve-mask.
■ Vaginal bleeding	consciousness	■ Anticipate need for intubation and mechanical ventilation.
■ Ruptured ectopic	■ Weakness	■ Establish IV access with two large-bore catheters (14-16
pregnancy or ovarian cyst	■ Rapid, weak, thready pulses	gauge) and begin fluid resuscitation with crystalloids
	■ Dysrhythmias	(e.g., normal saline solution).
Medical	■ Hypotension	■ Draw blood for laboratory studies (e.g., blood cultures,
■ Myocardial infarction	■ Narrowed pulse pressure	lactate, WBC).
■ Dehydration	■ Cool, clammy skin (warm	■ Control any external bleeding with direct pressure or
■ Addisonian crisis	skin in early onset of septic	pressure dressing.
■ Diabetes insipidus	and neurogenic shock)	■ Assess for life-threatening injuries (e.g., pericardial
■ Sepsis	■ Tachypnea, dyspnea, or	tamponade, liver laceration, tension pneumothorax).
■ Diabetes mellitus	shallow, irregular	■ Consider vasopressor therapy if hypotension persists
■ Pulmonary embolus	respirations	after fluid resuscitation.
	■ Decreased O₂ saturation	■ Insert an indwelling bladder catheter and nasogastric tube.
Trauma	■ Extreme thirst	■ Administer antibiotic therapy if sepsis is suspected.
■ Ruptured or lacerated	■ Nausea and vomiting	■ Treat dysrhythmias.
vessel or organ (e.g.,		
spleen)		

Continued

S

Table 80 Emergency Management: Shock—cont'd

Etiology*	Assessment Findings	Interventions
■ Fractures, spinal injury ■ Multiorgan injury	■ Chills ■ Pallor ■ Cyanosis ■ Obvious hemorrhage or injury ■ Temperature dysregulation	**Ongoing Monitoring** ■ Level of consciousness ■ Vital signs, including pulse oximetry; peripheral pulses, capillary refill, skin color and temperature ■ Respiratory status ■ Cardiac rhythm ■ Urine output

ABCs, Airway, breathing, circulation; *WBC*, white blood cell.

*See Table 67-1, Lewis et al., *Medical-Surgical Nursing*, ed. 8, p. 1718 for additional etiologies of shock.

with a natural airway or an endotracheal tube, oxygen delivery must be optimized.

- Supplemental oxygen with or without mechanical ventilation may be necessary to support the delivery of oxygen to maintain an arterial oxygen saturation of 90% or greater (PaO_2 >60 mm Hg) to avoid hypoxemia (see Artificial Airways: Endotracheal Tubes, p. 699, Oxygen Therapy, p. 743, and Mechanical Ventilation, p. 736). The mean arterial pressure and circulating blood volume are optimized with fluid replacement and drug therapy (see Tables 67-8 and 67-9 in Lewis et al., *Medical-Surgical Nursing,* ed. 8, pp. 1730 and 1731 to 1732).

In addition to general management of shock, there are specific interventions for different types of shock (Table 81). Drugs used in the treatment of shock are presented in Table 67-9, Lewis et al., *Medical-Surgical Nursing,* ed. 8, pp. 1731 to 1732.

Nursing Management

Goals

The patient with shock will have evidence of adequate tissue perfusion, restoration of normal or baseline BP, return/recovery of organ function, and avoidance of complications from prolonged states of hypoperfusion.

See NCP 67-1 for the patient in shock, Lewis et al., *Medical-Surgical Nursing,* ed. 8, pp. 1736 to 1737.

Nursing Diagnoses

- Ineffective peripheral tissue perfusion
- Risk for decreased cardiac tissue perfusion
- Risk for ineffective cerebral tissue perfusion
- Risk for ineffective gastrointestinal perfusion
- Risk for ineffective renal perfusion
- Ineffective breathing pattern
- Decreased cardiac output
- Fear
- Anxiety

Nursing Interventions

To prevent shock, you need to identify persons who are at risk. In general, patients who are older, those with debilitating diseases, and those who are immunocompromised are at increased risk. Any person who sustains surgical or accidental trauma is at risk of shock resulting from hemorrhage, spinal cord injury, and burn injuries.

Your role in shock involves (1) monitoring the patient's ongoing physical and emotional status, (2) identifying trends to detect changes in the patient's condition, (3) planning and implementing nursing interventions and therapy, (4) evaluating the patient's

Table 81 Collaborative Care: Specific Strategies for the Treatment of Shock

	Oxygenation	Circulation	Drug Therapies	Supportive Therapies
Cardiogenic shock	Provide supplemental O_2 (e.g., nasal cannula, non-rebreather mask) Intubation/mechanical ventilation, if necessary Monitor SvO_2 or $ScvO_2$	Restore blood flow with thrombolytics, angioplasty with stenting, emergent coronary revascularization Reduce workload of the heart with circulatory assist devices: IABP, VAD	Nitrates (e.g., nitroglycerin) Inotropes (e.g., dobutamine) Diuretics (e.g., furosemide) β-Adrenergic blockers (contraindicated with ↓ ejection fraction)	Correct dysrhythmias
Hypovolemic shock	Provide supplemental O_2 Monitor SvO_2 or $ScvO_2$	Restore fluid volume (e.g., blood/blood products, crystalloids) Rapid fluid replacement using two large-bore (14-16 gauge) peripheral IVs Endpoints of fluid resuscitation: CVP 15 mm Hg PAWP 10-12 mm Hg	No specific drug therapy	Correct the cause (e.g., stop bleeding, GI losses) Use warmed fluids

Septic shock	Provide supplemental O_2 Intubation/mechanical ventilation, if necessary Monitor SvO_2 or $ScvO_2$	Aggressive fluid resuscitation Endpoints of fluid resuscitation: CVP 15 mm Hg PAWP 10-12 mm Hg	Antibiotics as ordered Vasopressors (e.g., dopamine) Inotropes (e.g., dobutamine) Anticoagulants (e.g., low-molecular-weight heparin)	Obtain cultures (e.g., blood, wound) before beginning antibiotics Monitor temperature Control blood glucose Stress ulcer prophylaxis
Neurogenic shock	Maintain patent airway Provide supplemental O_2 Intubation/mechanical ventilation, if necessary	Cautious administration of fluids	Vasopressors (e.g., phenylephrine) Atropine (for bradycardia)	Minimize spinal cord trauma with stabilization Monitor temperature

Continued

S

Table 81   **Collaborative Care: Specific Strategies for the Treatment of Shock—cont'd**

	Oxygenation	Circulation	Drug Therapies	Supportive Therapies
Anaphylactic shock	Maintain patent airway Optimize oxygenation with supplemental O_2 Intubation/mechanical ventilation, if necessary	Aggressive fluid resuscitation with colloids	Antihistamines (e.g., diphenhydramine) Epinephrine (subcutaneous, IV, nebulized) Bronchodilators: nebulized (e.g., albuterol) Corticosteroids (if hypotension persists)	Identify and remove offending cause Prevention via avoidance of known allergens Premedication with history of prior sensitivity (e.g., contrast media)
Obstructive shock	Maintain patent airway Provide supplemental O_2 Intubation/mechanical ventilation, if necessary	Restore circulation by treating cause of obstruction Fluid resuscitation may provide temporary improvement in CO and BP	No specific drug therapy	Treat cause of obstruction (e.g., pericardiocentesis for cardiac tamponade, needle decompression or chest tube insertion for tension pneumothorax, embolectomy for pulmonary embolism)

CO, Cardiac output; *CVP*, central venous pressure; *GI*, gastrointestinal; *IABP*, intraaortic balloon pump; *PAWP*, pulmonary artery wedge pressure; *VAD*, ventricular assist device.

response to therapy, (5) providing emotional support to the patient and caregiver, and (6) collaborating with other members of the health team to coordinate care.

Do not overlook or underestimate the effects of fear and anxiety on the patient and caregiver when faced with a critical, life-threatening situation. Fear, anxiety, and pain may aggravate respiratory distress and increase the release of catecholamines.

- Provide medications to decrease anxiety and pain as appropriate. Continuous infusions of a benzodiazepine (e.g., lorazepam [Ativan]) and an opioid or anesthetic (e.g., morphine, propofol [Diprivan]) are extremely helpful in decreasing anxiety and pain.
- Talk to the patient and encourage the caregiver to talk to the patient, even if the patient is intubated, sedated, or appears comatose. Hearing is often the last sense to be reduced, and even if the patient cannot respond, he or she may still be able to hear. If the intubated patient is capable of writing, provide a "magic slate" or a pencil and paper.
- Do not overlook the patient's spiritual needs. One way to provide support is to offer to call a member of the clergy rather than wait for the patient or caregiver to express a wish for spiritual counseling.

Caregivers can have a therapeutic effect on the patient. To perform this role, they need to be supportive and comforting. Encourage caregivers to perform simple comfort measures if desired. Provide privacy and assure the patient and caregivers that assistance is readily available if needed. If the prognosis becomes increasingly grave, you must support the patient's caregiver when making difficult decisions such as withdrawing life support. Rehabilitation of the patient who has experienced critical illness necessitates correction of the precipitating cause and prevention or early treatment of complications. Continue to monitor the patient for indications of complications throughout recovery including decreased range of motion, decreased physical endurance, renal failure following acute tubular necrosis, and the development of fibrotic lung disease because of ARDS. Patients recovering from shock may require diverse services after discharge. These can include admission to transitional care units (e.g., for mechanical ventilation weaning), rehabilitation centers (inpatient or outpatient), or home health care agencies. Anticipate and facilitate a safe transition from the hospital to home starting when the patient is admitted to the hospital.

SICKLE CELL DISEASE

Description

Sickle cell disease (SCD) is a group of inherited, autosomal recessive disorders characterized by the presence of an abnormal form of hemoglobin (Hb) in the erythrocyte. This abnormal hemoglobin, *hemoglobin S* (Hb S), causes the erythrocyte to stiffen and elongate, taking on a sickle shape in response to low oxygen (O_2) levels.

SCD is usually identified during infancy or early childhood. It is an incurable disease that is often fatal by middle age from renal, pulmonary failure, and/or stroke. The disease affects more than 50,000 Americans and is predominant in African Americans, occurring in an estimated prevalence of 1 in about 400 live births. It can also affect persons of Mediterranean, Caribbean, South and Central American, Arabian, or East Indian ancestry.

Pathophysiology

Types of SCD include sickle cell anemia, sickle cell-thalassemia, sickle cell Hb C disease, and sickle cell trait. *Sickle cell anemia* is the most severe of the SCD syndromes. It occurs when a person is homozygous for hemoglobin S (Hb SS); the person has inherited Hb S from both parents.

Sickle cell-thalassemia and *sickle cell Hb C* occur when a person inherits Hb S from one parent and another type of abnormal hemoglobin (e.g., thalassemia or hemoglobin C) from the other parent. Both of these forms of SCD are less common and less severe than sickle cell anemia.

Sickle cell trait occurs when a person is heterozygous for hemoglobin S (Hb AS); the person has inherited hemoglobin S from one parent and normal hemoglobin (hemoglobin A) from the other parent. Sickle cell trait is typically a very mild to asymptomatic condition.

The major pathophysiologic event of SCD is the sickling of erythrocytes. Sickling episodes are most commonly triggered by low O_2 tension in the blood. Hypoxia or deoxygenation of the erythrocytes can be caused by viral or bacterial infection (most common factor), high altitude, emotional stress, surgery, and blood loss. Other triggering events include dehydration, increased hydrogen ion concentration (acidosis), decreased plasma volume, or low body temperature. A sickling episode can also occur without an obvious cause.

- Sickled erythrocytes become rigid and take on an elongated, crescent shape. Sickled cells are unable to easily pass through capillaries or other small vessels and can cause vascular occlusion, leading to acute or chronic tissue injury. The resulting hemostasis promotes a self-perpetuating cycle of local hypoxia, deoxygenation of more erythrocytes, and more sickling.

- Circulating sickled cells are hemolyzed by the spleen, leading to anemia. Initially the sickling of cells is reversible with reoxygenation, but eventually the condition becomes irreversible because of cell membrane damage from recurrent sickling.

Sickle cell crisis is a severe, painful, acute exacerbation of RBC sickling causing a vaso-occlusive crisis. As blood flow is impaired by sickled cells, vasospasm occurs, further restricting blood flow. Tissue ischemia, infarction, and necrosis eventually occur from lack of oxygen. Shock is a possible life-threatening consequence because of severe oxygen depletion of the tissues and a reduction of the circulating fluid volume. Sickle cell crisis can begin suddenly and persist for days to weeks.

- The frequency, extent, and severity of sickling episodes are highly variable and unpredictable, but they largely depend on the percentage of Hb S present. Individuals with sickle cell anemia have the most severe form because erythrocytes contain a high percentage of Hb S.

Clinical Manifestations

The effects of SCD vary greatly from person to person. Many people with sickle cell anemia are in reasonably good health most of the time. However, they may have chronic health problems and pain because of organ tissue hypoxia and damage (e.g., involving the kidneys and/or liver). The typical patient is anemic but asymptomatic except during sickling episodes.

- Because most individuals with sickle cell anemia have dark skin, pallor is more readily detected by examining the mucous membranes. The skin may have a grayish cast. Because of the hemolysis, jaundice is common and patients are prone to gallstones (cholelithiasis).
- The primary symptom associated with sickling is pain. During sickle cell crisis the pain is quite severe as a result of tissue ischemia. The back, chest, extremities, and abdomen are most commonly affected. Pain episodes are accompanied by fever, swelling, tenderness, tachypnea, hypertension, and nausea and vomiting.

Complications

With repeated episodes of sickling there is gradual involvement of all body systems, especially the spleen, lungs, kidneys, and brain.

- Infection is a major cause of morbidity and mortality in patients with sickle cell disease. Pneumonia is the most common infection.
- The spleen becomes infarcted, dysfunctional, and small because of repeated scarring.
- *Acute chest syndrome* describes pulmonary complications that include pneumonia, tissue infarction, and fat embolism, resulting in pulmonary hypertension, MI, and ultimately cor pulmonale.
- The kidneys may be injured from the lack of oxygen, resulting in renal failure.
- Stroke can result from thrombosis and infarction of cerebral blood vessels.
- The heart may become ischemic and enlarged, leading to heart failure.
- Retinal vessel obstruction may result in hemorrhage, scarring, retinal detachment, and blindness.
- Bone changes may include osteoporosis and osteosclerosis after infarction. Chronic leg ulcers can result from hypoxia.

Diagnostic Studies
- Peripheral blood smear may reveal sickled cells and abnormal reticulocytes.
- Sickle hemoglobin can be diagnosed by the sickling test, which uses RBCs (in vitro) and exposes them to a deoxygenation agent.
- Findings of hemolysis (jaundice, elevated serum bilirubin levels) and abnormal laboratory test results (see Table 9, p. 32) may be present.
- X-ray, magnetic resonance imaging (MRI), and Doppler studies may be indicated to assess for bone and joint deformities, stroke, and deep vein thromboses, respectively.

Nursing and Collaborative Management
Care is directed toward alleviating the symptoms from complications of the disease, minimizing end-organ damage, and promptly treating serious sequelae, such as acute chest syndrome. Teach patients with SCD to avoid high altitudes, maintain adequate fluid intake, and treat infections promptly.

- Pneumovax, *Haemophilus influenzae,* influenza, and hepatitis immunizations should be administered.
- Chronic leg ulcers may be treated with bed rest, antibiotics, warm saline soaks, mechanical or enzyme debridement, and grafting if necessary.

- Sickle cell crises may require hospitalization. O_2 may be administered to treat hypoxia and control sickling. Rest may be instituted to reduce metabolic requirements and fluids and electrolytes are administered to reduce blood viscosity and maintain renal function.
- Transfusion therapy is indicated when an aplastic crisis occurs. These patients, like those with thalassemia major, may require chelation therapy to reduce transfusion-produced iron overload.
- During an acute crisis, optimal pain control usually includes large doses of continuous (rather than as-needed [prn]) opioid analgesics along with breakthrough analgesia, often in the form of patient-controlled analgesia (PCA).
- Infection must be treated. Patients with acute chest syndrome are treated with broad-spectrum antibiotics, O_2 therapy, and fluid therapy.
- Although many antisickling agents have been tried, hydroxyurea (Hydrea) is the only one shown to be clinically beneficial. This drug increases the production of hemoglobin F (fetal hemoglobin), which is accompanied by a reduction in hemolysis, an increase in hemoglobin concentration, and a decrease in sickled cells and painful crises.
- Hematopoietic stem cell transplantation (HSCT) is the only available treatment that can cure some patients with SCD. Recent advances in gene therapy technology provide some promise for the future treatment of SCD.

▼ **Patient and Caregiver Teaching**

Patient teaching and support is important in the long-term care of the patient. The patient and caregiver need to understand the basis of the disease and the reasons for supportive care.

- Teach the patient ways to avoid crises, which include taking steps to reduce the chance of developing hypoxia, such as avoiding high altitudes and seeking medical attention quickly to counteract problems including upper respiratory tract infections.
- Also teach about pain control because the pain during a crisis may be severe and often requires considerable analgesia.

SJÖGREN'S SYNDROME

Sjögren's syndrome is a relatively common autoimmune disease that targets moisture-producing glands, leading to the common symptoms of xerostomia (dry mouth) and keratoconjunctivitis sicca (dry eyes). The nose, throat, airways, and skin can also become dry. The disease can affect other glands as well, including those in the stomach, pancreas, and intestines. The disease is usually diagnosed in women after age 40 years.

In *primary Sjögren's syndrome,* symptoms can be traced to problems with the lacrimal and salivary glands. The patient with primary disease is likely to have antibodies against the cytoplasmic antigens SS-A and SS-B, as well as antinuclear antibody (ANA). The patient with *secondary Sjögren's syndrome* typically has had another autoimmune disease (e.g., rheumatoid arthritis, systemic lupus erythematosus) before Sjögren's develops.

- Sjögren's syndrome appears to be caused by genetic and environmental factors. The trigger may be a viral or bacterial infection that adversely stimulates the immune system, causing lymphocytes to attack and damage the lacrimal and salivary glands.

Decreased tearing leads to a "gritty" sensation in the eyes, burning, blurred vision, and photosensitivity. Dry mouth produces buccal membrane fissures, altered sense of taste, dysphagia, and increased frequency of mouth infections or dental caries.

- Dry skin and rashes, joint and muscle pain, and thyroid problems may also be present.
- Autoimmune thyroid disorders are common, including Graves' disease or Hashimoto's thyroiditis.
- The disease may become more generalized and involve the lymph nodes, bone marrow, and visceral organs (pseudolymphoma). The risk of developing lymphoma is high in Sjögren's syndrome.

Ophthalmologic examination (Schirmer's test), salivary flow rates, and lower lip biopsy of minor salivary glands confirm the diagnosis.

Treatment is symptomatic, including instillation of artificial tears as often as necessary to maintain adequate hydration and lubrication, surgical occlusion of the puncta lacrimalia, and increased fluids with meals.

- Dental hygiene is important. Pilocarpine (Salagen) and cevimeline (Evoxac) can be used to treat symptoms of dry mouth.
- Increased humidity at home may reduce respiratory infections. Vaginal lubrication with a water-soluble product such as KY jelly may increase comfort during intercourse.

SPINAL CORD INJURY

Description

The population at highest risk for spinal cord injury (SCI) is young adult men between the ages of 16 and 30 years. The causes of SCI frequently include motor vehicle crashes, falls, violence, and sports injuries.

SCIs are classified by the mechanism of injury, level of injury, and completeness or degree of injury. The major mechanisms of injury are flexion, hyperextension, flexion-rotation, extension-rotation, and compression. The level of injury may be cervical, thoracic, or lumbar. Cervical and lumbar injuries are the most common because these levels are associated with the greatest flexibility and movement.

The degree of spinal cord involvement may be either complete or incomplete (partial).

- *Complete cord involvement* results in total loss of sensory and motor function below the level of the lesion (injury). If the cervical cord is involved, paralysis of all four extremities occurs, resulting in *tetraplegia* (paralysis of both arms and legs). If the thoracic or lumbar cord is damaged, the result is *paraplegia* (paralysis and loss of sensation in the legs).
- *Incomplete cord involvement* (partial transection) results in a mixed loss of voluntary motor activity and sensation and leaves some tracts intact. The degree of sensory and motor loss varies depending on the level of the lesion and reflects the specific nerve tracts damaged and those spared.

Pathophysiology

Penetrating trauma, such as gunshot and stab wounds, can result in tearing and transection of the spinal cord. The initial mechanical disruption of axons as a result of stretch or laceration is referred to as the *primary injury*. *Secondary injury* refers to the ongoing, progressive damage that occurs after the initial injury.

- There are several theories on what causes ongoing damage at the molecular and cellular level, including free radical formation, uncontrolled calcium influx, ischemia, and lipid peroxidation. At the molecular level, *apoptosis* (cell death) occurs and may continue sometimes for weeks or months after the initial injury. Thus the complete cord damage (previously thought to be transection) in severe trauma is related to autodestruction of the cord.

Hemorrhagic areas in the center of the spinal cord appear within 1 hour, and by 4 hours there may be infarction in the gray matter.

This ongoing destructive process makes it critical that initial care and management of the patient with a spinal cord injury be initiated as soon as possible to limit further destruction of the spinal cord.

Figure 13 illustrates the cascade of events causing secondary injury following traumatic spinal cord injury. The resulting hypoxia reduces oxygen tension below the level that meets the metabolic needs of the spinal cord. Lactate metabolites and an increase in vasoactive substances, including norepinephrine, serotonin, and dopamine, are noted. At high levels, these vasoactive substances cause vasospasms and hypoxia, leading to subsequent necrosis. Unfortunately, the spinal cord has minimal ability to adapt to vasospasm.

- Because secondary injury processes occur over time, the extent of injury and prognosis for recovery are most accurately determined at 72 hours or more after injury.

Spinal and Neurogenic Shock. About 50% of people with acute SCI experience a temporary neurologic syndrome known as *spinal shock* that is characterized by decreased reflexes, loss of sensation, and flaccid paralysis below the level of the injury. This syndrome lasts days to months and may mask postinjury neurologic function. Active rehabilitation may begin in the presence of spinal shock.

Neurogenic shock results from the loss of vasomotor tone caused by injury and is characterized by hypotension and bradycardia. Loss of sympathetic innervation causes peripheral vasodilation, venous pooling, and decreased cardiac output. These effects are generally associated with a cervical or high thoracic injury.

Clinical Manifestations

Manifestations of SCI are related to the level and degree of injury. The patient with an incomplete lesion may demonstrate a mixture of symptoms—the higher the injury, the more serious the effects because of the proximity of the cervical cord to the medulla and brainstem. Movement and rehabilitation potential related to specific locations of the SCI are described in Table 61-3, Lewis et al., *Medical-Surgical Nursing,* ed. 8, p. 1550. In general, sensory function closely parallels motor function at all levels.

Complications

Respiratory system. Cervical injury or fracture above the level of C4 presents with a total loss of respiratory muscle function. Mechanical ventilation is required to keep the patient alive. Injury below the level of C4 can result in diaphragmatic breathing with respiratory insufficiency and hypoventilation.

Cardiovascular system. Any cord injury above the level of T6 greatly decreases the influence of the sympathetic nervous system.

PATHOPHYSIOLOGY MAP

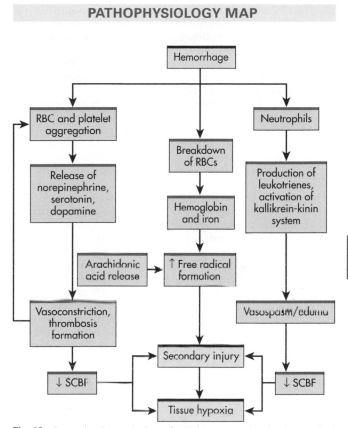

Fig. 13. Cascade of metabolic and cellular events that leads to spinal cord ischemia and hypoxia of secondary injury. *RBCs*, red blood cells; *SCBF*, spinal cord blood flow.

Bradycardia and peripheral vasodilation result. Cardiac monitoring is necessary.

Urinary system. Urinary retention is common in acute spinal cord injuries and spinal shock. While the patient is in spinal shock, the bladder is atonic and becomes overdistended. An indwelling catheter is inserted to drain the bladder. In the postacute phase the bladder may become hyperirritable, with a loss of inhibition from the brain resulting in reflex emptying.

Gastrointestinal system. If the cord injury has occurred above the level of T5, the primary problems are related to hypomotility. Decreased GI activity contributes to the development of a paralytic ileus and gastric distention. A nasogastric (NG) tube for intermittent suctioning may relieve the gastric distention. Histamine H_2-receptor blockers and proton pump inhibitors are frequently used to prevent the development of stress ulcers.

Loss of voluntary neurologic control over the bowel results in a *neurogenic* bowel. With an injury level of T12 or below, the bowel is areflexic and sphincter tone is decreased, resulting in constipation. As reflexes return, the bowel becomes reflexic, sphincter tone is enhanced, and reflex emptying occurs. Bowel programs can be used to manage both types of neurogenic bowel.

Integumentary system. A major consequence of lack of movement is the potential for skin breakdown over bony prominences in areas of decreased sensation. Pressure ulcers can occur quickly and lead to major infection or sepsis.

Peripheral vascular problems. Deep vein thrombosis (DVT) is a common problem accompanying SCI in the first 3 months. Pulmonary embolism is one of the leading causes of death in patients with SCI. Techniques for assessment of DVT include Doppler examination, impedance plethysmography, and measuring of leg and thigh girth.

Autonomic dysreflexia is a massive uncompensated cardiovascular reaction mediated by the sympathetic nervous system. It occurs in response to visceral stimulation after spinal shock is resolved in patients with spinal cord lesions at T6 or higher.

- The condition is a life-threatening situation that requires immediate resolution. If resolution does not occur, this condition can lead to status epilepticus, myocardial infarction, stroke, and even death.
- The most common precipitating cause is a distended bladder or rectum, although any sensory stimulation may cause autonomic dysreflexia.
- Manifestations include hypertension (up to 300 mm Hg systolic), blurred vision, throbbing headache, marked diaphoresis above the level of the lesion, bradycardia (30 to 40 beats per minute), piloerection (erection of body hair), nasal congestion, and nausea. It is important that you measure the blood pressure (BP) when a patient with an SCI complains of a headache.
- You should elevate the head of the bed 45 degrees or sit the patient upright, notify the physician, and assess the cause of the reaction. Implement interventions to relieve the cause immediately (e.g., relieving bladder or bowel distention,

removal of all skin stimuli). If symptoms persist after the source has been relieved, an α-adrenergic blocker (e.g., phentolamine [Regitine]) or an arterial vasodilator (e.g., nifedipine [Procardia]) is administered.

- Teach the patient and caregiver the causes and symptoms of autonomic dysreflexia (see Table 61-7, Lewis et al., *Medical-Surgical Nursing,* ed. 8, p. 1559). They must understand the life-threatening nature of this dysfunction and must know how to relieve the cause.

Diagnostic Studies

- CT scan is the gold standard in diagnosing injury stability, location and degree of bony injury, and degree of spinal canal compromise. Cervical x-rays are obtained when CT scan is not readily available.
- MRI is used to assess soft tissue and neural changes in patients with unexplained neurologic deficit or worsening of neurologic status.
- Comprehensive neurologic examination is done along with assessment of head, chest, and abdomen for additional injuries or trauma.
- Patients with cervical injuries who demonstrate altered mental status may need vertebral angiography to rule out vertebral artery damage.

Collaborative Care

For injury at the cervical level, all body systems must be maintained until the full extent of the damage can be evaluated. A thorough assessment is done to specifically evaluate the degree of deficit and establish the level and degree of injury. The patient may go directly to surgery after initial immobilization and assessment or to the intensive care unit (ICU) for monitoring and management.

Nonoperative Stablization

Nonoperative treatments are focused on stabilization of the injured spinal segment and decompression, either through traction or realignment, to prevent secondary spinal cord damage caused by repeated contusion or compression.

Surgical Therapy

When cord compression is certain or the neurologic disorder progresses, benefits may be seen following immediate surgery. Surgery stabilizes the spinal column. Early cord decompression may result in reduced secondary injury to the spinal cord and therefore improved outcomes. Other criteria for early surgery include (1) evidence of cord compression, (2) progressive neurologic deficit, (3) compound fracture of the vertebrae, (4) bony fragments (may dislodge and penetrate the cord), and (5) penetrating wounds of the spinal cord or surrounding structures.

- More common surgical procedures include decompression laminectomy by anterior cervical and thoracic approaches with fusion, posterior laminectomy with the use of acrylic wire mesh and fusion, and the insertion of stabilizing rods (e.g., Harrington rods for the correction and stabilization of thoracic deformities).

Drug Therapy

The administration of high-dose steroids within 8 hours of injury for patients with acute SCI is practiced by most physicians. The use of methylprednisolone (MP) is contraindicated in penetrating trauma to the spinal cord and should be used with caution in the elderly population. MP, a blocker of lipid peroxidation byproducts, is thought to improve blood flow and reduce edema in the spinal cord.

- Vasopressor agents such as dopamine (Intropin) are used in the acute phase as adjuvants to treatment. These agents maintain mean arterial pressure at a level >90 mm Hg so that perfusion to the spinal cord is improved.

Nursing Management

Goals

The patient with an SCI will maintain an optimal level of neurologic functioning; have minimal or no complications of immobility; learn new skills, gain new knowledge, and acquire new behaviors to be able to care for self or successfully direct others to do so; and return to home and the community at an optimal level of functioning.

See NCP 61-1 for the patient with an SCI, Lewis et al., *Medical-Surgical Nursing,* ed. 8, pp. 1554 to 1555.

Nursing Diagnoses

- Ineffective breathing pattern
- Impaired skin integrity
- Constipation
- Impaired urinary elimination
- Impaired physical mobility
- Risk for autonomic dysreflexia
- Ineffective coping

Nursing Interventions

High cervical injury resulting from flexion-rotation is the most complex SCI and is discussed in this section. Interventions for this type of injury can be modified for patients with less severe problems.

Immobilization. Proper immobilization of the neck involves maintenance of a neutral position. The body should always be correctly aligned, and turning should be performed so that the patient is moved as a unit (e.g., logrolling) to prevent movement of the spine. For cervical injuries, skeletal traction is used less frequently with the development of better surgical stabilization. When skeletal traction is used, realignment or reduction of the injury is usually provided by Crutchfield, Vinke, Gardner-Wells, or other types of skull tongs.

- Infection at the sites of tong insertion is a potential problem. Preventive care includes cleansing the sites twice each day with normal saline solution and applying an antibiotic ointment that acts as a mechanical barrier to the bacteria.
- Special beds are often used to provide frequent turning to prevent pressure sores and cardiopulmonary complications.

After cervical fusion or other stabilization surgery, a hard cervical collar or sternal-occipital-mandibular immobilizer brace can be worn until the fusion becomes solid. In a stable injury for which surgery is not done, a halo fixation apparatus may be applied.

Respiratory dysfunction. If the patient is exhausted from labored breathing or arterial blood gases (ABGs) deteriorate (indicating inadequate oxygenation), endotracheal intubation or tracheostomy and mechanical ventilation should be initiated. (See Artificial Airways: Endotracheal Tubes, p. 699, Tracheostomy, p. 754, and Mechanical Ventilation, p. 736.) Respiratory arrest is a possibility that requires careful monitoring and prompt action should it occur. Pneumonia and atelectasis are potential problems because of reduced vital capacity and the loss of intercostal and abdominal muscle function.

- Regularly assess breath sounds, ABGs, tidal volume, vital capacity, skin color, breathing patterns (especially the use of accessory muscles), subjective comments about the ability to breathe, and the amount and color of sputum.
- In addition to monitoring, you can intervene in maintaining ventilation by the administration of oxygen (O_2) until ABGs stabilize, chest physiotherapy and assisted coughing, incentive spirometry, and tracheal suctioning.

Cardiovascular instability. If bradycardia is symptomatic, an anticholinergic medication such as atropine is administered. A temporary pacemaker may be inserted in some instances (see Pacemakers, p. 749). Hypotension is managed with a vasopressor agent, such as dopamine, and fluid replacement.

- Sequential compression devices or compression gradient stockings can be used to prevent thromboemboli and promote venous return.
- Perform range-of-motion (ROM) exercises and heel-cord stretching regularly. Assess the thighs and calves of the legs every shift for the signs of DVT.
- Monitor the patient for indications of hypovolemic shock secondary to hemorrhage.

Fluid and nutritional maintenance. During the first 48 to 72 hours after the injury, the GI tract may stop functioning (paralytic ileus) and an NG tube must be inserted.

- Once bowel sounds are present or flatus is passed, oral food and fluids can be introduced gradually. Because of severe catabolism, a high-protein, high-calorie diet is necessary for energy and tissue repair.
- In patients with high cervical cord injuries, evaluate swallowing before starting oral feedings. If the patient is unable to resume eating, enteral or parenteral nutrition (PN) may be started to provide nutritional support.

Bowel and bladder management

- An indwelling catheter is usually inserted as soon as possible after injury. Its patency must be ensured by irrigation and frequent inspection. Strict aseptic technique for catheter care is essential to avoid introducing infection.
- Urinary tract infections (UTIs) are a common problem. The best method for preventing UTIs is regular and complete bladder drainage.
- Constipation is generally a problem during spinal shock because no voluntary or involuntary (reflex) evacuation of the bowels occurs. A bowel program should be started during acute care. This consists of a rectal stimulant (suppository or mini-enema) inserted daily at a regular time of day followed by gentle digital stimulation or manual evacuation.

Temperature control. Because there is no vasoconstriction, piloerection, or heat loss through perspiration below the level of injury, temperature control is largely external to the patient. Therefore you must monitor the environment closely to maintain an appropriate temperature. Monitor body temperature regularly.

Stress ulcers. Stress ulcers are a problem because of the physiologic response to severe trauma, psychologic stress, and high-dose corticosteroids. Peak incidence is 6 to 14 days after injury. Test stool and gastric contents daily for blood, and observe hematocrit for a slow drop. When corticosteroids are given, administer with antacids or food. Histamine H_2-receptor blockers (e.g., ranitidine

[Zantac]) or proton pump inhibitors (e.g., omeprazole [Prilosec]), may be given prophylactically to decrease hydrochloric acid secretion.

Sensory deprivation. You must compensate for the patient's absent sensations to prevent sensory deprivation. Do this by stimulating the patient above the level of injury. Conversation, music, strong aromas, and interesting flavors should be a part of nursing care. Provide prism glasses so the patient can read and watch television. Make every effort to prevent the patient from withdrawing from the environment.

Reflexes. Once spinal shock is resolved, reflexes often return with hyperactive and exaggerated responses. Penile erections can occur from a variety of stimuli, causing embarrassment and discomfort. Spasms ranging from mild twitches to convulsive movements below the level of the lesion may also occur. Reflex activity may be interpreted by the patient or caregiver as a return of function. You must tactfully explain the reason for the activity. Spasms may be controlled with antispasmodic medications, such as baclofen (Lioresal), dantrolene (Dantrium), or tizanidine (Zanaflex).

Rehabilitation. Physiologic and psychologic rehabilitation is complex and involved. Many of the problems identified in the acute period become chronic and continue throughout life. Rehabilitation focuses on refined retraining of physiologic processes and extensive patient, caregiver, and family teaching about how to manage the physiologic and life changes resulting from injury.

SPINAL CORD TUMORS

Description

Tumors that affect the spinal cord account for 0.5% to 1% of all neoplasms. These tumors are classified as primary (arising from some component of cord, dura, nerves, or vessels) or secondary (from primary growths in the breast, prostate, lung, kidney, and other sites).

- Spinal cord tumors are further classified as *extradural tumors* (outside the spinal cord), *intradural-extramedullary tumors* (within the dura but outside the actual spinal cord), and *intradural-intramedullary tumors* (within the spinal cord itself) (see Fig. 61-13 and Table 61-15, Lewis and others, *Medical-Surgical Nursing,* ed. 8, p. 1564).
- Approximately 90% of all spinal tumors are extradural.

Because many of these tumors are slow growing, their symptoms stem from the mechanical effects of slow compression and irritation of nerve roots, displacement of the cord, or gradual obstruction of the vascular supply. Slowness of growth does not cause autode-struction as in traumatic lesions. Therefore complete functional restoration is possible when the tumor is removed, with the exception of intradural-intramedullary tumors.

Clinical Manifestations

The most common early symptom of a spinal cord tumor outside the cord is pain in the back with a radiation of pain simulating intercostal neuralgia, angina, or herpes zoster. The location of the pain depends on the level of compression. The pain worsens with activity, coughing, straining, and lying down.

- Sensory disruption is later manifested by coldness, numbness, and tingling in an extremity or several extremities, slowly progressing upward until it reaches the level of the lesion.
- Impaired sensation of pain, temperature, and light touch precedes a deficit in vibration and position sense that may progress to complete anesthesia.
- Motor weakness accompanies sensory disturbances and consists of slowly increasing clumsiness, weakness, and spasticity. The sensory and motor disturbances are ipsilateral to the lesion.
- Bladder disturbances are marked by urgency with difficulty in starting the flow and progressing to retention with overflow incontinence.

Manifestations of intradural spinal tumor develop as progressive damage to the long spinal tracts, producing paralysis, sensory loss, and bladder dysfunction. Pain can be severe as a result of the compression of spinal roots or vertebrae.

Diagnostic Studies

Extradural tumors are seen early on routine spinal x-rays, whereas intradural and intramedullary tumors require magnetic resonance imaging (MRI) or computed tomography (CT) scans for detection. Cerebrospinal fluid (CSF) analysis may reveal tumor cells.

Nursing and Collaborative Management

More than 85% of primary neoplasms are benign and can be completely resected; 90% of patients recover without residual problems.

Compression of the spinal cord is an emergency. Relief of the ischemia related to the compression is the goal of therapy. Corticosteroids, usually dexamethasone (Decadron) in large doses, are generally prescribed immediately to relieve tumor-related edema.

Treatment for nearly all spinal cord tumors is surgical removal. The exception is the metastatic tumor that is sensitive to radiation and that has caused only minimal neurologic deficits in the patient. In general, extradural or intradural-extramedullary tumors can be completely removed surgically.

Radiation therapy after surgery is fairly effective. Chemotherapy may be used in conjunction with radiation therapy.

- Depending on the amount of neurologic dysfunction exhibited, the patient may need to be cared for as though recovering from a spinal cord injury. Rehabilitation of patients with spinal cord tumors is also similar to spinal cord injury rehabilitation.

SPLEEN DISORDERS

The spleen can be affected by many illnesses, most of which can cause some degree of splenomegaly *(enlarged spleen)*. Some of the many causes of splenomegaly include sickle cell disease, infections, cirrhosis, heart failure (HF), and polycythemia vera. The term *hypersplenism* refers to the occurrence of splenomegaly and peripheral cytopenias (anemia, leukopenia, thrombocytopenia).

- The degree of splenic enlargement varies with the disease. For example, massive splenic enlargement occurs with chronic myelogenous leukemia and thalassemia major, whereas mild splenic enlargement occurs with HF and systemic lupus erythematosus. When the spleen enlarges, its normal filtering and sequestering capacity increases. Consequently, there is often a reduction in the number of circulating blood cells.

A slight to moderate enlargement of the spleen is usually asymptomatic and found during a routine examination of the abdomen. Massive splenomegaly can be well tolerated, but patients may complain of abdominal discomfort and early satiety. In addition to physical examination, other techniques to assess spleen size include Tc-sulfur colloid liver-spleen scan, computed tomography (CT) or PET scan, magnetic resonance imaging (MRI), and ultrasound scan.

Occasionally laparoscopy or open laparotomy and splenectomy are indicated in the evaluation or treatment of splenomegaly. Splenectomy can have a dramatic effect in increasing peripheral red blood cell (RBC), white blood cell (WBC), and platelet counts. Another indication for splenectomy is splenic rupture. The spleen may rupture from trauma, inadvertent tearing during other surgical procedures, and diseases such as mononucleosis, malaria, and lymphoid neoplasms.

Nursing responsibilities for patients with spleen disorders vary depending on the nature of the problem.

- Splenomegaly may be painful and require analgesic administration; care in moving, turning, and positioning; and evaluation of lung expansion, because spleen enlargement may impair diaphragmatic excursion.
- If anemia, thrombocytopenia, or leukopenia develops from splenic enlargement, nursing measures must be instituted to support the patient and prevent life-threatening complications.
- After splenectomy the patient must be observed for hemorrhage, which can lead to shock, fever, and abdominal distention.
- Postsplenectomy patients may develop immunologic deficiencies and have a lifelong risk for infection from encapsulated organisms, such as pneumococcus. This risk is reduced by immunization with polyvalent pneumococcal vaccine (Pneumovax).

STOMACH CANCER

Description
Stomach (gastric) cancer is an adenocarcinoma of the stomach wall. The rate of stomach cancer has been steadily declining in the United States since the 1930s. Most individuals are over age 65 when diagnosed. More than 50% have advanced metastatic disease at the time of diagnosis. The 5-year survival rate is less than 30% in those with advanced disease and 80% in patients with early stage cancer confined to the stomach.

Pathophysiology
Many factors have been implicated in stomach cancer. Stomach cancer probably begins with a nonspecific mucosal injury as a result of autoimmune-related inflammation, repeated exposure to irritants such as bile, antiinflammatory agents or tobacco use. Stomach cancer has also been associated with diets containing smoked foods, salted fish and meat, and pickled vegetables. *Helicobacter pylori* infection, especially at an early age, is considered a risk factor for stomach cancer. Other predisposing factors are obesity, family history, atrophic gastritis, pernicious anemia, adenomatous and hyperplastic polyps, and achlorhydria. Whole grains

and fresh fruits and vegetables are associated with reduced rates of stomach cancer.

Stomach cancer spreads by direct extension and typically infiltrates rapidly to the surrounding tissue and liver. Seeding of tumor cells into the peritoneal cavity may occur later in the disease.

Clinical Manifestations

Stomach cancers often spread to adjacent organs before any distressing symptoms such as indigestion or dysphagia occur. Clinical manifestations include unexplained weight loss, lack of appetite, abdominal discomfort or pain, signs and symptoms of anemia, or indigestion.

- Anemia commonly occurs with chronic blood loss as the lesion erodes the stomach mucosa. The patient appears pale and weak with fatigue, dizziness, weakness, and positive occult stools.
- Pain and discomfort may be alleviated by belching and the use of antacids, antisecretory agents, and diet modifications similar to peptic ulcer disease. Manifestations include vague epigastric fullness with feelings of early satiety after meals. Weight loss, dysphagia, and constipation frequently accompany epigastric distress.

A mass may be often felt in the epigastrium. Supraclavicular lymph nodes that are hard and enlarged are suggestive of metastasis via the thoracic duct. The presence of ascites is a poor prognostic sign.

Diagnostic Studies

- Endoscopic examination with biopsy of the stomach is the best diagnostic tool.
- Endoscopic ultrasound and computed tomography (CT) and PET scan can be used to stage the disease.
- Blood studies detect anemia and its severity and also elevations in liver enzymes and serum amylase may indicate liver and pancreatic involvement.

Collaborative Care

Treatment of choice is surgical removal of the tumor. Surgical procedures used are similar to those used for peptic ulcer disease (see Peptic Ulcer Disease, p. 493).

- Preoperative management focuses on the correction of nutritional deficits and transfusions of packed red blood cells (RBCs) to treat anemia. Gastric decompression may be necessary if gastric outlet obstruction is present, and special preparation of the bowel is needed if the tumor has involved the colon.

Therapy for localized stomach cancer includes surgical resection followed by fluorouracil (5-FU) and radiotherapy or pre- and post-operative epirubicin (Ellence), cisplatin (Platinol), and continuous infusion fluorouracil without radiotherapy (see Chemotherapy, p. 717). Radiation therapy may be used as a palliative measure to decrease tumor mass and provide temporary relief of obstruction.

Nursing Management
Goals
The patient with stomach cancer will experience minimal discomfort, achieve optimal nutritional status, and maintain a degree of spiritual and psychologic well-being appropriate to the disease stage.

Nursing Diagnoses
- Imbalanced nutrition: less than body requirements
- Activity intolerance
- Anxiety
- Acute pain
- Grieving

Nursing Interventions
Your role in the early detection of stomach cancer is focused on the identification of patients at risk such as those with pernicious anemia or achlorhydria or those who smoke.

When diagnostic tests confirm the presence of malignancy, offer emotional and physical support, provide information, and clarify test results. The preoperative teaching plan is similar to that for peptic ulcer disease surgery (see Peptic Ulcer Disease, p. 493).

Postoperative care is also similar to that following a Billroth I or II procedure for peptic ulcer disease. Closely observe the patient for signs of fluids leaking at the site of anastomosis, as evidenced by an elevation in temperature and increasing dyspnea. If a total gastrectomy is done, dumping syndrome may occur (see pp. 498–499 under Peptic Ulcer Disease).

- Postoperative wound healing may be impaired because of inadequate dietary intake. This necessitates intravenous (IV) or oral replacement of C, D, K, and B-complex vitamins and IM or intranasal administration of cobalamin.

When chemotherapy is prescribed, provide information regarding the actions and side effects of the drugs. For the patient receiving radiation therapy your role is to provide detailed instructions, reassure the patient, and ensure completion of the designated number of treatments. Teach the patient about skin care, the need for good nutrition and fluid intake during therapy, and appropriate use of antiemetic drugs.

▼ Patient and Caregiver Teaching

Before discharge, instruct the patient and caregivers about comfort measures and the use of analgesics; additional considerations include:

- Teach wound care, if needed, to the primary caregiver in the home situation.
- Dressings, special equipment, or special services that may be required for the patient's continued care at home.
- Provide a list of community agencies that are available for assistance.

STROKE

Description

Stroke occurs when there is ischemia to a part of the brain or hemorrhage into the brain that results in brain cell death. Functions, such as movement, sensation, or emotions, that were controlled by the affected brain area are lost or impaired. The severity of the loss of function varies according to the location and extent of the brain area involved.

- Stroke is the third most common cause of death. Strokes are considered a major public health problem in the United States in terms of mortality and morbidity, since an estimated 800,000 persons experience strokes annually.
- More than 275,000 deaths occur annually from stroke. After an initial stroke, 34% of men and 38% of women will die within 1 year. The percentage is higher for people 65 years old.
- Of those who survive, 50% to 70% will be functionally independent and 15% to 30% will live with permanent disability.

Risk factors associated with stroke can be divided into nonmodifiable and modifiable.

- *Nonmodifiable risk factors* include age, race, and heredity. African Americans experience a higher incidence of stroke, which is associated with an increased incidence of hypertension, obesity, and diabetes mellitus (DM). African American men from the South are almost four times more likely to die from a stroke than Southern white men. Persons with a family history of stroke or transient ischemic attacks (TIAs) are also at higher risk for stroke.

- *Modifiable risk factors* are hypertension, cardiovascular disease, DM, obesity, sickle cell disease, and certain lifestyle habits, such as cigarette smoking, a diet high in fat, and heavy alcohol consumption. Hypertension is the single most important modifiable risk factor, and its treatment can reduce the risk of stroke by up to 50%.

Transient Ischemic Attack

A transient ischemic attack (TIA) is a transient episode of neurologic dysfunction caused by focal brain, spinal cord, or retinal ischemia, but without acute infarction of the brain. Clinical symptoms typically last less than one hour. TIAs may be caused by microemboli that temporarily block the blood flow and are a warning sign of progressive cerebrovascular disease.

Most TIAs resolve. However, encourage patients to go to the emergency room at symptom onset since once a TIA starts, one does not know if it will persist and become a true stroke or resolve. In general, one third of individuals who experience a TIA will not experience another event, one third will have additional TIAs, and one third will progress to stroke.

TIA signs and symptoms depend on the blood vessel involved and the brain area that is ischemic.

- If the carotid system is involved, patients may have a temporary loss of vision in one eye, transient hemiparesis, numbness or loss of sensation, or a sudden inability to speak.
- Signs of a TIA involving the vertebrobasilar system may include tinnitus, vertigo, darkened or blurred vision, ptosis, dysphagia, ataxia, and unilateral or bilateral numbness or weakness.

Evaluation must be done to confirm that signs and symptoms of a TIA are not related to other brain lesions, such as a developing subdural hematoma or an increasing tumor mass.

- Computed tomography (CT) of the brain without contrast is the most important initial diagnostic study. Cardiac monitoring and tests may reveal an underlying cardiac condition that is responsible for clot formation.
- Medications that prevent platelet aggregation, such as aspirin, ticlopidine (Ticlid), clopidogrel (Plavix), dipyridamole (Persantine), combined dipyridamole and aspirin (Aggrenox), and anticoagulant medications (e.g., oral warfarin [Coumadin]), may be prescribed for long-term therapy after a TIA.

Types of Strokes

Strokes are classified as ischemic or hemorrhagic based on their underlying pathophysiology (Table 82 and Fig. 14).

- An *ischemic stroke* results from a decreased blood flow to the brain secondary to partial or complete occlusion of an artery. This type of stroke accounts for approximately 80% of all strokes. Ischemic strokes are further divided into thrombotic and embolic. A transient ischemic attack is usually a precursor to ischemic stroke.
- A *hemorrhagic stroke* results from bleeding into the brain tissue itself (intracerebral or intraparenchymal hemorrhage) or into the subarachnoid space or ventricles (subarachnoid hemorrhage). These account for 15% of all strokes.

Pathophysiology

Thrombotic stroke. Thrombosis results from the formation of a blood clot that causes narrowing of the lumen of a blood vessel with eventual occlusion and infarction. It is the most common cause of stroke.

- Two thirds of thrombotic strokes are associated with hypertension or DM; both of these conditions accelerate the atherosclerotic process.

Thrombotic strokes may be preceded by a TIA. The extent of the stroke depends on rapidity of onset, size of lesion, and presence of collateral circulation.

- Most patients do not have a decreased level of consciousness in the first 24 hours unless it is caused by a brainstem stroke or other conditions, such as seizures, increased intracranial pressure, or hemorrhage.
- Ischemic stroke symptoms may progress in the first 72 hours as infarction and cerebral edema increase.

Embolic stroke. Cerebral embolism is the occlusion of a cerebral artery by an embolus, resulting in necrosis and edema of the area supplied by the involved blood vessel. Embolism is the second most common cause of stroke.

The majority of emboli originate in the heart. The emboli travel to the cerebral circulation and lodge where a vessel narrows. Emboli are associated with heart conditions such as atrial fibrillation, myocardial infarction (MI), and inflammatory and valvular heart conditions.

- Onset of an embolic stroke is usually sudden and may or may not be related to activity. The patient usually remains conscious, although a headache may develop.
- Recurrence is common unless the underlying cause is aggressively treated.

Table 82   **Types of Stroke**

Type	Gender/Age	Warning/Onset	Course/Prognosis
Ischemic			
Thrombotic	Men more than women Oldest median age	*Warning:* TIA (30%–50% of cases) *Onset:* Often during or after sleep	Stepwise progression, signs and symptoms develop slowly, usually some improvement, recurrence in 20%–25% of survivors
Embolic	Men more than women	*Warning:* TIA (uncommon) *Onset:* Lack of relationship to activity, sudden onset	Single event, signs and symptoms develop quickly, usually some improvement, recurrence common without aggressive treatment of underlying disease
Hemorrhagic			
Intracerebral	Slightly higher in women	*Warning:* Headache (25% of cases) *Onset:* Activity (often)	Progression over 24 hr; poor prognosis, fatality more likely with presence of coma
Subarachnoid	Slightly higher in women Youngest median age	*Warning:* Headache (common) *Onset:* Activity (often), sudden onset, most commonly related to head trauma	Usually single sudden event, fatality more likely with presence of coma

TIA, Transient ischemic attack.

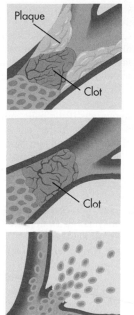

Thrombotic stroke. The process of clot formation (thrombosis) results in a narrowing of the lumen, which blocks the passage of the blood through the artery.

Embolic stroke. An embolus is a blood clot or other debris circulating in the blood. When it reaches an artery in the brain that is too narrow to pass through, it lodges there and blocks the flow of blood.

Hemorrhagic stroke. A burst blood vessel may allow blood to seep into and damage brain tissues until clotting shuts off the leak.

Fig. 14. Major types of stroke.

Hemorrhagic stroke. **Intracerebral hemorrhage** is bleeding within the brain caused by a rupture of a vessel. Hypertension is the most important cause of intracerebral hemorrhage. Other causes include vascular malformations, coagulation disorders, anticoagulant drugs, trauma, and ruptured aneurysms.

- Hemorrhage commonly occurs during periods of activity. There is most often a sudden onset of symptoms, and progression occurs over minutes to hours as a result of ongoing bleeding.
- Symptoms include neurologic deficits, headache, nausea, vomiting, decreased level of consciousness, and hypertension. Extent of the symptoms varies depending on the amount and duration of bleeding.
- Prognosis of patients with intracerebral hemorrhage is poor, with 40% to 80% of patients dying within 30 days, and 50% of the deaths occurring within the first 48 hours.

Subarachnoid hemorrhage occurs when there is intracranial bleeding into the cerebrospinal fluid-filled space between the arachnoid and pia mater membranes on the surface of the brain. Subarachnoid hemorrhage is commonly caused by rupture of a cerebral aneurysm (congenital or acquired weakness and ballooning of vessels). Other causes of subarachnoid hemorrhage include arteriovenous malformations (AVMs), trauma, and illicit drug (cocaine) abuse.

- The patient may have warning symptoms if the ballooning artery applies pressure to brain tissue, or minor warning symptoms may result from leaking of an aneurysm before major rupture. Sudden onset of a severe headache that is different from a previous headache and typically the "worst headache of one's life" is a characteristic symptom of a ruptured aneurysm.
- Loss of consciousness may or may not occur, and the patient's level of consciousness may range from alert to comatose, depending on the severity of the bleeding.
- Other symptoms include focal neurologic deficits (including cranial nerve deficits), nausea, vomiting, seizures, and stiff neck.
- Despite improvements in surgical techniques and management, many patients with subarachnoid hemorrhage die or are left with significant disability.

Clinical Manifestations

Manifestations seen with specific cerebral artery involvement are listed in Table 58-2, Lewis et al., *Medical-Surgical Nursing*, ed. 8, p. 1464. Figure 15 illustrates manifestations of right- and left-sided stroke.

Motor function. Motor deficits are the most obvious effect of stroke. Because the pyramidal pathway crosses at the level of the medulla, a lesion on one side of the brain affects motor function on the opposite side of the brain (contralateral). This destruction can result in loss of skilled voluntary movements *(akinesia),* impairment of integration of movements, and alterations in muscle tone and reflex activity.

- Hyporeflexia that initially occurs with stroke progresses to hyperreflexia for most patients.

Communication. The left hemisphere is dominant for language skills in all right-handed persons and most left-handed persons.

- Language disorders involve the expression and comprehension of written or spoken words. The patient may experience *aphasia* (total loss of comprehension and use of language)

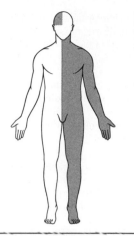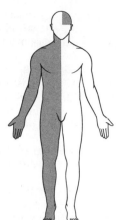

Right-brain damage (stroke on right side of the brain)	**Left-brain damage** (stroke on left side of the brain)
• Paralyzed left side: hemiplegia	• Paralyzed right side: hemiplegia
• Left-sided neglect	• Impaired speech/language aphasias
• Spatial-perceptual deficits	
• Tends to deny or minimize problems	• Impaired right/left discrimination
	• Slow performance, cautious
• Rapid performance, short attention span	• Aware of deficits: depression, anxiety
• Impulsive, safety problems	• Impaired comprehension related to language, math
• Impaired judgment	
• Impaired time concepts	

Fig. 15. Manifestations of right- and left-brain stroke.

when a stroke damages the dominant hemisphere of the brain.

- Patterns of aphasia may differ as the stroke affects different portions of the brain. Aphasia may be classified as nonfluent (minimal speech activity with slow speech that requires obvious effort) or fluent (speech is present but contains little meaningful communication).

- Most stroke patients also experience *dysarthria*, a disturbance in the muscular control of speech.

Affect. Patients with a stroke may have difficulty expressing their emotions; emotional responses may be exaggerated or unpredictable.

Additional manifestations include impairment of memory and judgment, deficits in spatial-perceptual orientation, and transient problems with bowel and bladder function.

Diagnostic Studies

When symptoms of a stroke occur, diagnostic studies are done to confirm that it is a stroke (and not another brain lesion, such as a subdural hematoma) and to identify the likely cause of the stroke. Tests also guide decisions about therapy to prevent secondary stroke.

- CT scan, the primary diagnostic test, can indicate lesion size and location and differentiate between ischemic and hemorrhagic stroke.
- CT angiography (CTA) provides visualization of cerebral blood vessels and an estimate of perfusion. CTA also detects filling defects in the cerebral arteries.
- Magnetic resonance imaging (MRI) is used to determine the extent of brain injury.
- Magnetic resonance angiography (MRA) can detect vascular lesions and blockages similar to CTA.
- Angiography can identify cervical and cerebrovascular occlusion, atherosclerotic plaques, and malformation of vessels.
- Intraarterial digital subtraction angiography (DSA) involves injection of a contrast agent to visualize vessels in the neck and the circle of Willis.
- Transcranial Doppler (TCD) ultrasonography has been effective in detecting microemboli and vasospasm in the major cerebral arteries.
- If the suspected cause of the stroke includes emboli from the heart, diagnostic cardiac tests should be done.

The LICOX system may be used as a diagnostic tool for evaluating the progression of stroke. LICOX measures brain oxygenation and temperature.

Collaborative Care

Prevention

The goals of stroke prevention include management of modifiable risk factors to prevent a stroke. Health promotion focuses on (1) healthy diet, (2) weight control, (3) regular exercise, (4) no smoking, (5) limiting alcohol consumption, and (6) routine health assessments. Patients with known risk factors such as diabetes mellitus, hypertension, obesity, high serum lipids, or cardiac dysfunction require close management.

- Measures to prevent the development of a thrombus or embolus are used in patients with TIAs as they are at high risk for stroke. Antiplatelet drugs are usually the chosen treatment to prevent stroke in patients who have had a TIA. Aspirin at a dose of 81 to 325 mg/day is the most frequently used antiplatelet agent. Other drugs include ticlopidine (Ticlid), clopidogrel (Plavix), dipyridamole (Persantine), and combined dipyridamole and aspirin (Aggrenox). Oral anticoagulation using warfarin is the treatment of choice for individuals with atrial fibrillation who have had a TIA.
- Statins (simvastatin [Zocor], lovastatin [Mevacor]) have also been shown to be effective in the prevention of stroke for individuals who have experienced a TIA in the past.
- Surgical therapy for the patient with TIAs from carotid disease includes carotid endarterectomy, transluminal angioplasty, stenting, and extracranial-intracranial (EC-IC) bypass.

Acute Care: Ischemic Stroke

The goals of acute care are preservation of life, prevention of further brain damage, and reduction of disability. Treatment changes as the patient progresses from the acute to the rehabilitation phase.

- Acute care begins with managing the airway, breathing, and circulation (the ABCs). Oxygen administration, artificial airway insertion, intubation, and mechanical ventilation may be required. Table 58-6, Lewis et al., *Medical-Surgical Nursing,* ed. 8, p. 1468 outlines emergency management of the patient with a stroke.
- Elevated BP is common immediately after a stroke and may be a protective response to maintain cerebral perfusion. Immediately following ischemic stroke, use of drugs to lower BP is recommended only if BP is markedly increased (mean arterial pressure >130 mm Hg or systolic pressure >220 mm Hg).
- Fluid and electrolyte balance must be controlled carefully. Although the goal is to maintain perfusion to the brain, overhydration may compromise perfusion by increasing cerebral edema. Adequate fluid intake during acute care by means of oral or intravenous (IV) administration or tube feedings should be 1500 to 2000 mL/day. Urine output is monitored.
- Management of increased intracranial pressure (ICP) focuses on improving venous drainage, including elevation of the head of the bed as ordered, maintaining head and neck in alignment, and avoiding hip flexion.

- Cooling blankets may be used cautiously to lower temperature. Closely monitor the patient's temperature. Aggressive management of temperature during the first 24 hours after a stroke is most effective in preventing detrimental outcomes.
- Other measures include pain management, avoidance of hypervolemia, and management of constipation. Diuretic medications, such as mannitol (Osmitrol) and furosemide (Lasix), may be used to decrease cerebral edema.

Drug therapy. Recombinant tissue plasminogen activator (tPA) administered IV is used to reestablish blood flow and prevent cell death for patients with ischemic strokes. This drug must be administered within 3 to 4.5 hours of the onset of clinical signs. Patients are screened carefully before tPA can be given, including a CT or MRI scan to rule out hemorrhagic stroke, blood tests for coagulation disorders, and screening for recent history of GI bleeding, head trauma, or major surgery.

- During infusion the patient's vital signs are monitored to assess for improvement or deterioration related to intracerebral hemorrhage.
- Control of blood pressure (BP) is critical during treatment and for 24 hours after treatment.
- Aspirin may be intiated within 24 to 48 hours of an ischemic stroke. Other platelet inhibitors and anticoagulants may also be used to prevent further clot formation. Platelet inhibitors include aspirin, ticlopidine (Ticlid), clopidogrel (Plavix), and dipyridamole (Persantine). Common anticoagulants include heparin and warfarin (Coumadin).

Surgical therapy. The mechanical embolus removal in cerebral ischemia (MERCI) retriever allows physicians to go inside the blocked artery of patients who are experiencing ischemic strokes.

Acute Care: Hemorrhagic Stroke

Drug therapy. Anticoagulants and platelet inhibitors are contraindicated in patients with hemorrhagic strokes. The main drug therapy for patients with hemorrhagic stroke is the management of hypertension. Oral and IV agents may be used to maintain blood pressure within a normal to high-normal range (SBP <160 mm Hg).

- Seizure prophylaxis in the acute period after intracerebral and subarachnoid hemorrhages is recommended.

Surgical therapy. Surgical interventions for hemorrhagic stroke include immediate evacuation of aneurysm-induced hematomas or cerebellar hematomas >3 cm. Individuals who have an arteriovenous malformation (AVM) may experience a hemorrhagic stroke if the AVM ruptures.

- Treatment of arteriovenous malformation (AVM) is surgical resection and/or radiosurgery (i.e., gamma knife). Both may be preceded by interventional neuroradiology to embolize the blood vessels that supply the AVM.

Subarachnoid hemorrhage is usually caused by a ruptured aneurysm. Approximately 20% of patients will have multiple aneurysms. Treatment of an aneurysm involves clipping or coiling the aneurysm to prevent rebleeding.

- Following aneurysmal occlusion via clipping or coiling, hyperdynamic therapy (hemodilution induced-hypertension using vasoconstricting agents such as phenylephrine or dopamine [Intropin] and hypervolemia) may be instituted in an effort to increase the mean arterial pressure and increase cerebral perfusion. Volume expansion is achieved via crystalloid or colloid solution.
- The calcium channel blocker nimodipine (Nimotop) is given to patients with subarachnoid hemorrhage to decrease the effects of vasospasm and minimize cerebral damage.
- Subarachnoid and intracerebral hemorrhage can involve bleeding into the ventricles of the brain. Insertion of a ventriculostomy for cerebrospinal fluid drainage can result in dramatic improvement in these situations.

Rehabilitation Care

After the stroke has stabilized for 12 to 24 hours, care shifts from preserving life to lessening disability and attaining optimal function. Depending on the patient's status, rehabilitation potential, and available resources, the patient may be transferred to a rehabilitation facility or unit. Other options for rehabilitation include outpatient therapy or home care–based rehabilitation.

Nutritional Therapy

The nutritional needs of the patient require quick assessment and treatment. The patient may initially receive IV infusions to maintain fluid and electrolyte balance, as well as for administration of drugs. Patients with severe impairment may require enteral or parenteral nutrition support. Depending on the severity of the stroke, individual assessment and planning for nutrition are necessary.

- To assess swallowing ability, elevate the head of the bed to an upright position (unless contraindicated) and give the patient a small amount of crushed ice or ice water to swallow.

S

If the gag reflex is present and the patient is able to swallow safely, you may proceed with feeding.

- Place food on the unaffected side of the mouth. Feedings must be followed by scrupulous oral hygiene because food may collect on the affected side of the mouth.

Nursing Management

Goals

The patient who has experienced a stroke will maintain a stable or improved level of consciousness, attain maximum physical functioning, maintain stable body functions (e.g., bladder control), maximize communication abilities, attain maximum self-care abilities and skills, maintain adequate nutrition, avoid complications of stroke, and maintain effective personal and family coping.

See NCP 58-1 for the patient with a stroke, Lewis et al., *Medical-Surgical Nursing,* ed. 8, pp. 1473 to 1476.

Nursing Diagnoses

- Decreased intracranial adaptive capacity
- Ineffective airway clearance
- Impaired physical mobility
- Impaired verbal communication
- Impaired physical mobility
- Impaired urinary elimination
- Unilateral neglect
- Impaired swallowing
- Situational low self-esteem

Nursing Interventions

Respiratory system. During the acute phase of a stroke the nursing priority is management of respiratory function.

- An oropharyngeal airway may be used in comatose patients to hold the tongue in place, prevent airway obstruction, and make suctioning accessible. Interventions include frequent assessment of airway patency and function, suctioning, patient mobility, positioning of the patient to prevent aspiration, and encouragement of deep breathing.

Neurologic system. Monitor the patient's neurologic status closely to detect changes suggesting extension of the stroke, increased ICP, vasospasm, or recovery from stroke symptoms.

- The primary clinical assessment tool to evaluate and document neurological status in acute stroke patients is the NIH Stroke Scale (NIHSS). The stroke scale can serve as a measure of stroke severity (see NIHHS in Table 58-8, Lewis et al., *Medical-Surgical Nursing,* ed. 8, p. 1472).

- A decreasing level of consciousness may indicate increasing ICP. Closely monitor vital signs.

Cardiovascular system. Nursing goals for the cardiovascular system are aimed at maintaining homeostasis.

- Interventions include (1) monitoring vital signs frequently; (2) monitoring cardiac rhythms; (3) calculating intake and output, noting imbalances; (4) regulating IV infusions; (5) adjusting fluid intake to the individual needs of the patient; (6) monitoring lung sounds for crackles and rhonchi indicating pulmonary congestion; and (7) monitoring heart sounds for murmurs or for S_3 or S_4 heart sounds.
- After a stroke the patient is at risk for deep vein thrombosis in the weak or paralyzed lower extremity. The most effective prevention is to keep the patient moving. Teach active range-of-motion (ROM) exercises if the patient has voluntary movement in the affected extremity. For the patient with hemiplegia, passive ROM exercises should be done several times each day.
- Other measures to prevent DVT include positioning to minimize the effects of dependent edema and the use of elastic compression gradient stockings.

Musculoskeletal system. The goal for the musculoskeletal system is to maintain optimal function, which is accomplished by prevention of joint contractures and muscle atrophy.

- In the acute phase, ROM exercises and positioning are important interventions. Passive ROM exercise is begun on the first day of hospitalization. Muscle atrophy secondary to lack of innervation and inactivity can develop within 1 month after stroke.
- The paralyzed or weak side needs special attention when the patient is positioned. Position each joint higher than the joint proximal to it. Specific deformities on the affected side of the patient with stroke are shoulder adduction; flexion contractures of the hand, wrist, and elbow; external rotation of the hip; and plantar flexion of the foot.

Integumentary system. The patient's skin is particularly susceptible to breakdown because of the loss of sensation, diminished circulation, and immobility.

- Prevention of skin breakdown includes pressure relief by position changes, special mattresses, or wheelchair cushions; good skin hygiene; emollients applied to dry skin; and early mobility.
- An example of a position change schedule is side-backside, with a maximum duration of 2 hours for any position.

- Position the patient on the weak or paralyzed side for only 30 minutes.

Gastrointestinal system. The most common bowel problem is constipation. Depending on the patient's fluid balance status and swallowing ability, fluid intake should include 1800 to 2000 mL/day and fiber intake up to 25 g/day. Physical activity also promotes bowel function.

Laxatives, suppositories, or additional stool softeners may be ordered if the patient does not respond to increased fluid and fiber.

Urinary system. In the acute stage of stroke, the primary urinary problem is poor bladder control, resulting in incontinence.

- Efforts should be made to promote normal bladder function and avoid the use of an indwelling catheter.
- Long-term use of an indwelling catheter is associated with urinary tract infections and delayed bladder retraining. An intermittent catheterization program may be used for patients with urinary retention.

Communication. During the acute stage the nurse's role in meeting the psychologic needs of the patient is primarily supportive.

- An alert patient is usually anxious because of a lack of understanding of what has happened and the inability to communicate. If the patient cannot understand words, gestures may be used to support verbal cues. It is helpful to speak slowly and calmly use relatively simple words.

Sensory-perceptual alterations. Homonymous hemianopsia (blindness in the same half of each visual field) is a common problem after a stroke.

- Initially, help the patient to compensate by arranging the environment within the patient's perceptual field, such as arranging the food tray so that all food is on the right side or the left side to accommodate for field of vision.
- Later, the patient is instructed to consciously attend to the neglected side. The weak or paralyzed extremities are carefully noted for adequacy of dressing, hygiene, and trauma.
- Visual problems may include diplopia, loss of the corneal reflex, and ptosis, particularly if the stroke is in the vertebrobasilar distribution. Diplopia is often treated with the use of an eye patch. If the corneal reflex is absent, the patient is at risk for a corneal abrasion and should be observed closely and protected against eye injuries.

Coping. A stroke is usually a sudden, extremely stressful event for the patient, close family members, and significant others.

- Reactions vary considerably but may involve fear, apprehension, denial of severity of the stroke, depression, anger, and sorrow.
- During the acute phase of caring for the patient and family, nursing interventions designed to facilitate coping involve providing information and emotional support.
- Explanations to the patient about what has happened and diagnostic and therapeutic procedures should be clear and understandable. It is particularly challenging to keep the aphasic patient adequately informed.
- Because family members usually have not had time to prepare for the illness, they may need assistance in arranging care for family members or pets and arranging transportation and finances.

Home care and rehabilitation. The patient is usually discharged from the acute care setting to home, an intermediate or long-term care facility, or a rehabilitation facility. You have an excellent opportunity to prepare the patient and family for hospital discharge through education, demonstration and return demonstration, practice, and evaluation of self-care skills before discharge. Total care is considered in discharge planning in relation to medications, nutrition, mobility, exercises, hygiene, and toileting.

Follow-up care is carefully planned to permit continuing nursing, physical, occupational, and speech therapy, as well as medical care.

Rehabilitation requires a team approach so patient and caregiver can benefit from the combined, expert care of an interdisciplinary team. The team must communicate and coordinate care to achieve the patient's goals. You are in a good position to facilitate this process and are often the key to successful rehabilitation efforts.

The rehabilitation nurse assesses the patient, caregiver, and family with attention to (1) rehabilitation potential of the patient, (2) physical status of all body systems, (3) presence of complications caused by the stroke or other chronic conditions, (4) cognitive status of the patient, (5) family resources and support, and (6) expectations of the patient and caregiver related to the rehabilitation program.

Rehabilitation and long-term management of the stroke patient are further described in Chapter 58 of Lewis et al., *Medical-Surgical Nursing,* ed. 8.

▼ **Patient and Caregiver Teaching**
- Provide the caregiver with instruction and practice in the necessary areas of home care while the patient is hospitalized. This allows for support and encouragement, as well as opportunities for feedback. Adjustments in the home environment, such as

the removal of a door to accommodate a wheelchair, can be made before discharge.

- Your instruction related to home care should include exercise and ambulation techniques; dietary requirements; recognition of signs indicating the possibility of another stroke (e.g., headache, vertigo, numbness, visual disturbances); understanding of emotional lability and the possibility of depression; medication routine; and time, place, and frequency of follow-up activities, such as occupational therapy and physical therapy.
- Assist the caregiver to stay healthy after the patient is discharged, emphasize the importance of planning for respite or time away from caregiving activities on a regular basis.

SYNDROME OF INAPPROPRIATE ANTIDIURETIC HORMONE

Description

The syndrome of inappropriate antidiuretic hormone (SIADH) occurs with an overproduction or oversecretion of antidiuretic hormone (ADH). The most common cause is malignancy, especially small cell lung cancer. SIADH occurs more frequently in older adults.

The disorder is characterized by fluid retention, serum hypoosmolality, dilutional hyponatremia, hypochloremia, concentrated urine in the presence of normal or increased vascular volume, and normal renal function.

Clinical Manifestations

Excess ADH increases renal tubular permeability and reabsorption of water into the circulation. Consequently, extracellular fluid volume expands, plasma osmolality declines, glomerular filtration rate (GFR) rises, and sodium (Na^+) levels decline. Initially, the patient displays thirst, dyspnea on exertion, and fatigue.

- The patient experiences low urinary output and weight gain.
- As serum sodium levels fall (usually <120 mEq/L [120 mmol/L]), manifestations become more severe and include vomiting, abdominal cramps, muscle twitching, and seizures.

As plasma osmolality and serum Na^+ levels continue to decline, cerebral edema may occur, leading to lethargy, anorexia, confusion, headache, seizures, and coma.

- Other effects of hyponatremia include muscle cramps and weakness.

Diagnostic Studies

- Simultaneous measurements of urine and serum osmolality can diagnose SIADH. Serum osmolality level much lower than urine osmolality level indicates inappropriate excretion of concentrated urine in the presence of dilute serum.

Nursing and Collaborative Management

Treatment is directed at the underlying cause. Medications that stimulate the release of ADH should be avoided or discontinued. In mild cases the only treatment may be restriction of fluids to 800 to 1000 mL/day. In cases of severe hyponatremia, intravenous hypertonic saline solution (3% to 5%) may be administered. A loop diuretic such as furosemide (Lasix) may be used to promote diuresis, but only if the serum sodium is at least 125 mEq/L (125 mmol/L) because it may cause further sodium loss. Because furosemide increases potassium, calcium, and magnesium losses, supplements may be needed. In severe hyponatremia, a fluid restriction of 500 mL/day is indicated.

In chronic symptomatic SIADH, demeclocycline (Declomycin) may be used. This drug blocks the effect of ADH on renal collecting tubules, thereby allowing a more dilute urine and retention of sodium.

- When SIADH is chronic, teach the patient to self-manage treatment regimens. Fluids are restricted to 800 to 1000 mL per day. Ice chips or sugarless chewing gum can help decrease thirst. Assist the patient to plan fluid intake so liquid allowances are saved for social occasions if desired.
- The patient may be treated with a diuretic to remove excess fluid volume. Teach the patient to supplement the diet with sodium and potassium, especially if diuretics are prescribed.
- Solutions of containing electrolytes must be well diluted to prevent gastrointestinal (GI) irritation or damage. They are best taken at mealtime to allow mixing with and dilution by food. Teach the patient the symptoms of fluid and electrolyte imbalances, especially those involving sodium and potassium, so that responses to treatment can be monitored

SYPHILIS

Description

Syphilis is a sexually transmitted disease (STD) in which many organs and tissues can become infected by *Treponema pallidum,* a spirochete. Since 2000 syphilis rates have increased each year. The increased rate is mainly due to men who have sex with men.

Pathophysiology

The organism *T. pallidum* is thought to enter the body through very small breaks in the skin or mucous membranes. The infection causes the production of antibodies that also react with normal tissues. Its entry is facilitated by the minor abrasions that often occur during intercourse. It is extremely fragile and is easily destroyed by drying, heating, or washing.

- Not all people who are exposed to syphilis acquire the disease; about one third become infected after intercourse with an infected person.
- In addition to sexual contact, syphilis may be spread through contact with infectious lesions and through the sharing of needles among intravenous (IV) drug users.
- Congenital syphilis is transmitted from an infected mother to the fetus in utero after the tenth week of pregnancy.
- The incubation period for syphilis ranges from 10 to 90 days.

There is an association between syphilis and human immunodeficiency virus (HIV) infection. Persons at increased risk for acquiring syphilis are also at increased risk for acquiring HIV. Often, both infections may be present in the same person. Therefore the evaluation of all patients with syphilis should include serologic testing for HIV with the patient's consent. Conversely HIV patients should be tested at least annually for syphilis.

Clinical Manifestations

Syphilis has a variety of signs and symptoms that can mimic a number of other diseases. Consequently, it is more difficult to recognize syphilis than other STDs. If it is not treated, specific clinical stages are characteristic of the disease progression.

- In the *primary stage, chancres* (painless indurated lesions found on the penis, vulva, and lips and in the mouth, vagina, and rectum) are seen at the site of bacterial invasion. The chancre lasts 10 to 90 days. During this time the draining of the microorganisms into the lymph nodes causes regional lymphadenopathy. Genital ulcers may also be present. Without treatment the infection progresses to the secondary stage.
- In the *secondary stage,* syphilis is systemic. During this stage blood-borne bacteria spread to all major organ systems. Manifestations characteristic of this stage include flulike symptoms and generalized adenopathy. Cutaneous lesions

include a bilateral, symmetric rash usually involving the trunk, palms, and soles; mucous patches in the mouth, tongue, or cervix; and condylomata lata (moist papules) in the anal and genital area.

- *Latent* syphilis follows the secondary stage and is a period during which the immune system is able to suppress the infection. There are no signs or symptoms of syphilis during this time.
- The *late or tertiary stage* of syphilis is the most severe, which appears 3 to 20 years after initial infection. Because antibiotics can cure syphilis, manifestations of late syphilis are rare. When late syphilis does occur, however, it is responsible for significant morbidity and mortality. *Gummas* (destructive skin, bone, and soft tissue lesions associated with late syphilis) are probably caused by a severe hypersensitivity reaction to the microorganism. Within the cardiovascular system late syphilis may cause aneurysms, heart valve insufficiency, and heart failure. Within the central nervous system the presence of *T. pallidum* in cerebrospinal fluid (CSF) may cause manifestations of neurosyphilis.

Complications

Complications occur in late syphilis. The gummas of late syphilis may produce irreparable damage to bone, liver, or skin.

- In cardiovascular syphilis, the resulting aneurysm may press on structures such as the intercostal nerves, causing pain. Scarring of the aortic valve results in aortic valve insufficiency and eventually heart failure.
- Neurosyphilis is responsible for degeneration of the brain with mental deterioration. Problems related to sensory nerve involvement are a result of *tabes dorsalis* (progressive locomotor ataxia). There may be sudden attacks of pain anywhere in the body. Loss of vision and position sense in the feet and legs can also occur. Walking may become even more difficult as joint stability is lost.

Diagnostic Studies

- Detailed and accurate sexual history
- Darkfield microscopy and direct fluorescent antibody tests of lesion exudate or tissue can confirm the diagnosis.
- To screen for syphilis, Venereal Disease Research Laboratory (VDRL) and rapid plasma reagin (RPR) testing can detect nonspecific antitreponemal antibodies, usually positive 10 to 14 days after chancre appearance.

- To confirm a diagnosis of syphilis, the fluorescent treponemal antibody absorption (FTA-ABS) test and the *T. pallidum* particle agglutination (TP-PA) test can detect specific antitreponemal antibodies.

Collaborative Care

Management is aimed at the eradication of all syphilitic organisms. However, treatment cannot reverse damage that is already present in the late stage of the disease.

- Penicillin G benzathine (Bicillin) or aqueous penicillin G procaine remains the treatment of choice for all stages of syphilis. eTable 53-1 at http://evolve.elsevier.com/Lewis/ medsurg describes drug therapy for the various stages of syphilis from the Centers for Disease Control and Prevention STD guidelines.
- Patients having persistent or recurring symptoms after drug therapy has ended should be re-treated.
- It is important that all sexual contacts in the last 90 days be treated.
- Patients with neurosyphilis must be carefully monitored with periodic serologic testing, clinical evaluation at 6-month intervals, and repeat CSF examinations for at least 3 years.

Nursing Management: Syphilis

See Nursing Management: Sexually Transmitted Diseases, p. 570.

SYSTEMIC INFLAMMATORY RESPONSE SYNDROME (SIRS) AND MULTIPLE ORGAN DYSFUNCTION SYNDROME (MODS)

Description

Systemic inflammatory response syndrome (SIRS) is a systemic inflammatory response to a variety of insults, including infection (referred to as sepsis), ischemia, infarction, and injury. Generalized inflammation in organs remote from the initial insult characterizes SIRS. Many mechanisms can trigger a systemic inflammatory response, including:

- Mechanical tissue trauma: burns, crush injuries, surgical procedures
- Abscess formation: intraabdominal, extremities

- Ischemic or necrotic tissue: pancreatitis, vascular disease, myocardial infarction
- Microbial invasion: bacteria, viruses, fungi, parasites
- Endotoxin release: gram-negative and -positive bacteria
- Global perfusion deficits: post-cardiac resuscitation, shock states
- Regional perfusion deficits: distal perfusion deficits

Multiple organ dysfunction syndrome (MODS) is failure of two or more organ systems in an acutely ill patient such that homeostasis cannot be maintained without intervention. MODS results from SIRS, but the transition from SIRS to MODS does not occur in a clear-cut manner.

- Prognosis for the patient with MODS is poor, with estimated mortality rates at 70% to 80% when three or more organ systems fail.

Pathophysiology and Clinical Manifestations

When the inflammatory response is not controlled, consequences occur. These include activation of inflammatory cells and release of mediators, direct damage to the endothelium, and hypermetabolism.

- Vasodilation becomes excessive and leads to decreased systemic vascular resistance (SVR) and hypotension.
- An increase in vascular permeability allows mediators and protein to leak out of the endothelium and into the interstitial space.
- WBCs phagocytize the foreign debris, and the coagulation cascade is activated.
- Hypotension, decreased perfusion, microemboli, and redistributed or shunted blood flow eventually compromise organ perfusion.

The respiratory system is often the first system to show signs of dysfunction in SIRS and MODS. Inflammatory mediators have a direct effect on the pulmonary vasculature. Endothelial damage from the release of inflammatory mediators results in increased capillary permeability. Fluid then moves to the alveoli, causing alveolar edema. The alveoli collapse and the end result is acute respiratory distress syndrome (ARDS, see p. 13).

Cardiovascular changes include myocardial depression and massive vasodilation in response to increasing tissue demands. To compensate for hypotension, heart rate and stroke volume increase, but increased capillary permeability diminishes venous return and thus preload. Eventually, either perfusion of vital organs becomes insufficient or the cells are unable to use oxygen and their function is further compromised.

Neurologic dysfunction commonly manifests as mental status changes, and mental status changes can be an early sign of SIRS or MODS. Confusion, agitation, disorientation, lethargy, or coma may occur. Mental changes may be caused by hypoxemia, the direct effect of inflammatory mediators, or impaired perfusion.

Acute kidney injury (AKI) (also called acute renal failure [ARF]) is frequently seen in SIRS and MODS. Hypoperfusion and the effects of the mediators can cause ARF. An additional risk for ARF in this patient is the use of nephrotoxic antibiotics to treat gram-negative bacteremia.

In the early stages of SIRS and MODS, blood is shunted away from the gastrointestinal (GI) mucosa, making it highly vulnerable to ischemic injury. Decreased perfusion leads to a breakdown of the mucosal barrier, thereby increasing the risk for ulceration and GI bleeding.

- Breakdown of the mucosal barrier of the gut also results in the potential for bacterial movement from the GI tract into the circulation.
- GI motility often decreases in critical illness, causing abdominal distention and paralytic ileus.
- Metabolic changes are pronounced in SIRS and MODS. Both syndromes trigger a hypermetabolic response. The net result is a catabolic state, and lean body mass (muscle) is lost.
- The hypermetabolism may last for days and results in liver dysfunction.
- The liver is unable to synthesize albumin that is necessary to maintain plasma oncotic pressure, adding to the loss of intravascular fluid to the interstitial space.
- As the state of hypermetabolism persists, the patient is unable to convert lactate to glucose, and lactate accumulates (lactic acidosis). Eventually the liver is unable to maintain a glucose level and the patient becomes hypoglycemic.

Electrolyte imbalances are common and result from hormonal and metabolic changes and fluid shifts. These changes exacerbate mental status changes, neuromuscular dysfunction, and dysrhythmias.

- Release of antidiuretic hormone and aldosterone results in sodium and water retention; aldosterone increases urinary potassium loss, and catecholamines cause potassium to move into the cells, resulting in hypokalemia.
- Metabolic acidosis results from impaired tissue perfusion, hypoxia, a shift to anaerobic metabolism, and progressive renal dysfunction.

- Hypocalcemia, hypomagnesemia, and hypophosphatemia are common.

The clinical manifestations of MODS are presented in Tables 67-5 and 67-11, Lewis et al., *Medical-Surgical Nursing,* ed. 8, p. 1723 and pp. 1740 to 1741.

Nursing and Collaborative Management: SIRS and MODS

The most important goal in the management of SIRS and MODS is to prevent the progression of SIRS to MODS. A critical component of the nursing role is vigilant assessment and ongoing monitoring to detect early signs of deterioration or organ dysfunction.

Collaborative care of patients with MODS focuses on prevention and treatment of infection, maintenance of tissue oxygenation, nutritional and metabolic support, and appropriate support for individual failing organs.

- Aggressive infection control is essential to decrease the risk for hospital-acquired infections. Early, aggressive surgery is recommended to remove necrotic tissue (e.g., early debridement of burn tissue) that may provide a culture medium for microorganisms. Aggressive pulmonary management, including early ambulation, can reduce the risk of infection. Strict asepsis can decrease infectious related to intraarterial lines, endotracheal tubes, urinary catheters, IV lines, and other invasive devices or procedures.
- Hypoxemia frequently occurs in patients with SIRS or MODS. Interventions to decrease oxygen demand and increase oxygen delivery are essential. Sedation, mechanical ventilation, analgesia, and rest may decrease oxygen demand and should be considered.
- Hypermetabolism in SIRS or MODS can result in profound weight loss, cachexia, and further organ failure. Nutritional support is vital to preserve organ function. Providing early and adequate nutrition decreases morbidity and mortality. The use of the enteral route is preferred to parenteral nutrition.

Support of any failing organ is a primary goal of therapy. For example, the patient with ARDS requires aggressive oxygen therapy and mechanical ventilation. Renal failure may require dialysis or continuous renal replacement therapy.

SYSTEMIC LUPUS ERYTHEMATOSUS

Description

Systemic lupus erythematosus (SLE) is a multisystem inflammatory autoimmune disease. It typically affects the skin; joints; serous membranes (pleura, pericardium); and renal, hematologic, and neurologic systems. SLE is characterized by variability within and among persons, and its chronic unpredictable course is marked by alternating periods of exacerbations and remissions. Women are 10 times more likely to develop SLE than men, and it is observed more often in African Americans, Asian Americans, and Native Americans than in whites.

Pathophysiology

The etiology of SLE is unknown, but it is thought to result from interactions among genetic, hormonal, environmental, and immunologic factors. Multiple susceptibility genes from the HLA complex show associations with SLE, including HLA-DR3.

- Hormones are also known to play a role in the etiology of SLE. Onset or exacerbation of disease symptoms sometimes occurs after the onset of menarche, with the use of oral contraceptives, and during and after pregnancy. The disease tends to worsen in the immediate postpartum period.
- Environmental factors believed to contribute to the occurrence of SLE include sun exposure and sunburns and exposure to infectious agents and certain drugs such as procainamide (Pronestyl), hydralazine (Apresoline), and a number of antiseizure drugs.

SLE is characterized by the production of a large variety of autoantibodies against nucleic acids (e.g., single- and double-stranded deoxyribonucleic acid [DNA]), erythrocytes, coagulation proteins, lymphocytes, platelets, and many other self-proteins. Most characteristically the autoimmune reactions are directed against constituents of the cell nucleus (antinuclear antibodies [ANA]), particularly DNA. Circulating immune complexes containing antibody against DNA are deposited in the basement membranes of capillaries in the kidneys, heart, skin, brain, and joints. The overaggressive antibody response is also related to B- and T-cell hyperactivity. Specific manifestations of SLE depend on which cell types or organs are involved.

Clinical Manifestations and Complications

No characteristic pattern occurs in the progressive organ involvement. General complaints, including fever, weight loss, arthralgia, and excessive fatigue, may precede an exacerbation of disease activity.

Dermatologic manifestations. Cutaneous vascular lesions can appear in any location but are most likely to develop in sun-exposed areas. Severe skin reactions can occur in persons who are photosensitive. The classic butterfly rash over the cheeks and bridge of the nose occurs in 50% of patients with SLE.

- Ulcers of the oral or nasopharyngeal membranes can occur. Transient diffuse or patchy hair loss (alopecia) is common. The scalp becomes dry, scaly, and atrophied.

Musculoskeletal problems. Polyarthralgia with morning stiffness is often the patient's first complaint and may precede the onset of multisystem disease by many years. Arthritis occurs in 90% of all patients with SLE. Diffuse swelling is accompanied by joint and muscle pain.

- Lupus-related arthritis is generally nonerosive, but it may cause deformities such as swan neck, ulnar deviation, and subluxation with hyperlaxity of the joints.

Cardiopulmonary problems. Tachypnea and cough in patients with SLE are suggestive of restrictive lung disease. Cardiac involvement may include dysrhythmias resulting from fibrosis of the sinoatrial (SA) and atrioventricular (AV) nodes. This occurrence is an ominous sign of advanced disease.

- Clinical factors such as hypertension and hypercholesterolemia require aggressive therapy and careful monitoring.

Renal problems. Lupus nephritis (LN) occurs in about 50% of patients with SLE. Manifestations of renal involvement vary from mild proteinuria to rapid, progressive glomerulonephritis. Treatment typically includes corticosteroids, cytotoxic agents (cyclophosphamide [Cytoxan]), and immunosuppressive agents (azathioprine [Imuran], and cyclosporine. Mycophenolate mofetil [CellCept]) may be more effective and less toxic than cyclophosphamide, which has been the standard of treatment.

Nervous system problems. Centralized or focal seizures are the most common neurologic manifestation. They are generally controlled by corticosteroids or antiseizure drug therapy.

- Cognitive dysfunction may result from the deposition of immune complexes within the brain tissue. It is characterized by disordered thought processes, disorientation, memory deficits, and psychiatric symptoms, such as severe depression and psychosis. Occasionally a stroke or aseptic meningitis may be attributable to SLE. Headaches are common and can become severe during a flare (exacerbation).

Hematologic problems. The formation of antibodies against blood cells such as erythrocytes, leukocytes, thrombocytes, and coagulation factors is a common feature. Anemia, mild leukopenia, and thrombocytopenia are often present. Some patients develop a tendency toward coagulopathy involving either excessive bleeding or blood clot development.

Infection. Patients appear to have increased susceptibility to infections, possibly related to defects in their ability to phagocytize invading bacteria, deficiencies in the production of antibodies, and the immunosuppressive effect of many antiinflammatory drugs. Infection is a major cause of death, with pneumonia being the most common infection.

Diagnostic Studies

The diagnosis is based on the history, physical examination, and laboratory findings.

- SLE is characterized by the presence of ANA, which establishes the existence of an autoimmune disease. Other antibodies include anti-DNA, antineuronal, anticoagulant, anti-white blood cell (WBC), anti-red blood cell (RBC), antiplatelet, antiphospholipid, and antibasement membrane. The antibody tests that are the most specific for SLE include the anti–double-stranded DNA and the anti-Smith (Sm).
- Lupus erythematosus (LE) cell prep test is nonspecific for SLE and is positive in other rheumatic diseases.
- Erythrocyte sedimentation rate (ESR) and C-reactive protein (CRP) levels are not diagnostic of SLE but may be used to monitor disease activity.

Collaborative Care

A major challenge in SLE treatment is to manage the active phase of the disease while preventing complications of treatments that cause long-term tissue damage.

Drug Therapy

Nonsteroidal antiinflammatory drugs (NSAIDs) continue to be an important intervention, especially for patients with mild polyarthralgia or polyarthritis. Antimalarial agents such as hydroxychloroquine (Plaquenil) are also often used to treat fatigue and moderate skin and joint problems, as well as prevent flares.

Corticosteroid exposure should be limited, but tapering doses of intravenous (IV) methylprednisolone may be useful in controlling severe exacerbations of polyarthritis. Steroid-sparing immunosuppressants such as methotrexate can serve as an alternate treatment. Immunosuppressive drugs such as azathioprine (Imuran) and cyclophosphamide (Cytoxan) may be prescribed to reduce the need for long-term corticosteroid therapy or treat severe organ-system disease, such as lupus nephritis.

Nursing Management

Goals

The patient with SLE will have satisfactory pain relief, adhere to the therapeutic regimen to achieve maximum symptom management, demonstrate awareness of and avoid activities that induce disease exacerbation, and maintain optimal role function and a positive self-image.

See NCP 65-2 for the patient with systemic lupus erythematosus, Lewis et al., *Medical-Surgical Nursing,* ed. 8, pp. 1669 to 1670.

Nursing Diagnoses

- Fatigue
- Acute pain
- Impaired skin integrity
- Deficient knowledge

Nursing Interventions

Prevention of SLE is not possible at this time. The education of health professionals and the community should promote a clear understanding of the disease and earlier diagnosis and treatment.

During an exacerbation, patients may become abruptly and dramatically ill. Nursing interventions include accurately recording the severity of symptoms and documenting response to therapy. Specifically assess fever pattern, joint inflammation, limitation of motion, location and degree of discomfort, and fatigability.

- Monitor the patient's weight and fluid intake and output if corticosteroids are prescribed because of the fluid-retention effect of these drugs and the possibility of renal failure. Careful collection of 24-hour urine for protein and creatinine clearance may be ordered.
- Observe for signs of bleeding that result from drug therapy, such as pallor, skin bruising, petechiae, or tarry stools.
- Careful assessment of neurologic status includes observation for visual disturbances, headaches, personality changes, and forgetfulness. Psychosis may indicate central nervous system disease or may be the effect of corticosteroid therapy. Irritation of the nerves of the extremities (peripheral neuropathy) may produce numbness, tingling, and weakness of the hands and feet.
- Explain the nature of the disease, modes of therapy, and all diagnostic procedures. Emotional support for the patient and family is essential.

▼ **Patient and Caregiver Teaching**

The patient with SLE confronts many psychosocial issues. Emphasize health teaching and the importance of patient cooperation for successful home management. Help the patient understand that even strong adherence to the treatment plan is not a guarantee against exacerbation, because the course of the disease is unpredictable. However, a variety of factors may increase disease activity, such as fatigue, sun exposure, emotional stress, infection, drugs, and surgery. Also assist the patient and caregiver to eliminate or minimize exposure to precipitating factors. Patient and caregiver education is outlined in Table 83. Counsel the patient and caregiver that SLE has a good prognosis for the majority of persons.

- Many couples require pregnancy and sexual counseling. For the best outcome, pregnancy should be planned at a point when the disease activity is minimal.
- Pain and fatigue are cited most frequently as interfering with quality of life. Friends and relatives are confused by the patient's complaints of transient joint pain and overwhelming fatigue. Pacing techniques and relaxation therapy can help the patient remain involved in day-to-day activities.

Table 83	Patient and Caregiver Teaching Guide: Systemic Lupus Erythematosus

You should include the following information in the teaching plan for a patient with systemic lupus erythematosus and the caregiver:

Teaching related to the disease and appropriate management should include:

1. Disease process
2. Names of drugs, actions, side effects, dosage, administration
3. Pain management strategies
4. Energy conservation and pacing techniques
5. Therapeutic exercise, use of heat therapy (for arthralgia)
6. Avoidance of physical and emotional stress
7. Avoidance of exposure to individuals with infection
8. Avoidance of drying soaps, powders, household chemicals
9. Use of sunscreen protection (at least SPF 15) and protective clothing, with minimal sun exposure from 11:00 AM to 3:00 PM
10. Regular medical and laboratory follow-up
11. Marital and pregnancy counseling as needed
12. Community resources and health care agencies

SPF, Sun protection factor.

SYSTEMIC SCLEROSIS (SCLERODERMA)

Description

Systemic sclerosis (SS), or *scleroderma*, is a disorder of the connective tissue characterized by fibrotic, degenerative, and occasionally inflammatory changes in the skin, blood vessels, synovium, skeletal muscle, and internal organs. Two types of SS exist; one is the more common *limited cutaneous disease* (80%), and the second is *diffuse cutaneous disease*. Both forms are systemic with the degree and type of organ involvement and disease progression very different.

Although symptoms may begin at any time, the usual age at onset is between 30 and 50 years, with 75% of patients being women.

Pathophysiology

The exact cause of SS remains unknown. Collagen is overproduced and disrupts the normal functioning of organs such as the lungs, kidney, heart, and gastrointestinal (GI) tract. Disruption of the cell is followed by platelet aggregation and fibrosis. Immunologic dysfunction and vascular abnormalities are believed to play a role in the development of widespread systemic disease. Other risk factors include environmental occupational exposure to coal, plastics, and silica dust.

Clinical Manifestations

Manifestations range from a diffuse cutaneous thickening with rapidly progressive and widespread organ involvement to the more benign variant of limited cutaneous SS. The signs of limited disease appear on the face and hands, whereas diffuse disease initially involves the trunk and extremities. Clinical manifestations can be described by the acronym *CREST:* **C**alcinosis (painful calcium deposits in skin), **R**aynaud's phenomenon, **E**sophageal dysfunction (difficulty swallowing), **S**clerodactyly (tightening of the skin on the fingers), and **T**elangiectasia (red spots on the hands, face, and lips).

Raynaud's phenomenon (paroxysmal vasospasm of the digits) is the most common initial complaint in limited systemic sclerosis. Raynaud's phenomenon may precede the onset of systemic disease by months, years, or even decades (see Raynaud's Phenomenon, p. 539).

Symmetric painless swelling or thickening of the skin of the fingers and hands may progress to diffuse scleroderma of the trunk. In limited disease, skin thickening generally does not extend above the elbow or above the knee, although the face can be affected in some individuals. In more diffuse disease the skin loses elasticity and becomes taut and shiny, producing the typical expressionless facies with tightly pursed lips.

About 20% of people with systemic sclerosis develop secondary Sjögren's syndrome, a condition associated with dry eyes and dry mouth. Dysphagia, gum disease, and dental caries can result. Frequent reflux of gastric acid also can occur as a result of esophageal fibrosis.

Lung involvement includes pleural thickening, pulmonary fibrosis, pulmonary artery hypertension, and pulmonary function abnormalities.

Primary heart disease consists of pericarditis, pericardial effusion, and cardiac dysrhythmias. Myocardial fibrosis resulting in heart failure occurs most frequently in persons with diffuse SS.

Renal disease was previously a major cause of death in diffuse SS. Recent improvements in dialysis, bilateral nephrectomy in patients with uncontrollable hypertension, and kidney transplantation have offered some hope to patients with renal failure. In particular, use of angiotensin-converting enzyme (ACE) inhibitors (e.g., lisinopril [Prinivil]) has had marked impact on the ability to treat renal disease.

Diagnostic Studies

- Blood studies may reveal mild hemolytic anemia.
- Scleroderma antibody SCL-70 may be found in patients with diffuse disease. Anticentromere antibody is seen in many patients with CREST.
- If renal involvement is present, urinalysis may show proteinuria, microscopic hematuria, and casts.
- X-ray evidence of subcutaneous calcification, distal esophageal hypomotility, and/or bilateral pulmonary fibrosis is diagnostic of SS.
- Pulmonary function studies reveal decreased vital capacity and lung compliance.

Collaborative Care

Management of SS offers no specific treatment with long-term effects. Care is directed toward attempts to prevent or treat the secondary complications of involved organs.

Physical therapy helps maintain joint mobility and preserve muscle strength. Occupational therapy assists the patient in maintaining functional abilities. Gastroesophageal reflux may be treated by antacids and periodic dilation of the esophagus.

Drug Therapy

No specific drugs or combinations of drugs have shown to be effective. Vasoactive agents are often prescribed in early disease to manage Raynaud's phenomenon. Calcium channel blockers (nifedipine [Adalat, Procardia], diltiazem [Cardizem]) are a common treatment choice. Other vasoactive drugs include reserpine (Serpasil) and losartan (Cozaar). Tracleer (Bosentan), an endothelin receptor antagonist, and epoprostenol (Flolan), a vasodilator, may assist in preventing and treating digital ulcers while improving exercise capacity and heart and lung dynamics.

Topical agents may provide some relief from joint pain. Capsaicin cream may be useful not only as a local analgesic but also as a vasodilator. Other therapies are prescribed to address specific systemic problems, such as tetracycline for diarrhea resulting from bacterial overgrowth, and histamine H_2-receptor blockers (e.g., cimetidine [Tagamet]) and proton pump inhibitors (e.g., omeprazole [Prilosec]) for esophageal symptoms. An antihypertensive agent (e.g., captopril [Capoten], propranolol [Inderal], methyldopa [Aldomet]) may be used to treat hypertension with renal involvement, and a chemotherapeutic agent (e.g., cyclophosphamide [Cytoxan]) may be used for lung disease.

Nursing Management

Because prevention is not possible, nursing interventions often begin during hospitalization for diagnostic purposes. Emotional stress and cold ambient temperatures may aggravate Raynaud's phenomenon. Patients with SS should not have finger stick blood testing done because of compromised circulation and poor healing of the fingers. Help the patient to resolve feelings of helplessness by providing information about the illness and encouraging active participation in planning care.

- Hands and feet should be protected from cold exposure and possible burns or cuts that might heal slowly. Smoking should be avoided because of its vasoconstricting effect. Lotions may help to alleviate skin dryness and cracking but must be rubbed in for an unusually long time because of skin thickness.
- Dysphagia may be reduced by eating small, frequent meals, chewing carefully and slowly, and drinking fluids. Heartburn may be minimized by using antacids 45 to 60 minutes after each meal and by sitting upright for at least 2 hours after eating.
- Job modifications are often necessary because stair climbing, typing, writing, and cold exposure may pose particular problems.

- Some people need to wear gloves to protect fingertip ulcers and provide extra warmth. Sensitive areas on the fingertips resulting from ulcers may require padded utensils or special assistive devices to reduce discomfort.
- Daily oral hygiene must be emphasized, or neglect may lead to increased tooth and gingival problems.
- Biofeedback training and relaxation techniques may be used to reduce tension and improve sleeping habits.

The patient must actively carry out therapeutic exercises at home. Reinforce the use of moist heat applications, the use of assistive devices, and the organization of activities to preserve strength and reduce disability. Sexual dysfunction resulting from body changes, pain, muscular weakness, limited mobility, decreased self-esteem, and decreased vaginal secretions may require sensitive counseling by the nurse.

TESTICULAR CANCER

Description
Testicular cancer is rare, but it is the most common type of cancer in young men between 15 and 34 years of age. Testicular tumors are more common in men who have had undescended testicles (cryptorchidism) or a family history of testicular cancer or anomalies.

- Other predisposing factors include orchitis, human immunodeficiency virus (HIV) infection, maternal exposure to diethylstilbestrol (DES), and testicular cancer in the contralateral testis.
- Most testicular cancers develop from embryonic germ cells and include seminomas and nonseminomas.

Clinical Manifestations
Testicular cancer may have a slow or rapid onset depending on the tumor.

- The patient may notice a painless lump in his scrotum, as well as scrotal swelling and a feeling of heaviness. The scrotal mass is usually nontender and very firm.
- Some patients complain of a dull ache or heavy sensation in the lower abdomen, perianal area, or scrotum.
- Manifestations associated with metastasis include back pain, cough, dyspnea, hemoptysis, dysphagia, alterations in vision or mental status, and seizures.

Diagnostic Studies

- Palpation of the scrotal contents is the first step
- Ultrasound of the testes
- Blood serum levels of α-fetoprotein (AFP), lactate dehydrogenase (LDH), and human chorionic gonadotropin (hCG) if testicular cancer is suspected.
- Chest x-ray and computed tomography (CT) scan of the abdomen and pelvis are done to detect metastasis.

Nursing and Collaborative Management

As with many forms of cancer, the patient's survival is closely associated with early tumor recognition. The scrotum is easily examined, and beginning tumors are usually palpable. Teach and encourage every man to perform a monthly testicular self-examination for the purpose of detecting testicular tumors or other scrotal abnormalities such as varicoceles. (See Table 55-9 and Fig. 55-10 for scrotum self-examination guidelines, Lewis et al., *Medical-Surgical Nursing*, ed. 8, p. 1397.)

- The man may indicate some reluctance to examine his own genitals, but with encouragement he can learn this simple procedure. He should be encouraged to do self-examinations frequently until he is comfortable with the procedure. The scrotum should be examined once each month.

Collaborative management generally involves an orchiectomy or a radical orchiectomy (surgical removal of the affected testis, spermatic cord, and regional lymph nodes). Retroperitoneal lymph node dissection and removal are also done to manage the disease in early stages.

- Postorchiectomy treatment involves surveillance, radiation therapy, or chemotherapy, depending on the stage of the cancer. Chemotherapy protocols use combination therapy of various agents including bleomycin (Blenoxane), etoposide (VePesid), ifosfamide (Ifex), and cisplatin (Platinol).

The prognosis for patients with testicular cancer has improved, and 95% of all patients obtain complete remission if the disease is detected in the early stages. All patients with testicular cancer, regardless of pathology or stage, require meticulous follow-up monitoring and regular physical examinations, chest x-ray, CT scan, and assessment of hCG and AFP. The goal is to detect relapse when tumor burden is minimal.

- Because of the high risk for infertility, the cryopreservation of sperm in a sperm bank before treatment begins should be discussed and recommended for the man with testicular cancer.

TETANUS

Description

Tetanus (lockjaw) is an extremely severe polyradiculitis and poly-neuritis affecting spinal and cranial nerves. It results from the effects of a potent neurotoxin released by the anaerobic bacillus *Clostridium tetani*. The toxin interferes with the function of the reflex arc by blocking inhibitory transmitters at the presynaptic sites in the spinal cord and brainstem. The spores of the bacillus are present in soil, garden mold, and manure. Worldwide, the number of cases per year is estimated to be 1 million. In the United States the number of individuals under the age of 40 years with tetanus is increasing, most likely related to intravenous (IV) drug use.

Pathophysiology

C. tetani enters the body through a traumatic or suppurative wound, which provides an appropriate low-oxygen environment for the organisms to mature and produce toxin. Other possible sources include dental infection, chronic otitis media, injections of heroin, human and animal bites, frostbite, open fractures, and gunshot wounds.

- Incubation period is usually 7 days but can range from 3 to 21 days, with symptoms frequently appearing after the original wound is healed. In general, the longer the incubation period, the milder the illness and the better the prognosis.

Clinical Manifestations

Initial manifestations of generalized tetanus include a feeling of stiffness in the jaw *(trismus)* or neck, a slight fever, and other symptoms of general infection. Generalized tonic spasms occur because of the lack of reciprocal innervation.

- As the disease progresses, the neck muscles, back, abdomen, and extremities become progressively rigid. In severe forms, continuous tonic convulsions may occur with *opisthotonos* (extreme arching of the back and retraction of the head). Laryngeal and respiratory spasms cause apnea and anoxia.

Additional effects are manifested by overstimulation of the sympathetic nervous system; these include profuse diaphoresis, labile hypertension, episodic tachycardia, hyperthermia, and dysrhythmias. The slightest noise, jarring motion, or bright light can set off a seizure. These seizures are agonizingly painful. Mortality is almost 100% in the severe form.

Nursing and Collaborative Management

Health teaching is aimed at ensuring tetanus prophylaxis, which is the most important factor influencing the incidence of this disease. Adults should receive a tetanus and diphtheria toxoid booster every 10 years.

- Teach the patient that immediate, thorough cleansing of all wounds with soap and water is important in prevention.
- If an open wound occurs and the patient has not been immunized within 5 years, the health care provider should be contacted so that a tetanus booster can be given.

Management includes administration of tetanus and diphtheria toxoid booster (Td) and tetanus immune globulin (TIG) in different sites before the onset of symptoms to neutralize circulating toxins. A much larger dose of TIG is given to patients with manifestations of clinical tetanus.

- Control of spasms is essential and is managed by deep sedation, usually with diazepam (Valium), barbiturates, and, in severe cases, neuromuscular blocking agents such as vecuronium that act to paralyze skeletal muscles.
- A 10- to 14-day course of penicillin, tetracycline, or doxycycline is recommended to inhibit further growth of *C. tetani*.
- Because of laryngospasm and potential need for neuromuscular blocking drugs, a tracheostomy is usually performed early and the patient is maintained on mechanical ventilation. Sedative agents and opioid analgesics are given concomitantly to all patients who are pharmacologically paralyzed. Any recognized wound should be debrided or an abscess drained. Antibiotics may be given to prevent secondary infections.

THALASSEMIA

Description

Thalassemia is a disease of decreased erythrocyte (red blood cell [RBC]) production resulting from an inadequate production of normal hemoglobin (Hb). Hemolysis also occurs in thalassemia.

- In contrast to iron deficiency anemia, in which heme synthesis is the problem, thalassemia involves a problem with the globin protein. Therefore the basic defect of thalassemia is abnormal Hb synthesis.

Pathophysiology

Thalassemias are a group of autosomal recessive genetic disorders commonly found in members of ethnic groups whose origins are near the Mediterranean Sea or equatorial regions of Asia, the Middle East, and Africa. An individual with thalassemia may have a heterozygous or homozygous form of the disease.

- A person who is heterozygous has one thalassemic gene and one normal gene. He or she is said to have *thalassemia minor* or *thalassemic trait,* which is a mild form of the disease.
- A homozygous person has two thalassemic genes, causing a severe condition known as *thalassemia major.*

Clinical Manifestations

- The patient with thalassemia minor is frequently asymptomatic, with mild to moderate anemia with microcytosis (small cells) and hypochromia (pale cells).
- The patient who has thalassemia major is pale and displays other general symptoms of anemia (see Anemia, p. 29). In addition, the person has marked splenomegaly, hepatomegaly, and jaundice from RBC hemolysis. Chronic bone marrow hyperplasia leads to expansion of the marrow space. This may cause thickening of the cranium and maxillary cavity.
- Thalassemia major is a life-threatening disease in which growth, both physical and mental, is often retarded.

Collaborative Care

The laboratory findings in thalassemia major are summarized in Table 9, p. 32.

- Thalassemia minor requires no treatment because the body adapts to the reduction of normal Hb.
- Symptoms of thalassemia major are managed with blood transfusions or exchange transfusions in conjunction with oral deferasirox (Exjade) or IV or subcutaneous deferoxamine (Desferal) (chelating agents that bind to iron) to reduce the iron overloading (hemochromatosis) that occurs with chronic transfusion therapy. Because RBCs are sequestered in the enlarged spleen, thalassemia may be treated by splenectomy.
- Although hematopoietic stem cell transplantation remains the only cure for patients with thalassemia, the risk of this procedure may outweigh its benefits.

THROMBOANGIITIS OBLITERANS (BUERGER'S DISEASE)

Thromboangiitis obliterans (Buerger's disease) is a nonatherosclerotic, segmental, recurrent inflammatory vasoocclusive disorder of the small- to medium-sized arteries and veins of the upper and lower extremities. The disorder occurs predominantly in young men (<40 years of age) with a long history of tobacco use, but without other CVD risk factors (e.g., hypertension, hyperlipidemia, diabetes mellitus).

- In Buerger's disease, an inflammatory process damages the blood vessel wall. Lymphocytes and giant cells infiltrate the vessel wall, accompanied by fibroblast proliferation. Ultimately, thrombosis and fibrosis occur in the vessel, causing tissue ischemia.
- The symptom complex of Buerger's disease is often confused with that of peripheral artery disease and other inflammatory or autoimmune diseases (e.g., scleroderma).
- Patients may have intermittent claudication of the feet, hands, or arms. As the disease progresses, pain while at rest and ischemic ulcerations develop.
- Signs and symptoms also can include color and temperature changes of the limbs, paresthesia, superficial vein thrombosis, and cold sensitivity.

There are no laboratory or diagnostic tests specific to Buerger's disease. Diagnosis is based on age of onset, history of tobacco use, clinical symptoms, involvement of distal vessels, presence of ischemic ulcerations, and exclusion of disorders, including diabetes mellitus, autoimmune disease, thrombophilia, and proximal source of emboli.

Treatment includes a complete cessation of tobacco use in any form. Conservative management includes the use of antibiotics to treat any infected ulcers and analgesics to manage the ischemic pain. Patients must avoid trauma to the extremities.

Painful ulcerations may require finger or toe amputations. Amputation below the knee may occur in severe cases. The amputation rate of patients who continue tobacco use is almost 3 times greater than for those who do not.

THROMBOCYTOPENIC PURPURA

Description

Immune thrombocytopenic purpura (ITP), the most common acquired thrombocytopenia, is a syndrome of abnormal destruction of circulating platelets. ITP is an autoimmune disease.

- In ITP, platelets are coated with antibodies. Although these platelets function normally, when they reach the spleen the antibody-coated platelets are recognized as foreign and destroyed by macrophages. Platelets normally survive 8 to 10 days, but in ITP survival is shortened.

- Chronic ITP occurs most commonly in women between 20 and 40 years old. Chronic ITP has a gradual onset, and transient remissions occur.

Thrombotic thrombocytopenic purpura (TTP) is an uncommon syndrome characterized by hemolytic anemia, thrombocytopenia, neurologic abnormalities, fever (in the absence of infection), and renal abnormalities. TTP is almost always associated with hemolytic-uremic syndrome (HUS).

- The disease is characterized by the enhanced agglutination of platelets, which form microthrombi that deposit in arterioles and capillaries.

- In most cases, the cause is a result of the deficiency of a plasma enzyme (ADAMTS13) that usually breaks down the von Willebrand (vWF) clotting factor into normal size.

- TTP is seen primarily in adults between the ages of 20 and 50 years old, with a slight female predominance.

- The syndrome may be idiopathic (autoimmune disorder against ADAMTS13), caused by certain drug toxicities (e.g., chemotherapy, cyclosporine, quinine, oral contraceptives, valacyclovir [Valtrex], clopidogrel [Plavix]), pregnancy/preeclampsia, infection, or the result of an autoimmune disorder such as systemic lupus erythematosus or scleroderma.

- TTP is a medical emergency because bleeding and clotting occur simultaneously.

Clinical Manifestations

Many patients with thrombocytopenia may be asymptomatic.

- The most common symptom is bleeding, usually mucosal or cutaneous. Mucosal bleeding may manifest as epistaxis and gingival bleeding, and large bullous hemorrhages may appear on the buccal mucosa. Bleeding into the skin is manifested as petechiae, purpura, or superficial ecchymoses.

When the platelet count is low, red blood cells (RBCs) may leak out of the blood vessels and into the skin to cause *petechiae*.

- When petechiae are numerous, the resulting reddish skin bruise is known as *purpura*.
- Larger purplish lesions caused by hemorrhage are called *ecchymoses*. Ecchymoses may be flat or raised; on occasion pain and tenderness are present.
- Prolonged bleeding after routine procedures, such as venipuncture or intramuscular (IM) injection, may indicate thrombocytopenia. Because bleeding may be internal, you must be aware of manifestations that reflect this type of blood loss, including weakness, fainting, dizziness, tachycardia, abdominal pain, and hypotension.

The major complication of thrombocytopenia is hemorrhage, which may be insidious or acute and internal or external. It may occur in any area of the body, including the joints, retina, and brain. Cerebral hemorrhage may be fatal. Insidious hemorrhage may first be detected by discovering the anemia that accompanies blood loss.

Diagnostic Studies

- Platelet count is decreased below 150,000/μL (150×10^9/L); spontaneous life-threatening hemorrhages (e.g., intracranial bleeding) may occur with counts < 20,000/μL (20×10^9/L).
- Bleeding time is prolonged.
- Specific assays for antigens help differentiate ITP from other types of thrombocytopenia.
- Bone marrow analysis may show normal or increased megakaryocytes (precursors of platelets); it is done to rule out leukemia, aplastic anemia, and other myeloproliferative disorders.
- Flow cytometry may detect antiplatelet antibodies.
- Hematocrit (Hct) and hemoglobin (Hb) levels are assessed for anemia.

Collaborative Care

Immune thrombocytopenic purpura. Multiple therapies are used to manage the patient with ITP. If the patient is asymptomatic, therapy may not be used unless the platelet count is <30,000/μL. Corticosteroids (e.g., prednisone) are used to suppress the phagocytic response of splenic macrophages. This alters the spleen's recognition of platelets and increases platelet life span. In addition, corticosteroids depress antibody formation and reduce capillary fragility and bleeding time.

Splenectomy may be indicated if the patient does not respond to prednisone initially or requires unacceptably high doses to maintain an adequate platelet count. Approximately 80% of patients benefit from splenectomy, which results in a complete or partial remission. Treatment may also include high doses of intravenous immunoglobulin (IVIG) in the patient who is unresponsive to corticosteroids or splenectomy. The immunoglobulin works by competing with the antiplatelet antibodies for macrophage receptors. IVIG raises the platelet count, but the beneficial effects may be temporary.

Romiplostim (Nplate) and eltrombopag (Promacta) are newer treatments for chronic ITP patients who have had an insufficient response to steroids, immunoglobulins, or splenectomy. They are thrombopoietin receptor agonists and increase platelet production.

- Immunosuppressive agents used in refractory cases include rituximab (Rituxan), cyclophosphamide (Cytoxan), azathioprine (Imuran), and mycophenolate mofetil (CellCept). High-dose cyclophosamide and combination chemotherapy are third-line therapy.
- Platelet transfusions are not indicated until the count is <10,000/µL (10 × 10^9/L) or if the patient is bleeding before a procedure.
- Aspirin and other medications that affect platelet function and development should be avoided.

Thrombotic thrombocytopenic purpura. TTP may be treated in a variety of ways. The first step is to treat the underlying disorder (e.g., infection) or remove the causative agent, if identified. If untreated, TTP usually results in irreversible renal failure and death. Plasma exchange or plasmapheresis may be needed to aggressively reverse the process. Treatment should be continued daily until the patient's platelet counts normalize and hemolysis has ceased.

Corticosteroids may be added to this treatment. Rituximab has been used for patients who are refractory to plasma exchange. Other immunosuppressants such as cyclosporine or cyclophosphamide may also be used. Splenectomy may be considered in patients who are refractory to plasma exchange or immnosuppression. The administration of platelets is generally contraindicated because it may lead to new vWF-platelet complexes and increased clotting.

Nursing Management
Goals
The patient with thrombocytopenia will have no gross or occult bleeding, maintain vascular integrity, and manage home care to prevent any complications related to an increased risk for bleeding.

See NCP 31-2 for the patient with thrombocytopenia, Lewis et al., *Medical-Surgical Nursing,* ed. 8, p. 683.

Nursing Diagnoses

- Impaired oral mucous membrane
- Risk for bleeding
- Deficient knowledge

Nursing Interventions

It is important for you to discourage excessive use of over-the-counter (OTC) medications known to be possible causes of acquired thrombocytopenia. Many medications contain aspirin as an ingredient. Aspirin reduces platelet adhesiveness, thus potentially contributing to bleeding.

Encourage persons to have a complete medical evaluation if manifestations of bleeding tendencies (e.g., prolonged epistaxis, petechiae) develop. In addition, be observant for early signs of thrombocytopenia in patients receiving cancer chemotherapy drugs.

The goal during acute episodes of thrombocytopenia is to prevent or control hemorrhage. In the patient with thrombocytopenia, bleeding is usually from superficial sites; deep bleeding (into the muscles, joints, and abdomen) usually occurs only when clotting factors are diminished. It is important to emphasize that a seemingly minor nosebleed or new petechiae may indicate potential hemorrhage and the health care provider should be notified.

- In a woman with thrombocytopenia, menstrual blood loss may exceed the usual amount and duration. Counting sanitary napkins or tampons used during menses is an important intervention to detect excess blood loss.
- Proper administration of platelet transfusions is an important nursing responsibility. Platelet concentrates, derived from fresh whole blood, can effectively increase the platelet level.
- All patients with ITP should be monitored for response to therapy.

▼ **Patient and Caregiver Teaching**

Teach the person with acquired thrombocytopenia to avoid causative agents when possible. If causative agents cannot be avoided (e.g., chemotherapy), the patient should learn to avoid injury or trauma during these periods and detect the clinical signs and symptoms of bleeding caused by thrombocytopenia.

- The patient with either ITP or acquired thrombocytopenia should have planned periodic medical evaluations to assess the patient's status and intercede in situations in which exacerbations and bleeding are likely to occur.
- The impact of either an acute or chronic condition on the patient's quality of life should also be addressed.

For a more complete listing of precautions that patients should take when their platelet count is low, see Table 31-16, Lewis et al., *Medical-Surgical Nursing,* ed. 8, p. 684.

THYROID CANCER

Description
Thyroid cancer is the most common endocrine-related cancer. An estimated 37,200 new cases of thyroid cancer occur annually. For most types of thyroid cancer effective treatment is available. Four main types of thyroid cancer are papillary, follicular, medullary, and anaplastic.

- Papillary thyroid cancer is the most common type, accounting for about 70% to 80% of all thyroid cancers. Papillary cancer tends to grow slowly and spreads initially to lymph nodes in the neck.
- Follicular thyroid cancer makes up about 10% to 15% of all thyroid cancers and tends to occur in older patients. Follicular cancer first grows into the cervical lymph nodes. Follicular cancer is more likely than papillary cancer to grow into blood vessels and from there to spread to the lungs and bones.
- Medullary thyroid cancer, which accounts for 5% to 10% of all thyroid cancers, is more likely to occur in families and be associated with other endocrine problems. It can be diagnosed by genetic testing. In family members of a person with medullary thyroid cancer, a positive test for *RET protooncogene* can lead to an early diagnosis of medullary thyroid cancer and treatment.
- Anaplastic thyroid cancer, which is found in <5% of patients with thyroid cancer, is the most advanced and aggressive thyroid cancer. It is the least likely to respond to treatment.

Clinical Manifestations
The primary sign of thyroid cancer is the presence of a painless, palpable nodule or nodules in an enlarged thyroid gland. Patients or health care providers discover most of these nodules during routine palpation of the neck. An estimated 5% to 10% of solitary thyroid nodules are malignant.

Diagnostic Studies
- In thyroid cancer, physical exam may reveal firm cervical masses, which are suggestive of lymph node metastasis. Thyroid

cancers can grow directly through the thyroid capsule to invade surrounding structures. Hemoptysis and airway obstruction may occur if the trachea is involved.

- Nodular thyroid gland enlargement or palpation of a mass requires further evaluation. Ultrasound is often the first test used. Computed tomography (CT), magnetic resonance imaging (MRI), and ultrasound-guided fine-needle aspiration (FNA) are other diagnostic options.
- A thyroid scan may be done to evaluate for a malignancy. The scan shows whether nodules on the thyroid are "hot" or "cold." If the nodule does not take up the radioactive iodine, it appears as "cold" and has a higher risk of being malignant.

Nursing and Collaborative Management

Surgical removal of the tumor is usually indicated for thyroid cancer. Surgical procedures may range from unilateral total lobectomy with removal of the isthmus to near total thyroidectomy with bilateral lobectomy. The latter choice is desirable because it is more likely to preserve the function of the parathyroid gland.

Many thyroid cancers are TSH dependent, and thyroid hormone in hyperphysiologic doses is often prescribed to inhibit pituitary secretion of TSH. Radiation therapy may be used as the primary treatment or as palliative treatment for patients with metastatic thyroid cancer.

Nursing care for the patient with thyroid tumors is similar to that of a patient undergoing thyroidectomy (see Hyperthyroidism, surgical therapy, p. 344). Because of the surgical site location as well as the potential for hypocalcemia, the patient requires frequent postoperative assessment. Assess the patient for airway obstruction, bleeding, and manifestations of hypocalcemia (tetany).

TRIGEMINAL NEURALGIA

Description

Trigeminal neuralgia (tic douloureux) is sudden, usually unilateral, severe, brief, stabbing, recurrent, episodes of pain in the distribution of the trigeminal nerve. It is a relatively uncommon cranial nerve disorder. It is seen twice as often in women as men. The majority of cases are in persons older than 40 years.

- Risk factors are multiple sclerosis and hypertension. Other factors that may result in neuralgia include herpes virus infection, infection of the teeth and jaw, and a brainstem infarct.

Pathophysiology

The trigeminal nerve is the fifth cranial nerve (CN V) and has both motor and sensory branches. The sensory branches, primarily the maxillary and mandibular branches, are involved.

- Although no specific cause has been identified, one theory is that compression of blood vessels, especially the superior cerebellar artery, occurs and results in chronic irritation of the trigeminal nerve at the root entry zone.
- The effectiveness of antiseizure drug therapy may be related to the ability of these drugs to stabilize the neuronal membrane and decrease paroxysmal afferent impulses of the nerve.

Clinical Manifestations

The classic feature of trigeminal neuralgia is an abrupt onset of paroxysms of excruciating pain described as burning or knifelike, or a lightning-like shock in the lips, upper or lower gums, cheek, forehead, or side of the nose.

- Intense pain, twitching, grimacing, and frequent blinking and tearing of the eye occur during the acute attack (giving rise to the term *tic*).
- The attacks are usually brief, lasting seconds to 2 or 3 minutes, and are generally unilateral.
- Recurrences are unpredictable; they may occur several times each day or weeks or months apart.
- After the refractory (pain-free) period, a phenomenon known as *clustering* can occur; it is characterized by a cycle of pain and refractoriness that continues for hours.

The painful episodes are usually initiated by a triggering mechanism of light cutaneous stimulation at specific points (trigger zones) along the distribution of the nerve branches.

- Precipitating stimuli include chewing, teeth brushing, a hot or cold blast of air on the face, washing the face, yawning, or even talking. Touch and tickle seem to predominate as causative triggers rather than pain or changes in temperature.
- As a result, the patient may not eat properly, neglect hygienic practices, wear a cloth over the face, and withdraw from interaction with other individuals. The patient may sleep excessively as a means of coping with the pain.

Diagnostic Studies

- Computed tomography (CT) scan to rule out any lesions, tumors, or vascular abnormalities.

- Magnetic resonance imaging (MRI) to rule out multiple sclerosis.
- Neurologic assessment including audiologic evaluation, although results are usually normal.

Collaborative Care

Drug Therapy

Carbamazepine (Tegretol) or oxcarbazepine (Trileptal) are the usual first-line therapy for trigeminal neuralgia. By acting on sodium channels, these drugs lengthen the time for neuron repolarization, resulting in decreased neuron firing. These antiseizure drugs may prevent an acute attack or promote remission of symptoms. Because drug therapy may not provide permanent pain relief, some patients may seek help from otolaryngologists or acupuncture and megavitamins.

- Nerve blocking with local anesthetics is a treatment option. Local nerve blocking results in complete anesthesia of the area supplied by the injected branches. Relief of pain is temporary, lasting 6 to 18 months.
- Biofeedback is another strategy for pain management. In addition to controlling the pain, the patient may experience a strong sense of personal control by mastering the technique and altering certain body functions.

Surgical Therapy

If a conservative approach including drug therapy is not effective, surgical therapy is available.

- *Glycerol rhizotomy* is a percutaneous procedure that consists of an injection of glycerol through the foramen ovale into the trigeminal cistern.
- *Percutaneous radiofrequency rhizotomy* (electrocoagulation) consists of placing a needle into the trigeminal rootlets that are adjacent to the pons and destroying the area by means of a radiofrequency current. This can result in facial numbness (although some degree of sensation may be retained) or trigeminal motor weakness.
- *Microvascular decompression* of the trigeminal nerve is performed by displacing and repositioning blood vessels that appear to be compressing the nerve at the root-entry zone where it exits the pons. This procedure relieves pain without residual sensory loss but is potentially dangerous, as is any surgery near the brainstem. Other procedures include gamma knife radiosurgery, retrogasserian rhizotomy, and suboccipital craniotomy.

Nursing Management

Monitor the patient's response to drug therapy and note any side effects. Strong opioids such as morphine should be used cautiously because of the potential for addiction over time. Alternative pain-relief measures, such as biofeedback, should be explored for the patient who is not a surgical candidate and whose pain is not controlled by other therapeutic measures. Careful assessment of pain, including history, pain relief, and drug dependency, can assist in selecting appropriate interventions.

Environmental management is essential during an acute period to lessen triggering stimuli. Keep the room at an even, moderate temperature and free of drafts. A private room is preferred during an acute period.

Instruct the patient about the importance of nutrition, hygiene, and oral care, conveying understanding if previous neglect is apparent.

- You should provide lukewarm water and soft cloths or cotton saturated with solutions not requiring rinsing for cleansing the face. A small, very soft-bristled toothbrush or a warm mouthwash assists in promoting oral care.
- Hygiene activities are best carried out when analgesia is at its peak.
- Food should be high in protein and calories and easy to chew. It should be served lukewarm and offered frequently. When oral intake is markedly reduced and the patient's nutritional status is compromised, a nasogastric (NG) tube can be inserted on the unaffected side for NG feedings.

For the patient who has had surgery, compare the patient's post-operative pain with the preoperative level. Frequently evaluate the corneal reflex, extraocular muscles, hearing, sensation, and facial nerve function. General postoperative nursing care after a craniotomy is appropriate if intracranial surgery is performed.

- After a percutaneous radiofrequency procedure, apply an ice pack to the jaw on the operative side for 3 to 5 hours. To avoid injuring the mouth, the patient should not chew on the operative side until sensation has returned.

▼ **Patient and Caregiver Teaching**

Regular follow-up care should be planned. The patient needs instruction regarding the dosage and side effects of medications. Encourage the patient to keep environmental stimuli to a moderate level and use stress reduction methods.

Long-term management after surgical intervention depends on the residual effects of the procedure used. If anesthesia is present or the corneal reflex is altered, the patient should be taught to

(1) chew on the unaffected side, (2) avoid hot foods or beverages that can burn the mucous membranes, (3) check the oral cavity after meals to remove food particles, (4) practice meticulous oral hygiene and continue with semiannual dental visits, (5) protect the face against extremes of temperature, (6) use an electric razor, (7) wear a protective eye shield, and (8) examine eye regularly for symptoms of infection or irritation.

- The patient may have developed protective practices to prevent pain and may need counseling or psychiatric assistance in the readjustment period, especially in reestablishing personal relationships.

TUBERCULOSIS

Description

Tuberculosis (TB) is an infectious disease caused by *Mycobacterium tuberculosis*. It usually involves the lungs, but it can also occur in other parts of the body.

TB is the world's second most common cause of death from infectious disease, after human immunodeficiency virus/acquired immunodeficiency syndrome (HIV/AIDS). In the United States persons at risk include the homeless, residents of inner-city neighborhoods, foreign-born persons, older adults, those in institutions (long-term care facilities, prisons), IV injecting drug users, persons at poverty level, and those with poor access to health care.

- The incidence of TB worldwide was declining until the mid 1980s when HIV disease emerged. Major factors contributing to this resurgence include TB high rates of TB among patients with HIV infection and the emergence of multidrug-resistant (MDR) strains of *M. tuberculosis*. TB rates are slowly declining again.
- Once a strain of *M. tuberculosis* develops resistance to isoniazid and rifampin, it is defined as multidrug-resistant tuberculosis (MDR-TB). Resistance can result from incorrect prescribing, lack of public health case management, and patient non-adherence to the prescribed regimen.

Pathophysiology

M. tuberculosis is a gram-positive, acid-fast bacillus that is usually spread from person to person via airborne droplets produced by speaking and coughing. Brief exposure to a few tubercle bacilli rarely causes an infection. TB is more commonly spread by repeated close contact (within 6 inches of the person's mouth) with the infected person.

- TB is not highly infectious, and transmission usually requires close, frequent, or prolonged exposure. The disease cannot be spread by hands, books, glasses, or dishes.
- Once inhaled, these small particles lodge in the bronchiole and alveolus. *M. tuberculosis* replicates slowly and spreads via the lymphatic system.
- The organisms find favorable environments for growth primarily in the upper lobes of the lungs, kidneys, epiphyses of the bone, cerebral cortex, and adrenal glands.

Classification

TB infection occurs when the bacteria are inhaled but there is an effective immune response and the bacteria become inactive. Most people have an effective immune response to encapsulate these organisms for the rest of their lives.

TB infection in a person who does not have the active TB disease is referred to as *latent TB infection* (LTBI). People with LTBI are not sick because the organisms are not active.

- An estimated 10 to 15 million Americans have LTBI. About 10% of them will develop active TB disease at some point in their lives. Therefore treatment of LTBI is important. A comparison of latent TB infection and TB disease is presented in Table 84.

TB disease is defined as active bacteria that multiply and cause clinically active disease. Certain individuals are at a higher risk of active disease, including those who are immunosuppressed for any reason or have diabetes mellitus. Dormant but viable *M. tuberculosis* organisms persist for years. Reactivation of LTBI can occur if the host's defense mechanisms become impaired.

Clinical Manifestations

In the early stages the patient is usually free of symptoms. People with LTBI have a positive skin test but are asymptomatic.

- Active TB disease may initially present with fatigue, malaise, anorexia, unexplained weight loss, low-grade fevers, and night sweats.

A characteristic pulmonary manifestation is a cough that becomes frequent and may produce mucopurulent sputum. Hemoptysis is not a common finding.

- Sometimes TB has more acute, sudden manifestations; the patient has a high fever, chills, generalized flulike symptoms, pleuritic pain, and a productive cough.
- The HIV-infected patient with TB often has atypical physical examinations and chest x-ray findings. Classic signs such as fever, cough, and weight loss may be attributed to *Pneu-*

| Table 84 | Comparison of Latent TB Infection and TB Disease |

Person with Latent TB Infection	Person with TB Disease
Has no symptoms	Has symptoms that may include: ■ a bad cough that lasts 3 weeks or longer ■ pain in the chest ■ coughing up blood or sputum ■ weakness or fatigue ■ weight loss ■ no appetite ■ chills ■ fever ■ sweating at night
Does not feel sick	Usually feels sick
Cannot spread TB bacteria to others	May spread TB bacteria to others
Usually has a skin test or blood test result indicating TB infection	Usually has a skin test or blood test result indicating TB infection
Has a normal chest x-ray and a negative sputum smear	May have an abnormal chest x-ray, or positive sputum smear or culture
Needs treatment for latent TB infection to prevent active TB disease	Needs treatment for active TB disease

Source: http://www.cdc.gov/tb/topic/basics/default.htm.

mocystis jiroveci or other HIV-associated opportunistic diseases. Clinical manifestations of respiratory problems in patients with HIV must be carefully investigated to determine the cause.

Complications

Large numbers of organisms can invade the bloodstream and spread to all body organs. This involvement of many organs simultaneously is called *miliary TB*. It can occur as a result of primary disease or reactivation of latent infection.

- The patient may be either acutely ill with fever, dyspnea, and cyanosis, or chronically ill with systemic manifestations of weight loss, fever, and gastrointestinal (GI) disturbance.

- Hepatomegaly, splenomegaly, and generalized lymphade-nopathy may also be present.

Pleural TB can result from either primary disease or reactivation of a latent infection. *Empyema* is less common than effusion but may occur from large numbers of tubercular organisms in the pleural space.

Acute pneumonia may result when large amounts of tubercle bacilli are discharged from granulomas into the lungs or lymph nodes.

- Manifestations are similar to those of bacterial pneumonia, including chills, fever, productive cough, pleuritic pain, and leukocytosis.

Diagnostic Studies

- Tuberculin skin test (TST): positive reaction indicates TB infection (latent or active). See Table 26-11 and Chapter 26, Lewis et al., *Medical-Surgical Nursing,* ed. 8, for guidelines in performing and interpreting TSTs.
- Chest x-ray: diagnosis cannot be based solely on x-ray because other diseases may mimic TB.
- Bacteriologic studies: stained sputum smears for acid-fast bacilli (AFB test) can identify tubercle bacilli; cultures to grow tubercle bacilli to confirm diagnosis.
- QuantiFERON-TB (QFT), a rapid diagnostic test using blood, is an option in detecting TB and may be used in place of TST in health care settings.

Collaborative Care

Most patients with TB are treated on an outpatient basis and continue to work and maintain their lifestyles with few changes. Hospitalization may be used for diagnostic evaluation and severely ill or debilitated patients.

Drug Therapy

The mainstay of TB treatment is drug therapy. Drug therapy is used to treat an individual with clinical disease, as well as prevent disease in an infected person. In view of the growing prevalence of multidrug-resistant TB, the patient with active TB should be managed aggressively. Treatment of previously untreated TB usually consists of a combination of at least four drugs to increase therapeutic effectiveness and decrease the development of *M. tuberculosis*–resistant strains. Four different regimen options have been identified by the Centers for Disease Control and Prevention (CDC) (see Tables 28-11 and 12, Lewis et al., *Medical-Surgical Nursing,* ed. 8, pp. 555-556).

- First-line drugs include isoniazid (INH), rifampin (Rifadin), pyrazinamide (PZA), ethambutol (Myambutol), rifabutin (Mycobutin), and rifapentine (Priftin). Combinations of isoniazid and rifampin and of isoniazid, rifampin, and pyrazinamide are available to simplify therapy.
- Second-line drugs are used primarily for the treatment of resistant strains or if the patient develops toxicity to the primary drugs. Newer second-line drugs include the quinolones (e.g., levofloxacin [Levaquin], moxifloxacin [Avelox], gatifloxacin [Tequin]).
- The preferred drug administration strategy for all patients with TB to ensure adherence is directly observed therapy (DOT). This involves providing the antituberculosis drugs directly to the patient and watching as he or she swallows the medications.
- Noncompliance is a major factor in the emergence of multidrug resistance and treatment failures. Many individuals do not adhere to the treatment program in spite of understanding that noncompliance can lead to reactivation of TB and multidrug-resistant TB. Drug therapy is usually continued for 6 to 9 months.
- The recommended length of 6 to 9 months of drug therapy also contributes to noncompliance.

Drug regimens should be adapted to the resistance pattern evident from sputum culture. In follow-up care for patients receiving long-term therapy, it is important to monitor drug effectiveness and the development of toxic side effects.

- Sputum specimens are usually initially obtained weekly and then monthly to assess effectiveness of medication.

Isoniazid is usually used in the treatment of latent TB infection to prevent the infection from developing into active disease.

Immunization with bacille Calmette-Guérin (BCG) vaccine to prevent tuberculosis is currently used in many parts of the world. However, efficacy of the vaccine is not clear, and development of an effective TB vaccine is an urgent worldwide public health priority.

Nursing Management
Goals
The patient with tuberculosis will comply with the therapeutic regimen, have no recurrence of disease, have normal pulmonary function, and take appropriate measures to prevent the spread of the disease.

Nursing Diagnoses
- Ineffective breathing pattern
- Imbalanced nutrition: less than body requirements
- Noncompliance
- Ineffective health maintenance
- Activity intolerance

Nursing Interventions

The ultimate goal related to TB in the United States is eradication.

- Selective screening programs in known high-risk groups are of value in detecting persons with TB.
- Chest x-rays to assess for the presence of TB in persons with a positive tuberculin skin test should be encouraged.
- Contacts of the individual who has TB should be identified and assessed for the possibility of infection and the need for prophylactic drug treatment.
- When an individual has respiratory symptoms such as cough, dyspnea, or productive sputum, especially if accompanied by night sweats and unexplained weight loss, you should assess for the presence of TB.

If hospitalization is needed for patients suspected of having TB, special measures should be taken.

- Airborne isolation is indicated until the patient has been taking adequate drug therapy for at least 2 weeks, has shown a clinical response to therapy, and has three negative AFB smears.
- High-efficiency particulate air (HEPA) masks molded to fit tightly around the nose and mouth are worn whenever entering the patient's room.

Follow-up care may be indicated during the subsequent 12 months after the medication regimen is completed; this includes bacteriologic studies and chest x-rays.

▼ **Patient and Caregiver Teaching**
- In the hospital the patient should be taught to cover the nose and mouth with paper tissue every time he or she coughs, sneezes, or produces sputum. The patient wears a standard isolation mask to prevent coughing tubercular organisms into the environment.
- Teach the patient so that the need for dedication to the prescribed medication regimen is fully understood by the patient and caregiver. Reassure the patient that TB can be cured if the regimen is followed.
- Because approximately 5% of individuals experience relapses, teach the patient to recognize symptoms that

indicate the recurrence of TB. If these symptoms occur, immediate medical attention should be sought.

- Also teach the patient about factors that could reactivate TB, such as immunosuppression and malignancy.

ULCERATIVE COLITIS

Description

Ulcerative colitis is an autoimmune disorder that, along with Crohn's disease, is referred to as *inflammatory bowel disease* (IBD). See Inflammatory Bowel Disease, p. 359 for the discussion of the disorder.

URETHRITIS

Urethritis is an inflammation of the urethra. Causes of urethritis include a bacterial or viral infection, trichomonal and monilial infection (especially in women), chlamydia, and gonorrhea (especially in men).

In men, purulent discharge usually indicates a gonococcal urethritis; a clear discharge typically signifies a nongonococcal urethritis.

- Urethritis also produces bothersome lower urinary tract symptoms, including dysuria, urgency, and frequent urination, similar to those seen with cystitis.

In women, urethritis is difficult to diagnose. It frequently produces bothersome lower urinary tract symptoms as described, but urethral discharge may not be present.

- Cultures on split urine collections (taken at beginning of urine flow and then midstream) or any urethral discharge may confirm a diagnosis of urethral infection.
- Treatment is based on identifying and treating the cause and providing symptomatic relief.
- Sulfamethoxazole with trimethoprim (Bactrim, Septra) and nitrofurantoin (Furadantin) are examples of medications used for bacterial infections. Metronidazole (Flagyl) and clotrimazole (Mycelex) may be used for trichomonal infection. Medications such as nystatin (Mycostatin) or fluconazole (Diflucan) may be prescribed for monilial infections. In chlamydial infections, doxycycline (Vibramycin) may be used.

U

- Women with negative urine cultures and no pyuria do not usually respond to antibiotics. Warm sitz baths may temporarily relieve bothersome symptoms.

Teach patients to avoid the use of vaginal deodorant sprays, properly cleanse the perineal area after bowel movements and urination, and avoid intercourse until symptoms subside. Also teach patients with sexually transmitted urethritis to refer their sex partners for evaluation and testing if they had sexual contact in the 60 days preceding onset of the symptoms or diagnosis.

URINARY INCONTINENCE AND RETENTION

Description

Urinary incontinence (UI), the uncontrolled leakage of urine, affects an estimated 17 million people in the United States. Although its prevalence is higher among older women and men, it is not a natural consequence of aging. An estimated 80% of incontinence can be cured or significantly improved.

Urinary retention is the inability to empty the bladder despite micturition or the accumulation of urine in the bladder because of an inability to urinate. In certain cases, it is associated with urinary leakage or postvoid dribbling called overflow UI.

- Acute urinary retention is the total inability to pass urine via micturition; it is a medical emergency. Chronic urinary retention is defined as incomplete bladder emptying despite urination.

Pathophysiology

UI can result from anything that interferes with bladder or urethral sphincter control.

- Causes can include confusion or depression, infection, atropic vaginitis, urinary retention, restricted mobility, fecal impaction, or drugs.
- UI disorders include stress, urge, overflow, and reflex incontinence. (For a complete description of UI, see Table 46-18, Lewis et al., *Medical-Surgical Nursing,* ed. 8, p. 1148.)
- Patients may have more than one type of incontinence.
- Urinary retention is caused by two different dysfunctions of the urinary system: bladder outlet obstruction and deficient detrusor (bladder muscle) contraction strength.
- Obstruction leads to urinary retention when the blockage is severe enough that the bladder can no longer evacuate its contents despite a detrusor contraction. A common cause of obstruction in men is an enlarged prostate.

- Common causes of deficient detrusor contraction strength are neurologic diseases affecting the sacral segments 2, 3, and 4; long-standing diabetes mellitus; overdistention; long-term alcoholism; and drugs (e.g., anticholinergic drugs).

Diagnostic Studies

- Focused history, physical assessment, and a voiding record provide information about the onset of UI, factors that provoke urinary leakage and associated conditions.
- Pelvic examination assesses for organ prolapse and evaluates pelvic floor muscle strength.
- Urinalysis identifies possible factors contributing to transient incontinence or urinary retention (e.g., urinary infection, diabetes mellitus).
- Postvoid residual (PVR) urine must be measured in the patient undergoing evaluation for urinary incontinence and retention. The PVR volume is obtained by asking the patient to urinate, followed by catheterization within a relatively brief period (preferably 10 to 20 minutes). Alternatively, an ultrasound can be used to estimate the residual volume.
- Urodynamic testing is indicated in selected cases of urinary incontinence and retention.
- Imaging studies of upper urinary tract (e.g., ultrasound) are obtained when retention or incontinence is associated with urinary tract infections or there is evidence of upper urinary tract involvement.

Collaborative Care: Urinary Incontinence

Transient, reversible factors are corrected initially, followed by management of the type of UI. In general, less invasive treatments are attempted before more invasive methods (e.g., surgery) are used.

Several behavioral therapies may be used to improve urinary continence.

- Pelvic floor muscle training (Kegel exercises) may help some patients manage stress, urge, or mixed UI.
- Biofeedback is used to assist the patient to identify, isolate, contract, and relax the pelvic muscles.

Drug Therapy

Drug therapy varies according to the type of incontinence.

- Drugs have a very limited role in the management of stress incontinence. α-Adrenergic agonists can be used to increase bladder sphincter tone and urethral resistance. Unfortunately, they exert a limited beneficial effect and are associated with adverse effects, including exacerbation of hypertension and tachycardia.

- Drugs play a more central role in the management of urge or reflex incontinence. Anticholinergic drugs and newer, more specific muscarinic receptor antagonists relax the bladder muscle and inhibit overactive detrusor contractions. These preparations include immediate- and extended-release tolterodine (Detrol, Detrol LA); immediate, extended, and transdermal oxybutynin (Ditropan, Ditropan XL, Oxytrol TDS); twice daily trospium chloride (Sanctura); extended-release solifenacine (VESIcare); and darifenacin (Enablex). Common side effects of anticholingergic drugs include dry mouth, constipation, and dyspepsia.

Surgical Therapy

Surgical techniques also vary according to the type of incontinence.

- Surgical correction of stress UI may reposition the urethra and/or create a backboard of support or otherwise stabilize the urethra and bladder neck to be more receptive to changes in intrabdominal pressure.
- Another technique for stress UI augments the urethral resistance of the intrinsic sphincter unit with a sling or periurethral injectables.
- Placement of a suburethral sling, using autologous fascia, cadaveric fascia, or a synthetic material, is also used to correct stress UI in women.
- An artificial urethral sphincter can be used in men with intrinsic sphincter deficiency and severe stress UI.
- Alternatively, one of several bulking agents can be injected underneath the mucosa of the urethra to correct stress UI in women or men.

Nursing Management: Urinary Incontinence

You need to recognize both the physical and the emotional problems associated with incontinence. The patient's dignity, privacy, and feelings of self-worth must be maintained or enhanced.

- This often includes a two-step approach involving containment devices to manage existing urinary leakage and a definitive plan of management designed to reduce or resolve the factors leading to incontinence.
- Emphasize consumption of an adequate volume of fluids and reduction or elimination of bladder irritants (particularly caffeine and alcohol) from the diet.
- Advise the patient to maintain a regular, flexible schedule of urination (usually every 2 to 3 hours while awake).

- Also advise patients to quit smoking, because it increases the risk of stress UI.
- Aggressive management of constipation, beginning with ensuring adequate fluid intake, increasing dietary fiber, light exercise, and judicious use of stool softeners, is recommended.
- Behavioral treatments include bladder retraining and pelvic floor muscle training. (A patient teaching guide for pelvic floor muscle exercise is found in Table 46-20, Lewis et al., *Medical-Surgical Nursing,* ed. 8, p. 1150.)
- Assess strategies the patient uses to contain UI and share information on products specifically designed to contain urine.
- In inpatient or long-term care facilities, nursing management of UI includes maximizing toilet access. This may take the form of offering the urinal or bedpan or assisting the patient to the bathroom every 2 to 3 hours or at scheduled times. Ensure that toilets are accessible to patients and there is adequate privacy to allow effective urine elimination.

Collaborative Care: Urinary Retention

Behavioral therapies also may be used in the management of urinary retention. Scheduled toileting and double voiding may be effective in chronic urinary retention with moderate postvoid residual volumes.

- Double voiding is an attempt to maximize bladder evacuation by having the patient urinate, sit on the toilet for 3 to 4 minutes, and urinate again before exiting the bathroom.
- If catheterization is required for acute or chronic urinary retention, intermittent catheterization is preferred. It allows the patient to remain free of an indwelling catheter with its associated risk of urinary tract infection (UTI) and urethral irritation.

Drug Therapy

Several drugs may be administered to promote bladder evacuation. For patients with obstruction at the level of the bladder neck, an α-adrenergic antagonist may be prescribed. These drugs relax the smooth muscle of the bladder neck, prostatic urethra, and possibly dual-innervated rhabdosphincter, diminishing urethral resistance.

Surgical Therapy

Surgical interventions are useful when managing urinary retention caused by obstruction. Transurethral or open surgical techniques are used to treat benign or malignant prostatic enlargement, bladder neck contracture, urethral strictures, or dyssynergia of the bladder neck in selected patients.

- Pelvic reconstruction using an abdominal or transvaginal approach can be used to correct bladder outlet obstruction in women with severe pelvic organ prolapse.

Unfortunately, surgery plays little role in the management of urinary retention caused by deficient detrusor contraction strength.

Nursing Management: Urinary Retention

Acute urinary retention is a medical emergency that requires prompt recognition and bladder drainage. You should insert a catheter (as prescribed) unless otherwise directed.

- The patient with acute urinary retention should be taught strategies to minimize risk, including avoiding intake of large volumes of fluid over a brief period.
- A patient unable to urinate is advised to drink a cup of coffee or brewed caffeinated tea to maximize urinary urgency and sit in a tub of warm water or take a warm shower and attempt to urinate while in the tub or shower.
- If this does not lead to successful urination, the patient is advised to seek immediate care.
- Patients with chronic urinary retention may be managed by behavioral methods, an indwelling or intermittent catheterization, surgery, or drugs.
- Scheduled toileting and double voiding are the primary behavioral interventions used for chronic retention.

URINARY TRACT CALCULI

Description

An estimated 500,000 people in the United States have *nephrolithiasis* (kidney stone disease). Except for struvite stones, associated with urinary tract infection (UTI), stone disorders are more common in men than women. The majority of patients are between 20 and 55 years old.

- The incidence is also higher in persons with a family history of stone formation. Recurrence of stones can occur in up to 50% of patients.
- Stone formation occurs more often in the summer months, thus supporting the role of dehydration in this process.
- The term *calculus* refers to the stone, and *lithiasis* refers to stone formation.

Pathophysiology

Many factors are involved in the incidence and type of stone formation, including metabolic, dietary, genetic, climatic, lifestyle, and occupational influences. Many theories have been proposed to explain the formation of stones in the urinary tract.

- Crystals, when in a supersaturated concentration, can precipitate and unite to form a stone. Keeping urine dilute and free flowing reduces the risk of recurrent stone formation in many individuals.
- Urinary pH, solute load, and inhibitors in the urine affect the formation of stones. The higher the pH, the less soluble are calcium and phosphate. The lower the pH, the less soluble are uric acid and cystine.

Other important factors in stone development include obstruction with urinary stasis and urinary infection with urea-splitting bacteria (e.g., *Proteus, Klebsiella, Pseudomonas,* and some species of staphylococci). These bacteria cause the urine to become alkaline and contribute to the formation of struvite (calcium-magnesium-ammonium phosphate) stones.

- Infected stones, entrapped in the kidney, may assume a staghorn configuration as they enlarge. These stones can lead to hydronephrosis, and loss of kidney function. Infected stones are frequent with an external urinary diversion, long-term indwelling catheter, neurogenic bladder, or urinary retention.
- There are five major categories of stones: calcium phosphate, calcium oxalate, uric acid, cystine, and struvite. Stone composition may be mixed, although calcium stones are the most common.

Clinical Manifestations

Urinary stones cause manifestations when they obstruct the urinary flow; symptoms include hematuria, abdominal or flank pain, and renal colic.

- The type of pain is determined by the location of the stone. If the stone is nonobstructing, pain may be absent. If it produces obstruction in a calyx or at the ureteropelvic junction (UPJ), the patient may experience dull costovertebral flank pain or even colic. Pain resulting from the passage of a calculus down the ureter is intense and colicky. The patient may be in mild shock with cool, moist skin. As a stone nears the ureterovesical junction (UVJ), pain will be felt in the lateral flank and sometimes down into the testicles, labia, or groin.
- Manifestations may also include those of a urinary infection with fever and chills.

Diagnostic Studies

- Serum calcium, phosphorus, sodium, potassium, bicarbonate, uric acid, and creatinine levels and blood urea nitrogen (BUN) are used to assess renal function and stone etiology.
- Urine pH checks for struvite stones and renal tubular necrosis (tendency to alkaline pH) and uric acid stones (tendency to acidic pH).
- X-ray of the abdomen and renal ultrasound will identify larger, radiopaque stones.
- Ultrasonography can be used to identify radiopaque or radiolucent calculi in the renal pelvis, calyx, or proximal ureter.
- Computed tomography (CT) scan differentiates a nonopaque stone from a tumor.
- Intravenous pyelogram (IVP) or retrograde pyelogram localizes the degree and site of obstruction or confirms the presence of a radiolucent stone, such as a uric acid (cystine calculus), or a staghorn calculus.

Collaborative Care

Evaluation and management of the patient with renal lithiasis consist of two concurrent approaches.

The *first approach* is directed toward management of the acute attack. This involves treating symptoms of pain, infection, or obstruction. Opioids are typically required at frequent intervals for relief of renal colic pain. Many stones pass spontaneously. However, stones larger than 4 mm in size are unlikely to pass through the ureter.

The *second approach* is evaluation of the cause of the stone formation and prevention of further stone development. Information obtained from the patient includes family history of stone formation, geographic residence, nutritional assessment (including intake of vitamins A and D), activity pattern (active or sedentary), history of periods of prolonged illness with immobilization or dehydration, and history of disease or surgery involving the gastrointestinal (GI) or genitourinary (GU) tract.

Adequate hydration, dietary sodium restrictions, dietary changes, and medications minimize urinary stone formation.

- Various medications are prescribed that prevent stone formation by altering urine pH, preventing excessive urinary excretion of a substance, or correcting a primary disease (e.g., hyperparathyroidism).

Treatment of struvite stones requires control of infection. Acetohydroxamic acid, an inhibitor of the chemical action caused by persistent bacteria, can retard struvite stone formation. If infection cannot be controlled, the stone may have to be removed surgically.

Indications for open surgical, endourologic, or lithotripsy stone removal include:

- Stones too large for spontaneous passage, associated with bacteriuria or symptomatic infection, or causing impaired renal function, persistent pain, nausea, or ileus
- An inability of the patient to be treated medically
- A patient with one kidney

Endourologic procedures include the use of endoscopes to access stones in the urinary tract. *Cystoscopy* can remove small stones in the bladder. For large stones, a *cystolitholapaxy* is performed using a lithotrite to crush stones. A *cystoscopic lithotripsy* uses an ultrasonic lithotrite to pulverize stones. Complications with these cystoscopic procedures include hemorrhage, retained stone fragments, and infection. Flexible *ureteroscopes* can be used to remove stones from the renal pelvis and upper urinary tract with the use of ultrasonic, laser, or electrohydraulic lithotripsy. The same types of lithotripsy can be used during a percutaneous nephrolithotomy by way of a nephroscope inserted through the skin into the kidney pelvis.

Lithotripsy is a procedure for eliminating calculi from the urinary tract. Specific lithotripsy techniques include percutaneous ultrasonic lithotripsy, electrohydraulic lithotripsy, laser lithotripsy, and extracorporeal shock wave lithotripsy. Extracorporeal shock wave lithotripsy and laser lithotripsy are the most common.

- In *laser lithotripsy*, probes are used to fragment lower ureteral and large bladder stones.
- In *extracorporeal shock wave lithotripsy*, a noninvasive procedure, the patient is anesthetized (spinal or general) and placed in a water bath. Fluoroscopy or ultrasound is used to focus the lithotriptor on the affected kidney, and a high-voltage spark generator produces high-energy acoustic shock waves that shatter the stone without damaging the surrounding tissues. The stone is broken down into fine sand, which is excreted into the patient's urine within a few days of the procedure.

Hematuria is common after lithotripsy procedures. A self-retaining ureteral stent is often placed after this outpatient procedure to promote passage of sand (shattered stone) and prevent obstruction caused by sand buildup in the ureter. The stent is often removed 2 weeks after lithotripsy.

- If a stone is large or positioned in the mid or distal ureter, additional treatment such as surgery may be necessary.

A small group of patients may need open surgical procedures, such as extremely obese patients or those with complex abnormalities in the calyces or at the UPJ. The type of open surgery depends on location of the stone.

- A *nephrolithotomy* is an incision into the kidney to remove a stone. A *pyelolithotomy* is an incision into the renal pelvis to remove a stone. If the stone is located in the ureter, a *ureterolithotomy* is performed. A *cystostomy* may be indicated for bladder calculi. For open surgery on the kidney or ureter, a flank incision directly below the diaphragm and across the side is usually the preferred approach.

Nutritional Therapy

A high fluid intake (at least 3000 mL/day) is recommended after an episode of urolithiasis to produce a urine output of at least 2 L/day and prevent stone formation.

- A high level of calcium in the diet, which was previously thought to contribute to kidney stones, may actually lower the risk by reducing the urinary excretion of oxalate, a common factor in many stones.
- Initial nutritional therapy should include limiting oxalate-rich foods, thereby reducing oxalate excretion. Foods high in calcium, oxalate, and purines are presented in Table 46-13, Lewis et al., *Medical-Surgical Nursing,* ed. 8, p. 1139.

Nursing Management

Goals

The patient with urinary tract calculi will have relief of pain, no urinary tract obstruction, and an understanding of measures to prevent further recurrence of stones.

See NCP 46-2 for the patient with acute renal lithiasis, Lewis et al., *Medical-Surgical Nursing,* ed. 8, p. 1140.

Nursing Diagnoses

- Acute pain
- Impaired urinary elimination
- Deficient knowledge

Nursing Interventions

Preventive measures related to the person who is on bed rest or is relatively immobile for a prolonged time include maintaining an adequate fluid intake, turning the patient every 2 hours, and helping the patient to sit or stand if possible to maximize urinary flow.

Pain management and patient comfort are primary nursing responsibilities when managing a person with an obstructing stone and renal colic.

- All urine voided by the patient should be strained through gauze or a special urine strainer in an effort to detect the stone.
- Ambulation may be encouraged to promote movement of the stone from the upper to lower urinary tract. The patient should not walk unattended when experiencing acute colic, particularly if opioid analgesics are being used.

▼ **Patient and Caregiver Teaching**
- Prevention of stone recurrence includes adequate fluid intake to produce a urine output of approximately 2 L/day.
- Dietary restriction of purines may be helpful for the patient at risk for developing uric acid stones. Reduced intake of oxalates may be indicated in the person with recurring calcium oxalate calculi.
- Teach the patient the dosage, scheduling, and potential side effects of medications used to reduce the risk of stone formation.
- Selected patients may be taught to self-monitor urinary pH, or they may be asked to measure urinary output.

URINARY TRACT INFECTIONS

Description

Urinary tract infections (UTIs) are the second most common bacterial disease and the most common bacterial infection in women. *Escherichia coli (E. coli)* is the most common pathogen causing a UTI.

- Bacterial counts in the urine of 10^5 colony-forming units per milliliter (CFU/mL) or higher typically indicate a UTI. However, bacterial counts as low as 10^2 to 10^3 CFU/mL in a person with symptoms are also indicative of UTI.
- Fungal and parasitic UTIs are uncommon and are seen most frequently in the patient who is immunosuppressed, has diabetes mellitus (DM), or has taken multiple courses of antibiotics.

Classification

UTIs may be broadly classified as upper and lower UTIs according to their location within the urinary system. Infection of the upper urinary tract (involving the renal parenchyma, pelvis, and ureters) typically causes fever, chills, and flank pain, whereas a UTI confined to the lower urinary tract does not usually have systemic manifestations.

Specific terms are used to further delineate UTI location. For example, *pyelonephritis* implies infection of the renal parenchyma and collecting system, *cystitis* indicates inflammation of the bladder wall, and *urethritis* is inflammation of the urethra. *Urosepsis* is a UTI that has spread into the systemic circulation and is a life-threatening condition requiring emergency treatment.

Classifying a UTI as uncomplicated or complicated is also useful.

- *Uncomplicated infections* are those that occur in an otherwise normal urinary tract and usually only involve the bladder.
- *Complicated infections* include the coexisting presence of obstruction, stones, or catheters; the existence of DM or neurologic diseases; or a recurrent infection. The individual with a complicated infection is at an increased risk of renal damage.
- A *recurrent UTI* is reinfection caused by a second pathogen in a person who experienced a previous infection that was successfully eradicated. If a recurrent UTI occurs because the original infection is not adequately eradicated, it is classified as unresolved bacteriuria or bacterial persistence.

Pathophysiology

The urinary tract above the urethra is normally sterile, and organisms that cause UTIs are usually introduced by way of the ascending route from the urethra. Other less common routes are through the bloodstream or lymphatic system. Most infections are caused by gram-negative aerobic bacilli normally found in the gastrointestinal (GI) tract. Table 85 lists predisposing factors for UTIs.

- A common factor contributing to ascending infection is urologic instrumentation (e.g., catheterization, cystoscopy). Instrumentation allows bacteria that are normally present at the opening of the urethra to enter the urethra or bladder.
- Sexual intercourse promotes "milking" of bacteria from the vagina and perineum and may cause minor urethral trauma that predisposes women to UTIs.
- Rarely do UTIs result from a hematogenous route, where blood-borne bacteria secondarily invade the kidneys, ureters, or bladder from elsewhere in the body.

An important source of UTIs is health care-associated infections (HAI) previously called *nosocomial* infections. The cause is often *E. coli* and, less frequently, *Pseudomonas* organisms. Catheter-acquired UTIs are the most common HAI infections and are caused by development of bacterial biofilms that are found on the inner surface of the catheter.

Table 85	Predisposing Factors to Urinary Tract Infections

Factors Increasing Urinary Stasis
- Intrinsic obstruction (stone, tumor of urinary tract, urethral stricture, BPH)
- Extrinsic obstruction (tumor, fibrosis compressing urinary tract)
- Urinary retention (including neurogenic bladder and low bladder wall compliance)
- Renal impairment

Foreign Bodies
- Urinary tract calculi
- Catheters (indwelling, external condom catheter, ureteral stent, nephrostomy tube, intermittent catheterization)
- Urinary tract instrumentation (cystoscopy, urodynamics)

Anatomic Factors
- Congenital defects leading to obstruction or urinary stasis
- Fistula (abnormal opening) exposing urinary stream to skin, vagina, or fecal stream
- Shorter female urethra and colonization from normal vaginal flora
- Obesity

Factors Compromising Immune Response
- Aging
- Human immunodeficiency virus infection
- Diabetes mellitus

Functional Disorders
- Constipation
- Voiding dysfunction with detrusor sphincter dyssynergia

Other Factors
- Pregnancy
- Hypoestrogenic state
- Multiple sex partners (women)
- Use of spermicidal agents or contraceptive diaphragm (women)
- Poor personal hygiene

BPH, Benign prostatic hyperplasia.

U

Clinical Manifestations

Lower urinary tract symptoms are seen in UTIs of both the upper and lower urinary tracts.

- Symptoms include dysuria, frequent urination (more often than every 2 hours), urgency, and suprapubic discomfort or pressure.
- The urine may contain grossly visible blood (hematuria) or sediment, giving it a cloudy appearance.
- Flank pain, chills, and the presence of a fever indicate an infection involving the upper urinary tract (pyelonephritis).

Older adults tend to experience nonlocalized abdominal discomfort rather than dysuria and suprapubic pain. Patients over 80 years old may experience a slight decline in temperature.

Multiple factors may produce lower urinary tract symptoms similar to a UTI. For example, patients with bladder tumors or those receiving intravesical chemotherapy or pelvic radiation usually experience urinary frequency, urgency, and dysuria. Interstitial cystitis also produces urinary symptoms that are sometimes confused with a UTI (see Interstitial Cystitis/Painful Bladder Syndrome, p. 368).

Diagnostic Studies

- Dipstick urinalysis is obtained initially to identify presence of nitrites (indicating bacteriuria), white blood cells (WBCs), and leukocyte esterase (an enzyme present in WBCs indicating pyuria).
- After confirmation of bacteriuria and pyuria, a urine culture with sensitivity may be obtained.
- An intravenous pyelogram (IVP) or computed tomography (CT) scan may be obtained when obstruction of the urinary system is suspected.
- Renal ultrasound is the preferred urinary tract imaging technique because it is noninvasive, easy to perform, and relatively inexpensive.

Collaborative Care

Drug Therapy

Once a UTI has been diagnosed, appropriate antimicrobial therapy is initiated. Uncomplicated cystitis can be treated by a short-term course of antibiotics, typically for 1 to 3 days. In contrast, complicated UTIs require longer-term treatment, lasting 7 to 14 days or even longer.

- Trimethoprim-sulfamethoxazole (TMP-SMX, Bactrim) or nitrofurantoin (Macrodantin) is often used to empirically treat uncomplicated or initial UTIs.

- Fluoroquinolones (e.g., ciprofloxacin [Cipro], levofloxacin [Levaquin], gatifloxacin [Tequin]) may be used to treat complicated UTIs.
- A number of over-the-counter (OTC) or prescription drugs may be used in combination with antibiotic agents to relieve the discomfort associated with a UTI. Phenazopyridine (Pyridium) provides a soothing effect on the urinary tract mucosa. It also stains the urine a reddish orange that may be mistaken for blood in the urine and that may permanently stain underclothing.
- Combination agents, such as Urised (methenamine, phenylsalicylate, atropine, hyoscyamine), may also be used to relieve symptoms. Patients taking these agents should be advised that they can tint the urine blue or green.

Prophylactic or suppressive antibiotics are sometimes administered to patients who experience repeated UTIs. Although suppressive therapy is often effective on a short-term basis, this strategy is limited because of the risk of antibiotic resistance.

Nursing Management

Goals

The patient with a UTI will have relief from bothersome lower urinary tract symptoms, prevention of upper urinary tract involvement, and prevention of recurrence.

See NCP 46-1 for the patient with a UTI, Lewis et al., *Medical-Surgical Nursing*, ed. 8, p. 1126.

Nursing Diagnoses/Collaborative Problem

- Impaired urinary elimination
- Readiness for enhanced self-health management
- Potential complication: urosepsis

Nursing Interventions

Health promotion activities, especially for individuals who are at increased risk for UTI, include teaching preventive measures such as (1) emptying the bladder regularly and completely, (2) evacuating the bowel regularly, (3) wiping the perineal area from front to back after urination and defecation, and (4) drinking an adequate amount of liquid each day.

- Daily intake of cranberry or cranberry essence tablets may reduce the risk of recurrent UTIs in women.
- You have a major role in the prevention of HAI infections with avoidance of unnecessary catheterization and early removal of indwelling catheters.

In most cases, acute intervention for a patient with a UTI includes adequate fluid intake. Fluid intake flushes out bacteria before they have a chance to colonize in the bladder. Caffeine, alcohol, citrus juices, chocolate, and highly spiced foods or beverages should be avoided because they are potential bladder irritants.

- Application of local heat to the suprapubic area or lower back may relieve the discomfort associated with a UTI. A warm shower or sitting in a tub of warm water filled above the waist can also be effective in providing temporary relief.

▼ **Patient and Caregiver Teaching**

Instruct the patient about the prescribed drug therapy including side effects. Emphasize the importance of taking the full course of antibiotics.

- Instruct the patient to watch for any changes in the color or consistency of the urine and a decrease in or cessation of symptoms as a sign of therapy effectiveness.
- Teach patients to promptly report any of the following to their health care provider: persistence of bothersome LUTS beyond the antibiotic treatment course, onset of flank pain, or fever.
- The patient should be counseled that persistence of bothersome lower urinary tract symptoms beyond the antibiotic treatment course or the onset of flank pain or fever should be reported promptly to the health care provider.
- Your responsibility is to teach the patient and caregiver about the need for ongoing care. This includes taking antimicrobial drugs as ordered, maintaining adequate daily fluid intake, regular voiding (approximately every 3 to 4 hours), urinating before and after intercourse, and temporarily discontinuing the use of a diaphragm.
- Help the patient understand the need for follow-up care if symptoms do not resolve, worsen, or return once treatment is completed.

VAGINAL, CERVICAL, AND VULVAR INFECTIONS

Definition

Infection and inflammation of the vagina, cervix, and vulva tend to occur when the natural defenses of the acid vaginal secretions (maintained by sufficient estrogen levels) and the presence of *Lactobacillus* are disrupted. A woman's resistance may also be decreased as a result of aging, poor nutrition, and the use of drugs (e.g., antibiotics, hormones) that alter the bacterial flora or mucosa.

Pathophysiology

Organisms gain entrance to these areas through contaminated hands, clothing, and douche tips and during intercourse, surgery, and childbirth. Table 86 presents the etiology, clinical manifestations, diagnostic methods, and collaborative care of common infections of the lower genital tract.

- Most lower genital tract infections are related to sexual intercourse. Vulvar infections, such as herpes and genital warts, can be sexually transmitted when no lesions are present (see Herpes, Genital, p. 315, and Warts, Genital, p. 693).
- Oral contraceptives, antibiotics, and corticosteroids may produce changes in the vagina pH and trigger an overgrowth of the organisms present. For example, *Candida albicans* may be present in small numbers in the vagina. An overgrowth of this organism causes vulvovaginitis.

Clinical Manifestations

- Abnormal vaginal discharge and reddened vulvar lesions are common.
- In addition to a thick, white, curdy discharge, women with vulvovaginal candidiasis (VVC) often experience intense itching and dysuria.
- The hallmark of bacterial vaginosis is the fishy odor of the discharge.
- Older women may develop gynecologic problems, such as lichen sclerosis, a condition associated with intense itching in the genital skin area. The lesions are white initially, although scratching produces changes in the appearance.

Diagnostic Studies

- History, physical examination, and sexual history.
- Culture of ulcerative lesions for herpes.
- Vulvar dystrophies are examined by colposcope with biopsy specimens taken.
- Microscopy and culture of vaginal discharge are done.
- Bacterial vaginosis, VVC, and trichomoniasis are diagnosed by a wet mount.
- For cervicitis, endocervical cultures are obtained for chlamydia and gonorrhea. If purulent discharge is observed coming from the cervix, endocervical cells may be taken to do a Gram stain.

Collaborative Care

Antibiotics taken as directed will cure bacterial infections. Antifungal preparations (in oral or cream preparations) are indicated

Table 86 Infections of the Lower Genital Tract

Infection/Etiology	Clinical Manifestations and Diagnostic Methods	Drug Therapy
Vulvovaginal Candidiasis (VVC) (Monilial Vaginitis)		
Candida albicans (fungus)	Commonly found in mouth, gastrointestinal tract, and vagina; pruritus; thick white curdy discharge; KOH microscopic examination—pseudohyphae; pH 4.0-4.7	Antifungal agents (e.g., Monistat, Gyne-Lotrimin, Mycelex (available over the counter) available in cream or suppository Fluconazole (Diflucan) 150 mg orally as single dose
Trichomonas Vaginitis		
Trichomonas vaginalis (protozoa)	Sexually transmitted; pruritus; frothy greenish or gray discharge; hemorrhagic spots on cervix or vaginal walls; saline microscopic examination—swimming trichomonads; pH >4.5	Metronidazole (Flagyl) 2 g orally in single dose or 500 mg orally twice a day for 7 days for patient and partner

Bacterial Vaginosis		
Gardnerella vaginalis *Corynebacterium vaginale*	Mode of transmission unclear; watery discharge with fishy odor; may or may not have other symptoms; saline microscopic examination—epithelial cells; pH >4.5	Metronidazole (Flagyl) 500 mg orally or clindamycin (Cleocin) 300 mg orally twice a day for 7 days or clindamycin (Clindesse) vaginal cream in single dose; examine and treat partner
Cervicitis		
Chlamydia trachomatis	Sexually transmitted; mucopurulent discharge with postcoital spotting from cervical inflammation; culture for chlamydia and gonorrhea	Azithromycin (Zithromax) 1 g orally as single dose or doxycycline 100 mg orally twice a day for 7 days; treat partner with same drugs
Severe Recurrent Vaginitis		
Candida albicans (most often)	May be indication of HIV infection; all women who are unresponsive to first-line treatment should be offered HIV testing	Drug appropriate to opportunistic organism

HIV, Human immunodeficiency virus; *KOH,* potassium hydroxide.

V

for VVC. Women with vaginal conditions or cervical infection should abstain from intercourse for at least 1 week. Douching should be avoided, because it disrupts the normal protective mechanisms within the vagina. Sexual partners must be evaluated and treated if the patient is diagnosed with trichomoniasis, chlamydia, gonorrhea, syphilis, or human immunodeficiency virus (HIV).

Treatment of vulvar dystrophies is symptomatic and involves controlling the itching and hence the scratching. Interrupting the "itch-scratch cycle" prevents further secondary damage to the skin.

Nursing Management

You have the opportunity to educate women about common genital conditions and how women can reduce their risks. Recognizing symptoms that indicate a problem helps women seek care in a timely manner. Discussing problems that concern the patient's genitals or sexual intercourse is frequently difficult. Use a nonjudgmental attitude to make women feel more comfortable while empowering them to ask questions.

- When a woman is diagnosed with a genital condition, ensure that she fully understands the directions for treatment. Taking the full course of medication is especially important to decrease the chance of relapse. Because genitals are such a private area, use of graphs and models is especially helpful for patient teaching.
- When a woman is using a vaginal medication such as an antifungal cream for the first time, show her the applicator and how to fill it. Also teach where and how the applicator should be inserted by using visual aids or models.

VALVULAR HEART DISEASE

Description

Valvular heart disease is defined according to the affected valve or valves (mitral, aortic, tricuspid, pulmonary) and the type of functional alteration (*stenosis* or *regurgitation*).

- The pressure on either side of an open valve is normally equal. However, in a stenotic valve the valve opening is smaller, impeding the forward flow of blood and creating a pressure difference on the two sides of the open valve. The degree of stenosis (constriction or narrowing) is reflected in the pressure differences (i.e., the higher the gradient, the greater the stenosis).

- In regurgitation (also called *valvular incompetence* or *insufficiency*) incomplete closure of valve leaflets results in a backward flow of blood.

Valvular disorders occur in children and adolescents primarily from congenital conditions. Aortic stenosis and mitral regurgitation are the common valve disorders in older adults. Other causes of valve disease in adults include disorders related to acquired immunodeficiency syndrome (AIDS) and the use of some antiparkinson drugs (e.g., pergolide [Permax]).

Clinical manifestations of valvular heart disease are presented in Table 87.

Mitral Valve Stenosis

Pathophysiology. Most cases of adult mitral stenosis result from rheumatic heart disease. Less common causes include congenital mitral stenosis, rheumatoid arthritis, and systemic lupus erythematosus (SLE).

- Rheumatic endocarditis causes scarring of valve leaflets and chordae tendineae. Contractures and adhesions develop between the commissures (the junctional areas).
- The stenotic mitral valve takes on a "fish mouth" shape because of the thickening and shortening of the structures of the mitral valve. Flow obstruction increases left atrial pressure and volume, resulting in increased pressure in the pulmonary vasculature and eventually the right ventricle.

Clinical manifestations. The primary symptom is exertional dyspnea due to reduced lung compliance. Fatigue and palpitations from atrial fibrillation may also occur. Heart sounds include a loud first heart sound and a low-pitched, rumbling diastolic murmur (best heard at the apex with the stethoscope bell). Other clinical manifestations are identified in Table 87.

Mitral Valve Regurgitation

Pathophysiology. Mitral valve function depends on the integrity of mitral leaflets, chordae tendineae, papillary muscles, left atrium (LA), and left ventricle (LV). Any defect in any of these structures can result in regurgitation. Myocardial infarction with left ventricular failure increases the risk for rupture of the chordae tendineae and acute mitral regurgitation (MR).

- Most cases of MR are caused by myocardial infarction, chronic rheumatic heart disease, mitral valve prolapse, ischemic papillary muscle dysfunction, and infectious endocarditis.
- MR allows blood to flow backward from the LV to the LA because of incomplete valve closure during systole. Both chambers of the left side of the heart work harder to preserve an adequate cardiac output (CO).

Table 87	Clinical Manifestations of Valvular Heart Disease

Type of Valvular Heart Disease	Clinical Manifestations
Mitral valve stenosis	Dyspnea on exertion, hemoptysis; fatigue; atrial fibrillation on ECG, palpitations, stroke; loud, accentuated S_1; low-pitched, rumbling diastolic murmur
Mitral valve regurgitation	*Acute*—generally poorly tolerated; new systolic murmur with pulmonary edema and cardiogenic shock developing rapidly *Chronic*—weakness, fatigue, exertional dyspnea, palpitations; an S_3 gallop, holosystolic or pansystolic murmur
Mitral valve prolapse	Palpitations, dyspnea, chest pain, activity intolerance, syncope; midsystolic click, late or holosystolic murmur
Aortic valve stenosis	Angina, syncope, dyspnea on exertion, heart failure; normal or soft S_1, diminished or absent S_2, systolic murmur, prominent S_4
Aortic valve regurgitation	*Acute*—abrupt onset of profound dyspnea, chest pain, left ventricular failure, and cardiogenic shock *Chronic*—fatigue, exertional dyspnea, orthopnea, PND; water-hammer pulse; heaving precordial impulse; diminished or absent S_1 S_3, or S_4; soft high-pitched diastolic murmur, Austin-Flint murmur
Tricuspid and pulmonic stenosis	*Tricuspid*—peripheral edema, ascites, hepatomegaly; diastolic low-pitched, decrescendo murmur with increased intensity during inspiration *Pulmonic*—fatigue, loud midsystolic murmur

ECG, Electrocardiogram; *PND*, paroxysmal nocturnal dyspnea.

- In chronic MR, the additional volume load results in left atrial enlargement and left ventricular dilation and hypertrophy.
- In acute MR, abrupt dilation of the LA or LV does not occur. The sudden increase in pressure and volume transmits to the pulmonary bed, resulting in pulmonary edema and cardiogenic shock.

Clinical manifestations. Patients with acute MR will have thready, peripheral pulses and cool, clammy extremities. A low CO may mask a new systolic murmur. Rapid assessment (e.g., cardiac catheterization) and intervention (e.g., valve repair or replacement) are critical for a positive outcome.

Patients with chronic MR may remain asymptomatic for many years until the development of some degree of left ventricular failure. Symptoms are identified in Table 87.

Mitral Valve Prolapse

Pathophysiology. Mitral valve prolapse (MVP) is an abnormality of the mitral valve leaflets and papillary muscles or chordae that allows the leaflets to prolapse, or buckle, back into the left atrium during systole. It is the most common form of valvular heart disease in the United States.

- MVP is usually benign, but serious complications can occur, including mitral regurgitation, infective endocarditis, sudden cardiac death, and cerebral ischemia.
- There is an increased familial incidence in some patients resulting from a connective tissue defect affecting only the valve, or as part of Marfan's syndrome or other hereditary conditions that influence the structure of collagen in the body.

Clinical manifestations. MVP encompasses a broad spectrum of severity. Most patients are asymptomatic and remain so for their entire lives. Clinical manifestations may include those identified in Table 87.

- Patients may or may not have chest pain. If chest pain occurs, they tend to occur in clusters, especially during periods of emotional stress. Chest pain may occasionally be accompanied by dyspnea, palpitations, and syncope. See Table 88 for a teaching plan for patients with MVP.

Aortic Valve Stenosis

Pathophysiology. Congenitally abnormal stenotic aortic valves are generally found in childhood, adolescence, or young adulthood. In older patients, aortic stenosis is a result of rheumatic fever or senile fibrocalcific degeneration that may have an etiology similar to coronary artery disease.

Table 88	Patient and Caregiver Teaching Guide: Mitral Valve Prolapse

When teaching the patient and/or caregiver management of mitral valve prolapse, you should:

1. Teach patient the importance of antibiotic prophylaxis for endocarditis before undergoing certain dental or surgical procedures if the patient has MVP with regurgitation (see Table 37-3, Lewis et al., *Medical-Surgical Nursing*, ed. 8, p. 844).
2. Instruct patient to take medications as prescribed (e.g., β-adrenergic blockers to control palpitations, chest pain).
3. Advise patient to adopt healthy eating habits and avoid caffeine because it is a stimulant and may exacerbate symptoms.
4. Counsel patient who uses diet pills or other over-the-counter drugs to check for common ingredients that are stimulants (e.g., caffeine, ephedrine), as these will exacerbate symptoms.
5. Help patient to develop and implement an exercise program to maintain optimal health.
6. Instruct patient to contact health care provider or Emergency Medical Services if symptoms develop or worsen (e.g., palpitations, fatigue, shortness of breath, anxiety).

MVP, Mitral valve prolapse.

- In rheumatic valvular disease, fusion of the commissures and secondary calcification cause the valve leaflets to stiffen and retract, resulting in stenosis. Isolated aortic valve stenosis is usually nonrheumatic in origin.
- Aortic stenosis causes obstruction of flow from the left ventricle to the aorta during systole. The effect is left ventricular hypertrophy and increased myocardial oxygen consumption because of the increased myocardial mass.
- As the disease progresses and compensatory mechanisms fail, reduced CO leads to pulmonary hypertension and heart failure.

Clinical manifestations. Symptoms of aortic stenosis develop when the valve orifice becomes about one third of its normal size and reflect left ventricular failure. Common symptoms are presented in Table 87. Prognosis is poor for a patient with symptoms and whose valve obstruction is not relieved.

Aortic Valve Regurgitation
Pathophysiology. Aortic regurgitation may be the result of primary disease of the aortic valve leaflets, the aortic root, or both.

- Acute aortic regurgitation is caused by infective endo-carditis, trauma, or aortic dissection and constitutes a life-threatening emergency.
- Chronic aortic regurgitation is generally the result of rheumatic heart disease, a congenital bicuspid aortic valve, syphilis, or chronic arthritic conditions such as ankylosing spondylitis or reactive arthritis.
- Aortic regurgitation causes retrograde blood flow from the ascending aorta into the LV, resulting in volume overload.
- Myocardial contractility eventually declines, and blood volumes increase in the LA and pulmonary bed. Ultimately, pulmonary hypertension and right ventricular failure develop.

Clinical manifestations. Clinical manifestations of acute and chronic aortic valve regurgitation are presented in Table 87.

Tricuspid and Pulmonic Valve Disease

Diseases of the tricuspid and pulmonic valves are uncommon, with stenosis occurring more frequently than regurgitation. Tricuspid stenosis results in right atrial enlargement and elevated systemic venous pressures. Pulmonic stenosis results in right ventricular hypertension and hypertrophy. Table 87 presents clinical manifestations of these valve diseases.

Diagnostic Studies: Valvular Heart Disease

- Chest x-ray reveals heart size, alterations in pulmonary circulation, and valve calcification.
- Electrocardiogram (ECG) shows variations in heart rate (HR), rhythm, and possible ischemia or chamber enlargement.
- Echocardiogram reveals valve structure, function, and heart chamber size.
- Transesophageal echocardiography and Doppler color-flow imaging help diagnose and monitor valvular heart disease progression.
- Cardiac catheterization detects chamber pressure changes and pressure gradients (differences) across the valves.

Collaborative Care: Valvular Heart Disease

An important aspect of conservative therapy is the prevention of recurrent rheumatic fever and infective endocarditis. Treatment depends on the valve involved and the severity of disease. It focuses on preventing exacerbations of heart failure, acute pulmonary edema, thromboembolism, and recurrent endocarditis. Heart failure is treated with vasodilators, positive inotropes, β-adrenergic blockers, diuretics, and a low-sodium diet.

- Anticoagulant therapy prevents and treats systemic or pulmonary emboli, and it is also used as a prophylactic measure in patients with atrial fibrillation.
- Dysrhythmias, especially atrial dysrhythmias, are common and treated with β-adrenergic blockers, digoxin, antidysrhythmic drugs, or electrical cardioversion.
- An alternative treatment for some patients with valvular heart disease is the *percutaneous transluminal balloon valvuloplasty* (PTBV) procedure. Balloon valvuloplasty is used for pulmonic, aortic, and mitral stenosis. The procedure, performed in the cardiac catheterization laboratory, involves threading a balloon-tipped catheter from the femoral artery to the stenotic valve so that the balloon may be inflated in an attempt to separate valve leaflets.
- The PTBV procedure is generally indicated for older adult patients and patients who are poor surgical candidates. PTBV has fewer complications than valve replacement.

Surgical Therapy

The type of surgery used for a particular patient depends on the valves involved, the pathology and severity of the disease, and the patient's clinical condition.

- Valve repair is typically the surgical procedure of choice. It is often used in mitral or tricuspid valvular heart disease and has a lower operative mortality rate than valve replacement.
- Mitral *commissurotomy* (valvulotomy) is the procedure of choice for patients with pure mitral stenosis. The open method of commissurotomy (which has largely replaced the older, less precise closed method) requires the use of cardiopulmonary bypass, removal of thrombi from the atrium, excision of the left atrial appendage, commissure incision, and, as indicated, separation of fused chordae, splitting of underlying papillary muscle, and debriding the calcified valve.
- Open surgical *valvuloplasty* involves repairing the valve or suturing the torn leaflets, chordae tendineae, and papillary muscles. It is primarily performed to treat mitral regurgitation or tricuspid regurgitation.
- Further repair or reconstruction of the valve may be necessary and can be achieved by *annuloplasty*, a procedure also used in cases of mitral or tricuspid regurgitation. Annuloplasty entails reconstruction of valve leaflets and the annulus, with or without the aid of prosthetic rings (e.g., Carpentier ring).

Prosthetic valves. Valve replacement may be required for mitral, aortic, tricuspid, and occasionally, pulmonic valvular disease. The surgical treatment of choice for combined aortic stenosis and aortic regurgitation is valve replacement.

- Prosthetic valves are categorized as *mechanical* or *biologic (tissue) valves.* Mechanical valves are made of combinations of metal alloys, pyrolite carbon, and Dacron. Biologic valves are constructed from bovine, porcine, and human (cadaver) cardiac tissue. Mechanical prosthetic valves are more durable and last longer than biologic tissue valves but have an increased risk of thromboembolism, and require long-term anticoagulant therapy. Biologic valves do not require anticoagulant therapy because of their low thrombogenicity. However, they are less durable and tend to cause early calcification, tissue degeneration, and stiffening of leaflets.
- Long-term anticoagulation is recommended for all patients with mechanical prostheses and for those with biologic valves who have atrial fibrillation. Some patients with biologic tissue valves or annuloplasty with prosthetic rings may need anticoagulation after the first few months after surgery
- The choice of valves depends on many factors. For example, if a patient cannot take anticoagulant therapy (e.g., women of childbearing age), a biologic valve is considered. A mechanical valve may be best for a younger patient because it is more durable and lasts longer. For patients older than 65 years, durability is less important than the risks of bleeding from anticoagulants so most receive a biologic valve.

Nursing Management
Goals
The patient with valve heart disease will have normal cardiac function, improved activity tolerance, and an understanding of the disease process and preventive measures.

See eNCP 37-1 for the patient with valve heart disease on the Evolve website at http://evolve.elsevier.com/Lewis/medsurg

Nursing Diagnoses
- Activity intolerance
- Excess fluid volume
- Decreased cardiac output
- Deficient knowledge

Nursing Interventions
Diagnosing and treating streptococcal infection and providing prophylactic antibiotics for patients with a history of rheumatic fever are critical to prevent acquired rheumatic valve disease. The

patient at risk for endocarditis and any patient with certain high-risk cardiac conditions must also receive prophylactic antibiotics.

- The patient must adhere to recommended therapies. The individual with a history of rheumatic fever, endocarditis, and congenital heart disease should know the symptoms of valvular heart disease so early medical treatment may begin.

A patient with progressive valvular heart disease may require hospitalization or outpatient care for the management of HF, endocarditis, embolic disease, or dysrhythmias. HF is the most common reason for ongoing medical care.

Your role is to implement and evaluate the effectiveness of therapeutic interventions.

- Design activities with the patient's limitations in mind. An appropriate exercise plan can increase cardiac tolerance. However, activities that regularly produce fatigue and dyspnea should be restricted.
- Your patient's activities of daily living plan should have an emphasis on conserving energy, setting priorities, and taking planned rest periods.
- Referral to a vocational counselor may be necessary if the patient has a physically or emotionally demanding job.
- Perform ongoing cardiac assessments to monitor the effectiveness of cardiac medications. Teaching regarding the actions and side effects of drugs is important to achieve compliance.
- The patient on anticoagulation therapy (e.g., warfarin [Coumadin]) after surgery for valve replacement must have the international normalized ratio (INR) checked regularly to determine adequacy of therapy.

▼ **Patient and Caregiver Teaching**

- Teach the patient when to seek medical care. Any manifestations of infection, HF, signs of bleeding, and any planned invasive or dental procedures require the patient to notify the health care provider.
- The patient must understand the importance of prophylactic antibiotic therapy to prevent endocarditis. If the valve disease was caused by rheumatic fever, ongoing prophylaxis to prevent recurrence is necessary.
- Strongly discourage tobacco use.
- Encourage patients to wear a Medic-Alert bracelet.

Emphasize that valve surgery is not a cure and that regular follow-up with a health care provider will be required.

VARICOSE VEINS

Description

Varicose veins (varicosities) are dilated, tortuous subcutaneous veins commonly found in the saphenous vein system. They may be small and innocuous or large and bulging.

- *Primary* varicose veins (idiopathic) are caused by a congenital weakness of the veins and are more common in women.
- *Secondary* varicosities typically result from a previous venous thromboembolism (VTE). Secondary varicose veins may also occur in the esophagus as varices, in the anorectal area as hemorrhoids, and as abnormal arteriovenous (AV) connections.

Pathophysiology

The etiology of varicose veins is caused by multiple factors. Risk factors include congenital weakness of the vein structure, use of oral contraceptives or hormone replacement therapy, increasing age, obesity, pregnancy, venous obstruction resulting from thrombosis or extrinsic pressure by tumors, or occupations that require prolonged standing.

- Although the exact etiology remains unknown, it is thought that the vein valve leaflets are stretched and become incompetent (do not fit together properly). Incompetent vein valves allow retrograde blood flow, particularly when standing, resulting in increased venous pressure and further venous distention.

Clinical Manifestations

Discomfort from varicose veins varies dramatically among people and tends to be worsened after episodes of superficial thrombophlebitis. The most common symptom is a heavy, achy pain after prolonged standing, which is relieved by walking or limb elevation. Some patients feel pressure or a cramplike, burning sensation. Swelling and/or nocturnal leg cramps may also occur.

Superficial thrombophlebitis is the most frequent complication of varicose veins and may occur spontaneously or after trauma, surgical procedures, or pregnancy.

Diagnostic Studies

- Duplex ultrasound is the most widely used test to diagnose deep varicose veins because it can detect obstruction and reflux in the venous system with considerable accuracy.
- Superficial varicose veins can be diagnosed by appearance.

Collaborative Care

Treatment is usually not indicated if varicose veins are only a cosmetic problem. If venous insufficiency develops, collaborative care involves rest with limb elevation, graduated compression stockings, and exercise, such as walking.

Sclerotherapy involves the injection of a substance that obliterates venous telangiectasis (i.e., spider veins) and small superficial varicose veins. Direct intravenous (IV) injection of a sclerosing agent such as hypertonic saline induces inflammation and results in eventual thrombosis of the vein. This procedure can be performed safely in an office setting and causes minimal discomfort. After injection the leg is wrapped with thigh-high graduated compression stockings or an elastic bandage for 24 to 72 hours to maintain pressure over the vein. Long-term use of compression stockings is advised to help prevent the development of further varicosities.

Noninvasive options for the treatment of isolated, small venous telangiectasis include laser therapy and high-intensity pulse-light therapy. These methods work by using heat or light to injure the vein endothelium and cause vessel sclerosis.

Surgical intervention is indicated for recurrent superficial vein thrombosis or when chronic venous insufficiency cannot be controlled with conservative therapy. Traditional surgical intervention involves ligation of the entire vein (usually the greater saphenous) and dissection and removal of its incompetent tributaries. An alternative, but time-consuming, technique is ambulatory phlebectomy, which involves pulling the varicosity through a "stab" incision followed by excision of the vein. A newer, less invasive procedure is endovenous ablation of the saphenous vein. Ablation involves the insertion of a catheter that emits energy. This causes collapse and sclerosis of the vein.

Nursing Management

Prevention is a key factor related to varicose veins. Teach the patient to avoid sitting or standing for long periods, maintain ideal body weight, take precautions against injury to the extremities, avoid wearing constrictive clothing, and walk daily.

After vein ligation surgery, encourage the patient to deep breathe, which helps promote venous return. Check the extremities regularly for color, movement, sensation, temperature, presence of edema, and pedal pulses. Bruising and discoloration are considered normal.

- Postoperatively, elevate the legs 15 degrees to limit edema. Apply graduated compression stockings and remove every 8 hours for short periods, and reapply.

Long-term management of varicose veins is directed toward improving circulation, relieving discomfort, improving cosmetic appearance, and avoiding complications such as superficial thrombophlebitis and ulceration. Varicose veins can recur in other veins after surgery.

▼ **Patient and Caregiver Teaching**

- Teach the patient the proper use and care of custom fitted graduated compression stockings. The patient should apply stockings in bed, before rising in the morning.
- Stress the importance of periodic positioning of the legs above the heart.
- The patient with a job that requires long periods of standing or sitting needs to frequently flex and extend their hips, legs, and ankles and change positions.

VENOUS THROMBOSIS

Description

Venous thrombosis is the formation of a thrombus in association with inflammation of the vein. It is the most common disorder of the veins and is classified as either superficial thrombophlebitis or deep vein thrombosis (DVT) (Table 89). *Venous thromboembolism (VTE)* is the preferred terminology and represents the spectrum of pathology from DVT to pulmonary embolism (PE).

Pathophysiology

Three important factors *(Virchow's triad)* in the etiology of venous thrombosis are venous stasis, damage of the endothelium (inner lining of the vein), and hypercoagulability of the blood. The patient at risk for venous thrombosis usually has predisposing conditions related to these three disorders.

Venous stasis occurs when the valves are dysfunctional or the muscles of the extremities are inactive. Venous stasis occurs more frequently in people who are obese, have chronic heart failure or atrial fibrillation, have been on long trips without regular exercise, undergo a prolonged surgical procedure, or are immobile for long periods (e.g., with spinal cord injuries or fractured hips).

Damage to the endothelium of the vein may be caused by direct (e.g., surgery, intravascular catheterization, trauma, fracture, burns) or indirect (chemotherapy, vasculitis, sepsis, diabetes) injury to the vessel. Damaged endothelium has decreased fibrinolytic properties, which facilitates thrombus development.

Table 89	Comparison of Superficial Vein Thrombosis and Venous Thromboembolism	
	Superficial Vein Thrombosis	**Venous Thromboembolism**
Usual location	Superficial arm veins (e.g., IV catheters) and superficial leg veins (e.g., varicosities)	Deep veins of arms (e.g., axillary, subclavian), legs (e.g., femoral), pelvis (e.g., iliac, inferior or superior vena cava), and pulmonary system
Clinical findings	Tenderness, redness, warmth, pain, inflammation, and induration along the course of the superficial vein; vein appears as a palpable cord; edema rarely occurs	Tenderness to pressure over involved vein, induration of overlying muscle, venous distention; edema; may have mild to moderate pain; deep reddish color to area because of venous congestion. NOTE: Some patients may have no obvious physical changes in the affected extremity
Sequelae	Usually benign; if untreated, venous thromboembolism may occur if clot extends to deep veins	Embolization to lungs (pulmonary embolism) may occur and may result in death;* pulmonary hypertension and chronic venous insufficiency with or without venous leg ulceration may develop

*See Chapter 28 for clinical findings related to pulmonary embolism.

Hypercoagulability of the blood occurs in many hematologic disorders, particularly polycythemia and severe anemias, as well as sepsis and various malignancies.

- Women who smoke, use oral contraceptives or hormone replacement therapy, are older than age 35 years, and have a family history of VTE are at extremely high risk to develop a thrombotic event.

Localized platelet aggregation and fibrin entrap RBCs, WBCs, and more platelets to form a thrombus. Thrombus formation results from the adherence of red blood cells (RBCs), white blood cells (WBCs), platelets, and fibrin. A frequent site of thrombus formation is the valve cusps of veins.

- As the thrombus enlarges, blood cells and fibrin collect behind it, producing a larger clot with a "tail" that eventually occludes the lumen of the vein.
- If a thrombus only partially occludes the vein, the thrombus becomes covered by endothelial cells and the thrombotic process stops.
- If the thrombus does not become detached, it undergoes lysis or becomes firmly organized and adherent within 5 to 7 days.
- The organized thrombi may detach and result an embolus that flows the venous circulation to the heart and lodges in the pulmonary circulation, becoming a pulmonary embolism (PE).

Clinical Manifestations

- The patient with *superficial thrombophlebitis* may have a palpable, firm, subcutaneous cordlike vein with the surrounding area tender to the touch, reddened, and warm. A mild systemic temperature elevation and leukocytosis may be present. Edema of the extremity may occur. The most common cause of superficial thrombophlebitis in the upper exremities is vein trauma caused by cannulation of a vein or IV therapy. Superficial thrombophlebitis in the lower extremities which involves one or more varicose veins, are more common in pregnant women and obese patients with limited mobility, or older patients with long-standing venous insufficiency.
- The patient with lower extremity VTE may have no symptoms or may have unilateral leg edema, pain, warm skin, erythema, and a temperature above 100.4° F (38° C). If the calf is involved it may be tender to palpation. A positive *Homans' sign,* pain on dorsiflexion of the foot when the leg is raised, is a classic but unreliable sign with frequent false positives. If the inferior vena cava is involved, symptoms may occur in the arms, neck, back, and face.

Complications

The most serious complications of VTE are PE, chronic venous insufficiency, and phlegmasia cerulea dolens. PE is a life-threatening complication of VTE (see Pulmonary Embolism, p. 531).

- *Chronic venous insufficiency* results from valvular destruction, allowing retrograde flow of venous blood. Persistent edema, increased pigmentation, secondary varicosities, ulceration, and cyanosis of the limb when it is placed in a dependent position may develop in a person with this complication. Signs and symptoms of chronic venous insufficiency often do not develop until several years after VTE.
- *Phlegmasia cerulea dolens* (swollen, blue, painful leg), a very rare complication, may develop in a patient in the advanced stages of cancer. It results from severe lower extremity VTE(s) that involve the major leg veins causing near-total occlusion of venous outflow. Patients typically experience sudden, massive swelling, deep pain, and intense cyanosis of the extremity.

Diagnostic Studies

- Platelet count, hemoglobin (Hb), hematocrit (Hct), D-dimer testing, and coagulation tests (bleeding time, prothrombin time [PT], partial thromboplastin time [PTT]) may be altered if underlying blood dyscrasias are present.
- Venous compression ultrasound evaluates deep femoral, popliteal, and posterior tibial veins.
- Duplex scanning and venous Doppler evaluation determine location and extent of venous thrombi.
- Venogram (phlebogram) can determine clot location.

Collaborative Care

Management of the patient with superficial thrombophlebitis involves the immediate removal of the IV catheter. If edema is present, elevate the extremity. Warm, moist heat may be used to relieve pain and treat inflammation.

- Oral nonsteroidal antiinflammatory drugs (NSAIDs) (e.g., diclofenac [Voltaren]), topical NSAIDs (e.g., diclofenac gel [Solaraze]), or topical heparin gel may be used.
- Systemic anticoagulants are not recommended for infusion-related superficial thrombophlebitis.
- Teach the patient to wear graduated compression stockings and perform mild exercise such as walking.
- In patients at risk for VTE, a variety of interventions are used.
- Early ambulation and foot and leg exercises for bed-ridden patients are the easiest and most cost-effective method to prevent VTE.
- Graduated compression stockings (e.g., TED hose) are used to apply pressure to the lower extremities and prevent

venous stasis. It is critical that you accurately measure the patient's legs, obtain the correct stocking size and length (thigh-high or knee-high), apply the stockings properly, and teach the patient and caregiver regarding proper use.

- Sequential compression devices (SCDs) are inflatable garments wrapped around the legs that apply intermittent external pressure to the lower extremities. They are often used in combination with graduated compression stockings and benefits are similar.

Anticoagulant therapy is routinely used for VTE prevention and treatment. The goal of anticoagulation therapy for VTE prophylaxis is to prevent clot formation; whereas the goals in the treatment of confirmed VTE are to prevent propagation of the clot, development of any new thrombi, and embolization.

Currently, four major classes of anticoagulants are available: (1) vitamin K antagonists, (2) indirect thrombin inhibitors, (3) direct thrombin inhibitors, and (4) factor Xa inhibitors (see Table 38-9 anticoagulant therapy, Lewis et al., *Medical-Surgical Nursing*, ed. 8, p. 886). The use of aspirin alone for VTE thromboprophylaxis is not recommended for any patient group. Anticoagulant therapy does not dissolve the clot. Lysis of the clot begins spontaneously through the body's intrinsic fibrinolytic system.

Although most patients are managed medically, a small number of patients undergo surgery. Surgical options include open venous thrombectomy and inferior vena cava interruption. Venous thrombectomy involves the removal of a thrombus through an incision in the vein.

Nursing Management
Goals
The patient with venous thrombosis will have pain relief, decreased edema, no skin ulceration, no bleeding complications, and no evidence of PE.
Nursing Diagnoses/Collaborative Problems
- Acute pain
- Ineffective health maintenance
- Risk for impaired skin integrity
- Potential complication: bleeding related to anticoagulant therapy
- Potential complication: pulmonary embolism
Nursing Interventions
Nursing care for the patient with VTE is directed toward the prevention of emboli formation and the reduction of inflammation. Because effective anticoagulation is essential, review with the patient any medications, vitamins, minerals, and dietary and herbal

supplements being taken that may interfere with anticoagulation therapy.

- Always check the results of appropriate tests before initiating, administering, or adjusting anticoagulant therapy.
- Bed rest with limb elevation may be prescribed for patients with an acute VTE. Early exercise after VTE results in a more rapid decrease in edema and limb pain. Teach the patient and caregiver the importance of exercise and assist the patient to ambulate several times a day.

▼ **Patient and Caregiver Teaching**

Focus discharge teaching on modification of VTE risk factors, use of graduated compression stockings, importance of monitoring laboratory values, medication instructions, and guidelines for follow-up.

- Once the edema is resolved, measure the patient for custom-fit, graduated compression stockings. Stocking use (or sleeves in the case of an upper extremity VTE) is recommended for at least 2 years after a VTE.
- If appropriate, tell the patient to stop smoking and avoid all nicotine products. Instruct the patient to avoid constrictive clothing.
- Patients need to avoid standing or sitting in a motionless, leg-dependent position. Encourage frequent knee flexion, ankle rotation, and active walking during long periods of sitting or standing, such as on car or airplane trips.
- Teach the patient and caregiver about signs and symptoms of PE such as sudden onset of dyspnea, tachypnea, and pleuritic chest pain.
- The patient and caregiver need thorough education regarding medication dosage, actions, and side effects, the need for routine blood tests, and what symptoms to report to the health care provider.
- Teach patients taking warfarin (Coumadin) not to vary their dietary intake of foods containing vitamin K (e.g., green leafy vegetables) and to avoid any supplements containing vitamin K. Encourage proper hydration to prevent additional hypercoagulability of the blood, which may occur with dehydration.
- Assist the patient to develop an exercise program with an emphasis on walking and swimming. Water exercise is particularly beneficial because of the gentle, even pressure of the water.

WARTS, GENITAL

Description

Genital warts (condylomata acuminata) are caused by the human papillomavirus (HPV). There are over 100 types of papillomaviruses, and about 40 of these affect the genital tract. HPV is a highly contagious sexually transmitted disease (STD) seen frequently in young, sexually active adults. Infection with HPV is the most common STD in the United States with an estimated 20 million Americans infected. Most individuals who have HPV do not know they are infected because symptoms are often not present.

Pathophysiology

Minor trauma during intercourse can cause abrasions that allow HPV to enter the body. The epithelial cells infected with HPV undergo transformation and proliferation to form a warty growth. The incubation period of the virus is generally 3 to 4 months.

HPV types appear to be harmless and self-limiting (e.g., types 6 and 11 commonly found in genital warts), whereas others are thought to have oncogenic (cancer-causing) potential (e.g., types 16 and 18).

Clinical Manifestations

- Genital warts are discrete, single, or multiple papillary growths that are white to gray and pink flesh colored.
- They may grow and join together to form large, cauliflower-like masses. Most patients have 1 to 10 lesions.
- In men, the warts may occur on the penis and scrotum, around the anus, or in the urethra.
- In women, the warts may be located on the vulva, vagina, and cervix and in the perianal area.
- Itching may occur with anogenital warts. Bleeding on defecation may occur with anal warts.
- An infected mother may transmit the condition to her newborn. Cesarean delivery is not routinely indicated unless the birth canal becomes blocked by massive warts.

W

Diagnostic Studies

A diagnosis is frequently made on the basis of the gross appearance of the lesions. HPV cannot currently be confirmed by culture. Serologic and cytologic testing can be used to rule out carcinomas or benign neoplasms. The HPV DNA test can

- Determine if women with abnormal Pap test results need further follow-up

- Identify women who are infected with high-risk HPV strains associated with cervical cancer.

Collaborative Care

The primary goal when treating visible genital warts is the removal of symptomatic warts which may not decrease infectivity. Genital warts are difficult to treat and often require multiple office visits with a variety of treatment modalities. Therapy may be modified if a patient has not improved after three treatments or if the warts have not completely disappeared after six treatments.

- A common treatment is the use of 80% to 90% trichloroacetic acid (TCA) or bichloroacetic acid (BCA) applied directly on the wart.
- Podophyllin resin (10% to 25%), a cytotoxic agent, is recommended for small external genital warts.
- Podofilox (Condylox) liquid or gel can be applied by the patient for 3 successive days followed by 4 days of no treatment.
- Imiquimod cream (Aldara), an immune response modifier, can be applied three times per week for up to 16 weeks or until lesions resolve.

If warts do not regress with these therapies, treatments such as cryotherapy with liquid nitrogen, electrocautery, laser therapy, intralesional use of α-interferon, and surgical excision may be indicated.

Because treatment does not destroy the virus, recurrences and reinfection are possible, and careful long-term follow-up care is advised.

Vaccines (i.e., Gardasil, Cervarix) are now available to protect against HPV types 6, 11, 16, and 18. These types cause most cases of cervical cancer and genital warts and some vaginal and vulvar cancers. The vaccine is given in three IM doses over a 6-month period and has few side effects.

Nursing Management: Genital Warts

See Nursing Management: Sexually Transmitted Diseases, p. 570.

PART TWO

Treatments and Procedures

AMPUTATION

Description

An estimated 1.7 million people in the United States are living with limb loss. The middle and older age groups have the highest incidence of amputation because of the effects of peripheral vascular disease, atherosclerosis, and vascular changes related to diabetes mellitus.

Clinical indications for an amputation depend on the underlying disease or trauma. Common indications for amputation include circulatory impairment resulting from a peripheral vascular disorder, traumatic and thermal injuries, malignant tumors, uncontrolled or widespread infection of the extremity (i.e., gas gangrene, osteomyelitis), and congenital disorders.

- The goal of amputation surgery is to preserve extremity length and function while removing all infected, pathologic, or ischemic tissue. (See Fig. 63-20 for the levels of amputation of the upper and lower extremities, Lewis et al., *Medical-Surgical Nursing,* ed. 8, p. 1611.)

Nursing Management

Control of causative illnesses such as peripheral vascular disease, diabetes mellitus (DM), chronic osteomyelitis, and skin ulcers can eliminate or delay the need for amputation.

- Teach patients with these conditions to carefully examine the lower extremities daily and report problems, such as change in skin color or temperature, decrease in or absence of sensation in the feet and/or toes, tingling, burning pain, or the presence of a lesion, to the health care provider.
- Instruction in proper safety precautions in recreational activities and the performance of potentially hazardous work is an important nursing responsibility, especially for the occupational health nurse.

It is important for you to recognize the tremendous psychologic and social implications of an amputation for the patient. The disruption in body image caused by an amputation often causes a patient to go through psychologic stages similar to the grieving process. Allow the patient to go through the grieving process. Also help the patient's caregiver to work through the transitional process to arrive at a realistic and positive attitude about the future.

Preoperative Care

Before surgery, reinforce information that the patient and caregiver have received about the reasons for the amputation, the proposed prosthesis, and the mobility-training program.

- The patient should receive instruction in the performance of upper extremity exercises such as push-ups in bed or the wheelchair to promote arm strength. This instruction is essential for crutch walking and gait training.
- If a compression bandage is to be used after surgery, instruct the patient about its purpose and how it will be applied. If an immediate prosthesis is planned, discuss general ambulation expectations.

Warn the patient that he or she might feel as though the amputated limb is still present after surgery. This phenomenon, termed *phantom limb sensation,* occurs in 90% of amputees. The patient may have feelings of coldness and heaviness or cramping, shooting, burning, or crushing pain.

- As recovery and ambulation progress, phantom limb sensation and pain usually subside, although the pain can become chronic.

Postoperative Care

Prevention and detection of complications are important during the postoperative period. Carefully monitor the patient's vital signs and dressing for hemorrhage in the operative area. Careful attention to sterile technique during dressing changes reduces the potential for wound infection.

- If an immediate postoperative prosthesis has been applied, careful surveillance of the surgical site is required. A surgical tourniquet must always be available for emergency use. If excessive bleeding occurs, notify the surgeon immediately.
- Not all patients are candidates for prostheses. The seriously ill or debilitated patient may not have the upper body strength or energy required to use a prosthesis. Mobility with a wheelchair may be the most realistic goal for this type of patient.

Flexion contractures may delay the rehabilitation process. The most common and debilitating contracture is hip flexion. Patients should avoid sitting in a chair for more than 1 hour with hips flexed or having pillows under the surgical extremity.

▼ Patient and Caregiver Teaching

As the patient's overall condition improves, an exercise regimen is normally started under the supervision of the health care provider and physical therapist.

- Active exercise and conditioning are essential in developing ambulation skills. Active range-of-motion exercises of all joints should be started as soon after surgery as the patient's pain level and medical status permit.

| Table 90 | Patient and Caregiver Teaching Guide: Following an Amputation | A |

You should include the following instructions when teaching the patient after an amputation:

1. Inspect the residual limb daily for signs of skin irritation, especially erythema, excoriation, and odor. Pay particular attention to areas prone to pressure.
2. Discontinue use of the prosthesis if an irritation develops. Have the area checked before resuming use of the prosthesis.
3. Wash the residual limb thoroughly each night with warm water and a bacteriostatic soap. Rinse thoroughly and dry gently. Expose the residual limb to air for 20 minutes.
4. Do not use any substance such as lotions, alcohol, powders, or oil on residual limb unless prescribed by the health care provider.
5. Wear only a residual limb sock that is in good condition and supplied by the prosthetist.
6. Change residual limb sock daily. Launder in a mild soap, squeeze, and lay flat to dry.
7. Use prescribed pain management techniques.
8. Perform ROM to all joints daily. Perform general strengthening exercises, including the upper extremities daily.
9. Do not elevate the residual limb on a pillow.
10. Lay prone with hip in extension for 30 minutes three or four times daily.

ROM, Range of motion.

- Crutch walking is started as soon as the patient is physically able. After an immediate postsurgical fitting, orders related to weight bearing must be carefully followed to avoid disruption of the skin flap and delay of the healing process.
- Before discharge, instruct the patient and caregiver related to residual limb care, ambulation, prevention of contractures, recognition of complications, exercise, and follow-up care. Table 90 outlines patient and caregiver teaching after an amputation.

ARTIFICIAL AIRWAYS: ENDOTRACHEAL TUBES

Description

An artificial airway is created by inserting a tube into the trachea, bypassing upper airway and laryngeal structures. The tube is placed into the trachea through the mouth or nose past the larynx *(endo-tracheal [ET] intubation)* or through a stoma in the neck *(trache-ostomy)*. ET intubation is more common in patients in the intensive care unit (ICU). ET intubation is more common in ICU patients than a tracheostomy. It is performed quickly and safely at the bedside. Fig. 16 shows the parts of an ET tube.

- Indications for ET intubation include (1) upper airway obstruction, (2) apnea, (3) high risk of aspiration, (4) inef-fective clearance of secretions, and (5) respiratory distress.

If *oral intubation* is selected, the ET tube is passed through the mouth and vocal cords and into the trachea with the aid of a laryn-goscope or bronchoscope.

- Oral ET intubation is the procedure of choice for most emer-gencies because the airway can be secured rapidly. Com-pared with the nasal route, a larger-diameter tube can be used for oral intubation. A larger-bore ET tube provides less airway resistance and easier performance of suctioning and fiberoptic bronchoscopy if needed.
- There are risks associated with oral ET intubation. It may be difficult to place an oral tube if head and neck mobility is limited (e.g., suspected spinal cord injury). Teeth can be chipped or inadvertently dislodged during the procedure. Salivation is increased and swallowing is difficult. Often a patient will obstruct the ET tube by biting down on it. Seda-tion along with a bite block or oropharyngeal airway can be used to avoid potential problems. The ET tube and bite block (if used) should be secured (separately) to the face. Mouth care is a challenge.

In *nasal ET intubation*, the ET is placed blindly (i.e., without seeing the larynx) through the nose, nasopharynx, and vocal cords.

- Nasal intubation is contraindicated in patients with facial fractures, suspected fractures at the base of the skull, and postoperatively after cranial surgeries.
- The nasal tube may be uncomfortable for some because it presses on the septum, whereas others may prefer it because there is no need for a bite block and mouth care is more easily accomplished.
- However, nasal ET tubes are more subject to kinking than oral tubes; the work of breathing is greater because the longer, narrower tube offers more airflow resistance; and suctioning and secretion removal are more difficult. Nasal tubes have been linked with increased incidence of sinus infection and ventilator-associated pneumonia.

Unless endotracheal intubation is emergent, consent for the pro-cedure is obtained. Tell the patient and caregiver the reason for ET

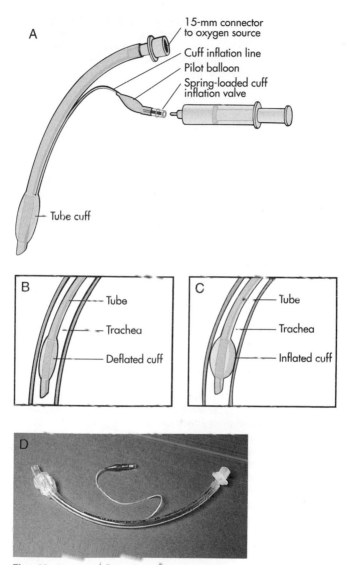

Fig. 16. Endotracheal tube, **A,** Parts of an endotracheal tube. **B,** Tube in place with cuff deflated. **C** Tube in place with the cuff inflated. **D,** Photo of tube before placement.

intubation, the steps that will occur in the procedure, and the patient's role in the procedure (if indicated). It is also important to explain that while intubated, the patient will not be able to speak, but that you will provide other means of communication. Also explain that the patient's hands may be restrained for safety purposes.

All patients undergoing intubation and receiving mechanical ventilation need to have a self-inflating *bag-valve-mask* (BVM) (e.g., *Ambu bag*) available and attached to O_2, suctioning equipment ready at the bedside, and IV access. The procedure for ET intubation is described in Lewis et al., *Medical-Surgical Nursing,* ed. 8, p. 1699.

Management of a patient with an artificial airway is often a shared responsibility between you and the respiratory therapist with specific management tasks determined by institutional policy. Nursing responsibilities for the patient with an artificial airway may include some or all of the following (1) maintaining correct tube placement, (2) maintaining proper cuff inflation, (3) monitoring oxygenation and ventilation, (4) maintaining tube patency, (5) assessing for complications, (6) providing oral care and maintaining skin integrity, and (7) fostering comfort and communication. A nursing care plan for the patient on a mechanical ventilator is available at http://evolve.elsevier.com/Lewis/medsurg.

Monitor the patient with an ET tube for proper placement at least every 2 to 4 hours. Observe for symmetric chest wall movement and auscultate to confirm bilateral breath sounds.

- It is an emergency if the ET tube is not positioned properly. If this occurs, stay with the patient, maintain the airway, support ventilation, and secure the appropriate assistance to immediately reposition the tube.
- It may be necessary to ventilate the patient with a BVM device (Ambu bag) and 100% O_2. If a malpositioned tube is not repositioned, no oxygen will be delivered to the lungs or the entire tidal volume will be delivered to one lung, placing the patient at risk for pneumothorax.

The cuff is an inflatable, pliable sleeve encircling the outer wall of the ET tube. The cuff stabilizes and seals the ET tube within the trachea and prevents the escape of ventilating gases. However, the cuff can cause tracheal damage.

- To avoid damage, inflate the cuff with air, and measure and monitor the cuff pressure. Normal arterial tracheal perfusion is estimated at 30 mm Hg. To ensure adequate tracheal perfusion, maintain cuff pressure at 20 to 25 mm Hg.

Measure and record cuff pressure after intubation and every 8 hours using the minimal occluding volume (MOV) technique or the minimal leak technique (MLT).

- The steps in the MOV technique for cuff inflation are as follows: (1) for the mechanically ventilated patient, place a stethoscope over the trachea and inflate the cuff to MOV by adding air until no air leak is heard at peak inspiratory pressure (end of ventilator inspiration); (2) for the spontaneously breathing patient, inflate until no sound is heard after a deep breath or after inhalation with a BVM; (3) use a manometer to verify that cuff pressure is between 20 and 25 mm Hg; and (4) record cuff pressure in the chart.

- If adequate cuff pressure cannot be maintained or larger volumes of air are needed to keep the cuff inflated, the cuff could be leaking or there could be tracheal dilation at the cuff site. In these situations, change the ET tube or notify the physician.

The procedure for MLT is similar with one exception. Remove a small amount of air from the cuff until a slight air leak is auscultated at peak inflation. Both techniques aim to prevent the risks of tracheal damage resulting from high cuff pressures.

- Closely monitor the patient with an ET for adequate oxygenation and ventilation by assessing clinical findings, arterial blood gases (ABGs), and other indicators of oxygenation status.

- You should not routinely suction a patient. It is important to routinely assess the patient to determine a need for suctioning. Indications for suctioning include (1) visible secretions in the ET tube, (2) sudden onset of respiratory distress, (3) suspected aspiration of secretions, (4) increase in peak airway pressures, (5) auscultation of adventitious breath sounds over the trachea and/or bronchi, (6) increase in respiratory rate and/or sustained coughing, and (7) sudden or gradual decrease in PaO_2 and/or SpO_2. See Table 91 for suctioning the patient with an artificial airway.

- With an oral ET tube in place, the patient's mouth is always open, and the lips, tongue, and gums should be moistened with saline or water swabs to prevent mucosal drying. Proper oral care provides comfort and prevents injury to the gums and plaque formation.

- Meticulous care is required to prevent skin breakdown on the face, lips, tongue, and/or nares because of pressure from the ET tube and/or bite block or from the method used to secure the ET tube to the patient's face. Reposition and retape the ET tube every 24 hours and as needed.

| Table 91 | **Suctioning Procedures for Patient on Mechanical Ventilator** |

General Measures
1. Gather all equipment.
2. Wash hands and don personal protective equipment.
3. Explain procedure and patient's role in assisting with secretion removal by coughing.
4. Monitor patient's cardiopulmonary status (e.g., vital signs, SpO_2, SvO_2, $ScvO_2$, ECG, level of consciousness) before, during, and after the procedure.
5. Turn on suction and set vacuum to 100-120 mm Hg.
6. Pause ventilator alarms.

Open-Suction Technique
1. Open sterile catheter package using the inside of the package as a sterile field. NOTE: Suction catheter should be no wider than half the diameter of the ET tube (e.g., for a 7-mm ET tube, select a 10-French suction catheter).
2. Fill the sterile solution container with sterile normal saline or water.
3. Don sterile gloves.
4. Pick up sterile suction catheter with dominant hand. Using nondominant hand, secure the connecting tube (to suction) to the suction catheter.
5. Check equipment for proper functioning by suctioning a small volume of sterile saline solution from the container. (Go to step 7.)

Closed-Suction Technique
6. Connect the suction tubing to the closed suction port.
7. Hyperoxygenate the patient for 30 sec using one of the following methods:
   Activate the suction hyperoxygenation setting on the ventilator using nondominant hand.
   Increase FIO_2 to 100%. NOTE: Remember to return FIO_2 to baseline level at the completion of the procedure.
   Disconnect the ventilator tubing from the ET tube and manually ventilate the patient with 100% O_2 using a BVM device.*
   Administer 5-6 breaths over 30 sec. NOTE: Use of a second person to deliver the manual breaths will significantly increase the tidal volume delivered.

Adapted from Chulay M: Suctioning: Endotracheal or tracheostomy tube. In Wiegand DL, Carlson KK, editors: *AACN procedure manual for critical care*, ed 5, St Louis, 2005, Mosby. *BVM*, Bag-valve-mask; *ECG*, electrocardiogram; *ET*, endotracheal, *FIO₂*, fraction of inspired oxygen.
*Attach a PEEP valve to the BVM for patients on >5 cm H_2O PEEP.

Table 91	Suctioning Procedures for Patient on Mechanical Ventilator—cont'd

8. With suction off, gently and quickly insert the catheter using the dominant hand. When you meet resistance, pull back ½ inch.

9. Apply continuous or intermittent suction using the nondominant thumb. Withdraw the catheter over 10 sec or less.

10. Hyperoxygenate for 30 sec as described in step 7.

11. If secretions remain and the patient has tolerated the procedure, perform two to three suction passes as described in steps 8 and 9. NOTE: Rinse the suction catheter with sterile saline solution between suctioning passes as needed.

12. Reconnect patient to ventilator (open-suction technique).

13. At the completion of ET tube suctioning, rinse the catheter and connecting tubing with the sterile saline solution.

14. Suction oral pharynx. NOTE: Use a separate catheter for this step when using the closed-suction technique.

15. Discard the suction catheter and rinse the connecting tubing with the sterile saline solution (open-suction technique).

16. Reset FIO₂ (if necessary) and ventilator alarms.

17. Reassess patient for signs of effective suctioning.

- For the nasally intubated patient, remove the old tape or ties and clean the skin around the ET tube with saline-soaked gauze or cotton swabs. For the orally intubated patient, remove the bite block (if present) and the old tape or ties.
- If the patient is anxious or uncooperative, it is recommended that two staff members should perform the repositioning procedure to prevent accidental dislodgement. Monitor the patient for any signs of respiratory distress throughout the procedure.

BIOLOGIC AND TARGETED THERAPY FOR CANCER TREATMENT

Description

Biologic and targeted therapy is used as a type of cancer treatment modality that can be effective alone or in combination with surgery, radiation therapy, and chemotherapy.

- *Biologic therapy,* or *biologic response modifier therapy,* consists of agents that modify the relationship between the host and tumor by altering the biologic response of the host to the tumor cell (Table 92).

- *Targeted therapy* includes drugs that interfere with cancer growth by targeting specific cellular receptors and pathways that are important in tumor growth (see Table 92). Targeted therapies are more selective for specific molecular targets than cytotoxic anticancer drugs. Thus they are able to kill cancer cells with less damage to normal cells compared with chemotherapy.

Targeted therapies include various tyrosine kinase inhibitors, monoclonal antibodies, angiogenesis inhibitors, and proteasome inhibitors.

- Tyrosine kinase inhibitors block an important enzyme that activates the signaling pathways that regulate cell proliferation and survival.
- Monoclonal antibodies bind to specific target cells and inhibit the internalization of receptor-antibody complexes and signaling pathways. They may also stimulate an immunologic response in the patient.
- Angiogenesis inhibitors work by preventing the mechanisms and pathways necessary for vascularization of tumors.
- Proteasomes are intracellular multienzyme complexes that degrade proteins. Proteasome inhibitors can cause these proteins to accumulate, thus leading to altered cell function.

Indications and side effects of biologic and targeted therapy are included in Table 92.

Nursing Management

The effects of biologic and targeted therapy occur acutely and are dose limited. Critical care nursing may be required for patients who experience capillary leak syndrome and pulmonary edema. Bone marrow depression that occurs with biologic therapy is usually more transient and less severe than that observed with chemotherapy.

- Fatigue associated with biologic therapy can be so severe that it can constitute a dose-limiting toxicity. Because these agents are increasingly combined with cytotoxic therapies, monitor the patient for combined and increased therapy-related effects.
- Acetaminophen administered before treatment and every 4 hours after treatment can help relieve the flulike syndrome associated with biologic agents. Intravenous (IV) meperidine (Demerol) has been used to control the severe chills associated with some biologic agents.

Table 92

DRUG THERAPY
Biologic and Targeted Therapy

Drug	Mechanism of Action	Indications	Side Effects
α-interferon (Roferon-A, Intron A)	Inhibits DNA and protein synthesis Suppresses cell proliferation Increases cytotoxic effects of natural killer (NK) cells	Hairy cell leukemia, chronic myelogenous leukemia, malignant melanoma, renal cell carcinoma, ovarian cancer, multiple myeloma, Kaposi sarcoma	Flulike syndrome (fever, chills, myalgia, headache), cognitive changes, fatigue, nausea, vomiting, anorexia, weight loss
interleukin-2 (aldesleukin [Proleukin])	Stimulates proliferation of T and B cells Activates NK cells	Metastatic renal cell cancer, metastatic melanoma	Same as above; capillary leak syndrome resulting in hypotension; bone marrow suppression
levamisole (Ergamisol)	Potentiates monocytes and macrophage function	Duke's stage C colon cancer (given in combination with 5-FU)	Diarrhea, metallic taste, nausea, fever, chills, mouth sores, headache
BCG vaccine (TheraCys)	Induces an immune response that prevents angiogenesis of tumor	In situ bladder cancer	Flulike syndrome, nausea, vomiting, rash, cough
Epidermal Growth Factor Receptor (EGFR)—Tyrosine Kinase Inhibitors			
cetuximab (Erbitux)	Inhibits EGFR	Colorectal cancer, head and neck cancer	Rash, infusion reactions, interstitial lung disease

Continued

B

Table 92

DRUG THERAPY
Biologic and Targeted Therapy—cont'd

Drug	Mechanism of Action	Indications	Side Effects
panitumumab (Vectibix)	Inhibits EGFR	Colorectal cancer that has metastasized following standard chemotherapy	Pulmonary fibrosis, severe skin rash complicated with infections, infusion reactions, interstitial lung disease
erlotinib (Tarceva)	Inhibits EGFR-TK	Non-small cell lung cancer	Rash, diarrhea, interstitial lung disease
gefitinib (Iressa)	Inhibits EGFR-TK	Non-small cell lung cancer	Rash, diarrhea, interstitial lung disease
lapatinib (Tykerb)	Inhibits EGFR-TK and binds receptor HER-2	Advanced or metastatic breast cancer	Cardiotoxicity, diarrhea, rash, nausea, vomiting, hand-foot syndrome
BCR-ABL Tyrosine Kinase Inhibitors			
imatinib (Gleevec)	Inhibits BCR-ABL tyrosine kinase	Chronic myeloid leukemia, GI stromal tumors (GIST)	Nausea, diarrhea, myalgia, fluid retention
nilotinib (Tasigna)	Inhibits BCR-ABL tyrosine kinase	Chronic myeloid leukemia	Neutropenia, thrombocytopenia, bleeding, nausea, fatigue, elevated lipase level, fever, rash, pruritus, diarrhea, pneumonia
dasatinib (Sprycel)	Inhibits BCR-ABL tyrosine kinase	Chronic myeloid leukemia	Myelosuppression, CNS or GI hemorrhage, fever, pleural effusion, pneumonia, cardiac failure, fluid retention, abdominal pain
CD 20 Monoclonal Antibodies			
rituximab (Rituxan)	Binds CD 20 antigen, causing cytotoxicity	Non-Hodgkin's lymphoma (B cell)	Fever, chills, nausea, headache, urticaria

B

Continued

ofatumumab (Arzerra)	Binds CD 20 antigen, causing cytotoxicity	Chronic lymphocytic leukemia	Increased risk for infection
ibritumomab tiuxetan/ yttrium-90 (Zevalin)	Binds CD 20 antigen, causing cytotoxicity and radiation injury	Non-Hodgkin's lymphoma (B cell)	Bone marrow suppression, fatigue, nausea, chills
tositumomab/^{131}I tositumomab (Bexxar)	Binds CD 20 antigen, causing immune attack and radiation injury	Non-Hodgkin's lymphoma (B cell)	Bone marrow suppression, fever, chills, nausea, headache
Angiogenesis Inhibitor			
bevacizumab (Avastin)	Binds vascular endothelial growth factor (VEGF), thereby inhibiting angiogenesis	Colorectal cancer, non–small cell lung cancer, renal cell carcinoma, breast cancer, and glioblastoma	Hypertension, colon bleeding and perforation, impaired wound healing, thromboembolism, diarrhea
pazcpanib (Votrient)	Same as above	Advanced renal cell carcinoma	Diarrhea, hypertension, hair depigmentation, nausea, anorexia, vomiting
Proteasome Inhibitor			
bortezomib (Velcade)	Inhibits proteasome activity, which functions to regulate cell growth	Multiple myeloma	Bone marrow suppression, nausea, vomiting, diarrhea, peripheral neuropathy, fatigue
Other Targeted Therapies			
gemtuzumab ozogamicin (Mylotarg)	Binds CD33 antigen (expressed on leukemic cells) to deliver cytotoxic drug into the DNA	Acute myeloid leukemia	Bone marrow suppression, fever, chills, nausea

Table 92

DRUG THERAPY
Biologic and Targeted Therapy—cont'd

Drug	Mechanism of Action	Indications	Side Effects
alemtuzumab (Campath)	Binds CD52 antigen (found on T and B cells, monocytes, NK cells, neutrophils)	Chronic lymphocytic leukemia (B cell), GIST	Bone marrow suppression, chills, fever, vomiting, diarrhea, fatigue
trastuzumab (Herceptin)	Binds human epidermal growth factor receptor 2 (HER-2)	Breast cancer (HER-2 positive)	Cardiotoxicity
sorafenib (Nexavar)	Inhibits several tyrosine kinases	Advanced renal cell carcinoma	Rash, diarrhea, hypertension; redness, pain, swelling, or blisters on hands/feet
sunitinib (Sutent)	Inhibits several tyrosine kinases	Advanced renal cell carcinoma, GIST	Fatigue, heart failure, hypertension
temsirolimus (Torisel)	Inhibits a specific protein known as the mammalian target of rapamycin (mTOR)	Advanced renal cell carcinoma	Hyperlipidemia (specifically triglycerides), hyperglycemia, interstitial lung disease, renal failure, rash, nausea, fatigue
everolimus (Afinitor)	Same as above	Advanced renal cell carcinoma	Mucositis, diarrhea, anorexia, edema, anemia, shortness of breath, coughing, nausea, vomiting, rash, fever

Other nursing measures include monitoring vital signs and temperature, planning for periods of rest for the patient, assisting with activities of daily living (ADLs), and monitoring for adequate oral intake.

CARDIOPULMONARY RESUSCITATION AND BASIC LIFE SUPPORT

C

Description

Cardiopulmonary resuscitation (CPR) is the process of externally supporting the circulation and respiration of a person who has a cardiac arrest. Resuscitation measures are divided into two components: *basic life support* (BLS) and *advanced cardiovascular life support* (ACLS). With the invention of the *automatic external defibrillator* (AED), BLS now includes early defibrillation that can be used by trained rescuers.

Basic Life Support

BLS involves the external support of circulation and ventilation for a patient with cardiac or respiratory arrest through CPR. The steps of BLS consist of a series of actions and skills performed by the rescuer or rescuers based on assessment findings.

- The first action performed by the rescuer on finding an adult victim is to assess for responsiveness. If the victim does not respond and the rescuer is alone, the rescuer should activate emergency medical services (EMS), get an AED (if available), return to the victim, and begin CPR. Survival from cardiac arrest is the highest when immediate CPR is provided and defibrillation occurs within 3 to 5 minutes.
- The next step in BLS is to assess the victim's airway to confirm the absence of breathing and establish a patent airway. The airway is opened by hyperextending the head with the head tilt-chin lift maneuver or, if a cervical spine injury is suspected, a jaw-thrust maneuver.
- If breathing is absent, or the victim is gasping occasionally, ventilation is provided by the rescuer with mouth-to-barrier (recommended) or mouth-to-mouth breathing. Ventilations are given with the victim's nostrils pinched and the rescuer's mouth placed around the victim's mouth to make a tight seal. Face-mask or bag-mask devices can also be used. If airflow is obstructed, the head should be repositioned and ventilation attempted. If the airway obstruction is not relieved, the rescuer should proceed with CPR.

- Health care providers are instructed to assess the pulse in victims who are unresponsive and not breathing. The carotid artery is used to determine the absence of a pulse, and if no pulse is palpated within 10 seconds, chest compression should be administered. *Chest compression* technique consists of hard, fast, and deep applications of pressure on the lower half of the sternum with the victim in a supine position on a flat, hard surface.
- Rescue breathing and chest compressions are combined for an effective resuscitation effort of the victim of cardiopulmonary arrest. *Hands-Only CPR* can be used to help adult victims who suddenly collapse from cardiac arrest outside of a health care setting. If you witness this event (as a bystander), you can select to provide chest compressions only or conventional CPR (described above). Both methods are effective when done in the first few minutes of an out-of-hospital cardiac arrest.
- When the AED or the ACLS team arrives, the victim's rhythm should be assessed. If the victim has a shockable rhythm (e.g., ventricular tachycardia or ventricular fibrillation), one shock should be delivered followed by five cycles of CPR before checking the rhythm. If the rhythm is not a shockable rhythm, CPR should be resumed and the rhythm rechecked every five cycles.

The guidelines for performing BLS with CPR are presented in Tables 93 and 94. Figures 1 through 5 in Appendix A of Lewis et al., *Medical-Surgical Nursing,* ed. 8, pp. 1788 to 1790 illustrate CPR techniques.

Table 93	Adult One-Rescuer Cardiopulmonary Resuscitation (CPR)

Assess
- Determine unresponsiveness:
  - Tap or gently shake shoulder.
  - Shout, "Are you all right?"

Activate Emergency Response System (ERS)*
- Activate ERS system (e.g., call 911) and get the AED (if available) (outside of hospital).
- Call a code and ask for the AED or crash cart (in the hospital).

Airway
Position the victim:
- Turn on back (if necessary) using logroll technique.

| Table 93 | **Adult One-Rescuer Cardiopulmonary Resuscitation (CPR)—cont'd** |

Open the airway using proper technique:
- Head tilt-chin lift maneuver (see Fig. A-2, Lewis et al., *Medical-Surgical Nursing,* ed. 8, p. 1788).
- Jaw-thrust maneuver if cervical spine injury is suspected (see Fig. 69-2, Lewis et al., *Medical-Surgical Nursing,* ed. 8, p. 1767).
- If unable to open airway using jaw-thrust maneuver, use head tilt-chin lift maneuver.

Breathing
1. Check for breathing:
   - LOOK for chest rising and falling.
   - LISTEN for air escaping during exhalation.
   - FEEL for flow of air on your face.
2. If victim is breathing adequately:
   - Continue to protect airway.
   - Place victim in recovery position (e.g., side-lying).
3. If victim is unresponsive and gasping occasionally or not breathing:
   - Provide two regular breaths each over 1 second.
   - Observe chest rise.
   - Allow for complete exhalation between breaths.
   - If unable to give two effective breaths:
     - Reposition victim to try to open airway.
     - Look for foreign body and, if seen, remove.
     - Reattempt to ventilate.
     - If ventilation is still unsuccessful, assess circulation.[†]
     - If adequate spontaneous breathing is restored and signs of circulation are present:
   - Maintain open airway.
   - Place victim in recovery position.

Circulation
Bystander Rescuer
Begin chest compressions after delivering two initial breaths or provide chest compressions only.
Health Care Professional
1. Assess for signs of circulation after delivery of the two initial breaths.
2. Feel for carotid pulse (5-10 seconds).
3. If victim has signs of circulation but is not breathing adequately, continue rescue breathing (1 breath/5-6 seconds) and recheck circulation every 2 minutes.
4. If there are no signs of circulation, expose the victim's chest and begin chest compressions.

Continued

C

Table 93	Adult One-Rescuer Cardiopulmonary Resuscitation (CPR)—cont'd

Compression/Ventilation

1. Compression-ventilation cycle:
   - Compression-ventilation ratio is 30:2.
2. Begin compressions:
   - Get into position for compressions at victim's side (by shoulders).
   - Place heel of one hand on the center of chest between the nipples.
   - Place heel of second hand on top of first.
   - Straighten arms and position shoulders directly over hands.
   - Push hard, deep, and fast.
   - Each compression should depress victim's sternum approximately 1½ to 2 inches.
   - Allow chest to rebound to normal position after each compression.
   - Perform compressions at the rate of 100 per minute.
   - Maintain correct position at all times and avoid interrupting chest compressions.
3. Provide ventilation:
   - Open airway using proper technique.
   - Deliver two slow regular breaths (1 second each) at the end of a cycle of 30 compressions.
   - Return hands to chest.
   - Find proper landmark and hand position.
   - Resume compressions.

Defibrillation

1. If witnessed arrest, use AED as soon as possible.
2. If unwitnessed arrest, deliver 5 cycles of CPR before using AED.
3. If rhythm is shockable, deliver one shock then resume CPR for 5 cycles before rechecking rhythm.
4. If the rhythm is not shockable, resume CPR and recheck rhythm every 5 cycles.

Continuation of CPR

- CPR should be continued between rhythm checks and shocks, and until ACLS providers arrive or the victim shows signs of movement.
- Do not interrupt CPR except in special circumstances.

Source: American Heart Association: *BLS for healthcare providers—student manual,* Dallas, TX, 2006, AHA.
*Rescuers should activate the ERS for unresponsive adults before beginning CPR, except in the case of drowning or a likely asphyxiation.
†Bystander rescuers are not taught to check for a pulse.
ACLS, Advanced cardiovascular life support; *AED,* Automatic external defibrillator.

Table 94	Adult Two-Rescuer Cardiopulmonary Resuscitation (CPR)

Assess/Activate Emergency Response System (ERS)*

One Rescuer

Determine unresponsiveness:

- Tap or gently shake shoulder.
- Shout, "Are you OK?"

Other Rescuer

- Activate ERS system (e.g., call 911 and get the AED [if available outside of hospital]).
- Call a code and ask for the AED or crash cart (in hospital).

Airway

Position the victim:

- Turn on back (if necessary) using logroll technique.

Open the airway using proper technique:

- Head tilt-chin lift maneuver (see Fig. A-2, Lewis et al., *Medical-Surgical Nursing,* ed. 8, p. 1788).
- Jaw-thrust maneuver if cervical spine injury is suspected (see Fig. 69-?, Lewis et al., *Medical-Surgical Nursing,* ed. 8, p. 1767).
- If unable to open airway using the jaw-thrust maneuver, use the head tilt-chin lift maneuver.

Breathing

1. Check for breathing:
   - LOOK for chest rising and falling.
   - LISTEN for air escaping during exhalation.
   - FEEL for flow of air on your face.
2. If victim is breathing adequately:
   - Continue to protect airway.
   - Place victim in recovery position (e.g., side-lying).
3. If victim is unresponsive and gasping occasionally or not breathing:
   - Provide two regular breaths each over 1 second.
   - Observe chest rise.
   - Allow for complete exhalation between breaths.
   - If unable to give two effective breaths:
     - Reposition victim to try to open airway.
     - Look for foreign body and, if seen, remove.
     - Reattempt to ventilate.
     - If ventilation is still unsuccessful, assess circulation.†
     - If adequate spontaneous breathing is restored and signs of circulation are present:
       - Maintain open airway.
       - Place victim in recovery position.

Continued

Table 94	Adult Two-Rescuer Cardiopulmonary Resuscitation (CPR)—cont'd

Circulation

Bystander Rescuer

Begin chest compressions after delivering two initial breaths or provide chest compressions only.

Health Care Professional

1. Assess for signs of circulation after delivery of the two initial breaths.
2. Feel for carotid pulse (5-10 seconds).
3. If victim has signs of circulation but is not breathing adequately, continue rescue breathing (1 breath/5-6 seconds) and recheck circulation every 2 minutes.
4. If there are no signs of circulation, say "No pulse" and prepare for chest compressions (e.g., expose the victim's chest).

Compression/Ventilation

Compression-Ventilation Cycle

Compression-ventilation ratio is 30:2.

Rescuer 1: Compressor

1. Get into position for compressions at victim's side (by shoulders).
2. Place heel of one hand on the center of chest between the nipples.
3. Place heel of second hand on top of first.
   - Straighten arms and position shoulders directly over hands.
4. Begin compressions.
   - Compressions should depress victim's sternum approximately $1\frac{1}{2}$ to 2 inches.
   - Allow chest to rebound to normal position after each compression.
   - Perform compressions hard, deep, and fast at the rate of 100 per minute.
   - Maintain correct position at all times and avoid interrupting chest compressions.

Rescuer 2: Ventilator

1. Get into position at victim's head.
2. Maintain an open airway.
3. Deliver two slow regular breaths (1 second each) at the end of a cycle of 30 compressions.
4. Ensure that chest is rising with each ventilation.
5. Monitor carotid pulse during compressions to verify effectiveness.

Table 94	Adult Two-Rescuer Cardiopulmonary Resuscitation (CPR)—cont'd

Switching
- Rescuers should change compressor and ventilator roles after 5 cycles of CPR (about every 2 minutes) to avoid compressor fatigue.
- Rescuers should exchange positions simultaneously with minimal delay (<5 seconds):
  - Ventilator moves to chest.
  - Compressor moves to head.

Defibrillation
1. If witnessed arrest, use AED as soon as possible.
2. If unwitnessed arrest, deliver 5 cycles of CPR before using AED.
3. If rhythm is shockable, deliver one shock then resume CPR for 5 cycles before rechecking rhythm.
4. If the rhythm is not shockable, resume CPR and recheck rhythm every 5 cycles.

Continuation of CPR
- CPR should be continued between rhythm checks and shocks, and until ACLS providers arrive or the victim shows signs of movement.
- Do not interrupt CPR except in special circumstances.

Source: American Heart Association: *BLS for healthcare providers— student manual,* Dallas, TX, 2006, AHA.
*Rescuers should activate the EMS for unresponsive adults before beginning CPR, except in the case of drowning or a likely asphyxiation.
†Bystander rescuers are not taught to check for a pulse.
AED, Automatic external defibrillator; *ACLS,* advanced cardiovascular life support.

CHEMOTHERAPY

Description

Chemotherapy is an effective treatment modality for cancer. It is a mainstay of cancer therapy used in the treatment of most solid tumors and hematologic malignancies (e.g., leukemias, lymphomas). The goal of chemotherapy is to eliminate or reduce the number of malignant cells present in the primary tumor and metastatic tumor site(s).

- The two major categories of chemotherapeutic drugs are cell cycle nonspecific and cell cycle phase-specific. These agents are often administered in combination with one another to maximize effectiveness by using agents that function by differing mechanisms and throughout the cell cycle.

Classification of Chemotherapeutic Drugs

Chemotherapy drugs are generally classified according to their molecular structure and mechanisms of action (Table 95).

Methods of Administration

The intravenous (IV) route is the most common route for chemotherapy. Major concerns with IV administration result from the irritant or vesicant characteristics of many chemotherapeutic agents.

- Irritants will damage the intima of the vein, causing phlebitis and sclerosis and limiting future peripheral venous access.
- Vesicants may cause severe local tissue breakdown and necrosis if inadvertently infiltrated into the skin.

To minimize these problems, a central vascular access device may be placed in large blood vessels to permit frequent, continuous, or intermittent administration of chemotherapy, thus avoiding multiple venipunctures. (See pp. 328 to 331 Lewis et al., *Medical-Surgical Nursing,* ed. 8.)

Regional chemotherapy delivers the drug directly to the tumor site. Examples of this type of administration include intraarterial, intraperitoneal, intrathecal (intraventricular), and intravesical bladder chemotherapy.

Effects of Chemotherapy

Chemotherapeutic agents cannot selectively distinguish between normal cells and cancer cells. Chemotherapy-induced side effects are caused by the destruction of normal cells that are rapidly proliferating such as those in the bone marrow, the lining of the gastrointestinal system, and the integumentary system (skin, hair, and nails). Effects of chemotherapy are caused by general cytotoxicity and organ-specific drug toxicities. Response of the body to the products of cellular destruction may cause fatigue, anorexia, and taste alterations.

The adverse effects of these drugs can be classified as acute, delayed, or chronic.

- *Acute toxicity* includes anaphylactic and hypersensitivity reactions, extravasation or a flare reaction, anticipatory nausea and vomiting, and dysrhythmias.

| Table 95 | DRUG THERAPY Classification of Chemotherapy Drugs |

Mechanisms of Action	Examples
Alkylating Agents *Cell Cycle Phase—Nonspecific Agents* Damage DNA by causing breaks in the double-stranded helix; if repair does not occur, cells will die immediately (cytocidal) or when they attempt to divide (cytostatic)	bendamustine (Treanda), busulfan (Myleran), chlorambucil (Leukeran), cyclophosphamide (Cytoxan, Neosar), dacarbazine (DTIC-Dome), ifosfamide (Ifex), mechlorethamine (Mustargen), melphalan (Alkeran), temozolomide (Temodar), thiotepa (Thioplex)
Nitrosoureas *Cell Cycle Phase—Nonspecific Agents* Like alkylating agents, break DNA helix, interfering with DNA replication; cross blood-brain barrier	carmustine (BiCNU, Gliadel), lomustine (CeeNU), streptozocin (Zanosar)
Platinum Drugs *Cell Cycle Phase—Nonspecific Agents* Bind to DNA and RNA, miscoding information and/or inhibiting DNA replication, and cells die	carboplatin (Paraplatin), cisplatin (Platinol-AQ), oxaliplatin (Eloxatin)
Antimetabolites *Cell Cycle Phase—Specific Agents* Mimic naturally occurring substances, thus interfering with enzyme function or DNA synthesis. Primarily act during S phase. Purine and pyrimidine are building blocks of nucleic acids needed for DNA and RNA synthesis	

Continued

Table 95	DRUG THERAPY Classification of Chemotherapy Drugs—cont'd

Mechanisms of Action	Examples
Antimetabolites—cont'd	
Cell Cycle Phase—Specific Agents—cont'd	
Interfere with purine metabolism	cladribine (Leustatin), clofarabine (Clolar), fludarabine (Fludara), mercaptopurine (Purinethol), nelarabine (Arranon), pentostatin (Nipent), thioguanine
Interfere with pyrimidine metabolism	capecitabine (Xeloda); cytarabine (Ara-C [Cytosar-U, DepoCyt]), floxuridine (FUDR), fluorouracil (5-FU [Adrucil]), gemcitabine (Gemzar)
Interfere with folic acid metabolism	methotrexate (Rheumatrex, Trexall), pemetrexed (Alimta)
Interfere with DNA synthesis	hydroxyurea (Hydrea, Droxia)
Antitumor Antibiotics	
Cell Cycle Phase—Nonspecific Agents	
Bind directly to DNA, thus inhibiting the synthesis of DNA and interfering with transcription of RNA	bleomycin (Blenoxane), dactinomycin (Cosmegen), daunorubicin (Cerubidine, DaunoXome), doxorubicin (Adriamycin, Rubex, Doxil), epirubicin (Ellence), idarubicin (Idamycin), mitomycin (Mutamycin), mitoxantrone (Novantrone), plicamycin (Mithracin), valrubicin (Valstar)
Mitotic Inhibitors	
Cell Cycle Phase—Specific Agents	
Taxanes	
Antimicrotubule agents that interfere with mitosis. Act during the late G2 phase and mitosis to stabilize microtubules, thus inhibiting cell division.	albumin-bound particles (Abraxane), docetaxel (Taxotere), paclitaxel (Taxol)

| Table 95 | **DRUG THERAPY**
Classification of Chemotherapy Drugs—cont'd |

Mechanisms of Action	Examples
Vinca Alkaloids	
Act in M phase to inhibit mitosis	vinblastine (Velban), vincristine (Oncovin), vinorelbine (Navelbine)
Others	
Microtubular inhibitor	estramustine (Emcyt), ixabepilone (Ixempra)
Topoisomerase Inhibitors *Cell Cycle Phase—Specific Agents*	
Inhibit the normal enzymes (topoisomerases) that function to make reversible breaks and repairs in DNA that allow for flexibility of DNA in replication	etoposide (VePesid), irinotecan (Camptosar), teniposide (Vumon), topotecan (Hycamtin)
Corticosteroids *Cell Cycle Phase—Nonspecific Agents*	
Disrupt the cell membrane and inhibit synthesis of protein; decrease circulating lymphocytes; inhibit mitosis; depress immune system; increase sense of well-being	cortisone (Cortone), dexamethasone (Decadron), hydrocortisone (Cortef), methylprednisolone (Medrol), prednisone
Hormone Therapy *Cell Cycle Phase—Nonspecific Agents* ***Antiestrogens***	
Selectively attach to estrogen receptors, causing down-regulation of them and inhibiting tumor growth; also known as SERMs (selective estrogen receptor modulators)	fulvestrant (Faslodex), raloxifene (Evista), tamoxifen (Nolvadex), toremifene (Fareston)

Continued

Table 95	**DRUG THERAPY** **Classification of Chemotherapy Drugs—cont'd**

Mechanisms of Action	Examples
Hormone Therapy—cont'd *Cell Cycle Phase—Nonspecific Agents—cont'd* **Estrogens**	
Interfere with hormone receptors and proteins	diethylstilbestrol (DES [Stilphostrol]), estradiol (Estrace), estramustine (Emcyt), estrogen (Menest)
Aromatase Inhibitors	
Inhibit aromatase, an enzyme that converts adrenal androgen to estrogen	anastrozole (Arimidex), exemestane (Aromasin), letrozole (Femara)
Miscellaneous	
Inhibits protein synthesis; enzyme derived from the yeast Erwinia used to deplete the supply of asparagines for leukemic cells that are dependent on an exogenous source of this amino acid	Erwinia asparaginase, l-asparaginase (Elspar)
Causes changes in DNA in leukemia cells and degrades the fusion protein PML-RAR-α	arsenic trioxide (Trisenox)
Suppresses mitosis at interphase; appears to alter preformed DNA, RNA, and protein	procarbazine (Matulane, Natulan)

Note: Many of these drugs are irritants or vesicants that require special attention during administration to avoid extravasation. It is important to know this information about a drug before administering it.

- *Delayed effects* are numerous and include delayed nausea and vomiting, mucositis, alopecia, skin rashes, bone marrow depression, altered bowel function, and a variety of neurotoxicities.
- *Chronic toxicities* involve damage to organs such as the heart, liver, kidneys, and lungs.

An extensive list of side effects and problems caused by chemotherapy and radiation therapy is provided in Table 16-12, Lewis et al., *Medical-Surgical Nursing,* ed. 8, pp. 281 to 282.

Nursing Management

You have an important role in identifying, reporting, and helping patients deal with the side effects of radiation and chemotherapy. Teach patients about their treatment regimen, supportive care options (e.g., antiemetics, antidiarrheals), and what to expect during the course of treatment to help decrease fear and anxiety. Encourage adherence and guide self-management.

- Myelosuppression is one of the most common effects of chemotherapy and can result in life-threatening and distressing effects, including infection, hemorrhage, and overwhelming fatigue. Monitor the complete blood count in patients receiving chemotherapy, particularly the neutrophil, platelet, and red blood cell (RBC) counts. White blood cell (WBC) growth factors are routinely used to reduce chemotherapy-induced neutropenia, and platelet transfusions are usually administered when platelet counts fall $<20,000/\mu L$ $(20 \times 10^9/L)$.

- Fatigue is a nearly universal symptom, affecting 70% to 100% of patients with cancer. You can help patients recognize that fatigue is a common effect of therapy. Ignoring fatigue may lead to an increase in symptoms. However, maintaining exercise and activity within tolerable limits is often helpful in managing fatigue. Guidelines for the evaluation and management of cancer related fatigue are available online at www.nccn.org.

The intestinal mucosa is one of the most sensitive tissues to chemotherapy, resulting in nausea and vomiting, diarrhea, mucositis, and anorexia—all of which can significantly affect the patient's hydration and nutritional status and sense of well-being. Assess patients with nausea and vomiting for signs and symptoms of dehydration and metabolic alkalosis. Record fluid intake to ensure that an adequate volume is being consumed and retained. Nausea and vomiting can be successfully managed with antiemetic regimens, dietary modification, and other nondrug interventions.

▼ **Patient and Caregiver Teaching**

Patient and caregiver teaching is an important part of your role related to chemotherapy.

- To decrease the fear and anxiety often associated with chemotherapy, tell the patient what to expect during a course of treatment.

- Explore the patient's attitude toward treatment so that any misconception or fear can be discussed.
- Inform the patient of the possible side effects of chemotherapy that may be experienced during treatment. Good nursing judgment is essential to determine the amount of information that the patient and caregiver can assimilate.
- Inform and reassure the patient that supportive care (e.g., antiemetic and antidiarrheal agents, hematopoietic growth factors) will be provided as needed.

CHEST TUBES AND PLEURAL DRAINAGE

Description

Chest tubes are inserted into the pleural space to remove air and fluid and allow the lung to re-expand.

Chest Tube Insertion

Chest tubes can be inserted in the emergency department (ED), at the patient's bedside, or in the operating room, depending on the situation. In the ED or at the bedside, the patient may be positioned seated on the edge of the bed with arms supported on a bedside table or supine with the midaxillary area of the affected side exposed.

- The area is cleansed with antiseptic solution and the chest wall is prepared with a local anesthetic. A small incision is made over a rib. The chest tube is then advanced up and over the top of the rib to avoid the intercostal nerves and blood vessels (Fig. 17).
- Insertion of a chest tube after thoracotomy takes place through a stab wound adjacent to the surgical incision. The chest tube is connected to a pleural drainage system. Two tubes may be connected to the same drainage unit with a Y-connector.
- The incision is closed with sutures and covered with a dressing. Insertion of a chest tube and its presence in the pleural space is painful. Monitor the patient's comfort at frequent intervals and use the appropriate pain relieving interventions.

Pleural Drainage

There are two types of pleural drainage systems. The first type consists of a flutter valve connected to a drainage bag. This simple apparatus is used for patients with chronic pleural effusions and simple pneumothorax.

C

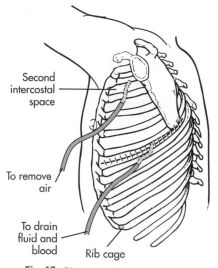

Second
intercostal
space

To remove
air

To drain
fluid and
blood   Rib cage

Fig. 17. Placement of chest tubes.

The second type is larger and has three basic compartments

- The first compartment, or collection chamber, receives fluid and air from the pleural space. The fluid stays in this chamber while the air vents to the second chamber. The second compartment, called the water-seal chamber, contains 2 cm of water, which acts as a one-way valve. Air enters from the collection chamber and bubbles up through the water. The water prevents backflow of air into the patient from the system.
- A third compartment, which is used to apply controlled suction to the system, is called the suction control chamber.

Initially, brisk bubbling of air occurs in this chamber when a pneumothorax is evacuated. During normal use, there will be intermittent bubbling during exhalation, coughing, or sneezing because of an increase in the patient's intrathoracic pressure. Eventually, the air leak will seal and the lung will be fully expanded

A variety of commercial, disposable, plastic chest drainage systems are available. One system is the Pleur-evac (Fig. 18).

Nursing Management: Chest Drainage

General guidelines for nursing care of the patient with chest tubes and water-seal drainage systems are presented in Table 28-23, Lewis et al., *Medical-Surgical Nursing,* ed. 8, p. 572.

Chest Tubes and Pleural Drainage

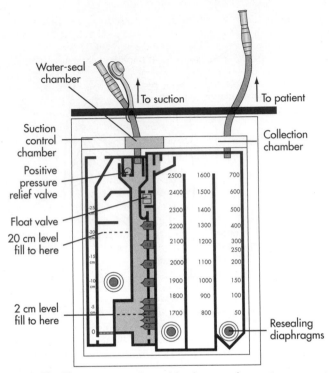

Fig. 18. Pleur-evac disposable chest suction system.

Drainage system:

- Keep all tubing coiled loosely below chest level. Do not let the patient lie on the tubing.
- Keep all connections among the chest tubes, drainage tubing, and drainage collector tight, and tape at connections.
- Keep the water-seal chamber and suction control chamber at appropriate water levels by adding sterile water as needed, because water loss by evaporation may occur.
- Mark the time of measurement and the fluid level on the chamber according to prescribed orders. Any change in the quantity or characteristics of drainage should be reported to the physician.
- Observe for air fluctuations and bubbling in the water-seal chamber. If no fluctuations are observed (rising with

inspiration and falling with expiration in a spontaneously breathing patient; the opposite occurs during positive pressure mechanical ventilation), the drainage system is blocked or the lungs are reexpanded. If bubbling increases, there may be an air leak.

- When bubbling is continuous and constant, to determine the source of the air leak momentarily clamp the tubing at successively distal points away from the patient until the bubbling ceases. When the bubbling ceases, you know the leak is above the clamp. Retaping the tubing connections or replacing the drainage apparatus may be necessary to prevent the air leak.

- High fluid levels in the water seal indicate residual negative pressure. The chest system may need to be vented by using the high-negativity release valve available on the drainage system to release residual pressure from the system.

- Never elevate the drainage system to the level of the patient's chest because this will cause fluid to drain back into the lungs.

- If the drainage system is overturned and the water seal is disrupted, return it to an upright position and encourage the patient to take a few deep breaths, followed by forced exhalations and cough maneuvers.

Do not strip chest tubes, as this dangerously increases intrapleural pressures. Drainage tubes may be milked upon physician order. *Milking:* alternately folding or squeezing and then releasing drainage tubing. Take 15-cm strips of the chest tube and squeeze and release starting close to the chest and repeating down the tube distally.

Patient's clinical status:

- Monitor the patient's clinical status. Vital signs should be taken frequently, lungs auscultated, and the chest wall observed for any abnormal chest movements.

- Assess for manifestations of reaccumulation of air and fluid in the chest ($\downarrow$ or absent breath sounds), significant bleeding (>100 mL/hr), chest drainage site infection (drainage, erythema, fever, $\uparrow$ WBC), or poor wound healing. Notify physician for management plan. Evaluate for subcutaneous emphysema at chest tube site.

- Encourage the patient to cough and breathe deeply periodically to facilitate lung expansion.

- Chest tubes are *not clamped routinely.* Clamps with rubber protection are kept at the bedside for special procedures such as changing the chest drainage system and assessment before removal of chest tubes.

- Chest tube malposition is the most common complication. Routine monitoring is done by the nurse to evaluate if the chest drainage is successful by observing for fluctuations in the water-seal chamber, listening for breath sounds over the lung fields, and measuring the amount of fluid drainage.
- Infection at the skin site is possible. Meticulous sterile technique during dressing changes can reduce the incidence of infected sites. Nursing care and patient teaching can minimize the risk of atelectasis and shoulder stiffness.

In addition to nursing assessment, chest x-ray is used to monitor tube position and lung re-expansion at intervals. If volumes from 1 to 1.5 L of pleural fluid are removed rapidly, re-expansion pulmonary edema or a vasovagal response with symptomatic hypotension can occur.

Chest Tube Removal

Chest tubes are removed when the lungs are reexpanded and fluid drainage has ceased. Suction is usually discontinued and gravity drainage is used for 24 hours before tube removal.

- The tube is removed by cutting the sutures; having the patient take a deep breath, exhale, and bear down (Valsalva maneuver); and then removing the tube.
- The site is covered with an airtight dressing, the pleura will seal itself off, and the wound heals in several days.
- The patient's condition is evaluated with a chest x-ray and close observation of respiratory function.

DIALYSIS

Description

Dialysis is a technique in which substances move from the blood through a semipermeable membrane and into a dialysis solution (dialysate). Dialysis is used to correct fluid and electrolyte imbalances and remove waste products in renal failure. It can also be used to treat drug overdoses.

The two methods of dialysis are *peritoneal dialysis* (PD) and *hemodialysis* (HD) (Table 96).

- In PD the peritoneal membrane acts as the semipermeable membrane.
- In HD an artificial membrane (usually made of cellulose-based or synthetic materials) is used as the semipermeable membrane and is in contact with the patient's blood.

Dialysis is begun when the patient's uremia can no longer be adequately treated with conservative medical management.

Table 96	Comparison of Peritoneal Dialysis and Hemodialysis

Peritoneal Dialysis (PD)

Advantages	Disadvantages
▪ Immediate initiation in almost any hospital ▪ Less complicated than HD ▪ Portable system with CAPD ▪ Fewer dietary restrictions ▪ Relatively short training time ▪ Usable in patient with vascular access problems ▪ Less cardiovascular stress ▪ Home dialysis possible ▪ Preferable for diabetic patient	▪ Bacterial or chemical peritonitis ▪ Protein loss into dialysate ▪ Exit site and tunnel infections ▪ Self-image problems with catheter placement ▪ Hyperglycemia ▪ Surgery for catheter placement ▪ Contraindication in patient with multiple abdominal surgeries, trauma, unrepaired hernia ▪ Requires completion of education program ▪ Catheter can migrate ▪ Best instituted with willing partner

Hemodialysis (HD)

Advantages	Disadvantages
▪ Rapid fluid removal ▪ Rapid removal of urea and creatinine ▪ Effective potassium removal ▪ Less protein loss ▪ Lowering of serum triglycerides ▪ Home dialysis possible ▪ Temporary access can be placed at bedside	▪ Vascular access problems ▪ Dietary and fluid restrictions ▪ Heparinization may be necessary ▪ Extensive equipment necessary ▪ Hypotension during dialysis ▪ Added blood loss that contributes to anemia ▪ Specially trained personnel necessary ▪ Surgery for permanent access placement ▪ Self-image problems with permanent access

D

Generally dialysis is initiated when the glomerular filtration rate (GFR) (or creatinine clearance) of the patient with kidney disease is <15 mL/min. This criterion can vary widely in different clinical situations, and the physician determines when to start dialysis based on the patient's clinical status. Certain uremic complications, including encephalopathy, neuropathies, uncontrollable hyperkalemia, pericarditis, and accelerated hypertension, indicate a need for immediate dialysis.

Dialysis is discussed in Lewis et al., *Medical-Surgical Nursing,* ed. 8, pp. 1181 to 1188.

EMERGENCY PATIENT: PRIMARY AND SECONDARY SURVEY

Recognition of life-threatening illness or injury is one of the most important aspects of emergency nursing. Initiation of interventions to reverse or prevent a crisis often is a priority before a diagnosis is made. This process begins with your first patient contact. Prompt identification of patients requiring immediate treatment and determination of appropriate interventions are essential nurse competencies.

- A *triage system* identifies and categorizes patients so the most critical are treated first. *Triage* is a French word meaning "to sort."
- The process is based on the premise that patients with a threat to life should be treated before other patients.

Initially, assess the patient for any threats to life (e.g., Is the patient dying?) or presence of a high risk situation (e.g., Is this a patient who should not wait to be seen?). After you complete the initial focused assessment to determine the presence of actual or potential threats to life, proceed with a more detailed assessment. A systematic approach to this assessment decreases the time required to identify potential threats to life and minimizes the risk of overlooking a life-threatening condition. A primary survey and a secondary survey are the approaches to use with trauma patients.

The **primary survey** focuses on airway, breathing, circulation, disability, and exposure/environmental control. It serves to identify life-threatening conditions so that appropriate interventions can be initiated. You may identify life-threatening conditions related to airway, breathing, circulation (ABCs), and disability (Table 97) at any point during the primary survey. When this occurs, start interventions immediately and before moving to the next step of the survey.

Table 97	Causes of Life-Threatening Conditions Identified During the Primary Survey*

Airway
- Inhalation injury
- Obstruction (partial or complete) from foreign bodies, debris (e.g., vomitus), or tongue
- Penetrating wounds and/or blunt trauma to upper airway structures

Breathing
- Anaphylaxis
- Flail chest with pulmonary contusion
- Hemothorax
- Pneumothorax (e.g., open, tension)

Circulation
- Direct cardiac injury (e.g., myocardial infarction, trauma)
- Pericardial tamponade
- Shock (e.g., massive burns, hypovolemia)
- Uncontrolled external hemorrhage
- Hypothermia

Disability
- Head injury
- Stroke

*List is not all-inclusive.

The secondary survey begins after addressing each step of the primary survey and initiating any lifesaving interventions. The **secondary survey** is a brief, systematic process that aims to identify *all* injuries (see Table 69-5, Lewis et al., *Medical Surgical Nursing* ed. 8, p. 1770).

ENTERAL NUTRITION

Enteral nutrition (EN, also known as *tube feeding*) is nutrition (e.g., a nutritionally balanced liquefied food or formula) provided through the GI tract via a tube, catheter, or stoma that delivers nutrients distal to the oral cavity.

Indications for EN as a supplemental form of nutrition include:
- The patient who has a functioning gastrointestinal (GI) tract but cannot take oral nourishment.
- Persons with anorexia, orofacial fractures, head and neck cancer, neurologic or psychiatric conditions that prevent

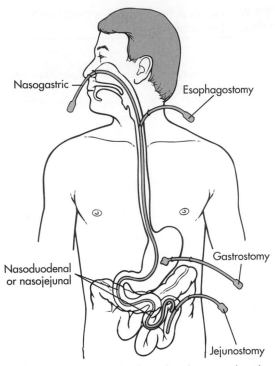

Fig. 19. Common enteral feeding tube placement locations.

oral intake, or extensive burns, or those who are receiving chemotherapy or radiation therapy.

EN is considered to be easily administered, safer, more physiologically efficient, and less expensive than parenteral nutrition. EN is used to provide nutrients by way of the GI tract either alone or as a supplement to oral or parenteral nutrition.

Figure 19 shows the location of commonly used enteral feeding tubes. These include:

- Nasogastric (NG) tube, which is most commonly used for short-term feeding problems
- Esophagostomy, gastrostomy, or jejunostomy tubes for feeding over an extended time
- Transpyloric (nasointestinal) tubes are used for feeding below the pyloric sphincter

Common delivery options are continuous infusion by pump, intermittent by gravity.

Use the following evidence-based principles for administration of tube feeding:

1. Elevate head of bed to a minimum of 30 degrees, but preferably 45 degrees to prevent aspiration.
2. Flush feeding tube with 30 mL of water every 4 hours during continuous feeding or before and after intermittent feeding.
3. Obtain x-ray confirmation to determine if a blindly placed nasogastric or orogastric tube (small- or large-bore) is properly positioned in the GI tract before administering feedings or medications.
4. Evaluate all enterally fed patients for risk of aspiration.
5. When possible, use a sterile, liquid EN formula rather than a powdered or reconstituted formula.
6. Use disposable gloves during the administration of EN.
7. Before administering medications, stop the enteral feeding formula and flush the tube with at least 15 mL of water.
8. Weigh the patient daily or several times a week, and maintain accurate intake and output records.

Give feedings at room or body temperature to decrease the likelihood of diarrhea and other GI complaints. Commercial formulas are preferable to blenderized foods for small-lumen tubes because of the risk of tube clogging, completeness of nutrition, and decreased risk of formula contamination.

Nursing considerations include the following:

- Assess for bowel sounds before feeding.
- Check an initial blood glucose level to assess glucose tolerance.
- Formulas that are reconstituted in advance should be immediately refrigerated and discarded within 24 hours of preparation.
- Label feedings with the date and time they are initially used.
- Administration sets (tubing) should be changed every 24 hours for open system enteral feedings; otherwise per manufacturer's guidelines.
- Assess the patient regularly for complications (e.g., aspiration, diarrhea, dehydration, hyperglycemia, constipation, fecal impaction).

The types of problems encountered in patients receiving tube feedings and corrective measures are presented in Table 40-12, Lewis et al., *Medical-Surgical Nursing,* ed. 8, p. 933. Additional information related to the nursing management of EN is presented in NCP 40-1 for the patient receiving enteral nutrition, Lewis et al., *Medical-Surgical Nursing,* ed. 8, p. 936.

HEIMLICH MANEUVER (ABDOMINAL THRUSTS)

Management of a foreign body airway obstruction depends on whether the person is conscious or unconscious (Table 98). Fig. 20 illustrates the Heimlich maneuver, which is an emergency procedure for dislodging an obstruction from the trachea to prevent asphyxiation. In rare instances when airway obstruction is not

Table 98	Management of the Adult Choking Victim

Conscious Adult Choking Victim
Assess Victim for Severe Airway Obstruction
If the victim displays any of the following signs of severe or complete airway obstruction, you must take immediate action:
- Poor or no air exchange
- Universal choking sign (victim clutches neck with hands)
- Unable to speak (Ask the victim, "Are you choking?")
- Weak, ineffective cough or no cough
- High-pitched sound or no sound while inhaling
- Increased difficulty breathing
- Possible cyanosis

Abdominal Thrusts (Heimlich Maneuver) with Standing/Sitting Victim (Fig. A-3 in Lewis et al., Medical-Surgical Nursing, ed. 8, p. 1789)
1. Stand or kneel behind victim and wrap arms around waist.
2. Make fist with one hand.
3. Place thumb side of fist against victim's abdomen. Position fist midline, slightly above navel and well below breastbone.
4. Grasp fist with other hand.
5. Press fist into victim's abdomen using quick upward thrusts. Each thrust should be a separate, distinct movement. Note: If victim is in the late stages of pregnancy or obese, chest thrusts should be used. Position hands (as described) over lower portion of the breastbone and apply quick backward thrusts.
6. Repeat thrusts until object is expelled or victim becomes unresponsive.

Unconscious Adult Choking Victim
Assessment
If you see a choking victim collapse and become unresponsive:
1. Activate the Emergency Response System (ERS).
2. Be sure victim is supine.

Table 98	Management of the Adult Choking Victim—cont'd

3. Perform tongue-jaw lift; look to see if a foreign body is visible and, if seen, remove it (see Fig. A-4 in Lewis et al., *Medical-Surgical Nursing*, ed. 8, p. 1789).
4. Open airway and attempt to ventilate:
   - Give two rescue breaths.
   - If breaths are unsuccessful in making victim's chest rise:
     - Reposition victim's head.
     - Reopen airway.
     - Reattempt to ventilate.
5. If efforts to ventilate are still unsuccessful, begin CPR (see Tables A-2 and A-3 in Lewis et al., *Medical-Surgical Nursing*, ed. 8, pp. 1791 to 1792).

Source: American Heart Association: *BLS for healthcare providers—student manual,* Dallas, TX, 2006, AHA.

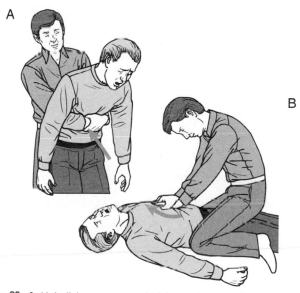

Fig. 20. A, Heimlich maneuver administered to conscious (standing) victim of foreign body airway obstruction. **B,** Heimlich maneuver administered to unconscious (lying) victim of foreign body airway obstruction—astride position.

relieved by methods in Table 98, additional procedures are necessary. These include transtracheal catheter ventilation and cricothyroidotomy, which should only be attempted by health care professionals experienced in these procedures.

MECHANICAL VENTILATION

Description

Mechanical ventilation is the process by which room air or oxygen-enriched air is moved in and out of the lungs by a mechanical ventilator. Mechanical ventilation is not curative. It is a means of supporting patients until they recover the ability to breathe independently, as a bridge to long-term mechanical ventilation, or until a decision is made to withdraw ventilatory support. Indications for mechanical ventilation include (1) apnea or an impending inability to breathe, (2) acute respiratory failure, (3) severe hypoxia, and (4) respiratory muscle fatigue.

Types of Mechanical Ventilators

The two major types of mechanical ventilation are negative pressure and positive pressure ventilation.

- Negative pressure ventilation involves the use of chambers that encase the chest or body and surround it with intermittent subatmospheric or negative pressure. Intermittent negative pressure around the chest wall causes the chest to be pulled outward. This reduces intrathoracic pressure. Air rushes in through the upper airway, which is outside the sealed chamber. Expiration is passive; the machine cycles off, allowing chest retraction. This type of ventilation is similar to normal ventilation in that decreased intrathoracic pressures produce inspiration and expiration is passive. Negative pressure ventilation delivers noninvasive ventilation and does not require an artificial airway.
- Several portable negative pressure ventilators are available for home use for patients with neuromuscular diseases, central nervous system disorders, diseases and injuries of the spinal cord, and severe chronic obstructive pulmonary disease (COPD). Negative pressure ventilators are not used extensively for acutely ill patients.
- Positive pressure ventilation (PPV) is the primary method used with acutely ill patients. During inspiration the ventilator pushes air into the lungs under positive pressure. Unlike spontaneous ventilation, intrathoracic pressure is raised during lung inflation rather than lowered. Expiration occurs

passively as in normal expiration. PPVs are categorized into volume and pressure ventilators.

See the detailed information on mechanical ventilation in eNCP 66-1 at http://evolve.elsevier.com/Lewis/medsurg. Nursing management of the patient receiving mechanical ventilation is available at http://evolve.elsevier.com/Lewis/medsurg.

O

OSTOMIES

Description

An *ostomy* is a surgical procedure that allows intestinal contents to pass from the bowel through an opening in the skin on the abdomen. The opening is called a *stoma,* and it is created when the intestine is brought through the abdominal wall and sutured to the skin.

An ostomy is used when the normal elimination route is no longer possible. For example, if the person has colorectal cancer, the diseased portion must be removed together with a certain margin of healthy tissue. Sometimes the tumor can be resected, leaving enough healthy tissue to immediately *anastomose* (reconnect) the two remaining ends of healthy bowel, and no ostomy is necessary. If the tumor involves the rectum and is large enough to necessitate the removal of the anal sphincters, the anus is sutured shut and a permanent ostomy is created.

Types of Ostomies

Ostomies are described according to location and type. For example, an ostomy in the ileum is called an *ileostomy* and an ostomy in the colon is called a *colostomy.* The ostomy is characterized by its anatomic site (e.g., sigmoid or transverse colostomy). The more distal the ostomy, the more the intestinal contents resemble feces that is eliminated from an intact colon and rectum. Locations for ostomies are shown in Fig. 21.

The major types of ostomies are end stoma, loop, and double-barrel ostomies.

- An *end stoma* is created by dividing the bowel and bringing the proximal end as a single stoma. The distal portion of the gastrointestinal (GI) tract is surgically removed, or the distal segment is sewn closed and left in the abdominal cavity. If the distal bowel is removed, then the stoma is permanent.
- A *loop stoma* is created by bringing a loop of bowel to the abdominal surface and then opening the anterior part of the bowel to provide fecal diversion. This results in one stoma with a proximal and distal opening and an intact posterior

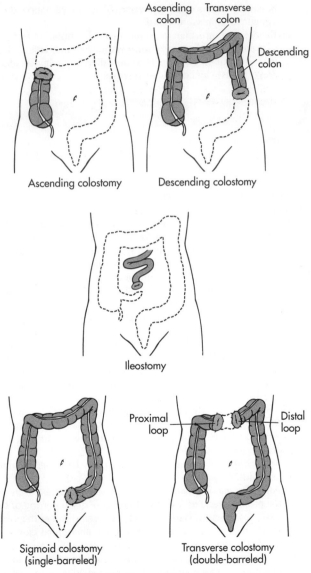

Fig. 21. Types of ostomies.

bowel wall that separates the two openings. This type of stoma is usually temporary.

- In a *double-barrel stoma* the bowel is divided, and both the proximal and distal ends are brought through the abdominal wall as two separate stomas (see Fig. 43-10, Lewis et al., *Medical-Surgical Nursing,* ed. 8, p. 1040). The proximal one is the functioning stoma; the distal, nonfunctioning stoma is referred to as the mucus fistula. The double-barreled stoma is usually temporary.

A comparison of colostomies and ileostomy is presented in Table 99. The actual procedures to perform ostomy surgeries are discussed in Lewis et al., *Medical-Surgical Nursing,* ed. 8, pp. 1039 to 1042.

Nursing Management

Preoperative care. Preoperative care that is unique to ostomy surgery includes (1) psychologic preparation for the ostomy; (2) selection of a flat site on the abdomen that allows secure attachment of the collection bag; and (3) selection of a stoma site that will be clearly visible to the patient to facilitate self-care. Psychologic preparation and emotional support are important as the person copes with the change in body image and a loss of control over elimination and its odors.

- If available, an experienced and competent clinician should visit the patient and caregiver and select the site where the ostomy should be positioned and mark the abdomen preoperatively. Stomas placed outside the rectus muscle increase the chance of developing a hernia. A flat site makes it much easier to create a good seal and avoid leakage from the bag.

Postoperative care. Postoperative nursing care includes assessment of the stoma and provision of an appropriate pouching system that protects the skin and contains drainage and odor. See NCP 43-3 for the patient with a colostomy or ileostomy, Lewis et al., *Medical-Surgical Nursing,* ed. 8, pp. 1043 to 1044.

The stoma should be pink. A dusky-blue stoma indicates ischemia, and a brown-black stoma indicates necrosis. Assess and document stoma color every 8 hours. There is mild to moderate swelling of the stoma the first 2 to 3 weeks after surgery.

The pouching system consists of a skin barrier and a bag or pouch to collect the feces. The skin barrier is a piece of pectin-based or karaya wafer that has a measurable thickness and hydrocolloid adhesive properties. The skin should be washed with mild soap, rinsed with warm water, and dried thoroughly before the barrier is applied.

- Pouches come as one- or two-piece systems. The one-piece system has the skin barrier attached, and the two-piece

Table 99 Comparison of Ileostomy and Colostomy

| | Ileostomy | Colostomy | | |
		Ascending	Transverse	Sigmoid
Stool consistency	Liquid to semiliquid	Semiliquid	Semiliquid to semiformed	Formed
Fluid requirement	Increased	Increased	Possibly increased	No change
Bowel regulation	No	No	No	Yes (if there is a history of a regular bowel pattern)
Pouch and skin barriers	Yes	Yes	Yes	Dependent on regulation
Irrigation	No	No	No	Possibly every 24-48 hr (if patient meets criteria)
Indications for surgery	Ulcerative colitis, Crohn's disease, diseased or injured colon, birth defect, familial polyposis, trauma, cancer	Perforating diverticulitis in lower colon; trauma; inoperable tumors of colon, rectum, or pelvis; rectovaginal fistula	Same as for ascending; birth defect	Cancer of the rectum or rectosigmoidal area; perforating diverticulum; trauma

system allows removal of the pouch without removing the skin barrier.

- An open-ended, transparent, plastic, odorproof pouch is used to observe the stoma and collect the drainage. The pouch must fit snugly to prevent leakage around the stoma.

- The volume, color, and consistency of the drainage are recorded. Each time the pouch is changed, the condition of the skin is observed for irritation. A pouch should never be placed directly on irritated skin without the use of a skin barrier.

Colostomy Care

- A colostomy in the ascending and transverse colon has semiliquid stools. Instruct the patient to use a drainable pouch. A colostomy in the sigmoid or descending colon has semiformed or formed stools and sometimes can be regulated by the irrigation method. The patient may or may not wear a drainage pouch. A nondrainable pouch should have a gas filter.

- For most patients with colostomies, there are few, if any, dietary restrictions. A well-balanced diet and adequate fluid intake are important. For foods and their effects on stomal output, see Table 43-30, Lewis et al., *Medical Surgical Nursing,* ed. 8, p. 1044.

Colostomy irrigations are used to stimulate emptying of the colon. Regularity is only possible when the stoma is in the distal colon or rectum. If control is achieved, there should be little or no spillage between irrigations, and the patient may need to wear only a pad or cover over the stoma. The procedure for colostomy irrigation is presented in Table 100.

▼ Patient and Caregiver Teaching

- The patient should be able to perform a pouch change, provide appropriate skin care, control odor, care for the stoma, and identify signs and symptoms of complications.

- The patient should know the importance of fluids and food in the diet, have the name and address of the United Ostomy Association (www.uoaa.org), and know when to seek health care.

- Home care and outpatient follow-up care by an enterostomal therapy (ET) nurse are highly recommended.

- Patients should be discharged with written pouch change instructions, teaching literature relevant to the type of stoma they have, a list of equipment they use (including names and phone numbers), a list of equipment retailers, outpatient

| Table 100 | Patient and Caregiver Teaching Guide: Colostomy Irrigation |

You should include the following instructions when teaching the patient and/or the caregiver to perform colostomy irrigation:

Equipment
- Lubricant
- Irrigation set (1000- to 2000-mL container, tubing with irrigating stoma cone, clamp)
- Irrigating sleeve with adhesive or belt
- Toilet tissue to clean around the stoma
- Disposal sack for soiled dressing

Procedure
1. Place 500 to 1000 mL of lukewarm water (not to exceed 105° F [40.5° C]) in container. The volume is titrated for the individual; use enough irrigant to distend the bowel but not enough to cause cramping pain. Most adults use 500 to 1000 mL of water.
2. Ensure comfortable position. Patient may sit in chair in front of toilet or on the toilet if the perineal wound is healed.
3. Clear tubing of all air by flushing it with fluid.
4. Hang container on hook or IV pole (18 to 24 inches) above stoma (about shoulder height).
5. Apply irrigating sleeve and place bottom end in toilet bowl.
6. Lubricate stoma cone, insert cone tip gently into the stoma, and hold tip securely in place.
7. Allow irrigation solution to flow in steadily for 5 to 10 minutes.
8. If cramping occurs, stop the flow of solution for a few seconds, leaving the cone in place.
9. Clamp the tubing and remove irrigating cone when the desired amount of irrigant has been delivered or the patient senses colonic distention.
10. Allow 30 to 45 minutes for the solution and feces to be expelled. Initial evacuation is usually complete in 10 to 15 minutes. Close off the irrigating sleeve at the bottom to allow ambulation.
11. Clean, rinse, and dry peristomal skin well.
12. Replace the colostomy drainage pouch or desired stoma covering.
13. Wash and rinse all equipment and hang to dry.

follow-up appointments with the surgeon and ET nurse, and the phone numbers of the surgeon and nurse.

See Table 43-29 for ostomy teaching guidelines, Lewis et al., *Medical-Surgical Nursing,* ed. 8, p. 1042.

Ileostomy Care

- Because regularity cannot be established, a pouch must be worn at all times. An open-ended, drainable pouch is preferable because drainage can be easily emptied. The drainable pouch is usually worn for 4 to 7 days before being changed unless leakage occurs.

- In the first 24 to 48 hours after surgery, the amount of drainage from the stoma may be negligible. Once peristalsis returns, the patient may experience a period of high volume output of 1000 to 1800 mL/day. Later on, the average amount can be 500 mL/day because the proximal small bowel adapts to absorb more fluid.

▼ **Patient and Caregiver Teaching**

Instruct the patient to drink at least 2 to 3 L of fluid daily and pay particular attention to excessive fluid losses from heat and sweating. Patients must learn signs and symptoms of fluid and electrolyte imbalance so that they can take appropriate action.

- A low-fiber diet is usually ordered initially. Fiber-containing foods are reintroduced gradually. A return to a normal, pre-surgical diet is the goal.

- The stoma may bleed easily when it is touched because it has a high vascular supply. Tell the patient that minimal oozing of blood is normal.

- Encourage the patient to share concerns and ask questions, provide information in a manner that is easily understood, recommend support services, and assist patients to develop confidence and competence in managing the stoma.

- Help the patient understand that sexual function or sexual activity may be affected, but sexuality does not have to be altered.

OXYGEN THERAPY

Description

Oxygen (O_2) therapy is frequently used in the treatment of chronic obstructive pulmonary disease (COPD) and other problems associated with hypoxemia. Long-term O_2 therapy (LTOT) improves survival, exercise capacity, cognitive performance, and sleep in hypoxemic patients.

Goals for O_2 therapy are to reduce the work of breathing, maintain the PaO_2, and/or reduce the workload on the heart. This is done by keeping the SaO_2 >90% during rest, sleep, and exertion, or PaO_2 >60 mm Hg.

O_2 is usually administered to treat hypoxemia caused by (1) respiratory disorders such as COPD, pulmonary hypertension, cor pulmonale, pneumonia, atelectasis, lung cancer, and pulmonary emboli; (2) cardiovascular disorders such as myocardial infarction, dysrhythmias, angina pectoris, and cardiogenic shock; and (3) central nervous system disorders such as overdose of opioids, head injury, and sleep disorders (sleep apnea).

Methods of Administration

Various methods of O_2 administration are used (Table 101). The method selected depends on factors such as the fraction of inspired O_2 concentration (FIO_2) and mobility of the patient, humidification required, patient cooperation, comfort, and cost.

- O_2 obtained from cylinders or wall systems is dry. Dry O_2 has an irritating effect on the mucous membranes and dries secretions. Therefore it is important that a high flow of O_2 delivering >35% to 50% oxygen be humidified when administered.

Complications

O_2 supports combustion and increases the rate of burning. This is why it is important that smoking be prohibited in the area in which O_2 is being used. A "No Smoking" sign should be prominently displayed where oxygen is in use. Also caution the patient against smoking cigarettes with an O_2 cannula in place.

The chemoreceptors in the respiratory center that control the drive to breathe respond to CO_2 and O_2. Normally CO_2 accumulation is the major stimulant of the respiratory center. Over time some COPD patients develop a tolerance for high CO_2 levels (the respiratory center loses its sensitivity to the elevated CO_2 levels). Theoretically for these individuals the "O_2 drive" to breathe is hypoxemia.

- It is critical to start O_2 at low flow rates until ABGs can be obtained. ABGs are used as a guide to determine what FIO_2 level is sufficient and can be tolerated. The patient's mental status and vital signs should be assessed before starting O_2 therapy and frequently thereafter.

Oxygen toxicity is a complication that can result from prolonged exposure to a high level of O_2. High concentrations of O_2 can result in a severe inflammatory response because of oxygen radicals and damaged alveolar-capillary membranes resulting in severe

Table 101	Methods of Oxygen Administration*

Description	Nursing Interventions
Low-Flow Delivery Devices *Nasal Cannula* Most commonly used device. Oxygen delivered via plastic nasal prongs. Safe and simple method that allows some freedom of movement and patient can eat, talk, or cough while wearing device. Useful for a patient requiring low O_2 concentrations. O_2 concentrations of 24% (at 1 L/min) to 44% (at 6 L/min) can be obtained.	Nasal cannula should be stabilized when caring for a restless patient. Amount of O_2 inhaled depends on room air and patient's breathing pattern. Most patients with COPD can tolerate 2 L/min via cannula. Assess patient's nares and ears for skin breakdown and may need to pad cannula where it sits on ears. If flow rates are >5 L/min, nasal membranes may dry and may cause pain in frontal sinuses.
Simple Face Mask Covers patient's nose and mouth. Used only for short periods, especially when transporting patients. Longer use is typically not tolerated as it is uncomfortable with tight seal and heat generated around nose/mouth from face. O_2 concentrations of 35%-50% can be achieved with flow rates of 6-12 L/min. Mask provides adequate humidification of inspired air.	Wash and dry under mask q2hr. Mask must fit snugly. Nasal cannula may be provided while patient is eating. Watch for pressure necrosis at top of ears from elastic straps if patient wears for a longer period of time. (Gauze or other padding may be used to alleviate this problem.)
Partial and Non-Rebreathing Masks Useful for short-term (24 hr) therapy for patients needing higher O_2 concentrations (60%-90% at 10-15 L/min).	Oxygen flow rate must be sufficient to keep bag from collapsing during inspiration to avoid CO_2 buildup.

Continued

| Table 101 | Methods of Oxygen Administration—cont'd |

Description	Nursing Interventions

Low-Flow Delivery Devices—cont'd
Partial and Non-Rebreathing Masks—cont'd

O_2 flows into reservoir bag and mask during inhalation.

This bag allows patient to rebreathe about first third of exhaled air (rich in O_2) in conjunction with flowing O_2.

Vents remain open on partial mask only; some facilities prefer this over non-rebreather as a safety issue.

If deflation occurs, liter flow needs to be increased to keep bag inflated.

Mask should fit snugly.

With non-rebreather masks, make sure valves are open during expiration and closed during inhalation to prevent drastic decrease in FIO_2.

Monitor patient closely because intubation may be next required intervention.

Oxygen-Conserving Cannula

Generally indicated for long-term O_2 therapy at home versus during hospitalization (e.g., pulmonary fibrosis, pulmonary hypertension).

May be "moustache" (Oxymizer) or "pendant" type.

Cannula has a built-in reservoir that $\uparrow$ O_2 concentration and allows patient to use lower flow, usually 30%-50%, which increases comfort, lowers cost, and can be increased with activities.

It can deliver up to 8 L/min of O_2.

May cause necrosis over tops of ears; can be padded.

Cannula cannot be cleaned; manufacturer recommends changing cannula every week.

It is more expensive than standard cannulas and requires evaluation with ABGs and oximetry to determine correct flow for patient.

Cannula is highly visible.

High-Flow Delivery Devices
Tracheostomy Collar

Collar attaches to neck with elastic strap and can deliver high humidity and O_2 via tracheostomy.

O_2 concentration is lost into atmosphere because collar does not fit tightly.

Secretions collect inside collar and around tracheostomy and collar should be removed and cleaned at least q4hr to prevent aspiration of fluid and infection.

| Table 101 | Methods of Oxygen Administration—cont'd |

Description	Nursing Interventions
Venturi device can be attached to flow meter and thus can deliver exact amounts of oxygen via collar.	Condensation occurs in tubing and needs to be periodically drained distally to tracheostomy.
Tracheostomy T Bar	
Almost identical to tracheostomy collar, but it has a vent and a T connector which allow an inline catheter (e.g., Ballard to be connected for suctioning).	It should be emptied as necessary.
	See tracheostomy collar above.
Tight fit allows better O_2 and humidity delivery than tracheostomy collar.	
Venturi Mask	
Mask can deliver precise, high flow rates of O_2.	Entrainment device on mask must be changed to deliver higher concentrations of O_2.
Lightweight plastic, cone-shaped device is fitted to face.	
Masks are available for delivery of 24%, 28%, 31%, 35%, 40%, and 50% O_2.	Air entrainment ports must not be occluded.
	Mask is uncomfortable and must be removed when patient eats.
Method is especially helpful for administering low, constant O_2 concentrations to patients with COPD.	Patient can talk but voice may be muffled.
Adaptors can be applied to increase humidification.	See other applicable nursing interventions under simple face mask above.

*Oxygen delivery devices are shown in Table 29-20, Lewis et al., *Medical-Surgical Nursing*, ed. 8, pp. 818-820.

pulmonary edema, shunting of blood, and hypoxemia. These individuals develop acute respiratory distress syndrome (ARDS).

- To prevent toxicity the amount of O_2 administered should be just enough to maintain the PaO_2 within a normal or acceptable range for the patient.

Infection can be a major hazard of O_2 administration. Heated nebulizers present the highest risk. Constant use of humidity supports bacterial growth, with *Pseudomonas aeruginosa* the most common infecting organism. Disposable equipment that operates

| Table 102 | Patient and Caregiver Teaching Guide: Home Oxygen Use |

The company that provides the prescribed oxygen therapy equipment will instruct the patient on equipment care. The following are some general instructions that you may include when teaching the patient and/or caregiver about the use of home oxygen.

Decreasing Risk for Infection
- Brush teeth or use mouthwash several times a day.
- Wash nasal cannula (prongs) with a liquid soap and thoroughly rinse 1 to 2 times a week.
- Replace cannula every 2 to 4 weeks.
- If you have a cold, replace the cannula after your symptoms pass.
- Always remove secretions that are coughed out.
- If you use an O_2 concentrator, every day unplug the unit and wipe down the cabinet with a damp cloth and dry.
- Ask the company providing the equipment how often the filter should be changed.

Safety Issues
- Post "No Smoking" warning signs outside the home.
- Oxygen will not "blow-up" but it will support combustion; it is a fuel for the flame/fire.
- Do not allow smoking in the home and do not smoke yourself while wearing O_2. Nasal cannulas and masks can catch fire and cause serious burns to face and airways.
- **Do not** use flammable liquids such as paint thinners, cleaning fluids, gasoline, kerosene, oil-based paints, aerosol sprays, etc. while using O_2. Do not use blankets or fabrics that carry a static charge, such as wool or synthetics.
- Inform your electrical company if you are using a concentrator so that in case of a power failure, they will know the medical urgency of restoring your power.

Adapted from www.YourLungHealth.org.

as a closed system should be used. Each hospital has a policy stating the required frequency of equipment changes based on the type of equipment used at that particular institution.

Chronic O_2 Therapy at Home

Improved survival occurs in patients with COPD who receive LTOT (>15 hours/day) to treat hypoxemia. The improved prognosis results from preventing disease progression and subsequent cor pulmonale. The benefits of long-term O_2 therapy include improved mental acuity, lung mechanics, sleep, and exercise tolerance; decreased hematocrit; and reduced pulmonary hypertension. The goal of O_2 therapy is to maintain SaO_2 >90% during rest, sleep, and exertion.

- Periodic reevaluations are necessary for the patient who is using chronic supplemental O_2. Generally the recommendation is that the patient should be reevaluated every 30 to 90 days during the first year of therapy and annually after that, as long as the patient remains stable.

▼ **Patient and Caregiver Teaching**

A home care guide for teaching the patient and family about home O_2 use is given in Table 102.

PACEMAKERS

Description

The artificial cardiac pacemaker is an electronic device used to pace the heart when the normal conduction pathway is damaged. The basic pacing circuit consists of a power source (battery-powered pulse generator), one or more conducting leads (pacing leads), and the myocardium. The electrical signal (stimulus) travels from the pacemaker, through the leads, to the wall of the myocardium. The myocardium is "captured" and stimulated to contract.

Types of Pacemakers

Permanent pacemakers are those that are implanted totally within the body, and *temporary pacemakers* are those that have the power source outside the body. The permanent pacemaker power source is implanted subcutaneously, usually over the pectoral muscle on the patient's nondominant side. It is attached to pacer leads, which are threaded transvenously (through a vein) to the right atrium and one or both ventricles. Indications for insertion of a permanent pacemaker are listed in Table 103.

There are three types of temporary pacemakers: transvenous, epicardial, and transcutaneous. Indications for temporary pacing are listed in Table 104.

- A transvenous pacemaker consists of a lead or leads that are threaded transvenously to the right atrium and/or right ventricle and attached to the external power source.
- Epicardial pacing involves attaching an atrial and ventricular pacing lead to the epicardium during heart surgery. The leads are passed through the chest wall and connected to the external power source.

Table 103	Indications for Permanent Pacemakers

- Acquired AV block
- Second-degree AV block
- Third-degree AV block
- Atrial fibrillation with a slow ventricular response
- Bundle branch block
- Cardiomyopathy
- Dilated
- Hypertrophic
- Heart failure
- SA node dysfunction
- Tachydysrhythmias (e.g., ventricular tachycardia)

AV, Atrioventricular; *SA*, sinoatrial.

Table 104	Indications for Temporary Pacemakers*

- Maintenance of adequate HR and rhythm during special circumstances such as surgery and postoperative recovery, cardiac catheterization or coronary angioplasty, during drug therapy that may cause bradycardia, and before implantation of a permanent pacemaker
- As prophylaxis after open heart surgery
- Acute anterior MI with second- or third-degree AV block or bundle branch block
- Acute inferior MI with symptomatic bradycardia and AV block
- Electrophysiologic studies to evaluate patient with bradydysrhythmias and tachydysrhythmias

AV, Atrioventricular; *HR*, heart rate; *MI*, myocardial infarction.
*List is not all-inclusive.

- A transcutaneous pacemaker is used to provide adequate heart rate and rhythm to the patient in an emergency situation and involves the use of external electrode pads that are connected to the external power source.

Patient Monitoring

Patients with temporary or permanent pacemakers will be monitored by electrocardiogram (ECG) to evaluate the status of the pacemaker. Pacemaker malfunction primarily involves a failure to sense or a failure to capture. *Failure to sense* occurs when the pacemaker fails to recognize spontaneous atrial or ventricular activity and fires inappropriately. Failure to sense is caused by pacer lead fracture (breakage), battery failure, sensing set too high, or electrode displacement. *Failure to capture* occurs when the electrical charge to the myocardium is insufficient to produce atrial or ventricular contraction. This can result in serious bradycardia or asystole. Failure to capture may be caused by pacer lead fracture, battery failure, electrode displacement, electrical charge set too low, or fibrosis at the electrode tip.

P

Table 105	Patient and Caregiver Teaching Guide: Pacemaker

Pacemaker

You should include the following instructions when teaching the patient and/or caregiver management of a pacemaker:

1. Maintain follow-up care with your primary care provider to begin regular pacemaker function checks.
2. Report any signs of infection at incision site (e.g., redness, swelling, drainage) or fever to your primary care provider immediately.
3. Keep incision dry for 4 days after implantation, or as ordered.
4. Avoid lifting arm on pacemaker side above shoulder until approved by your primary care provider.
5. Avoid direct blows to pacemaker site.
6. Avoid close proximity to high-output electric generators or large magnets such as an MRI scanner. These devices can interfere with the function of the pacemaker.
7. Microwave ovens are safe to use and do not interfere with pacemaker function.
8. Avoid standing near anti-theft devices in doorways of department stores and public libraries. You should walk through them at a normal pace.
9. Air travel is not restricted. Inform airport security of presence of pacemaker because it may set off the metal detector. If handheld screening wand is used, it should not be placed directly over the pacemaker. Manufacturer information may vary regarding the effect of metal detectors on the function of the pacemaker.
10. Monitor pulse and inform primary care provider if it drops below predetermined rate.
11. Carry pacemaker information card and a current list of your medications at all times.
12. Obtain and wear a Medic Alert ID or bracelet at all times.

MRI, Magnetic resonance imaging.

Nursing Management

Nursing interventions after pacemaker insertion include continuous
ECG monitoring to evaluate the function of the pacemaker, and
observation of the insertion site for signs of bleeding and to check
that the incision is intact. Note any temperature elevation. After
discharge, pacemaker function is checked on a regular basis to
detect problems with sensing or capturing.

- The patient with a newly implanted pacemaker and the caregiver may have questions about activity restrictions and
  fears concerning body image after the procedure.
- The goal of pacemaker therapy should be to enhance physiologic functioning and the quality of life. Emphasize this to
  the patient and caregiver, and provide specific advice on
  activity restrictions. Table 105 outlines patient and caregiver
  teaching for the patient with a pacemaker.

PARENTERAL NUTRITION

Description

Parenteral nutrition (PN) is the administration of nutrients by a
route (e.g., bloodstream) other than the gastrointestinal (GI) tract.
The goal of PN is to meet the patient's nutritional needs. Indications for PN include patients who are malnourished as a result of
medical treatment or disease processes (Table 106).

Administration of PN

PN may be administered as central PN or peripheral parenteral
nutrition. Both central and peripheral PN are used in a patient who
is not a candidate for enteral nutrition (EN).

- *Central PN* is indicated when long-term nutritional support
  is necessary or when the patient has high protein and caloric

Table 106	Common Indications for Parenteral Nutrition

- Chronic severe diarrhea and vomiting
- Complicated surgery or trauma
- Gastrointestinal obstruction
- Gastrointestinal tract anomalies and fistulae
- Intractable diarrhea
- Severe anorexia nervosa
- Severe malabsorption
- Short bowel syndrome

requirements. Central PN can also be given using peripherally inserted central catheters (PICCs) that are placed into the basilic or cephalic vein and then advanced into the distal end of the superior vena cava.

- *Peripheral parenteral nutrition* (PPN) is administered through a large, peripherally inserted catheter or vascular access device that uses a large vein. PPN is used when (1) nutritional support is needed for only a short time, (2) protein and caloric requirements are not high, (3) the risk of a central catheter is too great, or (4) parenteral support is used to supplement inadequate oral intake.

Commercially prepared PN base solutions are available. These base solutions contain dextrose and protein in the form of amino acids. The pharmacy adds the prescribed electrolytes (e.g., sodium, chloride, calcium, magnesium, phosphate), vitamins, and trace elements (e.g., zinc, copper, chromium, manganese) to customize the solution for the patient.

- A three-in-one or total nutrient admixture containing an intravenous (IV) fat emulsion, dextrose, and amino acids is widely used.
- All PN solutions should be prepared by a pharmacist or trained technician using strict aseptic techniques under a laminar flow hood. Nothing should be added to PN solutions after they are prepared by the pharmacy. The danger of drug incompatibilities and contamination is high.
- In general, PN solutions are good for 24 hours and must be refrigerated until 30 minutes before use.

Nursing Management

Because PN solutions are excellent media for microbial growth, it is essential that proper aseptic techniques be followed.

- Millipore filters should be placed on all parenteral lines: a 0.22-micron filter for parenteral solutions without fat emulsion and a 1.2-micron filter for parenteral solutions with fat emulsion.
- Filters and IV tubing are changed every 24 hours if PN with lipids is being administered and every 72 hours for PN with amino acids and dextrose. The tubing and the filter should be clearly labeled with the date and time they are put into use.
- Dressings covering the catheter site are changed according to institutional protocol, from every other day to once per week.
- Carefully observe the catheter site for signs of inflammation and infection. Phlebitis can readily occur in the vein as a

result of the hypertonic infusion, and the area can become infected. In immunosuppressed patients and patients receiving chemotherapy, corticosteroids, or antibiotics, signs of inflammation or infection can be subtle, if present at all.

■ If an infection is suspected during a dressing change, a culture specimen of the site and drainage should be sent for analysis and the health care provider should be notified immediately.

Hyperglycemia is a metabolic complication of PN. Blood glucose levels should be checked at the bedside every 4 to 6 hours with a glucose testing meter. Some increase in the blood glucose level is expected during the first few days after PN is started. Efforts are made to maintain a glucose range of 110 to 150 mg/dL. A sliding scale dose of insulin may be ordered to keep the glucose level in normal range.

An infusion pump must be used during administration of PN so that the infusion rate can be maintained, and an alarm will sound if the tubing becomes obstructed. You should periodically check the volume infused because pump malfunctions can alter the rate.

■ Sometimes fat emulsions are infused separately from the PN solution. The preferred delivery method is a continuous low volume, such as 20% lipids delivered over 12 hours, depending on patient needs.

■ Catheter-related infection and septicemia can occur. To determine the causative organism, cultures are performed of the catheter tip if the catheter has been removed or of the blood in the catheter if still in place. Blood cultures are drawn simultaneously from the catheter and a peripheral vein.

When the catheter is removed, the dressing should be changed daily until the wound heals. Encourage oral nourishment and maintain a careful record of intake. Additional information related to the nursing management of PN is presented in NCP 40-2 for the patient receiving parenteral nutrition, Lewis et al., *Medical-Surgical Nursing,* ed. 8, p. 939.

TRACHEOSTOMY

Description

A *tracheotomy* is a surgical incision into the trachea for the purpose of establishing an airway. A *tracheostomy* is the stoma (opening) that results from a tracheotomy. The standard surgical tracheostomy is usually performed in the operating room using general anesthesia. Therefore it was not typically an emergency procedure. A newer procedure, a *percutaneous tracheostomy,* can be performed emergently at the bedside using local anesthesia and some sedation/analgesia. It is a valid alternative to a surgically inserted tracheostomy, with less bleeding and fewer postoperative infections.

Indications for tracheostomy are to bypass an upper airway obstruction, facilitate the removal of secretions, permit long-term mechanical ventilation, and permit oral intake and speech in the patient requiring long-term mechanical ventilation. When compared with endotracheal tubes, tracheostomies have the following advantages:

- There is less risk of long-term damage to the airway.
- Patient comfort may be increased because no tube is present in the mouth.
- The patient can eat with a tracheostomy because the tube enters lower in the airway.
- Because the tube is more secure, patient mobility is increased.

When the patient can adequately exchange air and expectorate secretions, the tracheostomy tube can be removed. The stoma is closed with tape strips and covered with an occlusive dressing. Instruct the patient to splint the stoma with the fingers when coughing, swallowing, or speaking.

- Epithelial tissue begins to form in 24 to 48 hours, and the opening closes in several days. Surgical intervention to close a tracheostomy is not required.

Nursing Management

Goals

The patient with a tracheostomy will communicate needs, maintain a patent airway, have a normal white blood cell (WBC) count and temperature, and demonstrate satisfactory tracheostomy care.

See NCP 27-1 for the patient with a tracheostomy, Lewis et al., *Medical-Surgical Nursing,* ed. 8, pp. 532 to 534.

Nursing Diagnoses

- Ineffective airway clearance
- Impaired verbal communication
- Risk for aspiration
- Risk for infection
- Ineffective self-care management

Nursing Interventions

Before the tracheotomy, explain to the patient and family the purpose of the procedure and inform them that the patient will not be able to speak if an inflated cuff is used. A variety of tubes are available to meet patient needs (Fig. 22). Characteristics and

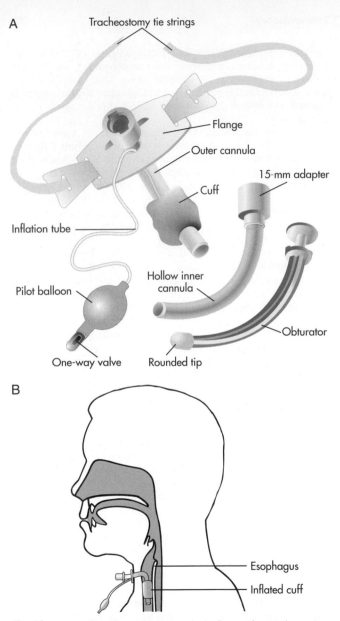

Fig. 22. Types of tracheostomy tubes. **A,** Parts of a tracheostomy tube. **B,** Tracheostomy tube inserted in airway with inflated cuff.

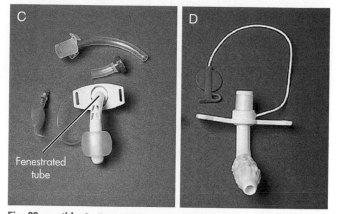

Fig. 22, cont'd. C, Fenestrated tracheostomy tube with cuff, inner cannula, decannulation plug, and pilot balloon. **D,** Tracheostomy tube with foam cuff and obturator (one cuff is deflated on tracheostomy tube).

nursing management of tracheostomies are described in Table 27-5, Lewis et al., *Medical-Surgical Nursing*, ed. 8, p 529

Care should be taken not to dislodge the tracheostomy tube during the first 5 to 7 days when the stoma is not mature (healed).

- Retention sutures are often placed in the tracheal cartilage when the tracheotomy is performed. You should tape the free ends to the skin in a place and manner that leaves them accessible if the tube is dislodged.

- Because tube replacement is difficult, several precautions are required: (1) a replacement tube of equal or smaller size is kept at the bedside, readily available for emergency reinsertion, (2) the first tube change is performed by a physician, usually no sooner than 7 days after the tracheotomy, and (3) tracheostomy tapes are not changed for at least 24 hours after the insertion procedure.

- If the tube is accidentally dislodged, immediately attempt to replace it. See the discussion of tube replacement techniques on p. 531 of Lewis et al., *Medical-Surgical Nursing*, ed. 8.

Care of the patient with a tracheostomy involves suctioning the airway to remove secretions, cleaning around the stoma, changing tracheostomy ties, and inner cannula care if a nondisposable inner cannula is used. See Table 107 for a detailed description of tracheostomy care.

Table 107	Tracheostomy Care

1. Explain procedure to patient.
2. Use tracheostomy care kit or collect necessary sterile equipment (e.g., suction catheter, gloves, water basin, drape, tracheostomy ties, tube brush or pipe cleaners, 4 × 4 gauze pads, hydrogen peroxide [3%] or mild soap, sterile water, and tracheostomy dressing [optional]). *Note:* Clean rather than sterile technique is used at home.
3. Position patient in semi-Fowler's position.
4. Assemble needed materials on bedside table next to patient.
5. Wash hands. Put on goggles and clean gloves.
6. Auscultate chest sounds. If rhonchi or coarse crackles are present, suction the patient if unable to cough up secretions (see Table 27-6, Lewis et al., *Medical-Surgical Nursing,* ed. 8, p. 530). Remove soiled dressing and clean gloves.
7. Open sterile equipment, pour sterile H_2O and hydrogen peroxide in basins, and put on sterile gloves. *Note:* Some manufacturers call for a mild soap to be used for cleaning.
8. Unlock and remove inner cannula, if present. Many tracheostomy tubes do not have inner cannulas. Care for these tubes includes all steps except for inner cannula care.
9. If disposable inner cannula is used, replace with new cannula. If a nondisposable cannula is used:
   a. Immerse inner cannula in 3% hydrogen peroxide and clean inside and outside of cannula using tube brush or pipe cleaners.
   b. Drain hydrogen peroxide from cannula. Immerse cannula in sterile water. Remove from sterile water and shake to dry.
   c. Insert inner cannula into outer cannula with the curved part downward and lock in place.
10. Remove dried secretions from stoma using 4 × 4 gauze pad soaked in sterile water. Gently pat area around the stoma dry. Be sure to clean under the tracheostomy faceplate, using cotton swabs to reach this area.
11. Maintain position of tracheal retention sutures, if present, by taping above and below the stoma.
12. Change tracheostomy ties. Use two-person change technique or secure new ties to flanges before removing the old ones. Tie tracheostomy ties securely with room for one finger between ties and skin (see Fig. 27-5 from Lewis et al., *Medical-Surgical Nursing,* ed. 8, p. 531). To prevent accidental tube removal, secure the tracheostomy tube by gently applying pressure to the flange of the tube during the tie changes. *Do not change tracheostomy ties for 24 hours after the tracheotomy procedure.*

Table 107	Tracheostomy Care—cont'd

13. As an alternative, some patients prefer tracheostomy ties made of Velcro, which are easier to adjust.
14. If drainage is excessive, place dressing around tube (see Fig. 27-5 from Lewis et al., *Medical-Surgical Nursing*, ed. 8, p. 531). A tracheostomy dressing or unlined gauze should be used. Do not cut the gauze because threads may be inhaled or wrapped around the tracheostomy tube. Change the dressing frequently. Wet dressings promote infection and stoma irritation.
15. Repeat care 3 times a day and as needed.

▼ **Patient and Caregiver Teaching**

- Assess ability of the patient and caregiver to provide care at home.
- Include instructions for tracheostomy tube care, stoma care, suctioning, airway care, and responding to emergencies.
- Make a referral to a home health care nurse to provide ongoing assistance and support.
- Teach patient and caregiver the signs and symptoms to report to health care professionals, such as changes in secretions (color and consistency) and elevated temperature.

U

URINARY CATHETERIZATION

Indications for short-term urinary catheterization are listed in Table 108. Two reasons that are not indications for catheterization are (1) routine acquisition of a urine specimen for laboratory analysis and (2) convenience of the nursing staff or the patient's family.

- Complications of long-term use (>30 days) of indwelling catheters include bladder spasms, periurethral abscess, pain, urinary tract infections (UTIs), urosepsis, urethral trauma/erosion, fistula/stricture formation, and stones.

Catheterization for sterile urine specimens may occasionally be indicated when patients have a history of complicated urinary infections. A catheter should be the final means of providing the patient with a dry environment for the prevention of skin breakdown and protection of dressings or skin lesions.

Scrupulous aseptic technique is mandatory when a urinary catheter is inserted. After insertion, nursing actions include maintaining catheter patency, managing fluid intake, providing for the comfort

Table 108	Indications for Urinary Catheterization

Indwelling Catheter
- Relief of urinary retention caused by lower urinary tract obstruction, paralysis, or inability to void
- Bladder decompression preoperatively and operatively for lower abdominal or pelvic surgery
- Facilitation of surgical repair of urethra and surrounding structures
- Splinting of ureters or urethra to facilitate healing after surgery or other trauma in area
- Accurate measurement of urinary output in critically ill patient
- Measurement of residual urine after urination (referred to as postvoid residual [PVR]) if portable ultrasound not available
- Contamination of stage III or IV pressure ulcers with urine that has impeded healing, despite appropriate personal care for the incontinence (indwelling)
- Terminal illness or severe impairment, which makes positioning or clothing changes uncomfortable, or which is associated with intractable pain (indwelling)

Straight (In-and-Out) Catheter
- Study of anatomic structures of urinary system
- Urodynamic testing
- Collection of sterile urine sample in selected situations
- Instillation of medications into bladder

and safety of the patient, and preventing infection. Concerns of the patient can include embarrassment related to exposure of the body, an altered body image, and fear concerning the care of the catheter that results in increased dependency.

- Catheters vary in construction materials, tip shape, and lumen size. Catheters are sized according to the French scale. Each French unit equals 0.33 mm of diameter. The diameter measured is the internal diameter of the catheter. The size used varies with the size of the individual and the purpose for catheterization.
- The most common route of catheterization is insertion of the catheter through the external meatus into the urethra, past the internal sphincter, and into the bladder.

Suprapubic catheterization is the simplest and oldest method of urinary diversion. The two methods of insertion of a suprapubic catheter into the bladder are (1) through a small incision in the abdominal wall and (2) by the use of a trocar. A suprapubic catheter is placed while the patient is under general anesthesia for another surgical procedure or at the bedside with a local anesthetic. The catheter may be sutured into place.

- The suprapubic catheter is used in temporary situations, such as bladder, prostate, and urethral surgery, and also used long term in selected patients.
- Nursing care includes taping the catheter to prevent dislodgement. The care of the tube and catheter is similar to that of the urethral catheter. A pectin-base skin barrier (e.g., Stomahesive) is effective around the insertion site in protecting the skin from breakdown.

The suprapubic catheter is prone to poor drainage because of mechanical obstruction of the catheter tip by the bladder wall, sediment, and clots. Nursing interventions to ensure the patency of the tube include (1) preventing tube kinking by coiling the excess tubing and maintaining gravity drainage, (2) having the patient turn from side to side, and (3) milking the tube. If these measures are not effective, the catheter is irrigated with sterile technique after a physician's order has been obtained.

- If the patient experiences bladder spasms that are difficult to control, urinary leakage may result. Oxybutynin (Ditropan) or other oral antispasmodics or belladonna and opium (B&O) suppositories may be prescribed to decrease bladder spasms.

An alternative approach to a long-term indwelling catheter is *intermittent catheterization,* also referred to as "straight" or "in and out" catheterization. It is being used with increasing frequency in conditions characterized by neurogenic bladder (e.g., spinal cord injuries, chronic neurologic diseases) or bladder outlet obstruction in men. This type of catheterization may also be used in the oliguric and anuric phases of acute kidney injury to reduce the possibility of infection from an indwelling catheter. Intermittent catheterization is also used postoperatively, often after a surgical procedure for female incontinence or following radioactive seed implantation into the prostate.

- The main goal of intermittent catheterization is to prevent urinary retention, stasis, and compromised blood supply to the bladder resulting from prolonged pressure.
- The technique consists of inserting a urethral catheter into the bladder every 3 to 5 hours. Some patients do intermittent catheterization only once or twice each day to measure residual urine and ensure an empty bladder.
- Instruct patients to wash and rinse the catheter and their hands with soap and water before and after catheterization. Lubricant is necessary for men and may make catheterization more comfortable for women.

- The catheter may be inserted by the patient or a care provider. The bladder is emptied, and the catheter is removed.
- In general, patients should change the catheter every 7 days.
- In the hospital, sterile technique is used for all urinary catheterizations. For home care, a clean technique that includes good hand washing with soap and water is used.
- Teach the patient to observe for signs of UTI so that treatment can be instituted early. If indicated, some patients are placed on a regimen of prophylactic antibiotics.

PART THREE

Reference Appendix

Abbreviations

ABG	arterial blood gas
ACE	angiotensin-converting enzyme
ACLS	advanced cardiac life support
ACS	acute coronary syndrome
ACTH	adrenocorticotropic hormone
ADH	antidiuretic hormone
AED	automatic external defibrillator
AIDS	acquired immunodeficiency syndrome
AKA	above-knee amputation
AKI	acute kidney injury
ALI	acute lung injury
ALL	acute lymphocytic leukemia
ALS	amyotrophic lateral sclerosis
AMI	acute myocardial infarction
ANA	antinuclear antibody
ANS	autonomic nervous system
AORN	Association of periOperative Room Nurses
APD	automated peritoneal dialysis
aPTT	activated partial thromboplastin time
ARDS	acute respiratory distress syndrome
ATN	acute tubular necrosis
BCLS	basic cardiac life support
BKA	below-knee amputation
BMI	body mass index
BMR	basal metabolic rate
BMT	bone marrow transplantation
BPH	benign prostatic hyperplasia
BSE	breast self-examination
BUN	blood urea nitrogen
CABG	coronary artery bypass graft
CAD	coronary artery disease, circulatory assist device
CAPD	continuous ambulatory peritoneal dialysis
CAVH	continuous arteriovenous hemofiltration
CBC	complete blood count
CCU	coronary care unit; critical care unit
CDC	Centers for Disease Control and Prevention
CIS	carcinoma in situ
CKD	chronic kidney disease
CLL	chronic lymphocytic leukemia
CML	chronic myelocytic leukemia
CMP	cardiomyopathy
CN	cranial nerve
CNS	central nervous system
CO	cardiac output
COPD	chronic obstructive pulmonary disease

Continued

Abbreviations—cont'd

CPAP	continuous positive airway pressure
CPR	cardiopulmonary resuscitation
CRRT	continuous renal replacement therapy
CRNA	certified registered nurse anesthetist
CSF	cerebrospinal fluid
CT	computed tomography
CVA	cerebrovascular accident; costovertebral angle
CVAD	central venous access device
CVI	chronic venous insufficiency
CVP	central venous pressure
D&C	dilation and curettage
DDD	degenerative disk disease
DI	diabetes insipidus
DIC	disseminated intravascular coagulation
DJD	degenerative joint disease
DKA	diabetic ketoacidosis
DM	diabetes mellitus; diastolic murmur
DRE	digital rectal examination
DVT	deep vein thrombosis
ECF	extracellular fluid
ECG	electrocardiogram
ED	emergency department, erectile dysfunction
EEG	electroencephalogram
EMG	electromyogram
EMS	emergency medical services
ENT	ear, nose, and throat
ERCP	endoscopic retrograde cholangiopancreatography
ERT	estrogen replacement therapy
ESR	erythrocyte sedimentation rate
ESRD	end-stage renal disease
ET	endotracheal
FEV	forced expiratory volume
FRC	functional residual capacity
FUO	fever of unknown origin
GCS	Glasgow Coma Scale
GERD	gastroesophageal reflux disease
GFR	glomerular filtration rate
GH	growth hormone
GI	glycemic index
GTT	glucose tolerance test
GU	genitourinary
GYN, Gyn	gynecological
H&P	history and physical examination
HAV	hepatitis A virus
Hb	hemoglobin

Abbreviations—cont'd

HBV	hepatitis B virus
Hb, Hgb	hemoglobin
Hct	hematocrit
HCV	hepatitis C virus
HD	hemodialysis, Huntington's disease
HDL	high-density lipoprotein
HF	heart failure
HIV	human immunodeficiency virus
HPV	human papillomavirus
HSCT	hematopoietic stem cell transplantation
I&D	incision and drainage
IABP	intraaortic balloon pumping
IBS	irritable bowel syndrome
ICP	intracranial pressure
IE	infective endocarditis
IFG	impaired fasting glucose
IGT	impaired glucose tolerance
INR	international normalized ratio
IOP	intraocular pressure
IPPB	intermittent positive pressure breathing
ITP	idiopathic thrombocytopenic purpura
IUD	intrauterine device
IV	intravenous
IVP	intravenous push; intravenous pyelogram
JVD	jugular venous distention
KUB	kidney, ureters, and bladder (x-ray)
KS	Kaposi sarcoma
KVO	keep vein open
LAD	left anterior descending
LDL	low-density lipoprotein
LGV	lymphogranuloma venereum
LLQ	left lower quadrant
LMN	lower motor neuron
LMP	last menstrual period
LOC	level of consciousness
LP	lumbar puncture
LUQ	left upper quadrant
LVH	left ventricular hypertrophy
MAP	mean arterial pressure
MD	muscular dystrophy
MDS	myelodysplastic syndrome
MG	myasthenia gravis
MI	myocardial infarction
MICU	medical intensive care unit
MODS	multiple organ dysfunction syndrome

Continued

Abbreviations—cont'd

MRB	manual resuscitation bag
MS	multiple sclerosis
MVP	mitral valve prolapse
NAFLD	nonalcoholic fatty liver disease
NANDA	North American Nursing Diagnosis Association
NAP	nursing assistive personnel
NASH	nonalcoholic steatohepatitis
NG	nasogastric
NHL	non-Hodgkin's lymphoma
NPO	nothing by mouth
NS	normal saline
NSR	normal sinus rhythm
OA	osteoarthritis
OD	right eye; optical density; overdose
OL	left eye
OOB	out of bed
OR	operating room
ORIF	open reduction and internal fixation
OSA	obstructive sleep apnea
OTC	over-the-counter
PA	posteroanterior; physician's assistant
PAC	premature atrial contraction
$PaCO_2$	partial pressure of carbon dioxide in arterial blood
PaO_2	partial pressure of oxygen in arterial blood
PACU	postanesthesia care unit
PAD	peripheral artery disease
PAP	pulmonary artery pressure
PAWP	pulmonary artery wedge pressure
PCA	patient-controlled analgesia
PCI	percutaneous coronary intervention
PCWP	pulmonary capillary wedge pressure
PD	Parkinson's disease, peritoneal dialysis
PE	pulmonary embolism; physical examination
PEEP	positive end-expiratory pressure
PEFR	peak expiratory flow rate
PERRLA	pupils equal, round, and reactive to light and accommodation
PET	positron emission tomography
PICC	percutaneously inserted central catheter
PID	pelvic inflammatory disease
PKD	polycystic kidney disease
PMH	past medical history
PMI	point of maximal impulse
PMS	premenstrual syndrome

Abbreviations—cont'd

PN	parenteral nutrition
PND	paroxysmal nocturnal dyspnea; postnasal drip
PNS	peripheral nervous system
PO, po	orally
POC	point-of-care
PPD	purified protein derivative
PSA	prostate-specific antigen
PSS	progressive systemic sclerosis
PT	prothrombin time
PTT	partial thromboplastin time
PVC	premature ventricular contraction
PUD	peptic ulcer disease
R/O	rule out
RA	rheumatoid arthritis
REM	rapid eye movement
RF	rheumatic fever
RHD	rheumatic heart disease
RLQ	right lower quadrant
RLS	restless legs syndrome
ROM	range of motion
ROS	review of systems
RS	Reiter's syndrome
RUQ	right upper quadrant
SA	sinoatrial
SCI	spinal cord injury
SCD	sickle cell disease, sudden cardiac death
SDP	sleep-disordered breathing
SICU	surgical intensive care unit
SIRS	systemic inflammatory response syndrome
SLE	systemic lupus erythematosus
SNS	sympathetic nervous system
SOB	shortness of breath
STD	sexually transmitted disease
STSG	split-thickness skin graft
SVR	systemic vascular resistance
SVT	superficial vein thrombosis
TAH	total abdominal hysterectomy
TB	tuberculosis
TBSA	total body surface area
TCDB	turn, cough, and deep breathe
TENS	transcutaneous electrical nerve stimulation
THR	total hip replacement
TIA	transient ischemic attack
TJC	The Joint Commission
TKO	to keep open

Continued

Abbreviations—cont'd

TPR	temperature, pulse, and respirations
TURP	transurethral resection of the prostate
UA	unstable angina
UGI	upper gastrointestinal
UI	urinary incontinence
UMN	upper motor neuron
URI	upper respiratory infection
UTI	urinary tract infection
VAD	venous access device, ventricular assist device
VD	venereal disease
VDH	valvular disease of the heart
VF	ventricular fibrillation
VS	vital signs
VT	ventricular tachycardia
VTE	venous thromboembolism
WHR	waist-to-hip ratio
WNL	within normal limits

THE JOINT COMMISSION
Official "Do Not Use" List[1]

Do Not Use	Potential Problem	Use Instead
U (unit)	Mistaken for "0" (zero), the number "4" (four) or "cc"	Write "unit"
IU (International Unit)	Mistaken for IV (intravenous) or the number 10 (ten)	Write "International Unit"
Q.D., QD, q.d., qd (daily)	Mistaken for each other	Write "daily"
Q.O.D., QOD, q.o.d., qod (every other day)	Period after the Q mistaken for "I" and the "O" mistaken for "I"	Write "every other day"
Trailing zero (X.0 mg)*	Decimal point is missed	Write X mg
Lack of leading zero (.X mg)		Write 0.X mg
MS	Can mean morphine sulfate or magnesium sulfate	Write "morphine sulfate" Write "magnesium sulfate"
MSO_4 and $MgSO_4$	Confused for one another	

© The Joint Commission, 2010. Reprinted with permission.

[1]Applies to all orders and all medication-related documentation that is handwritten (including free-text computer entry) or on pre-printed forms.

*Exception: A "trailing zero" may be used only where required to demonstrate the level of precision of the value being reported, such as for laboratory results, imaging studies that report size of lesions, or catheter/tube sizes. It may not be used in medication orders for other medication-related documentation.

Additional Abbreviations, Acronyms, and Symbols (For possible future inclusion in the Official "Do Not Use" List)

Do Not Use	Potential Problem	Use Instead
> (greater than) < (less than)	Misinterpreted as the number "7" (seven) or the letter "L" Confused for one another	Write "greater than" Write "less than"

Continued

**Additional Abbreviations, Acronyms, and Symbols
(For possible future inclusion in the Official
"Do Not Use" List)—cont'd**

Do Not Use	Potential Problem	Use Instead
Abbreviations for drug names	Misinterpreted due to similar abbreviations for multiple drugs	Write drug names in full
@	Mistaken for the number "2" (two)	Write "at"
cc	Mistaken for U (units) when poorly written	Write "mL" or "ml" or "milliliters" ("mL" is preferred)
μg	Mistaken for mg (milligrams) resulting in one thousand-fold overdose	Write "mcg" or "micrograms"

BLOOD GASES
Normal Values

	Arterial (Sea Level)
pH	7.35-7.45
PaO_2*	80-100 mm Hg
$PaCO_2$	32-48 mm Hg
HCO_3	22-26 mEq/L
O_2 saturation	>95%

*In a patient >60 years old, PaO_2 is equal to 80 mm Hg minus 1 mm Hg for every year over 60. Expected $PaO_2 = FIO_2 \times 5$.

Interpreting Arterial Blood Gases (ABGs)

1. Check pH
   $\uparrow$ = Alkalosis; $\downarrow$ = acidosis
2. Check $PaCO_2$
   $\uparrow$ = CO_2 retention (hypoventilation); respiratory acidosis or compensating for metabolic alkalosis
   $\downarrow$ = CO_2 blown off (hyperventilation); respiratory alkalosis or compensating for metabolic acidosis
3. Check HCO_3
   $\uparrow$ = Nonvolatile acid is lost; HCO_3 gained (metabolic alkalosis or compensating for respiratory acidosis)
   $\downarrow$ = Nonvolatile acid is added; HCO_3 is lost (metabolic acidosis or compensating for respiratory alkalosis)
4. Determine imbalance
5. Determine if compensation exists

Determining the Imbalance in ABGs

If: pH $\uparrow$ and $PaCO_2$ $\downarrow$ or pH $\downarrow$ and $PaCO_2$ $\uparrow$	**Then** respiratory disorder
If: pH $\uparrow$ and HCO_3 $\uparrow$ or pH $\downarrow$ and HCO_3 $\downarrow$	**Then** metabolic disorder
If: $PaCO_2$ $\uparrow$ and HCO_3 $\uparrow$ or $PaCO_2$ $\downarrow$ and HCO_3 $\downarrow$	**Then** compensation is occurring
If: $PaCO_2$ $\uparrow$ and HCO_3 $\downarrow$ or $PaCO_2$ $\downarrow$ and HCO_3 $\uparrow$	**Then** mixed imbalance

Laboratory Values

Test	Conventional Units	SI Units
Complete Blood Count		
Red blood cells (RBCs)	Male: 4.3-5.7 × 10⁶/μL Female: 3.8-5.1 × 10⁶/μL	Male: 4.3-5.7 × 10¹²/L Female: 3.8-5.1 × 10¹²/L
White blood cells (WBCs)	4.0-11.0 × 10³/μL	4.0-11.0 × 10⁹/L
Hemoglobin (Hb)	Male: 13.2-17.3 g/dL Female: 11.7-15.5 g/dL	Male: 132-173 g/L Female: 117-155 g/L
Hematocrit (Hct)	Male: 39%-50% Female: 35%-47%	Male: 0.39-0.50 Female: 0.35-0.47
Chemistry		
Albumin	3.5-5 g/dL	35-50 g/L
Alkaline phosphatase	38-126 U/L	0.65-2.14 μkat/L
Aspartate aminotransferase (AST)	10-30 U/L	0.17-0.51 μkat/L
Alanine aminotransferase (ALT)	10-40 U/L	0.17-0.68 μkat/L
Ammonia	15-45 mcg N/dL	11-32 μmol N/L
Amylase	30-122 U/L	0.51-2.07 μkat/L
Bilirubin		
Total	0.2-1.2 mg/dL	3.4-21.0 μmol/L
Direct	0.1-0.3 mg/dL	1.7-5.1 μmol/L
Indirect	0.1-1.0 mg/dL	1.7-17 μmol/L
Blood urea nitrogen (BUN)	10-30 mg/dL	1.8-7.1 mmol/L
Calcium (total)	8.6-10.2 mg/dL	2.15-2.55 mmol/L
Cholesterol	<200 mg/dL	<5.2 mmol/L
HDL	Male: >40 mg/dL Female: >50 mg/dL	>1.04 mmol/L >1.3 mmol/L

aPTT, Activated partial thromboplastin time; *FSP,* fibrin split products; *HDL,* high-density lipoprotein; *LDL,* low-density lipoprotein; *PT,* prothrombin time.

Laboratory Values—cont'd

Test	Conventional Units	SI Units
LDL	*Recommended:* <100 mg/dL *Near Optimal:* 100-129 mg/dL *Moderate risk for CAD:* 130-159 mg/dL *High risk for CAD:* >160 mg/dL	*Recommended:* <2.6 mmol/L *Near Optimal:* 2.6-3.34 mmol/L *Moderate risk for CAD:* 3.37-4.12 mmol/L *High risk for CAD:* >4.14 mmol/L
Chloride	96-106 mEq/L	96-106 mmol/L
HCO$_3$	23-29 mEq/L	23-29 mmol/L
Creatinine	0.5-1.5 mg/dL	44-133 µmol/L
Glucose	70-120 mg/dL	3.89-6.66 mmol/L
Iron	50-175 mcg/dL	9.0-31.3 µmol/L
Lactic dehydrogenase (LDH)	140-280 U/L	0.83-2.5 µkat/L
Lipase	31-186 U/L	0.5-3.2 µkat/L
Magnesium	1.5-2.5 mEq/l	0.75-1.25 mmol/l
Osmolality	275-295 mOsm/kg	275-295 mmol/kg
Phosphorus (phosphate)	2.4-4.4 mg/dL	0.78-1.42 mmol/L
Potassium	3.5-5.0 mEq/L	3.5-5.0 mmol/L
Protein (total)	6.4-8.3 g/dL	64-83 g/L
Sodium	135-145 mEq/L	135-145 mmol/L
Triglyceride	<150 mg/dL	<1.7 mmol/L
Coagulation		
Platelets	150-400 × 10^3/µL	150-400 × 10^9/L
PT	11-16 sec	Same as conventional unit
aPTT	25-35 sec	Same as conventional unit
FSP	<10 mcg/mL	<10 mg/L

Blood Products*

Description	Special Considerations	Indications for Use
Packed RBCs Packed RBCs are prepared from whole blood by sedimentation or centrifugation. One unit contains 250-350 mL.	Use of RBCs for treatment allows remaining components of blood (e.g., platelets, albumin, plasma) to be used for other purposes. There is less danger of fluid overload. Packed RBCs are preferred RBC source because they are more component specific. Leukocyte depletion (by the blood bank or filter) may be used to reduce hemolytic febrile reactions in patients who receive frequent transfusions.	Severe or symptomatic anemia, acute blood loss. In general, one unit of packed red blood cells can be expected to increase a patient's hemoglobin level by 1 g/dL or Hct by 30%.
Frozen RBCs Frozen RBCs are prepared from RBCs using glycerol for protection and frozen. They can be stored for 10 yr at −188.6° F (−87° C).	They must be used within 24 hr of thawing. Successive washings with saline solution remove majority of WBCs and plasma proteins.	Autotransfusion; stockpiling or rare donors for patients with alloantibodies. Infrequently used because filters remove most WBCs.

Continued

Platelets

Platelets are prepared from fresh whole blood within 4 hr after collection. One unit contains 30-60 mL of platelet concentrate.

Multiple units of platelets can be obtained from one donor by plateletpheresis. They can be kept at room temperature for 1-5 days depending on type of collection and storage bag used. Bag should be agitated periodically. Expected increase is 10,000/µL/U. Failure to have a rise may result from fever, sepsis, splenomegaly, or DIC. For patients who receive frequent transfusions or do not respond to previous platelet transfusions, may give leukocyte reduced, HLA, or type specific to prevent alloimmunization to HLA antigens.

Bleeding caused by thrombocytopenia; may be contraindicated in thrombotic thrombocytopenic purpura and heparin-induced thrombocytopenia except in life-threatening hemorrhage.

Fresh Frozen Plasma

Liquid portion of whole blood is separated from cells and frozen. One unit contains 200-250 mL. Plasma is rich in clotting factors but contains no platelets. It may be stored for 1 yr. It must be used within 2 hr after thawing.

Use of plasma in treating hypovolemic shock is being replaced by pure preparations such as albumin and plasma expanders.

Bleeding caused by deficiency in clotting factors (e.g., DIC, hemorrhage, massive transfusion, liver disease, vitamin K deficiency, excess warfarin).

Blood Products*—cont'd

Description	Special Considerations	Indications for Use
Albumin Albumin is prepared from plasma. It can be stored for 5 yr. It is available in 5% or 25% solution.	Albumin 25 g/100 mL is osmotically equal to 500 mL of plasma. Hyperosmolar solution acts by moving water from extravascular to intravascular space. It is heat treated and does not transmit viruses.	Hypovolemic shock, hypoalbuminemia
Cryoprecipitates and Commercial Concentrates Cryoprecipitate is prepared from fresh frozen plasma, with 10-20 mL/bag. It can be stored for 1 yr. Once thawed, must be used.	See Table 31-19.	Replacement of clotting factors, especially factor VIII, von Willebrand disease, and fibrinogen

DIC, Disseminated intravascular coagulation; *Hct,* hematocrit; *HLA,* human leukocyte antigen; *RBCs,* red blood cells; *WBCs,* white blood cells.
*Component therapy has replaced the use of whole blood, which accounts for less than 10% of all transfusions. Granulocyte transfusions are not included here because they are rarely used.

BREATH SOUNDS
Normal Sounds

Type	Normal Site	Duration, I/E Ratio	Characteristics
Vesicular	Peripheral lung	I > E 3:1	Soft, low-pitched, gentle, rustling sounds; heard over all lung areas except major bronchi; abnormal when heard over the large airways
Bronchovesicular	Sternal border of the major bronchi	I = E 1:1	Medium pitch and intensity; heard anteriorly over the mainstem bronchi on either side of the sternum and posteriorly between the scapulae; abnormal if heard over peripheral lung fields
Bronchial	Trachea and bronchi	I < E 2:3	Louder, higher pitched; resembles air blowing through a hollow pipe; abnormal if heard over peripheral lung

E, Expiration; *I,* inspiration.

BREATH SOUNDS
Adventitious Sounds (Abnormal Sounds)

Characteristics	Possible Clinical Condition
Fine Crackles (Formerly Called Rales)	
Series of short-duration, discontinuous, high-pitched sounds heard just before the end of inspiration; similar sound to that made by rolling hair between fingers just behind ear	Idiopathic pulmonary fibrosis, interstitial edema (early pulmonary edema), alveolar filling (pneumonia), loss of lung volume (atelectasis), early phase of heart failure
Coarse Crackles	
Series of long-duration, discontinuous, low-pitched sounds caused by air passing through airway intermittently occluded by mucus, unstable bronchial wall, or fold of mucosa; evident on inspiration and, at times, expiration	Heart failure, pulmonary edema, pneumonia with severe congestion, chronic obstructive pulmonary disease (COPD)
Rhonchi	
Continuous rumbling, snoring, or rattling sounds from obstruction of large airways with secretions; most prominent on expiration	COPD, cystic fibrosis, pneumonia, bronchiectasis
Wheezes	
Continuous high-pitched squeaking or musical sound caused by rapid vibration of bronchial walls; first evident on expiration but possibly evident on inspiration as obstruction of airway increases	Bronchospasm (caused by asthma), airway obstruction (caused by foreign body, tumor), COPD
Pleural Friction Rub	
Creaking or grating sound from roughened, inflamed surfaces of the pleura rubbing together; evident during inspiration, expiration, or both	Pleurisy, pneumonia, pulmonary infarct

Commonly Used Formulas

Parameter	Formula	Normal Range
Anion gap	$Na - (HCO_2 + Cl)$	8-16 mEq/L
Body mass index (BMI)	$\dfrac{\text{Weight in pounds}}{\text{Height in inches}^2} \times 703$	18.5-24.9 kg/m^2
Cardiac index (CI)	CO/Body surface area (BSA)	2.2-4.0 L/min/m^2
Cardiac output (CO)	$HR \times SV$	4-8 L/min
Cerebral perfusion pressure (CPP)	MAP-ICP	80-100 mm Hg
Ejection fraction (EF)	$\dfrac{SV}{\text{End-diastolic volume}} \times 100$	60% or greater
Heart rate (HR)		60-80 beats/min
Mean arterial pressure (MAP)	$\dfrac{2(DBP) + SBP}{3}$	70-105 mm Hg
Stroke volume (SV)	$\dfrac{CO}{HR}$	60-150 mL/beat

DBP, Diastolic blood pressure; *ICP*, intracranial pressure; *SBP*, systolic blood pressure.

Commonly Used Herbs

Name	Uses Based on Scientific Evidence	Comments
Aloe	Constipation	Use no longer than 7 days for constipation
		May cause electrolyte imbalances
		May lower blood glucose
Black cohosh	Menopausal symptoms	Generally safe when used for up to 6 months in healthy, nonpregnant women
		May lower blood pressure
Echinacea	Treatment of upper respiratory infections	Use with caution in patients with conditions affecting immune system
		May lead to liver inflammation
		Short-term use is recommended
Evening primrose	Eczema, skin irritation	Contraindicated in individuals with seizure disorders
Feverfew	Migraine headache prevention	May increase risk of bleeding
		Long-term users may experience withdrawal symptoms
Garlic	High cholesterol	May increase risk of bleeding
		May lower blood glucose
Ginkgo biloba	Intermittent claudication	Generally well tolerated in recommended dosages for up to 6 months
		May increase risk of bleeding
		May affect blood glucose levels
Ginseng (*Panax* species, including Asian and American ginseng)	Improve mental performance	May lower blood glucose levels
	Lower blood glucose in type 2 diabetes mellitus	May reduce effectiveness of warfarin
		Avoid in patients with hormone-sensitive conditions such as breast cancer
		Generally safe when used for up to 3 months

Hawthorn	Mild to moderate heart failure	May add to the effects of cardiac glycosides, antihypertensives, and cholesterol-lowering drugs
Kava	Anxiety	Avoid in patients with liver problems and patients taking medications that affect liver
		May increase sedation caused by some herbs or supplements
		Use cautiously with herbs or supplements that are metabolized by kidneys
Milk thistle	Hepatitis caused by viruses or alcohol	May lower blood glucose levels
	Cirrhosis	May interfere with liver's cytochrome P450 enzyme system
St. John's wort	Short-term treatment of mild to moderate depression	May lead to serious interactions with herbs, supplements, OTC drugs, or prescription drugs
		May lead to increased side effects when taken with other antidepressants
		Advise patients to consult health care professional before self-medicating with St. John's wort
Valerian	Insomnia	Generally safe in recommended dosages for up to 4-6 weeks
		Chronic use may result in insomnia

Advise patients who are pregnant or lactating to consult a health care practitioner before using any herbs. There is limited scientific evidence for the use of most herbs during pregnancy or lactation.
OTC, Over-the-counter.
Source: www.naturalstandard.com

Characteristics of Common Dysrhythmias

Pattern	Rate and Rhythm	P Wave	PR Interval	QRS Complex
Normal sinus rhythm (NSR)	60-100 beats/min and regular	Normal	Normal	Normal
Sinus bradycardia	<60 beats/min and regular	Normal	Normal	Normal
Sinus tachycardia	101-200 beats/min and regular	Normal	Normal	Normal
Premature atrial contraction (PAC)	Usually 60-100 beats/min and irregular	Abnormal shape	Normal	Normal (usually)
Paroxysmal supraventricular tachycardia (PSVT)	150-220 beats/min and regular	Abnormal shape, may be hidden in the preceding T wave	Normal or shortened	Normal (usually)
Atrial flutter	Atrial: 200-350 beats/min and regular. Ventricular: > or <100 beats/min and may be regular or irregular	Flutter (F) waves (sawtoothed pattern); more flutter waves than QRS complexes; may occur in a 2:1, 3:1, 4:1, etc. pattern	Not measurable	Normal (usually)
Atrial fibrillation	Atrial: 350-600 beats/min and irregular. Ventricular: > or <100 beats/min and irregular	Fibrillatory (f) waves	Not measurable	Normal (usually)
Junctional dysrhythmias	40-180 beats/min and regular	Inverted, may be hidden in QRS complex	Variable	Normal (usually)
First-degree AV block	Normal and regular	Normal	>0.20 sec	Normal

Second-degree AV block				
Type 1 (Mobitz 1, Wenckebach heart block)	*Atrial:* Normal and regular; *Ventricular:* Slower and irregular	Normal	Progressive lengthening	Normal QRS width, with pattern of one nonconducted (blocked) QRS complex
Type II (Mobitz II heart block)	*Atrial:* Usually normal and regular; *Ventricular:* Slower and regular or irregular	More P waves than QRS complexes (e.g., 2:1, 3:1)	Normal or prolonged	Widened QRS, preceded by two or more P waves, with nonconducted (blocked) QRS complex
Third-degree AV block (complete heart block)	*Atrial:* Regular but may appear irregular due to P waves hidden in QRS complexes; *Ventricular:* 20-60 beats/min and regular	Normal, but no connection with QRS complex	Variable	Normal or widened, no relationship with P waves
Premature ventricular contraction (PVC)	Underlying rhythm can be any rate; regular or irregular rhythm; PVCs occur at variable rates	Not usually visible; hidden in the PVC	Not measurable	Wide and distorted
Ventricular tachycardia (VT)	150-250 beats/min and regular or irregular	Not usually visible	Not measurable	Wide and distorted
Accelerated idioventricular rhythm	40-100 beats/min and regular	Not usually visible	Not measurable	Wide and distorted
Ventricular fibrillation (VF)	Not measurable and irregular	Absent	Not measurable	Not measurable

AV, Atrioventricular.

ELECTROCARDIOGRAM (ECG) MONITORING: WAVEFORM AND NORMAL SINUS RHYTHM

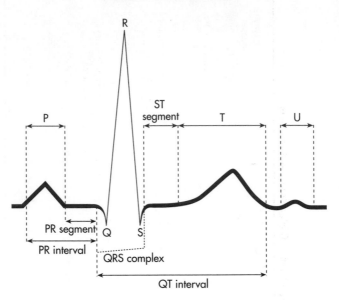

Definition and Sources of Variation in ECG Waveforms and Intervals*

Description	Normal Duration (sec)	Source of Possible Variation
P wave Represents time for the passage of the electrical impulse through the atrium causing atrial depolarization (contraction); should be upright	0.06-0.12	Disturbance in conduction within atria
PR interval Measured from beginning of P wave to beginning of QRS complex; represents time taken for impulse to spread through the atria, AV node and bundle of His, the bundle branches, and Purkinje fibers, to a point immediately preceding ventricular contraction	0.12-0.20	Disturbance in conduction usually in AV node, bundle of His, or bundle branches but can be in atria as well
QRS interval Measured from beginning to end of QRS complex; represents time taken for depolarization (contraction) of both ventricles (systole)	<0.12	Disturbance in conduction in bundle branches or in ventricles

Continued

Definition and Sources of Variation in ECG Waveforms and Intervals*—cont'd

Description	Normal Duration (sec)	Source of Possible Variation
ST segment Measured from the S wave of the QRS complex to the beginning of the T wave; represents the time between ventricular depolarization and repolarization (diastole); should be isoelectric (flat)	0.12	Disturbances usually caused by ischemia or infarction
T wave Represents time for ventricular repolarization; should be upright	0.16	Disturbances usually caused by electrolyte imbalances, ischemia, or infarction
QT interval Measured from beginning of QRS complex to end of T wave; represents time taken for entire electrical depolarization and repolarization of the ventricles	0.34-0.43	Disturbances usually affecting repolarization more than depolarization and caused by drugs, electrolyte imbalances, and changes in heart rate

AV, Atrioventricular; *ECG*, electrocardiogram.
*Heart rate influences the duration of these intervals, especially those of the PR and QT intervals (e.g., QT interval decreases in duration as HR increases).

Glasgow Coma Scale

Category of Response	Appropriate Stimulus	Response	Score
Eyes Open	Approach to bedside	Spontaneous response	4
	Verbal command	Opening of eyes to name or command	3
	Pain	Lack of opening of eyes to previous stimuli but opening to pain	2
		Lack of opening of eyes to any stimulus	1
		Untestable*	U
Best Verbal Response	Verbal questioning with maximum arousal	Appropriate orientation; conversant; correct identification of self, place, year, and month	5
		Confusion; conversant, but disorientation in one or more spheres	4
		Inappropriate or disorganized use of words (e.g., cursing), lack of sustained conversation	3
		Incomprehensible words, sounds (e.g., moaning)	2
		Lack of sound, even with painful stimuli	1
		Untestable*	U
Best Motor Response	Verbal command (e.g., "raise your arm, hold up two fingers")	Obedience of command	6
		Localization of pain, lack of obedience but presence of attempts to remove offending stimulus	5
	Pain (pressure on proximal nail bed)	Flexion withdrawal,* flexion of arm in response to pain without abnormal flex on posture	4
		Abnormal flexion, flexing of arm at elbow and pronation, making a fist	3
		Abnormal extension, extension of arm at elbow usually with adduction and internal rotation of arm at shoulder	2
		Lack of response	1
		Untestable*	U

*Added to the original scale by some centers.

HEART SOUNDS
Auscultatory Sites

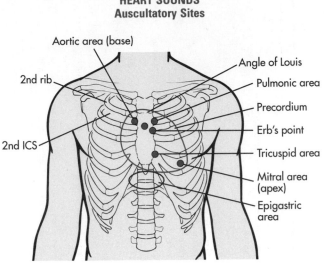

Characteristics of Heart Sounds

Sound	Auscultation Site	Clinical Occurrence
S_1 (M_1, T_1)	Apex	Closing of mitral and tricuspid valves; signals the beginning of systole
S_2 (A_2 P_2)	A_2 at second ICS, RSB; P_2 at second ICS, LSB	Closing of aortic and pulmonic valves; signals the beginning of diastole
S_2 physiologic split	Second ICS, LSB (pulmonic area)	Can be normal and is a split sound that corresponds with the respiratory cycle caused by a normal delay of pulmonic valve during inspiration; can be abnormal if heard during expiration or if it is constant during the respiratory cycle; accentuated during exercise or in individuals with thin chest walls; heard most often in children and young adults
S_3 (ventricular gallop)	Apex	Low-intensity vibration of the ventricular wall usually associated with decreased compliance of the ventricles during filling; heard closely after S_2; common in children and young adults and during last trimester of pregnancy
S_4 (atrial gallop)	Apex	Low-frequency vibration caused by atrial filling and contraction against increased resistance in ventricle; precedes S_1 of next cycle; may be normal in infants, children, and athletes; pathologic in patients with heart disease

Continued

Characteristics of Heart Sounds—cont'd

Sound	Auscultation Site	Clinical Occurrence
Murmurs	Heard with stethoscope lifted just off chest wall	Produced by turbulent blood flow across diseased heart valves. They are graded on a 6-point Roman numeral scale of loudness and recorded as a ratio. The numerator is the intensity of the murmur and the denominator is always VI, which indicates that the six-point scale is being used. A I/VI indicates a murmur that is barely audible, heard only in a quiet room and then not easily; a VI/VI indicates a murmur that can be heard with stethoscope lifted off chest wall.
Pericardial friction rubs	Usually heard best at the apex, with patient upright and leaning forward, and following expiration	Caused by friction that occurs when inflamed surfaces of pericardium (pericarditis) move against each other. They are high-pitched, scratchy sounds that may be transient or intermittent and may last several hours to days.

ICS, Intercostal space; *LSB,* left sternal border; *RSB,* right sternal border.

MEDICATION ADMINISTRATION
Equivalent Weights and Measures

Metric	Apothecary	Household
Weight		
1 kg	2.2 pounds	
1000 mg = 1 g	gr xv	
60 or 65 mg	gr i	
30 mg	gr ss (one half)	
0.4 mg	$\frac{1}{150}$ gr	
1 mcg = 0.0001 mg		
Volume		
1000 mL= 1 L	Approx. 1 quart	Approx. 1 quart
1 L distilled water weighs	1 kg	
500 mL	Approx. 1 pint	16 ounces
240 or 250 mL	viii (8 ounces)	1 cup
30 mL	i (1 fluid ounce)	2 tbs
15 mL	iv (4 fluid drams)	1 tbs
4 to 5 mL	i (1 fluid dram)	1 tsp
1 mL	Minims xv or xvi	

Intravenous (IV) Site Complications

	Infiltration	Phlebitis
Assessment		
Color	Pale	Red
Temperature	Cool to cold	Warm to hot
Swelling	Rounded	Cordlike vein path
Pain	Yes, usually	Yes
Flow	Slowed or stopped	No change or may be slowed
Nursing Actions		
	Tourniquet proximally (flow continues—infiltration)	Discontinue IV; usually call IV team
	Lower bag (blood in tubing—no infiltration)	Note irritating solution (diazepam [Valium], cephalothin sodium [Keflin], potassium chloride [KCl] running too fast)
	Discontinue IV	
	Call IV team	
	Get order for warm compresses and elevate part	Warm compresses; elevate and immobilize part

Drug Calculations

Ratio and proportion:

1. To set up a ratio and proportion, put on the right-hand side what you already have or what you already know (e.g., 1000 mg: 1 mL).
2. On the left-hand side put X, or what you want to know (e.g., 750 mg: X).
3. The equation should look like this: 750 mg: X = 1000 mg: 1 mL
4. Multiply the two inside numbers. Multiply the two outside numbers.

$$1000X = 750$$

5. Solve for X:

$$X = \frac{750}{1000} = 0.75 \text{ mL}$$

IV Drip Rate

$$\frac{\text{Total number of milliliters to be infused}}{\text{Total number of minutes infusion is to run}} \times \text{Drop factor} = \text{Rate (drops per minute)}$$

Techniques of Administration
Angles of Injection

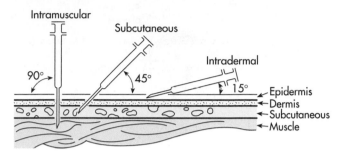

Injection Sites
Subcutaneous

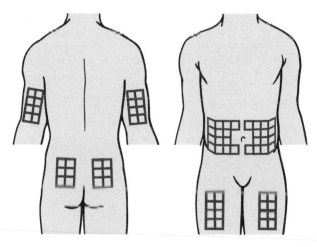

Intramuscular: Deltoid Muscle

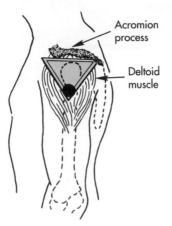

Acromion process

Deltoid muscle

Intramuscular: Dorsogluteal Muscle

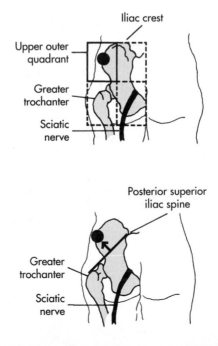

Iliac crest

Upper outer quadrant

Greater trochanter

Sciatic nerve

Posterior superior iliac spine

Greater trochanter

Sciatic nerve

Intramuscular: Vastus Lateralis Muscle

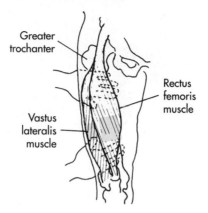

Intramuscular: Ventrogluteal Muscle

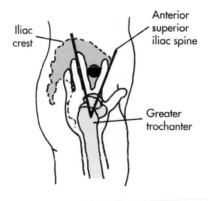

Z-Track Technique

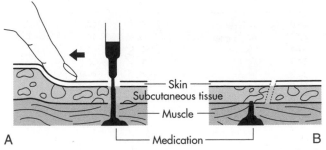

A, In Z-track injection, skin is pulled laterally, and then injection is administered. **B,** After needle is withdrawn, the skin is released. This technique helps prevent medication from leaking.

Intermittent IV Drug Administration

Peripheral Vein Intermittent Infusion Device

1. Irrigate device with 1 mL of normal saline.
2. Administer prescribed medication.
3. Irrigate device with 1 mL of normal saline after medication administration is completed.
4. If policy, perform a final irrigation with 1 mL of heparin solution (100 units of heparin per milliliter).

Central Vein Intermittent Infusion Device

1. Irrigate device with 2 to 5 mL of normal saline (volume depends on type of infusion catheter and agency policy).
2. Administer prescribed medication.
3. Irrigate device with 2 to 5 mL of normal saline when medication administration is completed.
4. Irrigate device with 2 to 5 mL of heparin solution (100 units of heparin per milliliter).

Temperature Conversion Factors

°C	°F	°C	°F	°C	°F
34.0	93.2	37.2	99.0	40.2	104.4
34.2	93.6	37.4	99.3	40.4	104.7
34.4	93.9	37.6	99.7	40.6	105.2
34.6	94.3	37.8	100.0	40.8	105.4
34.8	94.6	38.0	100.4	41.0	105.9
35.0	95.0	38.2	100.8	41.2	106.1
35.2	95.4	38.4	101.1	41.4	106.5
35.4	95.7	38.6	101.5	41.6	106.8
35.6	96.1	38.8	101.8	41.8	107.2
35.8	96.4	39.0	102.2	42.0	107.6
36.0	96.8	39.2	102.6	42.2	108.0
36.2	97.2	39.4	102.9	42.4	108.3
36.4	97.5	39.6	103.3	42.6	108.7
36.6	97.9	39.8	103.6	42.8	109.0
36.8	98.2	40.0	104.0	43.0	109.4
37.0	98.6	—	—	—	—

°C = Temperature in Celsius (centigrade) degrees. $(°C \times 9/5) + 32 = °F$.
°F = Temperature in Fahrenheit degrees. $(°F - 32) \times 5/9 = °C$.

TNM Classification System

Primary Tumor (T)

T_0 No evidence of primary tumor

T_{is} Carcinoma in situ

T_{1-4} Ascending degrees of increase in tumor size and involvement

T_x Tumor cannot be measured or found

Regional Lymph Nodes (N)

N_0 No evidence of disease in lymph nodes

N_{1-4} Ascending degrees of nodal involvement

N_x Regional lymph nodes unable to be assessed clinically

Distant Metastases (M)

M_0 No evidence of distant metastases

M_{1-4} Ascending degrees of metastatic involvement of the host, including distant nodes

M_x Cannot be determined

Note: For examples of TNM classification system applied to diseases, see Fig. 31-14 and Table 28-18.

English/Spanish Common Medical Terms

Hints for Pronunciation of Spanish Words
1. h is silent.
2. j is pronounced as h.
3. ll is pronounced as a y sound.
4. r is pronounced with a trilled sound, and rr is trilled even more.
5. v is pronounced with a b sound.
6. A y by itself is pronounced with a long e sound.
7. Accent marks over the vowel indicate the syllable that is to be stressed.

Introductory

I am _____.	Soy _____.
What is your name?	¿Cómo se llama usted?
I would like to examine you now.	Quisiera examinarlo (a) ahora.

General

How do you feel?	¿Cómo se siente?
Good	Bien
Bad	Mal
Do you feel better today?	¿Se siente mejor hoy?
Where do you work?	¿Dónde trabaja? (¿Cuál es su profesión o trabajo?) (¿Qué hace usted?)
Are you allergic to anything?	¿Es usted alérgico(a) a algo?
Medications, foods, insect bites?	¿Medicinas, alimentos, picaduras de insectos?
Do you take any medications?	¿Toma usted algunas medicinas?
Do you have any drug allergies?	¿Es usted alérgico(a) a algún médicamento?
Do you have a history of:	¿Ha sufrido antes:
Heart disease?	del corazón?
Diabetes?	de diabetes?
Epilepsy?	de epilepsia?
Bronchitis?	de bronquitis?
Emphysema?	de enfisema?
Asthma?	de asma?

Pain

Have you any pain?	¿Tiene dolor?
Where is the pain?	¿Dónde le duele?
Do you have any pain here?	¿Le duele aquí?
How severe is the pain?	¿Qué tan fuerte es el dolor?

English/Spanish Common Medical Terms—cont'd

Mild, moderate, sharp, or severe?	¿Ligero, moderado, agudo, severo?
What were you doing when the pain started?	¿Qué estaba haciendo cuando le comenzó el dolor?
Have you ever had this pain before?	¿Ha tenido este dolor antes?
Do you have a pain in your side?	¿Tiene usted dolor en el costado?
Is it worse now?	¿Es peor ahora?
Does it still pain you?	¿Le duele todavía?
Did you feel much pain at the time?	¿Sintió mucho dolor entonces?
Show me where.	Muéstreme dónde.
Does it hurt when I press here?	¿Le duele cuando aprieto aquí?

Head

Head	La cabeza
Face	La cara
Eye	El ojo

Ears/Nose/Throat

Ears	Los oídos
Eardrum	El tímpano
Laryngitis	La laringitis
Lip	El labio
Mouth	La boca
Nose	La naríz
Tongue	La lengua

Cardiovascular

Heart	El corazón
Heart attack	El ataque del corazón
Heart disease	La enfermedad del corazón
Heart murmur	El soplo del corazón
High blood pressure	Presión alta

Respiratory

Chest	El pecho
Lungs	Los pulmones

Gastrointestinal

Abdomen	El abdomen
Intestines/bowels	Los intestinos
Liver	El hígado
Nausea	Náusea
Gastric ulcer	La úlcera gástrica

Continued

English/Spanish Common Medical Terms—cont'd

Gastrointestinal—cont'd

Stomach	El estómago, la panza, la barriga
Stomachache	El dolor de estómago

Genitourinary

Genitals	Los genitales
Kidney	El riñón
Penis	El pene, el miembro
Urine	La orina

Musculoskeletal

Ankle	El tobillo
Arm	El brazo
Back	La espalda
Bones	Los huesos
Elbow	El codo
Finger	El dedo
Foot	El pie
Fracture	La fractura
Hand	La mano
Hip	La cadera
Knee	La rodilla
Leg	La pierna
Muscles	Los músculos
Rib	La costilla
Shoulder	El hombro
Thigh	El muslo

Neurologic

Brain	El cerebro
Dizziness	El vértigo, el mareo
Epilepsy	La epilepsia
Fainting spell	El desmayo
Unconsciousness	Pérdida del conocimiento (inconsciente, sin sentido)

Endocrine/Reproductive

Uterus	El útero, la matríz
Vagina	La vagina

Urinalysis

Test	Normal	Abnormal Finding	Possible Etiology and Significance
Color	Amber yellow	Dark, smoky color	Hematuria
		Yellow-brown to olive green	Excessive bilirubin
		Orange-red or orange-brown	Phenazopyridine (Pyridium)
		Cloudiness of freshly voided urine	Infection
		Colorless urine	Excessive fluid intake, renal disease, or diabetes insipidus
Odor	Aromatic	Urine allowed to stand	Becomes ammonia-like in odor
		Unpleasant odor	Urinary tract infection
Protein	Random protein (dipstick): 0-trace 24-hr protein (quantitative): <150 mg/day	Persistent proteinuria	Characteristic of acute and chronic renal disease, especially involving glomeruli; heart failure In absence of disease: high-protein diet, strenuous exercise, dehydration, fever, emotional stress, contamination by vaginal secretions
Glucose	None	Glycosuria	Diabetes mellitus, low renal threshold for glucose reabsorption (if blood glucose level is normal), pituitary disorders
Ketones	None	Present	Altered carbohydrate and fat metabolism in diabetes mellitus and starvation; dehydration, vomiting, severe diarrhea
Bilirubin	None	Present	Liver disorders. May appear before jaundice is visible.

Continued

Urinalysis—cont'd

Test	Normal	Abnormal Finding	Possible Etiology and Significance
Specific gravity	1.003-1.030 Maximum concentrating ability of kidney in morning urine (1.025-1.030)	Low	Dilute urine; excessive diuresis; diabetes insipidus
		High	Dehydration, albuminuria, glycosuria
		Fixed at about 1.010	Renal inability to concentrate urine; end-stage renal disease
Osmolality	300-1300 mOsm/kg (300-1300 mmol/kg)	<300 mOsm/kg	Tubular dysfunction. Kidney lost ability to concentrate or dilute urine. (Not part of routine urinalysis)
		>1300 mOsm/kg	
pH	4.0-8.0 (average, 6.0)	>8.0	Urinary tract infection; urine allowed to stand at room temperature (bacteria decompose urea to ammonia)
		<4.0	Respiratory or metabolic acidosis
RBC	0-4/hpf	>4/hpf	Calculi, cystitis, neoplasm, glomerulonephritis, tuberculosis, kidney biopsy, trauma
WBC	0-5/hpf	>5/hpf	Urinary tract infection or inflammation
Casts	None Occasional hyaline	Present	Molds of the renal tubules that may contain protein, WBCs, RBCs, or bacteria. Noncellular casts (hyaline in appearance) occasionally found in normal urine
Culture for organisms	No organisms in bladder <10⁴ organisms/mL result of normal urethral flora	Bacteria counts >10⁵/mL	Urinary tract infection. Most common organisms are *Escherichia coli,* enterococci, *Klebsiella, Proteus,* and streptococci.

hpf, High-powered field; *RBC,* red blood cells; *WBC,* white blood cells.

INDEX

Page numbers followed by *b*, *t*, and *f* indicate boxes, tables, and figures, respectively.